Textbook of
ENDODONTICS

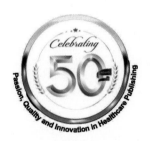

Textbook of
ENDODONTICS

FOURTH EDITION

Nisha Garg MDS
Professor
Department of Conservative Dentistry and Endodontics
Bhojia Dental College and Hospital
Baddi, Himachal Pradesh, India

Amit Garg MDS
Professor and Head
Department of Oral and Maxillofacial Surgery
Rayat and Bahra Dental College and Hospital
Mohali, Punjab, India

Foreword
Mohammad Hossein Nekoofar

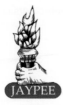

JAYPEE BROTHERS MEDICAL PUBLISHERS
The Health Sciences Publisher
New Delhi | London | Panama

Jaypee Brothers Medical Publishers (P) Ltd

Headquarters

Jaypee Brothers Medical Publishers (P) Ltd
4838/24, Ansari Road, Daryaganj
New Delhi 110 002, India
Phone: +91-11-43574357
Fax: +91-11-43574314
Email: jaypee@jaypeebrothers.com

Overseas offices

J.P. Medical Ltd
83, Victoria Street, London
SW1H 0HW (UK)
Phone: +44 20 3170 8910
Fax: +44 (0)20 3008 618
Email: info@jpmedpub.com

Jaypee Brothers Medical Publishers (P) Ltd
17/1-B Babar Road, Block-B, Shyamoli
Mohammadpur, Dhaka-1207
Bangladesh
Mobile: +08801912003485
Email: jaypeedhaka@gmail.com

Jaypee-Highlights Medical Publishers Inc
City of Knowledge, Bld. 235, 2nd Floor,
Clayton, Panama City, Panama
Phone: +1 507-301-0496
Fax: +1 507-301-0499
Email: cservice@jphmedical.com

Jaypee Brothers Medical Publishers (P) Ltd
Bhotahity, Kathmandu, Nepal
Phone: +977-9741283608
Email: kathmandu@jaypeebrothers.com

Website: www.jaypeebrothers.com
Website: www.jaypeedigital.com

Textbook of Endodontics

First Edition: 2007

Second Edition: 2010

Third Edition: 2014

Fourth Edition: **2019**

ISBN: 978-93-5270-535-1

Printed at : Ajanta Offset & Packagings Ltd., Fbd., Haryana

Dedicated to

Prisha
and
Vedant

CONTRIBUTORS

Akash Dupper MDS
Professor
Department of Conservative Dentistry
and Endodontics
Sri Sukhmani Dental College and
Hospital
Mohali, Punjab, India
Chapter: 4

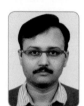

Ajay Chhabra MDS
Principal
Department of Conservative Dentistry
and Endodontics
Bhojia Dental College and Hospital
Baddi, Himachal Pradesh, India
Chapter: 21

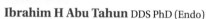

Amit Garg MDS
Professor and Head
Department of Oral and Maxillofacial
Surgery
Rayat and Bahra Dental College and
Hospital
Mohali, Punjab, India
Chapters: 7, 8, 10, 12

Amita MDS
Professor
Department of Conservative Dentistry
and Endodontics
BRS Dental College and Hospital
Panchkula, Haryana, India
Chapter: 26

Anil Chandra MDS
Professor
Department of Conservative Dentistry
and Endodontics
King George Medical College
Lucknow, Uttar Pradesh, India
Chapter: 15

Anil Dhingra MDS
Professor and Head
Department of Conservative Dentistry
and Endodontics
Seema Dental College and Hospital
Rishikesh, Uttarakhand, India
Chapter: 14

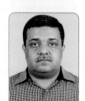

Avninder Kaur MDS
Professor and Head
Department of Pediatric and Preventive
Dentistry
Bhojia Dental College and Hospital
Baddi, Himachal Pradesh, India
Chapter: 36

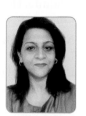

Ibrahim H Abu Tahun DDS PhD (Endo)
Associate Professor
Department of Conservative Dentistry,
School of Dentistry
University of Jordan
Amman, Jordan
Chapter: 2

Jaidev Singh Dhillon MDS
Former Principal and Head
Department of Conservative Dentistry
and Endodontics
Gian Sagar Dental College and Hospital
Rajpura, Punjab, India
Chapter: 18

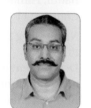

Jaydev MDS
Assistant Professor
Department of Conservative Dentistry
and Endodontics
Panineeya Mahavidyalaya Institute of
Dental Sciences and Research Center
Hyderabad, Telangana, India
Chapter: 24

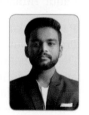

JS Mann MDS
Associate Professor and Head
Department of Conservative Dentistry
and Endodontics
Government Dental College and Hospital
Patiala, Punjab, India
Chapter: 19

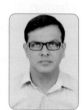

Manav Nayar MDS
Member
Royal College of Dental Surgeons of
Ontario
Consultant Endodontist
Napa Dental
Ontario, Canada
Chapter: 17

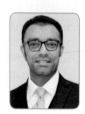

Manoj Hans MDS
Professor
Department of Conservative Dentistry
and Endodontics
KD Dental College and Hospital
Mathura, Uttar Pradesh, India
Chapter: 6
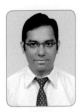

Navjot Singh Khurana MDS
Lecturer
Department of Conservative Dentistry
and Endodontics
Government Dental College
Patiala, Punjab, India
Chapter: 14

Navkesh Singh MDS
Senior Lecturer
Department of Conservative Dentistry
and Endodontics
Bhojia Dental College and Hospital
Baddi, Himachal Pradesh, India
Chapter: 11
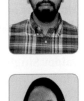

Nisha Garg MDS
Professor
Department of Conservative Dentistry
and Endodontics
Bhojia Dental College and Hospital
Baddi, Himachal Pradesh, India
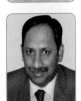

P Karunakar MDS
Professor and Head
Department of Conservative Dentistry
and Endodontics
Panineeya Mahavidyalaya Institute of
Dental Sciences and Research Center
Hyderabad, Telangana, India
Chapter: 19
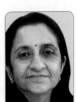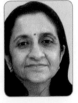

Poonam Bogra MDS
Professor
Department of Conservative Dentistry
and Endodontics
DAV Dental College
Yamunanagar, Haryana, India
Chapters: 5, 15, 37

Puneet Jindal MDS
Ex-Senior Resident
Post Graduate Institute of Medical
Education and Research
Chandigarh, India
Chapters: 37
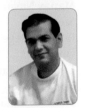

Rakesh Singla MDS
Professor and Head
Department of Conservative Dentistry
and Endodontics
Jan Nayak Ch Devi Lal Dental College
Sirsa, Haryana, India
Chapters: 13, 21, 29
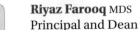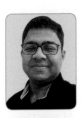

Riyaz Farooq MDS
Principal and Dean
Government Dental College and Hospital
Srinagar, Jammu and Kashmir, India
Chapter: 20
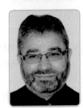

RS Kang MDS
Former Associate Professor and Head
Department of Conservative Dentistry
and Endodontics
Government Dental College and Hospital
Patiala, Punjab, India
Chapter: 13
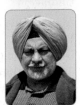

Ruhani Bhatia
Senior Lecturer
Department of Conservative Dentistry
and Endodontics
Bhojia Dental College and Hospital
Baddi, Himachal Pradesh, India
Chapter: 28
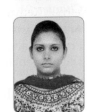

Sameer Makkar MDS
Professor and Head
Conservative Dentistry and Endodontics
Swami Devi Dyal Hospital and
Dental College
Panchkula, Haryana, India
Chapter: 16
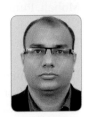

Sanjay Jain MDS
Ex-Professor and PG Guide
Consultant Periodontist
Pune, Maharashtra, India
Chapter: 34
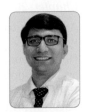

Sanjay Miglani MDS FISDR
Department of Conservative Dentistry
and Endodontics
Faculty of Dentistry
Jamia Millia Islamia (A Central
University)
Jamia Nagar, New Delhi, India
Chapter: 14
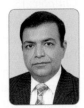

Savita Thakur MDS
Ex-Senior Lecturer
Department of Conservative Dentistry
and Endodontics
Bhojia Dental College and Hospital
Baddi, Himachal Pradesh, India
Chapter: 28

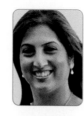

Sheenam Markan MDS
Reader
Department of Conservative Dentistry
and Endodontics
Bhojia Dental College and Hospital
Baddi, Himachal Pradesh, India
Chapter: 25

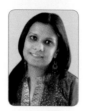

Tom JM Dienya BDS MDSc (Endo)
Chairman
Department of Conservative and
Prosthetic Dentistry
School of Dental Sciences
University of Nairboi
Nairboi, Kenya
Chapter: 13

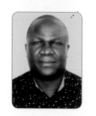

Vijay Singh Babloo MDS
Professor and Head
Department of Conservative Dentistry
and Endodontics
DAV Dental College and Hospital
Yamunanagar, Haryana, India
Chapter: 27

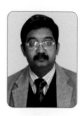

Viresh Chopra MDS
Faculty of ARD (Adult Restorative
Dentistry)
Department of Conservative Dentistry
and Endodontics
Oman Dental College
Muscat, Oman
Chapter: 23

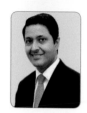

Yoshitsugu Terauchi DDD PhD
Lecturer
Tokyo Medical and
Dental University
Japan
Chapter: 24

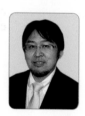

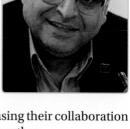

As dentists, especially endodontists, we are continuous students in this vast, ever-changing field. It has been predicted by the American Clinical and Climatological Association that by the year 2020 medical knowledge will double every 73 days. Facing this big data problem is why the approach of this textbook is a suitable choice for a variety of readers differing in background, knowledge and experience. By incorporating both new and latter studies in areas, such as vital pulp therapy, bioactive ceramics, laser, microbiology, and regenerative endodontics, this textbook acts as an efficient instructional manuscript keeping practitioners updated in comprehensive clinical decision making.

In addition to its recognition of almost all the important advances in today's endodontics world, the element that also captured my attention greatly, was the utilization of illustration and color to smoothly guide the reader through otherwise very intricate and complex material. This brought me back to the Indian festival of colors in all its beauty. Dr Nisha Garg and Dr Amit Garg have truly captured the soul of their roots in the books setting, whilst tastefully showcasing their collaboration with globally admired scholars in what could only have been achieved by great minds coming together.

If given the chance, I would gladly take the steps toward translating *Textbook of Endodontics* to Persian, in order to give my fellow Iranian colleagues and students the opportunity to take advantage of this comprehensive, well-compiled piece.

I wish all the best for Dr Nisha Garg and Dr Amit Garg, as I see a clear, bright future for both of them in the forth in coming endeavors.

Mohammad Hossein Nekoofar
DDs MSc Diplomate of Iranian Board of Endodontics PhD (Cardiff UK)
Department of Endodontics
School of Dentistry
Department of Tissue Engineering and Applied Cell Sciences
School of Advanced Technologies in Medicine
Tehran University of Medical Sciences
Honorary Senior Clinical Lecturer
School of Dentistry
College of Biomedical and Life Sciences
Cardiff University, UK

Member of Editorial Board of International Endodontic Journal
Immediate Past-President of Iranian Association of Endodontists

PREFACE TO THE FOURTH EDITION

In presenting the fourth edition of *Textbook of Endodontics*, we would like to express our appreciation in the kindly manner in which the earlier editions were accepted by dental students and professionals across the country.

The scope of book is simple yet comprehensive that serves as an introductory for dental students and a refresher source for general practitioners. This book attempts to incorporate most recent advances in endodontics while at the same time not losing the sight of basics; therefore, making the study of endodontics easier and interesting. We could not have achieved the current level of success without the help of students and our colleagues who always motivate us to deliver our best.

In an attempt to improve this book further, many eminent personalities were invited to edit, write and modify the important chapters in the form of text and photographs. We would especially thank Drs Jaidev Dhillon, Ajay Chhabra, Anil Dhingra, Jaydev, Puneet Jindal, Navjot Singh Khurana, Viresh Chopra, Manoj Hans, and Sanjay Jain, for providing us clinical case photographs and radiographs for better understanding of the subject.

We are indebted to Dr Poonam Bogra for writing important chapters biofilm and smear layer in endodontics for the book. We are especially thankful to Dr Poonam Bogra for editing chapters, access cavity preparation, regenerative endodontics, and cleaning and shaping.

We fall lack of words to thank Dr Vijay Singh Babloo for critically evaluating the chapter post-endodontic restorations, Dr Sameer Makkar for irrigation and disinfection, Dr Karunakar for obturation, Dr Riyaz for MTA, and Dr Ibrahim Abu Tahun for editing chapter pulp and periapical tissues. We are especially grateful to Dr Rakesh Singla for critical evaluation and being always present throughout the duration of our project.

We are thankful to Dr Sanjay Miglani for editing the chapter internal anatomy, Dr Tom JM Dienya for endodontic instruments, Dr Avninder Kaur for vital pulp therapy, Dr Savita Thakur for editing management of traumatic injuries, and Dr Manav Nayar for working length determination. We are especially thankful to Dr Yoshitsugu Terauchi for sharing his device for removal of the separarted instrument.

We are thankful to Dr RS Kang and Dr JS Mann, for their constant support, motivation and encouragement. We wish to thank for critical evaluation and profound comments by our colleagues Drs Pranav, Shabnam, Alka and Mohit; and postgraduates, for their 'ready to help' attitude and positive criticism which helped in improvement of the book.

We offer our humble gratitude and sincere thanks to Mr Vikram Bhojia (Secretary, Bhojia Trust) for providing healthy and encouraging environment for our work.

We are grateful to companies Dentsply, Coltene Whaledent, Sybron Endo, and 3M ESPE for providing high-resolution images of products related to endodontics.

It is hoped that all these modifications will be appreciated and render the book still more valuable basis for endodontic practice.

We are specially thankful to our kids, Prisha and Vedant, for their understanding, patience and support throughout this project.

We are very grateful to the whole team of M/s Jaypee Brothers Medical Publishers (P) Ltd, who helped and guided us, especially Shri Jitendar P Vij (Group Chairman), Mr Ankit Vij (Managing Director), Mr MS Mani (Group President), Ms Ritu Sharma (Director–Content Strategy), Ms Sunita Katla (Executive Assistant to Group Chairman and Publishing Manager), Ms Pooja Bhandari (Production Head), Ms Samina Khan (Executive Assistant to Director–Content Strategy), Dr Pinky Chauhan (Development Editor), Ms Seema Dogra (Cover Visualizer), Gopal Singh Kirola (Graphic Designer), and their team members, for all their support and work on this project and make it a success. Without their cooperation, we could not have completed this project.

Nisha Garg
Amit Garg

The amount of literature available in dentistry today is vast. Endodontics being no exception. However, during both our graduation as well as postgraduation, we always felt the need for a book which would help us to revise and update our knowledge. When we were doing undergraduation, there were no Indian authored books on endodontics. We were thus motivated to frame a specialized, precise, concise, easy to read and remember yet, up-to-date *Textbook of Endodontics*.

The line diagrams are in an expressive interpretation of endodontic procedures, which are worked upon and simplified to render them more comprehensive and comparable with real photographs. These illustrations (around 1,200) are easy to remember and reproduce during examinations.

Emphasis is laid upon the language which is simple, understandable and exclusively designed for undergraduates, postgraduates, general practitioners and teachers in the field.

It took us more than three years to accomplish the arduous task of writing this book. This thrust for knowledge led us to link everywhere, where we could Medline journals, books and more.

Nevertheless, a never-ending approach and internal craving of mind and soul finally resulted in publication of the book. God perhaps gave us some ability and showered his light on us, guiding us for this task.

Till the last week before the publication of the book, we were frantically looking for loopholes, missing information and any important updates we might have missed out. To the best of our knowledge, we did everything we could. But for knowledge, one life is not enough. The sky is the limit.

We await the response of this first edition, which would improve us in the next editions to come.

Nisha Garg
Amit Garg

CONTENTS

CHAPTER

1 Introduction

Chapter Outline

- Scope of Endodontics
- History of Endodontics
- Contemporary Endodontics

Endodontics is the branch of dentistry which deals with diseases of dental pulp and periradicular tissues. *En* is a Greek word for "inside" and *odont* is Greek word for "tooth."

Endodontics is the branch of dentistry which deals with morphology, physiology, and pathology of human pulp and periradicular tissues.

Study of endodontics involves basic knowledge of pulp biology, etiology, diagnosis, treatment, and prevention of the diseases and injuries of the pulp and associated periradicular tissues **(Fig. 1.1)**.

Scope of Endodontics

- Diagnosis and differential diagnosis of orofacial pain of pulpal and periradicular origin

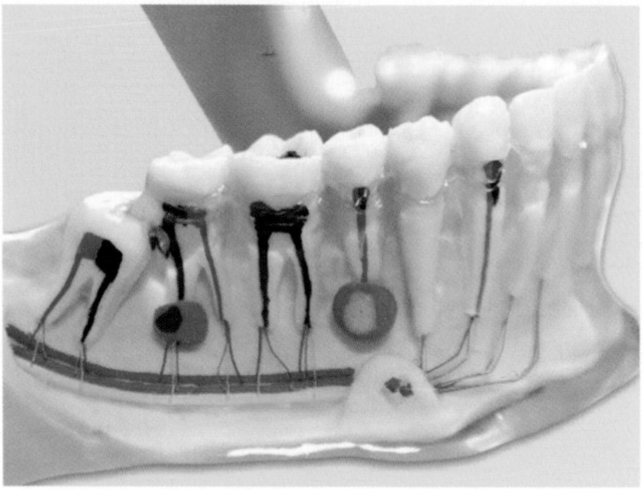

Fig. 1.1 Model of teeth showing pulp along with endodontic lesions of the teeth.

- Vital pulp therapy like pulp capping, pulpotomy, apexogenesis, and apexification
- Nonsurgical treatment of root canal system
- Surgical removal of periapical pathology of pulpal origin
- Bleaching of discolored teeth
- Retreatment of endodontic failure cases
- Restorations of endodotically treated teeth with coronal restoration and post and core
- Intentional replantation
- Replantation of avulsed tooth
- Hemisection, bicuspidization and root resection
- Endodontic implants

History of Endodontics (Table 1.1)

Endodontics has been practiced as early as 2nd or 3rd century BC. The history of endodontics begins in 17th century, and since then, many advances, developments, and research work has been done continuously.

Advances in endodontics have been made continuously, especially after Pierre Fauchard (1678–1761) (founder of modern dentistry) described the pulp very precisely in his textbook "Le Chirurgien Dentiste."

Later in 1725, Lazare Riviere introduced the use of clove oil as sedative, and in 1746, Pierre Fauchard demonstrated the removal of pulp tissue. Dr. Grossman, the pioneer of endodontics, divided the evolution of endodontics in four eras from 1776 to 1976, each consisting of 50 years.

Prescience	1776–1826
Age of discovery	1826–1876
Dark age	1876–1926
The renaissance	1926–1976
Innovation era	1977–till date

Table 1.1: History of endodontics

1725	Lazare Riviere	Introduced clove oil for sedative property
1728	Pierre Fauchard	First described the pulp tissue
1746	Pierre Fauchard	Described removal of pulp tissue
1820	Leonard Koecker	Cauterized exposed pulp with heated instrument and protected it with lead foil
1836	S Spooner	Suggested arsenic trioxide for pulp devitalization
1838	Edwin Maynard	Introduced first root canal instrument
1847	Edwin Truman	Introduced gutta-percha as a filling material
1864	SC Barnum	Prepared a thin rubber leaf to isolate the tooth during filling
1867	Bowman	Used gutta-percha cones for filling of root canals
1867	Magitot	Use of electric current for testing pulp vitality
1890	Gramm	Introduced gold plated copper points for filling
1891	Otto Walkhoff	introduced camphorated chlorophenol as a medication
1895	Roentgen	Introduced formocresol
1914	Callahan	Introduction of lateral compaction technique
1918	Cluster	Use of electrical current for determination of working length
1920	BW Hermann	Introduced calcium hydroxide
1936	Walker	Sodium hypochlorite
1942	Suzuki	Presented scientific study on apex locator
1944	Johnson	Introduced profile instrument system
1957	Nygaard-Ostby	Introduced EDTA
1958	Ingle and Levine	Gave standardizations and guidelines for endodontic instruments
1961	Sparser	Walking bleach technique
1962	Sunada	Calculated electrical resistance between periodontium and oral mucous membrane
1971	Weichman-Johnson	Use of lasers
1979	Mullaney et al.	Use of step-back technique
1979	McSpadden	McSpadden technique (thermomechanical compaction)
1980	Marshall and Pappin	Introduction of crown-down technique
1985–1986	Roane, Sabala, and Powell	Introduction of balanced force technique
1988	Munro	Introduced first commercial bleaching product
1989	Haywood and Heymann	Nightguard vital bleaching
1993	Torabinejad	Introduced MTA
2004	Pentron clinical laboratory	Introduced Resilon

Abbreviations: EDTA: ethylenediaminetetra acetic acid; MTA: mineral trioxide aggregate.

Prescience (1776–1826): In this era, endodontic therapy was concerned with crude modalities like abscesses being treated with poultices or leeches and pulps being cauterized using hot instruments.

Age of discovery (1826–1876): In this era, the development of anesthesia, gutta-percha, and barbed broaches happened. The medications were created for treating pulpal infections, and the cements and pastes were discovered to fill them.

Dark age (1876–1926): Inspite of introduction of X-rays and general anesthesia, extraction of tooth was the choice of treatment than endodontics because theory of the focal infection was the main concern at that time.

The renaissance (1926–1976): In this era, endodontics was established as science and therapy, forming its golden era. It showed the improvement in anesthesia and radiographs for better treatment results. The theory of focal infection was also fading out, resulting in more of endodontics being practiced. In 1943, because of growing interest in endodontics, the AAE, that is, the American Association of Endodontists was formed.

Innovation era: It is the period from 1977 onwards in which tremendous advancements at very fast rate are being introduced in the endodontics. The better vision, better techniques of biomechanical preparations, and obturation are being developed resulting in the simpler, easier, and faster endodontics with more predictable results.

Also the concept of single visit endodontics is now globally accepted in contrast to multiple visits.

▐ Contemporary Endodontics

Over the past two decades, knowledge of endodontic disease has improved like microbial biofilms, etiology of persistent infection and factors affecting prognosis of endodontic treatment. Management and prognosis in endodontics has improved because of advancements in materials, equipment, and techniques including nickel–titanium files, apex locators, obturating materials, magnification, and endodontic microsurgery. Contemporary culture-independent molecular techniques have exposed a more diverse microflora along with microflora of endodontic failure cases. Now, it has been established that rubber dam is mandatory for endodontic procedures. If patient or dentist is allergic to latex, alternatives to latex like silicone-based dams are recommended. Modern endodontic diagnostic and treatment procedures utilize magnification, like dental loupes, microscopes, and endoscopes, which can provide magnification of up to ×25 times. Magnification helps to

- ❑ Locate and negotiate root canals
- ❑ Visualize calcified root canals
- ❑ Detect missed canals and remove fractured instruments
- ❑ Visualize tooth fractures
- ❑ Perform endodontic microsurgery

Conventional pulp tests (cold, heat, and electrical tests) assess conduction of nerves in the pulp, so these are not vitality but sensibility tests. The results from thermal and electric tests are not quantitative and do not indicate the level of health or disease of the pulp.

But contemporary tests assess pulpal blood flow (laser Doppler flowmetry test), or oxygen saturation levels in the blood (pulse oximetry). Nowadays, digital radiography comes with many advantages like reduced radiation dose to patient, quick viewing of images, data storage, elimination of developing/fixing procedures, etc.

Cone beam computed tomography (CBCT) is a three-dimensional imaging technique designed to overcome the limitations of radiographs. It produces undistorted and accurate images of target area. CBCT detects endodontic lesions before they become visible on conventional radiographs. Earlier, pulp capping involved the use of calcium hydroxide, but now it is being replaced with mineral trioxide aggregate (MTA) which has better sealing characteristics, biocompatibility and form more predictable reparative dentine bridge than calcium hydroxide. For cleaning and shaping, newer rotary NiTi files are replacing 2% stainless steel files. These files have different cross-sectional shape, taper, tip sizes, and presence or absence of radial lands. These are used in crown-down technique to

- ❑ Prevent pushing debris and necrotic tissue apically
- ❑ Eliminate coronal interferences, thus reducing the risk of iatrogenic errors
- ❑ Facilitate irrigants to reach apical area

Traditionally, working length was determined by radiograph, paper point method, etc., but now, electronic apex locator (EAL) are used which give consistently reliable results. Earlier, silver points and lateral compaction technique was preferred for obturation, but nowadays, contemporary warm gutta-percha and thermoplasticized technique are employed to obturate the root canals. Since ages, zinc-oxide–eugenol-based sealers have been used in endodontics but now a days new adhesive, silicone and calcium phosphate-based root canal sealers have tried with desirable results **(Figs. 1.2A to D).** Earlier, prognosis of endodontic treatment was evaluated as a "success" or a "failure." These terms can be vague as they may be defined differently by the patient or the clinician. For example, a patient may feel symptom free endodontic treatment; however, a sinus may be present with periapical radiolucency. Contemporary endodontics uses the terms "healed," "healing," or "diseased" to describe the

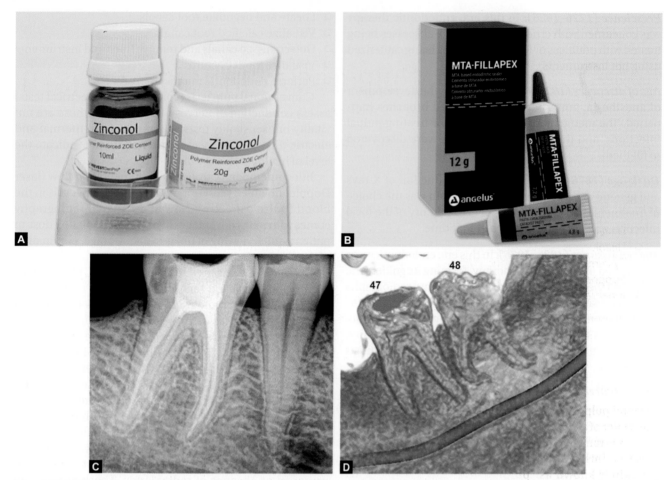

Figs. 1.2A to D Showing (A) Traditionally used Zinc oxide Eugenol sealer; (B) MTA based root canal sealer; (C) 2D radiographic image of teeth and (D) 3D image of teeth and surrounding tissues in CBCT.

outcome of treatment depending upon radiographic, clinical, and histological evaluation. Chance of a healed outcome after contemporary surgical endodontics can be as high as 95%.

Questions

1. Define endodontics. What is scope of endodontics?
2. Write short note on history of endodontics.

Pulp and Periradicular Tissue

▎Introduction

Dental pulp is soft tissue of mesenchymal origin located in center of a tooth. It consists of specialized cells, odontoblasts arranged peripherally in direct contact with dentin matrix. This close relationship between odontoblasts and dentin is known as "pulp–dentin complex" **(Fig. 2.1)**.

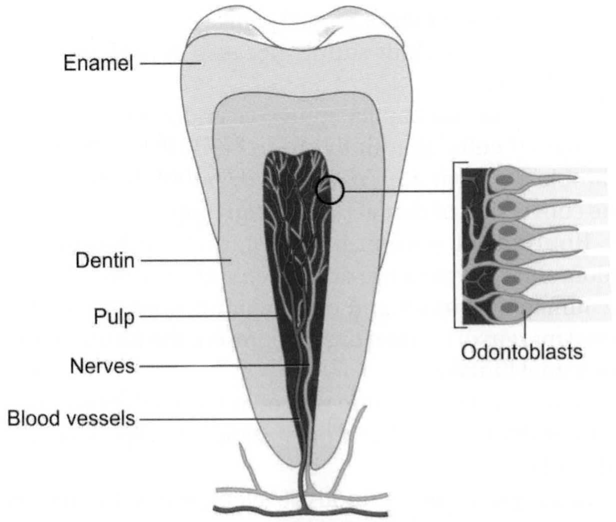

Connective tissue of pulp consists of cells, ground substance, fibers, interstitial fluid, odontoblasts, fibroblasts, and other cellular components. It has soft gelatinous consistency. Pulp is a microcirculatory system consisting of arterioles and venules as the largest vascular component. Due to lack of true collateral circulation, pulp is dependent upon few arterioles entering through the foramen. In this chapter, we would discuss the comprehensive description of pulp embryology, anatomy, histology, physiology, and pulp changes with age.

Fig. 2.1 Schematic representation of pulp-dentin complex. The pulp dentin junction shows that peripheral nerve endings of pulp extend into the dentinal tubules.

Labels: Enamel, Dentin, Pulp, Nerves, Blood vessels, Odontoblasts

Features of pulp, which distinguish it from tissue found elsewhere in the body:
- Pulp is surrounded by rigid walls and so is unable to expand in response to injury as a part of inflammatory process. Therefore, pulpal tissue is susceptible to change in pressure affecting the pain threshold
- There is minimal collateral blood supply to pulp tissue which reduces its capacity for repair following injury
- Due to presence of the specialized cells (odontoblasts and other cells which can differentiate into hard tissue secreting cells), pulp retains its ability to form dentin throughout life
- Innervation of pulp tissue is both simple and complex. Simple in that there are only free nerve endings and consequently the pulp lacks proprioception. Complex because of innervation of the odontoblast processes which produces a high level of sensitivity to thermal and chemical change

Development of Dental Pulp

Initiation of tooth development begins at 37 days of development with formation of a continuous horseshoe-band of thickened epithelium in the location of upper and lower jaws called as primary epithelial band. Each band of epithelium forms two subdivisions:

1. Dental lamina
2. Vestibular lamina

Dental Lamina

❑ Dental lamina appears as a thickening of the oral epithelium adjacent to condensation of ectomesenchyme
❑ In this, 20 knob-like areas appear, which form tooth buds for the 20 primary teeth. These areas appear at different timings. First ones to form are in mandibular anterior region
❑ Dental lamina begins to function at 6th prenatal week and continues to 15th year of birth. Successional lamina is the lamina from which permanent teeth develop

Tooth development is a continuous process, which can be divided into three stages:

1. Bud stage   2. Cap stage   3. Bell stage

1. **Bud stage (Fig. 2.2)**: It is initial stage where epithelial cells of dental lamina proliferate and produce a bud-like projection into adjacent ectomesenchyme
2. **Cap stage (Fig. 2.3)**: It is formed when cells of dental lamina proliferate to form a concavity which produces cap-like appearance. It shows outer and inner enamel epithelia and stellate reticulum. Rim of the enamel organ, that is, where inner and outer enamel epithelia are joined is called cervical loop
3. **Bell stage**: As the cells of loop proliferate, enamel organ assumes bell stage **(Fig. 2.4)**. Differentiation of epithelial and mesenchymal cells into ameloblasts and odontoblasts occur during bell stage. Pulp is initially called as dental papilla; it is designated as pulp only

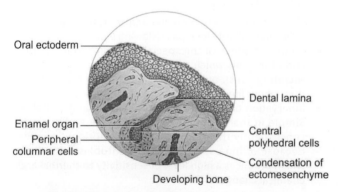

Fig. 2.2 Development of tooth showing bud stage.

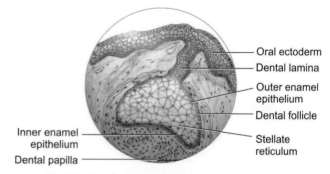

Fig. 2.3 Development of tooth showing cap stage.

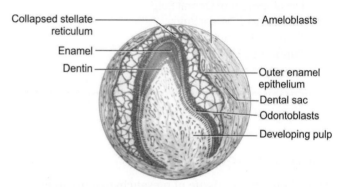

Fig. 2.4 Development of tooth showing bell stage.

when dentin forms around it. The differentiation of odontoblasts from undifferentiated ectomesenchymal cells is accomplished by interaction of cell and signaling molecules mediated through basal lamina and extracellular matrix. Dental papilla has high cell density and rich vascular supply because of proliferation of cells in it

Cells of dental papilla appear as undifferentiated mesenchymal cells; gradually these cells differentiate into fibroblasts. Formation of dentin by odontoblasts heralds the conversion of dental papilla into pulp.

Boundary between inner enamel epithelium and odontoblast form future dentinoenamel junction.

Junction of inner and outer enamel epithelium at the basal margin of enamel organ represent the future cementoenamel junction.

As the crown formation with enamel and dentin deposition continues, growth and organization of pulp vasculature takes place.

At the same time, as tooth develops, unmyelinated sensory nerves and autonomic nerves grow into pulpal tissue. Myelinated fibers develop and mature at a slower rate and plexus of Raschkow does not develop until after tooth has erupted.

Histology of Dental Pulp

Pulp can be distinguished into following four distinct zones from dentinopulpal junction toward center of the tooth (**Fig. 2.5**):

Zones of pulp are:
- Odontoblastic layer at the pulp periphery
- Cell free zone of Weil
- Cell rich zone
- Pulp core

Microscopic zones in pulp	
Zones—from outer to inner zone	Description
Odontoblastic layer (peripheral zone)	a. Consist of cell bodies and cytoplasmic processes. Odontoblastic cell bodies form odontoblastic zone, whereas the odontoblastic processes are located in predentin matrix b. Capillaries, nerve fibers (unmyelinated), and dendritic cells are found around the odontoblasts
Cell-free zone (Weil zone)	a. Central to odontoblasts is subodontoblastic layer b. 40 µm wide, it contains plexuses of capillaries and nerve fiber ramifications c. Not present in developing teeth but prominent in coronal pulp after development
Cell-rich zone	a. Contains fibroblasts, undifferentiated cells, macrophages, and capillaries b. Capillaries form extensive vascular system
Pulpal-core (central zone)	a. Acts as a support system for peripheral pulp because it contains blood vessels and nerves b. Principal cells are fibroblasts with collagen as ground substance

Contents of the pulp
- Cells
  - Odontoblasts
  - Fibroblasts
  - Undifferentiated mesenchymal cells
  - *Defense cells*
    - Macrophages
    - Plasma cells
    - Mast cells

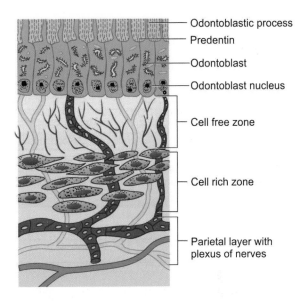

Fig. 2.5　Schematic representation of zones of pulp.

- Matrix
  - *Collagen fibers*
    - Type 1
    - Type 2
  - *Ground substance*
    - Glycosaminoglycans
    - Glycoproteins
    - Water
- Blood vessels: Arterioles, venules, capillaries
- Lymphatics: Draining to submandibular, submental, and deep cervical nodes
- Nerves
  - Subodontoblastic plexus of Raschkow
  - Sensory afferent from Vth nerve and superior cervical ganglion

Structural or Cellular Elements

Odontoblasts (Fig. 2.6)

☐ These are first type of cells which come across when pulp is approached from dentin
☐ Number of odontoblasts ranges from 59,000 to 76,000 per square millimeter in coronal dentin, with a lesser number in root dentin
☐ Cell bodies of odontoblasts appear tall, pseudostratified columnar in coronal pulp, single row of cuboidal cells in radicular pulp, and flattened squamous type in apical part
☐ Morphology of odontoblasts reflects their functional activity which ranges from an active synthetic phase to a quiescent phase
☐ Ultrastructure of odontoblast shows large nucleus which may contain up to four nucleoli

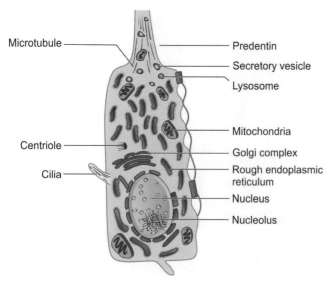

Fig. 2.6 Line diagram showing odontoblasts.

❑ Nucleus is situated at basal end. Golgi bodies are located centrally. Mitochondria, rough endoplasmic reticulum (RER), and ribosomes are distributed throughout the cell body
❑ Odontoblasts synthesize mainly Type 1 collagen, proteoglycans. They also secrete sialoproteins, alkaline phosphatase, phosphophoryn (phosphoprotein involved in extracellular mineralization)
❑ Irritated odontoblast secretes collagen, amorphous material, and large crystals into tubule lumen which result in decreased permeability to irritating substance

During dentin formation in crown, odontoblasts are pushed inwards to form periphery of the pulp chamber. This circumference is smaller than circumference at DEJ (Dentinoenamel junction) making odontoblasts to pack in pseudostratified fashion in coronal pulp.
  Space in root is not compressed, so odontoblasts maintain their cuboidal or columnar shape in root area.

POINTS TO REMEMBER

Similar characteristic features of odontoblasts, osteoblasts, and cementoblasts
• They all produce matrix composed of collagen fibers and proteoglycans capable of undergoing mineralization
• All exhibit highly ordered RER, Golgi complex, mitochondria, secretory granules, rich in RNA with prominent nucleoli

Difference between odontoblasts, osteoblasts, and cementoblasts
• Odontoblasts are columnar in shape while osteoblasts and cementoblast are polygonal in shape
• Odontoblasts leave behind cellular processes to form dentinal tubules while osteoblasts and cementoblast are trapped in matrix as osteocytes and cementocytes

Fibroblasts (Fig. 2.7)

❑ Fibroblast are found in the greatest numbers in pulp
❑ "Baume" refers them to mesenchymal cells/pulpoblasts or pulpocytes in their progressive levels of maturation
❑ These are spindle-shaped cells which secrete extracellular components like collagen and ground substance
❑ These cells have dual function
  • Formation and maintenance of fibrous component and ground substance of the connective tissue
  • Degradation and ingestion of excess collagen by action of lysosomal enzymes
❑ Fibroblasts of pulp are much like "***Peter Pan***" because they "never grow up" and remain in relatively undifferentiated state

Reserve Cells/Undifferentiated Mesenchymal Cells

❑ Undifferentiated mesenchymal cells are descendants of undifferentiated cells of dental papilla which can dedifferentiate and then redifferentiate into many cell types like odontoblasts and fibroblasts depending upon the stimulus
❑ These are found throughout the cell-rich and pulp core area
❑ They appear as large polyhedral cells possessing a large, lightly stained, centrally placed nucleus with abundant cytoplasm and peripheral cytoplasm extensions
❑ In older pulps, the number of undifferentiated mesenchymal cells diminishes, along with number of other cells in the pulp core. This reduces regenerative potential of the pulp

Defense Cells (Fig. 2.8)

❑ ***Histiocytes and macrophages:*** They originate from undifferentiated mesenchymal cells or monocytes.

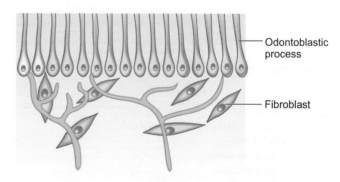

Fig. 2.7 Histology of pulp showing fibroblasts.

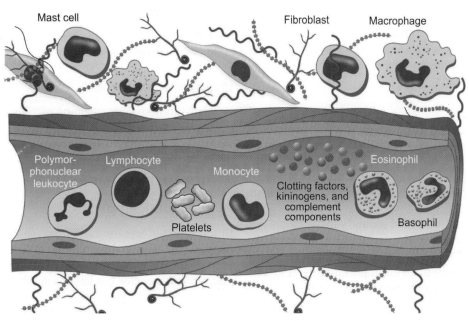

Fig. 2.8 Schematic representation of defense cells of pulp.

These cells appear as large oval or spindle shape and are involved in the elimination of dead cells, debris, bacteria and foreign bodies, etc.

- **Polymorphonuclear leukocytes:** Most common form of leukocyte is neutrophil, though it is not present in healthy pulp. These cells are mainly found in cases of microabscess formation. They are effective in destroying and phagocytizing the bacteria and dead cells
- **Lymphocytes:** These are found extravascularly in normal pulps. They appear at the site of inflammation after invasion by neutrophils. These cells are associated with injury and resultant immune response. Thus their presence indicates presence of persistent irritation
- **Mast cells:** On stimulation, degranulation of mast cells releases histamine which causes vasodilatation, increased vessel permeability and thus allowing fluids and leukocytes to escape

Extracellular Components

Extracellular components include fibers and the ground substance of pulp:

Fibers

- Principally Type 1 and Type 3 collagen fibers are found. Type 1 (55%) are present as thick striated fibrils, mainly responsible for pulp architecture. Type 3 (45%) are thinner fibrils and contribute to the elasticity of pulp. Overall collagen content of the pulp increases with age but the ratio between Type 1 and Type 3 remains stable
- Collagen is synthesized and secreted by odontoblasts and fibroblasts. Fibers produced by these cells differ in the degree of cross-linkage and variation in hydroxyline content. Fibers secreted by fibroblasts do not calcify
- Collagen with age becomes coarser and can lead to formation of pulp stones
- In peripheral pulp, collagen fibers have unique arrangement forming *von Korff's fibers*. These are corkscrew like originating between odontoblasts and pass into dentin matrix

Reticular fibers termed *argyrophilic fibers* are common in young pulps. A small number of oxytalan fibers occur in the pulp. There are no elastic fibers in the pulp except those present in large blood vessels.

Clinical Tips

Fibers are more numerous in radicular pulp than coronal and greatest concentration of collagen occurs in the most apical portion of pulp. Thus engaging pulp with a barbed broach in apical area offers removal of the tissue intact than engaging the broach coronally, where the pulp is more gelatinous and liable to tear.

Ground Substance

Ground substance of the pulp is a structureless mass with gel-like consistency forming bulk of pulp. *Chief components of ground substance* are
- Glycosaminoglycans
- Glycoproteins
- Water (90%)

   Depolymerization by enzymes produced by microorganisms found in pulpal inflammation may change ground substance of the pulp. Alexander et al. in 1980 found that these enzymes can degrade the ground substance of the pulp by disrupting the glycosaminoglycan–collagen linkage.

   Alterations in composition of ground substance caused by age or disease interfere with metabolism, reduced cellular function, and irregularities in mineral deposition. Thus, ground substance plays an important role in health and diseases of the pulp and dentin.

Functions of ground substance
- Forms the bulk of the pulp
- Supports the cells
- Acts as medium for transport of nutrients from vasculature to the cells and of metabolites from cells to the vasculature

■ Systemic Factors Affecting Pulp

Vitamin Deficiency

Vitamin C deficiency causes shrivelling of fibroblasts. Since fibroblasts don't develop fully, fibers produced by them are shorter, thinner, and less dense resulting in increase in permeability and bleeding tendency.

Steroids

Prolonged use of steroids
- Inhibits collagen synthesis
- Affects odontoblasts and thus inhibit dentinogenesis and reparative dentin formation
- Reduction in number of fibroblasts

Thyroid Deficiency

- It reduces vascularity of pulp
- Causes hypermineralization of bone and dentin
- Rapid deposition of dentin results in smaller pulp cavity

Diabetes

- Causes degenerative and inflammatory changes in pulp

Viral Infection

- Systemic viral infection can result in injury to odontoblasts and pulp inflammation

Hypoparathyroidism

- It can interfere mineralization of roots of teeth which are not fully formed
- Affected teeth have shorter roots than normal teeth

■ Supportive Elements

Pulpal Blood Supply

Blood flow reflects the functional capacity of an organ. Normal rate of pulpal blood flow is 20–60 mL/min/100 g pulp tissue. It is higher than that of surrounding oral tissues and skeletal muscles but lower than that of heart, kidney, or spleen.

   Teeth are supplied by branches of maxillary artery **(Flowchart 2.1)**. Blood vessels enter the pulp via apical and accessory foramina. One or two arterioles enter the apical foramen with sensory and sympathetic nerve bundles. Arterioles course up through radicular pulp and give off branches which spread laterally toward the odontoblasts layer and form capillary plexus. As they pass into coronal pulp, they diverge toward dentin, diminish in size and give rise to capillary network in subodontoblastic region **(Fig. 2.9)**. This network provides odontoblasts with rich source of metabolites.

   Blood passes from capillary plexus into venules which constitute efferent (exit) side of pulpal circulation and are slightly larger than corresponding arterioles. Venules enlarge as they merge and advance toward the apical foramen **(Flowchart 2.2)**. Efferent vessels are thin walled and show only scanty smooth muscle.

Lymphatic Vessels (Flowchart 2.3)

Lymphatic vessels arise as small, blind, thin-walled vessels in coronal region of the pulp and pass apically through middle and radicular parts of pulp. They exit via one or two large vessels through the apical foramen.

Lymphatic vessels can be differentiated from small venules in the following ways:
- Lack of continuity in vessel walls
- Absence of RBC in their lumina

Regulation of Pulpal Blood Flow

Walls of arterioles and venules are associated with smooth muscles which are innervated by unmyelinated

Flowchart 2.1 Arterial supply of teeth.

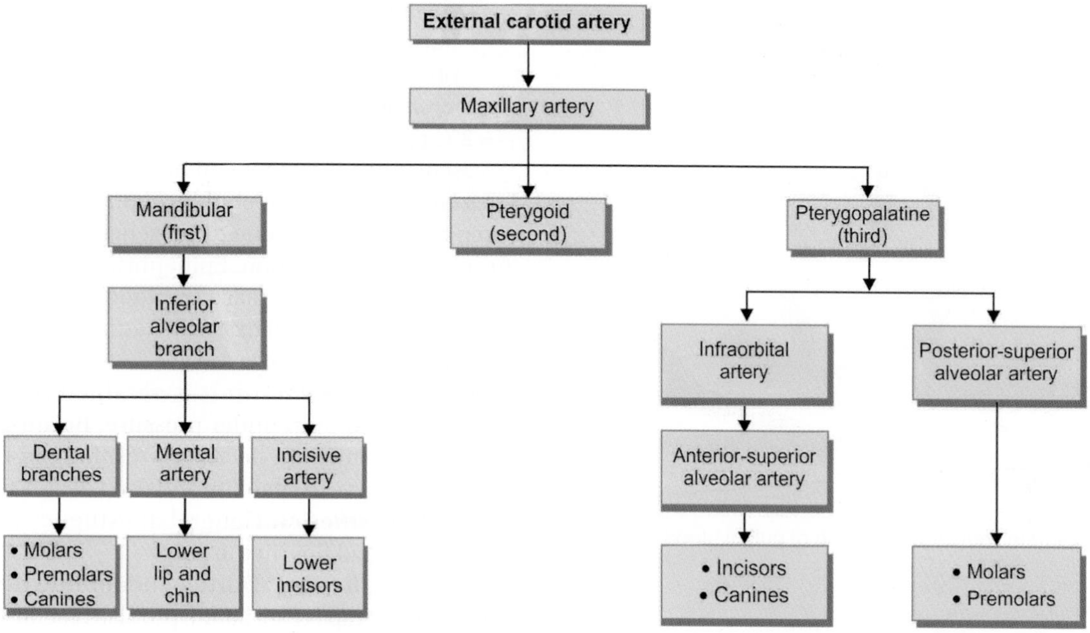

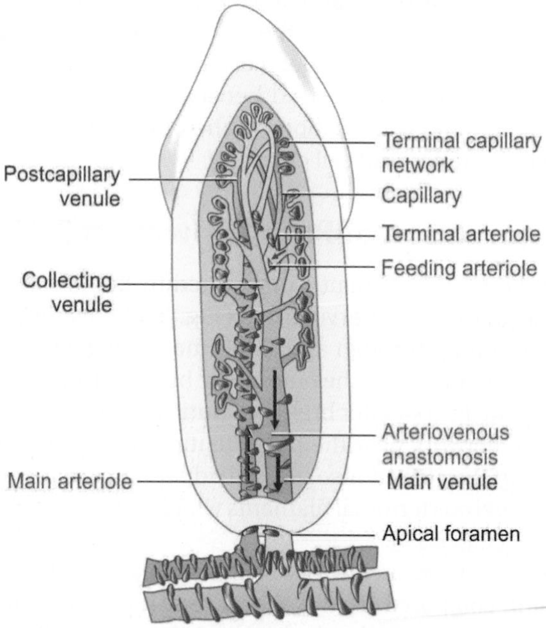

```
External carotid artery
        |
  Maxillary artery
        |
  +-----+--------------------+
  |                |                    |
Mandibular    Pterygoid        Pterygopalatine
(first)       (second)         (third)
  |                                 |
Inferior                  +---------+-----------+
alveolar            Infraorbital    Posterior-superior
branch              artery          alveolar artery
  |                      |                 |
+---+---+      Anterior-superior      • Molars
|   |   |      alveolar artery        • Premolars
Dental Mental Incisive       |
branches artery artery       |
|      |      |        • Incisors
• Molars Lower Lower    • Canines
• Premolars lip and incisors
• Canines chin
```

Flowchart 2.2 Venous drainage of teeth.

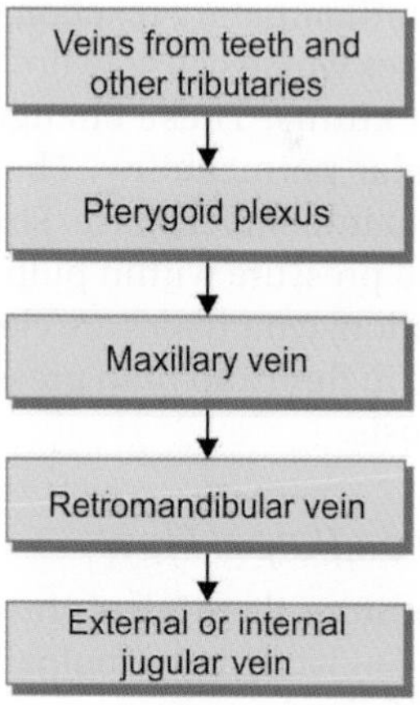

```
Veins from teeth and other tributaries
        |
Pterygoid plexus
        |
Maxillary vein
        |
Retromandibular vein
        |
External or internal jugular vein
```

Fig. 2.9 Diagram showing circulation of pulp.

Labels: Postcapillary venule, Collecting venule, Main arteriole, Terminal capillary network, Capillary, Terminal arteriole, Feeding arteriole, Arteriovenous anastomosis, Main venule, Apical foramen

Flowchart 2.3 Lymphatic drainage of teeth.

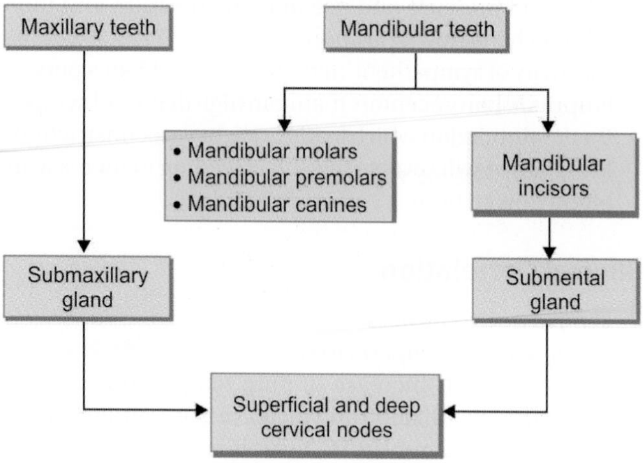

```
Maxillary teeth        Mandibular teeth
     |              +--------+--------+
     |         • Mandibular molars   Mandibular
     |         • Mandibular premolars incisors
     |         • Mandibular canines     |
Submaxillary                          Submental
gland                                 gland
     |                                   |
     +----> Superficial and deep <-------+
              cervical nodes
```

sympathetic fibers. When stimulated by stimulus (e.g., epinephrine containing local anesthetics), muscle fibers contract resulting in decrease in blood supply (**Fig. 2.10**).

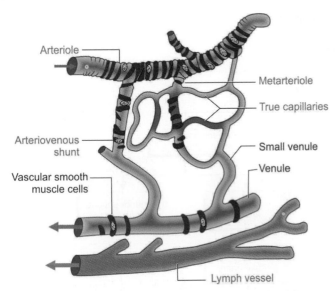

Arteriole
Metarteriole
True capillaries
Arteriovenous shunt
Small venule
Venule
Vascular smooth muscle cells
Lymph vessel

Fig. 2.10 Diagram showing regulation of pulpal blood flow.

Pulpal Response to Inflammation

Whenever there is inflammatory reaction, there is release of lysosomal enzymes which cause hydrolysis of collagen and the release of kinins. These changes further lead to increased vascular permeability. The escaping fluid accumulates in pulp interstitial space. Since space in the pulp is confined, so pressure within pulp chamber rises. In severe inflammation, lymphatics are closed resulting in continued increase in fluid and pulp pressure which may result in pulp necrosis.

Effect of Posture on Pulpal Flow

In normal upright posture, there is less pressure effect in the structures of head. On lying down, pulpal blood pressure elevates because of following reasons:
❑ Removal of gravitational effect: It causes increase in pulpal blood pressure and rise in tissue pressure and thus pain on lying down position
❑ Inactivity of sympathetic nervous system: When a person is upright, baroreceptors maintain high degree of sympathetic stimulation which leads to slight vasoconstriction. Lying down will reverse this effect leading to increase in blood flow to pulp

Clinical Correlation

❑ *Temperature changes*
  • *Increase in temperature:*
    – A 10–15°C increase in pulp temperature causes arteriolar dilation and increase in intrapulpal pressure of 2.5 mmHg/°C, but it is transient in nature

    – Irreversible changes occur when vasodilation is sustained by heating the pulp to 45°C for prolonged periods, resulting in persistent increase in pulp pressure
  • *Decrease in temperature:* Temperature lower than –2°C causes pathological changes in pulp tissue like vascular engorgement and necrosis
❑ *Local anesthetics:* Effect of local anesthetics on pulp vasculature is mainly due to presence of vasoconstrictor in anesthetic solution. Epinephrine present in local anesthetic causes decrease in blood flow in the pulp which is due to stimulation of α-adrenergic receptors located in pulpal blood vessels
❑ *Intrapulpal anesthesia:* It is obtained by injecting anesthesia into pulp under pressure. Because of this, pulp microcirculation decreases resulting in transient increase in nerve excitability and then decrease to zero
❑ *General anesthetics:* General anesthetics affect the velocity of blood flow in the pulp
❑ *Endodontic therapy:* During endodontic therapy, if only coronal pulp is extirpated, profuse bleeding occurs, whereas removal of pulp close to apex results in less bleeding. This is because of larger diameter of blood vessels in central part of the pulp
❑ *Aging:* With increasing age, pulp shows decrease in vascularity, increase in fibrosis, narrowing of diameter of blood vessels, and decrease in circulation. Finally, circulation gets impaired because of atherosclerotic changes and calcifications in the blood vessel leading to cell atrophy and cell death

▌ Innervation of Pulp (Flowchart 2.4)

Dental pulp is abundantly innervated by both sensory as well as autonomic nerve fibers **(Fig. 2.11)**. Nerve fibers enter the pulp through apical foramen along with blood vessels. After entering the pulp, nerve bundles run coronally and divide into smaller branches until a single axons form a dense network near the pulp–dentin margin, termed as *plexus of Raschkow*. Also the individual axons may branch into numerous terminal filaments which enter the dentinal tubules **(Fig. 2.12)**.

Sensory nerves are encased in myelin sheath. Myelin sheath is mainly composed of fatty substances or lipids and proteins. Myelin appears to be internal proliferation of Schwann cells. Unmyelinated fibers are surrounded by single layer of Schwann cells, but in these myelin spirals are absent. Unmyelinated fibers are surrounded by single layer of Schwann cells and are generally found in autonomic nervous system.

Nerve fibers are classified according to their diameter, velocity of conduction, and function.

Fibers having largest diameter are classified as A-fibers while those having smallest diameter are classified as

Flowchart 2.4 Nerve supply of teeth.

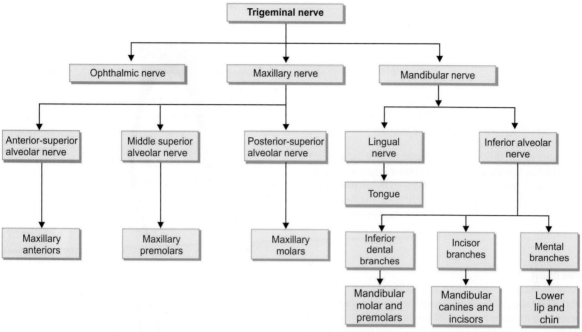

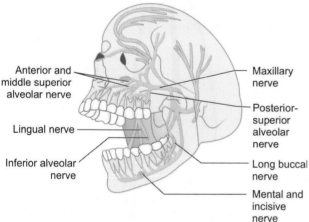

Fig. 2.11 Nerve supply of teeth.

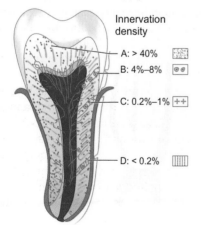

Fig. 2.12 Diagram showing nerve density at different areas of the tooth.

C-fibers (**Fig. 2.13**). Aδ fibers are faster conducting and are responsible for localized, sharp dentinal pain. C-fibers are slower conducting and are responsible for dull and throbbing pain.

Electrical pulp tester stimulates Aδ fibers first because of their lower threshold. As the intensity of stimulus is increased along with Aδ fibers, some of the C-fibers also get stimulated resulting in strong unpleasant sensation.

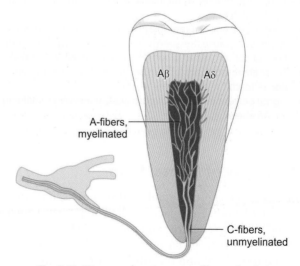

Fig. 2.13 Diagram showing nerve fibers of pulp.

Difference between Aδ and C-fibers

Aδ fibers	C-fibers
• Diameter 2–5 μm	• Diameter 0.3–1.2 μm
• High conduction velocity (6–30 m/s)	• Slow conduction velocity (0.5–2 m/s)
• Myelinated axons	• Unmyelinated fine sensory fibers
• Pain is well localized	• Not localized
• Low threshold	• High threshold
• Sharp, quick, and pricking pain	• Dull and lingering pain
• Direct innervation theory, Odontoblastic theory, and Hydrodynamic theory explain how A delta fibers are stimulated	• Inflammation accompanied with tissue injury results in increase in tissue pressure and chemical mediators which in turns stimulate C-fibers

Aδ nerve fibers

- Most of myelinated nerve fibers are Aδ fibers
- At the odontoblastic layer, they lose their myelin sheath and anastomose forming network of nerves called "plexuses of Raschkow." They send free nerve endings into dentinal tubules
- Diameter of these fibers ranges from 2 to 5 μm and conduction velocity 6–30 m/s
- These are large fibers with fast conduction velocities
- Pain transmitted through these fibers is perceived as sharp, quick, and momentary type
- Pain disappears quickly on removal of stimulus

C-nerve fibers

- C-nerve fibers are small unmyelinated fine sensory afferent nerves
- They have slow conduction velocities and high threshold
- Diameter ranges from 0.3 to 1.2 μm and conduction velocity 0.5–2 m/s
- They are stimulated by intense cold or hot stimuli or mechanical stimulation
- Even in presence of radiographic lesion, C-fibers can show response because these are more resistant to hypoxic conditions or compromised blood flow as compared to Aδ fibers
- These are responsible for pain occurring during instrumentation of teeth
- Eighty percent of nerves of pulp are C-fibers and remaining are Aδ fibers

Anatomy of Dental Pulp

Pulp lies in the center of tooth and shapes itself to miniature form of tooth. This space is called pulp cavity which is divided into pulp chamber and root canal **(Fig. 2.14)**.

In the anterior teeth, the pulp chamber gradually merges into the root canal and this division becomes indistinct **(Fig. 2.15)**. But in case of multirooted teeth, there is a single pulp chamber and usually two to four root canals **(Figs. 2.16**

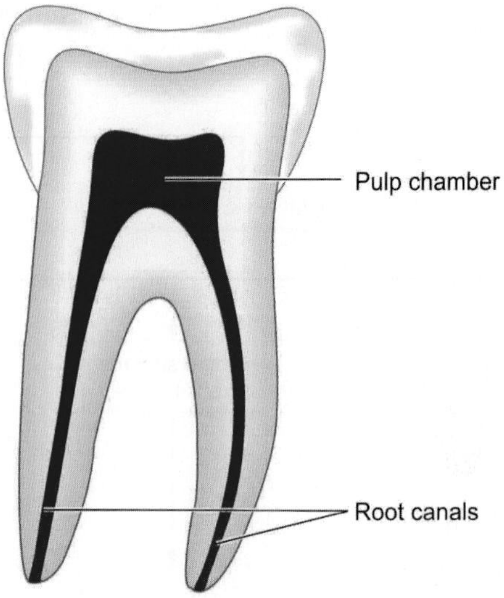

Fig. 2.14 Diagram showing pulp cavity.

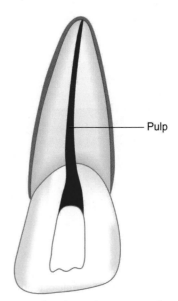

Fig. 2.15 Diagram showing pulp anatomy of anterior tooth.

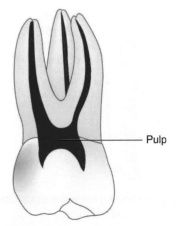

Fig. 2.16 Diagram showing pulp cavity of maxillary molar.

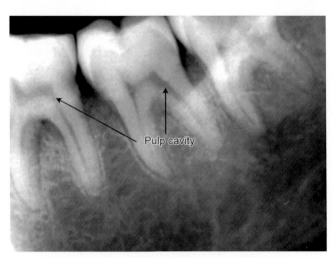

Fig. 2.17 Radiographic appearance of pulp cavity.

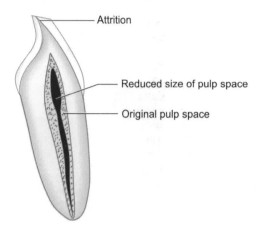

Fig. 2.19 Reduction in size of pulp cavity because of formation of secondary and tertiary dentin.

and 2.17). As the external morphology of the tooth varies from person to person, so does the internal morphology of crown and the root.

Pulp Chamber

It reflects the external form of enamel at the time of eruption, but anatomy is less sharply defined. Roof of pulp chamber consists of dentin covering the pulp chamber occlusally.

Canal orifices are openings in the floor of pulp chamber leading into the root canals (**Fig. 2.18**).

Because of caries, irritants, and advancing age, pulp chamber shows reduction in size due to deposition of secondary or tertiary dentin (**Fig. 2.19**).

Root Canal

Root canal is portion of pulp cavity which extends from canal orifice to apical foramen. Shape of root canal varies with size, shape, number of the roots in different teeth. A straight root canal throughout the entire length of root is uncommon. Curvature is found commonly along root length which can be gradual or sharp (**Fig. 2.20**). In most cases, numbers of root canals correspond to number of roots but a root may have more than one canal.

According to Orban, shape of the canal can be determined by shape of the root. Root canals can be round, tapering elliptical, broad, thin, etc.

"Meyer" stated that roots which are round and cone shaped usually contain one canal but roots which are elliptical with flat or concave surface frequently have more than one canals (**Fig. 2.21**).

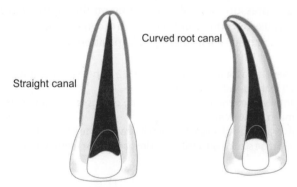

Fig. 2.20 Straight and curved root canal.

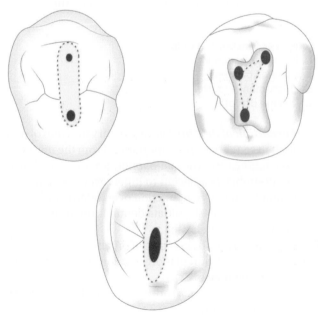

Fig. 2.18 Diagram showing opening of canal orifices in the pulp chamber.

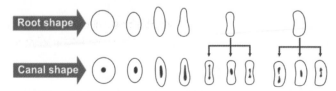

Fig. 2.21 Diagram showing relationship between shape of root and number of root canals

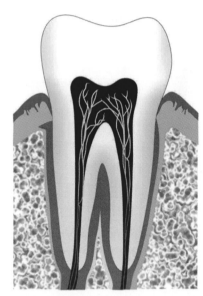

Fig. 2.22 Diagram showing that nerves and blood vessels enter or leave the tooth via apical foramen.

Apical foramen is an aperture at or near the apex of a root through which nerves and blood vessels of the pulp enter or leave the pulp cavity **(Fig. 2.22)**. In young newly erupted teeth, it is wide open, but as the root develops, apical foramen becomes narrower. Inner surface of the apex is lined with the cementum which may extend for a short distance into the root canal. Thus we can say that CDJ (Cementodentinal junction) does not necessarily occur at apical end of root but may occur within the main root canal **(Figs. 2.23A to C)**.

Multiple foramina are found in multirooted teeth. Majority of single rooted teeth have single canal which terminate in a single foramina. Change in shape and location of foramen can occur during posteruptive phase due to functional forces (tongue pressure, mesial drift) acting on the tooth. These forces cause resorption and deposition of cementum on walls of foramen resulting in shifting of its position.

- There are a total of 52 pulp organs, 32 in the permanent, and 20 in the deciduous teeth
- Total volume of all permanent pulp organs is 0.38 cm³ with mean of 0.02 cm³
- Average size of apical foramen in maxillary teeth is 0.4 mm
- Average size of apical foramen in mandibular teeth is 0.3 mm

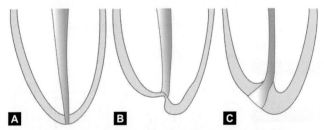

Figs. 2.23A to C Diagram showing cementodentinal junction (CDJ).

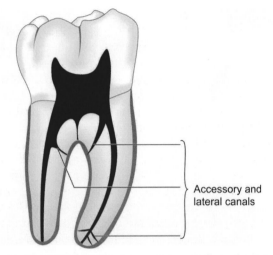

Fig. 2.24 Diagram showing accessory and lateral canals.

Accessory canals: These are the lateral branches of main canal that form communication between pulp and periodontium. Accessory canals contain connective tissue and vessels and can be seen anywhere from furcation to apex but tend to be more common in apical third of posterior teeth **(Fig. 2.24)**.

Mechanism of formation:
- Accessory canals occur in areas of premature loss of root sheath cells because these cells induce formation of odontoblasts
- In areas where developing root encounters a blood vessel. When dentin is forming; hard tissue may develop around a blood vessel resulting in accessory canal formation

▌Functions of Pulp

Pulp lives for dentin and the dentin lives by the grace of the pulp.

Four basic functions of pulp:
1. Formation of dentin
2. Nutrition of dentin
3. Innervation of tooth
4. Defense of tooth

1. *Formation of dentin:* It is the primary function of pulp both in sequence and importance. From the mesodermal aggregation (dental papilla) arises special layer of odontoblasts adjacent to inner layer of ectodermal enamel organ. On interaction of ectoderm and mesoderm, odontoblasts initiate dentin formation
   Pulp primarily helps in
   - Synthesis and secretion of organic matrix
   - Initial transport of inorganic components to newly formed matrix
   - Creating an environment favorable for matrix mineralization

2. ***Nutrition of dentin:*** Nutrients exchange across capillaries into pulpal interstitial fluid. This fluid travels into the dentin through the network of tubules formed by the odontoblasts to contain their processes
3. ***Innervation of tooth:*** Pulp and dentin show innervation due to presence of fluid movement between dentinal tubules and peripheral receptors and thus to sensory nerves of the pulp
4. ***Defense of tooth:*** Odontoblasts form dentin in response to injury in form of caries, attrition, trauma, or restorative procedure. Formation of reparative dentin and sclerotic dentin form the defense mechanisms of the tooth. Formation of reparative dentin occurs at the rate of 1.5 µm/day. Quantity and quality of formed reparative dentin is directly related to severity and duration of injury to pulp.

Pulp also shows an inflammatory and immunologic response in an attempt to neutralize or eliminate invasion of microorganisms and their byproducts in dentin.

Age Changes in the Pulp

Pulp-like other connective tissues undergoes changes with time. These changes can be natural or may be result of injury such as caries, trauma, or restorative dental procedure. Regardless of the cause, the pulp shows changes in appearance (morphogenic) and functions (physiologic).

Morphologic Changes

- Reduction of tubular diameter due to continuous deposition of intratubular dentin
- Reduction in pulp volume due to increase in secondary dentin deposition **(Fig. 2.25)**. It gives root canal a very thin or obliterated appearance
- Presence of dystrophic calcification and pulp stones **(Fig. 2.26)**

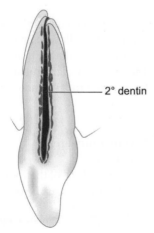

Fig. 2.25 Reduction in size of pulp volume due to increased secondary dentin deposition.

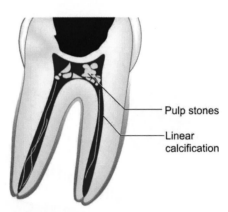

Fig. 2.26 Diagram showing pulp stones and reduced size of pulp cavity with advancing age.

- Decrease in the number of pulp cells. Cell density decreases to 50% by age of 70
- Decrease in sensitivity due to degeneration and loss of myelinated and unmyelinated axons
- Reduction in number of blood vessels, displaying arteriosclerotic changes
- Presence of collagen in pulp becomes more apparent because of formation of collagen bundles. Recent studies have shown that collagen content does not increase with age but stabilizes after completion of tooth formation

Physiologic Changes

- Decrease in dentin permeability giving protective environment to the pulp
- Reduced ability of pulp to react to the irritants and repair itself

Pulpal Calcifications/Pulp Stones/ Denticles

Pulp stones are nodular calcified masses present in mature teeth. Larger calcifications are called denticles. Sometimes denticles become extremely large, almost obliterating the pulp chamber or the root canal. Incidence of pulp stones increases with age, but they are also found in young age.

Classification of pulp stone
- According to structure
  - True
  - False
- According to size
  - Fine
  - Diffuse
- According to location
  - Free
  - Attached
  - Embedded

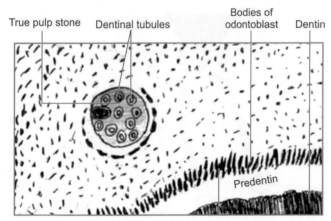

Fig. 2.27 Schematic representation of true denticles.

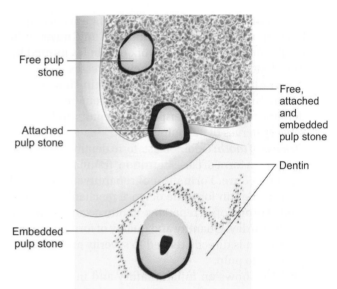

Fig. 2.28 Schematic representation of free, attached, and embedded pulp stones.

According to Structure

True Denticle (Fig. 2.27)

A true denticle is made up of dentin and is lined by odontoblasts. These are rare and usually located close to apical foramen. Development of true denticle is caused by inclusions of remnants of epithelial root sheath within the pulp. These epithelial remnants induce the cells of pulp to differentiate into odontoblast which form dentin masses.

False Denticles

Appear as concentric layers of calcified tissue. These appear within bundles of collagen fibers. They may arise around vessels. Calcification of thrombi in blood vessels, called phleboliths, may also serve as nidi for false denticles. All denticles begin as small nodules but increase in size by incremental growth on their surface.

According to Size

According to size, pulp stones can be fine and diffuse mineralizations. Diffuse calcifications are also known as fibrillar or linear calcifications because of their longitudinal orientation. These can be found in any area but more frequently found in radicular pulp. These are aligned close to blood vessels, nerves, or collagen bundles. These are not visible on radiographs because of their size and dispersion.

According to Location (Fig. 2.28)

❑ *Free denticles* are like islands, that is, entirely surrounded by pulp tissue
❑ *Attached denticles* are free pulp stones which partially fuse to continuously growing dentin
❑ *Embedded denticles* are attached stones that are now entirely surrounded by dentin

Clinical Significance of Pulp Stones

Presence of pulp stones may alter the internal anatomy of the pulp cavity, making the access opening of tooth difficult. They may deflect or engage the tip of exploring instrument. Since the pulp stone can originate in response to chronic irritation, the pulp chamber which appears to have diffuse and obscure outline may represent a large number of irregular pulp stones which may indicate chronic irritation of the pulp.

▮ Periradicular Tissue (Fig. 2.29)

Periradicular tissue consists of cementum, periodontal ligament, and alveolar bone.

Cementum

Cementum is a hard, avascular connective tissue that covers roots of the teeth. It is light yellow in color and can be differentiated from enamel by its darker hue and lack of luster. It is very permeable to dyes and chemical agents, from the pulp canal and the external root surface.

Types

Two main types of cementum are:
1. *Acellular cementum*
   a. Covers the cervical third of the root
   b. Forms before tooth reaches the occlusal plane
   c. It does not contain cells
   d. Thickness varies between 30 and 230 μm
   e. Abundance of Sharpey's fibers
   f. Main function is anchorage

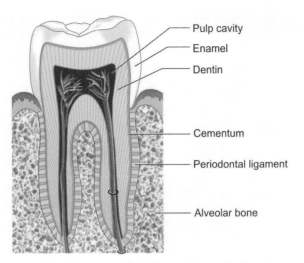

Fig. 2.29 Schematic representation of periradicular tissue.

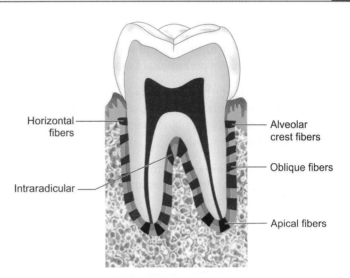

Fig. 2.30 Principal fibers of periodontal ligament.

2. ***Cellular cementum***
   a. Forms after tooth reaches the occlusal plane
   b. It contains cells
   c. Less calcified than acellular cementum
   d. Sharpey's fibers are present in lesser number as compared to acellular cementum
   e. Mainly found in apical third and inter-radicular region
   f. Main function is adaptation

Periodontal Ligament (Fig. 2.30)

Periodontal ligament is a unique structure as it forms a link between alveolar bone and cementum. It is continuous with connective tissue of the gingiva and communicates with the marrow spaces through vascular channels in the bone. Periodontal ligament houses the fibers, cells, and other structural elements like blood vessels and nerves.

Periodontal ligament comprises of the following components:
❑ Periodontal fibers
❑ Cells
❑ Blood vessels
❑ Nerves

Periodontal Fibers

The most important component of periodontal ligament is principal fibers. These fibers are composed mainly of collagen Type 1. Apart from the principal fibers, oxytalan and elastic fibers are also present. The principal fibers are present in six arrangements.

Horizontal group: These fibers are arranged horizontally emerging from alveolar bone and attached to the root cementum.

Alveolar crest group: These fibers arise from the alveolar crest in fan like manner and attach to the root cementum. These fibers prevent the extrusion of the tooth.

Oblique fibers: These fibers make the largest group in periodontal ligament. They extend from cementum to bone obliquely. They bear the occlusal forces and transmit them to alveolar bone.

Trans-septal fibers: These fibers run from the cementum of one tooth to the cementum of another tooth crossing over the alveolar crest.

Apical fibers: These fibers are present around the root apex.

Inter-radicular fibers: These fibers are present in furcation areas of multirooted teeth.

Cells

The cells present in periodontal ligament are:
❑ Fibroblast
❑ Macrophages
❑ Mast cells
❑ Neutrophils
❑ Lymphocytes
❑ Plasma cells
❑ Epithelial cell rests of Malassez

Nerve Fibers

The nerve fibers present in periodontal ligament are either of myelinated or non-myelinated type.

Blood Vessels

The periodontal ligament receives blood supply from the gingival, alveolar, and apical vessels.

Functions

Supportive: Tooth is supported and suspended in alveolar socket with the help of periodontal ligament.

Nutritive: Periodontal ligament has very rich blood supply. So, it supplies nutrients to adjoining structures like cementum, bone, and gingiva via blood vessels. It also provides lymphatic drainage.

Protective: These fibers perform the function of protection absorbing the occlusal forces and transmitting to the underlying alveolar bone.

Formative: The cells of PDL (periodontal ligament) help in formation of surrounding structures like alveolar bone and cementum.

Resorptive: The resorptive function is also accomplished with the cells like osteoclasts, cementoclasts, and fibroblasts provided by periodontal ligament.

Alveolar Bone (Fig. 2.31)

Bone is specialized connective tissue which comprises of inorganic phases that is very well designed for its role as load bearing structure of the body.

Cells

Cells present in bone are:
- Osteocytes
- Osteoblasts
- Osteoclasts

Intercellular Matrix

Bone consists of two-third inorganic matter and one-third organic matter. Inorganic matter is composed mainly of minerals calcium and phosphate along with hydroxyapatite, carbonate, citrate, etc. while organic matrix is composed mainly of collagen Type 1 (90%).

Bone consists of two plates of compact bone separated by spongy bone in between. In some area, there is no spongy bone. The spaces between trabeculae of spongy bone are filled with marrow which consists of hemopoietic tissue in early life and fatty tissue later in life. Bone is a dynamic tissue continuously forming and resorbing in response to functional needs. Both local as well as hormonal factors play an important role in metabolism of bone. In healthy conditions, the crest of alveolar bone lies approximately 2–3 mm apical to the cementoenamel junction, but it comes

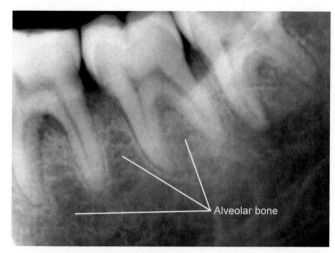

Fig. 2.31 Radiographic appearance of alveolar bone.

to lie more apically in periodontal diseases. In periapical diseases, it gets resorbed easily.

Question

1. Write short notes on:
   - Zones of dental pulp
   - Odontoblasts
   - Accessory and lateral canals
   - Innervation of pulp
   - Functions of pulp
   - Age changes in the pulp
   - Pulp stones/denticles/pulpal calcifications

Bibliography

1. Bender IB. Reversible and irreversible painful pulpitides: diagnosis and treatment. Aust Endod J 2000;26:10–4.
2. Bjørndal L, Mjör IA. Pulp-dentin biology in restorative dentistry. Part 4: Dental caries—Characteristics of lesions and pulpal reactions. Quintessence Int 2001;32:717–36.
3. Czarnecki RT, Schilder H. A histological evaluation of the human pulp in teeth with varying degrees of periodontal disease. J Endod 1979;5:242–53.
4. Di Nicolo R, Guedes-Pinto AC, Carvalho YR. Histopathology of the pulp of primary molars with active and arrested dentinal caries. J Clin Pediatr Dent 2000;25:47–9.
5. D'Souza R, Brown LR, Newland JR, Levy BM, Lachman LB. Detection and characterization of interleukin-1 in human dental pulps. Arch Oral Biol 1989;34:307–313.
6. Michaelson PL, Holland GR. Is pulpitis painful? Int Endod J 2002;35:829–32.

Pathologies of Pulp and Periapex

Introduction

Dental pulp consists of vascular connective tissue contained within the rigid dentin walls. It is the principal source of pain in oral cavity and also a major site of attention in endodontics and restorative procedures. Thus, knowledge of pulp is essential not only for providing dental treatment but also to know the rationale behind the treatment provided.

Important features of pulp (Fig. 3.1):
- It is a coherent soft tissue, surrounded by dentin which limits the area for expansion and restricts its ability to tolerate edema
- Odontoblasts present in pulp have ability to form dentin in response to caries and irritants
- Pulp has almost total lack of collateral circulation. This limits its ability to cope with bacteria, necrotic tissue, and inflammation
- It gives radiographic appearance as radiolucent line

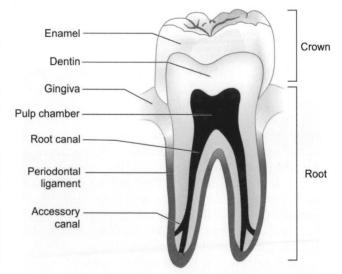

Enamel
Dentin
Gingiva
Pulp chamber
Root canal
Periodontal ligament
Accessory canal

Crown
Root

Fig. 3.1 Relation of pulp with its surrounding structures.

Etiology of Pulpal Diseases

- ❑ Classification of etiology according to *WEINE* beginning with the most common irritant
  - • ***Bacterial:*** Most common cause of pulpal injury is bacteria or their by-products which may enter the pulp through a break in dentin from
    - – Caries **(Figs. 3.2 and 3.3)**
    - – Accidental exposure
    - – Fracture
    - – Percolation around a restoration
    - – Extension of infection from gingival sulcus
    - – Periodontal pocket and abscess **(Fig. 3.4)**
    - – Anachoresis (process by which microorganisms get carried by the bloodstream from another source and localize on inflamed tissue)
  - • ***Traumatic***
    - – Acute trauma like fracture, luxation, or avulsion of tooth **(Fig. 3.5)**
    - – Chronic trauma including parafunctional habits like bruxism
  - • ***Iatrogenic***: Pulp inflammation resulting from clinician's own procedures is referred to as dentistogenic pulpitis. Iatrogenic causes of pulp pathologies can be
    - – *Thermal changes* caused during tooth preparation, restoration, bleaching of enamel, electrosurgical procedures, etc.

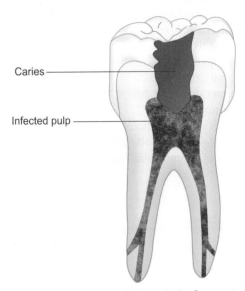

Fig. 3.2 Dental caries results in pulpal inflammation.

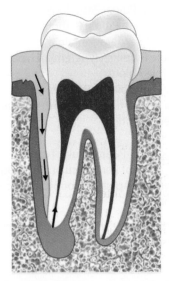

Fig. 3.4 Periodontal pocket or abscess can cause pulpal inflammation via portals of communication like apical foramen or lateral canals.

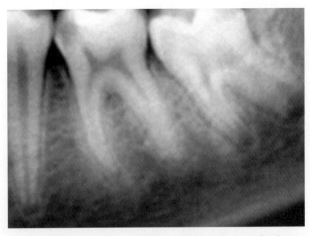

Fig. 3.3 Radiograph showing carious exposure of pulp in first molar.

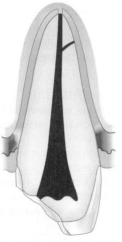

Fig. 3.5 Fracture of tooth can also cause pulpal inflammation.

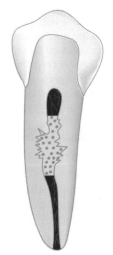

Fig. 3.6 Line diagram showing internal resorption of tooth.

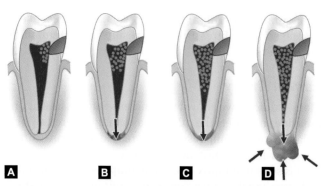

Figs. 3.7A to D Schematic representation of gradual pulpal response to dental caries.

– Orthodontic movement
– Periodontal curettage
– Periapical curettage
– Use of chemicals like temporary and permanent restorations, liners, bases, and use of cavity desiccants such as alcohol
• *Idiopathic*
  – Aging
  – Resorption; internal or external **(Fig. 3.6)**

Radiation injury to pulp
• Pulp cells exposed to ionizing radiation may become necrotic, show vascular damage and the interference in mitosis of cells
• Irradiation affects salivary glands resulting in decreased salivary flow, thereby increased predisposition to dental caries and pulpal involvement
• Effects of radiation damage to teeth depend on dose, source, type of radiation, exposure factor, and stage of tooth development at the time of irradiation

▌Progression of Pulpal Pathologies

Pulp reacts to above mentioned irritants same as other connective tissues. A normal pulp gives mild-to-moderate response to pulp tests and this response subsides on removal of stimulus. Degree of inflammation is proportional to the intensity and severity of the tissue damage. For example, slight irritation like incipient caries or shallow tooth preparation causes little or no pulpal inflammation, whereas extensive operative procedures may lead to severe pulpal inflammation.

Depending on condition of pulp, severity and duration of irritant, host response, pulp may respond from mild inflammation to pulp necrosis. These changes may not be accompanied by pain and thus may proceed unnoticed.

Pulpal reaction to microbial irritation (Figs. 3.7A to D)

Microorganisms present in carious enamel and dentin
↓
Penetration of microorganisms in deeper layers of carious dentin
↓
Pulp is affected before actual invasion of bacteria via their toxic by-products
↓
By-products cause local chronic cell infiltration
↓
When actual pulp exposure occurs, pulp tissue gets locally infiltrated by PMNs to form an area of liquefaction necrosis at the site of exposure
↓
Eventually necrosis spreads all across the pulp and periapical tissue resulting in severe inflammatory lesion

Pulp Inflammation and Its Sequelae

Traditional theory which explained pulpal inflammation and its sequelae was referred to as strangulation theory. Strangulation theory is no longer accepted and a current theory explains the sequelae of pulpal inflammation.

Strangulation Theory

It says that on irritation, there is local inflammation in pulp, which results in vasodilation, increased capillary pressure and permeability. These result in increased filtration from capillaries into tissues, thus increased tissue pressure. By this, thin vessel walls get compressed resulting in decreased blood flow and increased venous pressure. This results in vicious cycle, because increase in venous pressure further increases capillary pressure. Consequently, choking/

strangulation of pulpal blood vessels occur because of increased tissue pressure. This results in ischemia and further necrosis.

Current Theory

Many studies have shown that increase of pressure in one area does not affect the other areas of pulp. Therefore local inflammation in pulp results in increased tissue pressure in inflamed area and not the entire pulp cavity.

It is seen that injury to coronal pulp results in local disturbance, but if injury is severe, it results in complete stasis of blood vessels in and near the injured area. Net absorption of fluid into capillaries in adjacent uninflamed area results in increased lymphatic drainage thus keeping the pulpal volume almost constant.

Limited increase in pressure within affected pulpal area is explained by the following mechanism:
- Increased pressure in inflamed area favors net absorption of interstitial fluids from adjacent capillaries in uninflamed tissues
- Increased interstitial tissue pressure lowers the transcapillary hydrostatic pressure difference, thus opposes further filtration
- Increased interstitial fluid pressure increases lymphatic drainage
- Break in endothelium of pulpal capillaries facilitate exchange mechanism

Infectious sequelae of pulpitis include apical periodontitis, periapical abscess/cellulitis, and osteomyelitis of the jaw (**Fig. 3.8**). Spread from maxillary teeth may cause purulent sinusitis, meningitis, brain abscess, orbital cellulitis, and cavernous sinus thrombosis. Spread from mandibular teeth may cause Ludwig's angina, parapharyngeal abscess, mediastinitis, pericarditis, and empyema (**Fig. 3.9**).

POINTS TO REMEMBER

Degree and nature of inflammatory response caused by microbial irritants depends upon
- Host resistance
- Virulence of microorganisms
- Duration of exposure
- Lymphatic drainage
- Amount of circulation in affected area
- Opportunity of release of inflammatory fluids

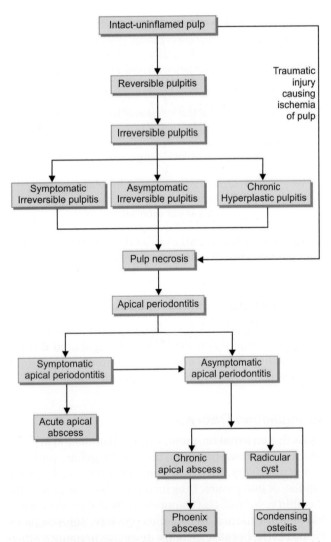

Fig. 3.8 Sequel of pulpal inflammation.

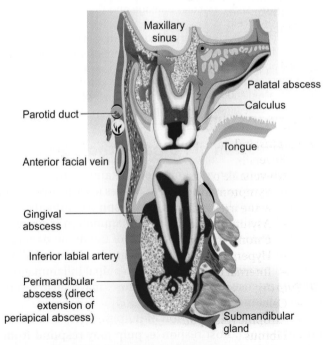

Fig. 3.9 Pulpal inflammation and its sequelae.

Diagnosis of Pulpal Pathology

- *Subjective symptoms:* Most common symptom is pain
- *Objective symptoms:*
  - Visual and tactile inspection—3Cs
    - Color
    - Contour
    - Consistency
  - Thermal tests:
    - *Heat tests:* Use of
      - Warm air
      - Hot water
      - Hot burnisher
      - Hot gutta-percha stick
    - *Cold tests:*
      - Ethyl chloride spray
      - Ice pencils
      - CO_2 snow (temperature $-78°C$)
  - Electrical pulp testing
  - Radiographs
  - Anesthetic tests
  - Test cavity

  Recent advances in diagnostic aids for pulp pathologies include
- Laser Doppler flowmetry
- Liquid crystal testing
- Hughes probeye camera
- Infrared thermography
- Thermocouples
- Pulse oximetry
- Dual wavelength spectrophotometry
- Plethysmography
- Xenon-133 radioisotopes

Classification of Pulpal Pathologies

Grossman's Clinical Classification

- *Pulpitis:* Inflammatory disease of dental pulp
  - Reversible pulpitis
  - Irreversible pulpitis
    - Symptomatic irreversible(previously known as acute irreversible pulpitis)
    - Asymptomatic irreversible(previously known as chronic irreversible pulpitis)
    - Hyperplastic pulpitis
    - Internal resorption
- *Pulp degeneration*
  - Calcific (radiographic diagnosis)
  - Atrophic (histopathological diagnosis)
  - Fibrous
- *Necrosis*

Baume's Classification

Based on clinical symptoms:
- Asymptomatic, vital pulp which has been injured or involved by deep caries for which pulp capping may be done
- Pulp with history of pain which is amenable to pharmacotherapy
- Pulp indicated for extirpation and immediate root filling
- Necrosed pulp involving infection of radicular dentin accessible to antiseptic root canal therapy

Seltzer and Bender's Classification

Based on clinical tests of pulp and histological diagnosis:

Treatable without Pulp Extirpation and Endodontic Treatment

- Intact uninflamed pulp
- Transition stage
- Atrophic pulp
- Acute pulpitis
- Chronic partial pulpitis without necrosis

Untreatable without Pulp Extirpation and Endodontic Treatment

- Chronic partial pulpitis with necrosis
- Chronic total pulpitis
- Total pulp necrosis

Ingle's Classification

Inflammatory Changes

- Hyper-reactive pulpalgia
  - Hypersensitivity
  - Hyperemia
- Acute pulpalgia
  - Incipient (may be reversible)
  - Moderate (may be referred)
  - Advanced (relieved by cold)
- Chronic pulpalgia
- Hyperplastic pulpitis
- Pulp necrosis

Retrogressive Changes

- Atrophic pulposis
- Calcific pulposis

Barodontalgia/Aerodontalgia

It is pain experienced in a recently restored tooth during low atmospheric pressure. Pain is experienced either during ascent or descent. Chronic pulpitis which appears asymptomatic in normal conditions may manifests as pain at high altitude because of low pressure. It is generally seen in altitude over 5,000 ft but more likely to be observed in 10,000 ft and above.

Rauch classified barodontalgia according to chief complaint:

Class I: In acute pulpitis, sharp pain occurs for a moment on ascent.

Class II: In chronic pulpitis, dull throbbing pain occurs on ascent.

Class III: In necrotic pulp, dull throbbing pain occurs on descent but it is asymptomatic on ascent.

Class IV: In periapical cyst or abscess, severe and persistent pain occurs with both ascent and descent

Possible mechanism of barodontalgia:
- Direct ischemia resulting from inflammation itself
- Indirect ischemia resulting from increased intrapulpal pressure due to vasodilatation and fluid diffusion to the tissue
- Due to expansion of intrapulpal gas which is a by-product of acids, bases, and enzymes of inflamed tissues
- Due to leakage of gas through vessels because of decreased gas solubility

Reversible Pulpitis/Hyperemia/ Hyperactive Pulpalgia

This is the first stage of pulpitis giving sharp hypersensitive response to cold, but pain subsides on removal of the stimulus. Patient may describe symptoms of momentary pain and is unable to locate the source of pain. This stage can last for months or years.

Definition

Reversible pulpitis is mild-to-moderate inflammatory condition of pulp caused by noxious stimuli in which the pulp is capable of returning to normal state following removal of stimuli.

It is an indication of peripheral Aδ-fiber stimulation. Determination of reversibility is the clinical judgment which is influenced by history of patient and clinical evaluation.

Etiology

In normal circumstances, enamel and cementum act as impermeable barrier to block the patency of dentinal tubules. When a stimulus interrupts this natural barrier, dentinal tubules become permeable, causing inflammation of pulp. Etiological factors can be
- Dental caries
- Trauma: Acute or chronic occlusal trauma

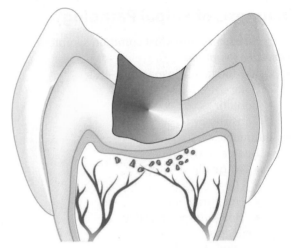
Fig. 3.10 Insertion of deep restoration causing pulp inflammation.

- Thermal injury:
  - Tooth preparation with dull bur without coolant
  - Overheating during polishing of a restoration
  - Keeping bur in contact with teeth too long
- Chemical stimulus—like sweet or sour foodstuff

Symptoms

- Characterized by sharp momentary pain, commonly caused by cold stimuli
- Pain does not occur spontaneously and does not continue after removal of irritant
- Following insertion of a deep restoration **(Fig. 3.10)**, patient may complain mild sensitivity to temperature changes, especially cold. Such sensitivity may last for a week or longer but gradually, it subsides. This sensitivity is symptom of reversible pulpitis

Histopathology

- It shows hyperemia to mild-to-moderate inflammatory changes
- Evidence of disruption of odontoblastic layer
- Formation of reparative dentin
- Dilated blood vessels
- Extravasation of edema fluid
- Presence of immunologically competent chronic inflammatory and occasionally acute cells

Diagnosis

- ***Pain:*** It is sharp but of short duration, usually caused by cold, sweet, and sour stimuli. Pain ceases after removal of stimulus
- ***Visual examination and history:*** It may reveal caries, recent restoration, traumatic occlusion, and undetected fracture

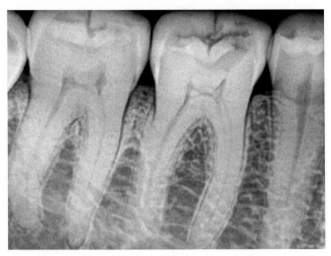

Fig. 3.11 Mandibular left first molar had deep occlusal caries and the patient complained of sensitivity to sweets and cold liquids. There was no discomfort on biting or percussion. The tooth was hyper-responsive to cold with no lingering pain. *Diagnosis: reversible pulpitis; normal apical tissues.* Treatment provided was excavation of caries followed by placement of a permanent restoration.

- *Radiographic examination:*
  - Shows normal PDL and lamina dura, i.e., normal periapical tissue
  - Presence of deep dental caries or restoration **(Fig. 3.11)**
- *Percussion test:* Tooth is normal to percussion and palpation without any mobility
- *Vitality test:* Pulp responds readily to cold stimuli.

Differential Diagnosis

- In reversible pulpitis, pain disappears on removal of stimuli, whereas in irreversible pulpitis, pain stays longer even after removal of stimulus
- Patient's description of pain, character, and duration leads to the diagnosis

Treatment

- The best treatment of reversible pulpitis is prevention
- Usually, a sedative dressing is placed, followed by permanent restoration when symptoms completely subside
- Periodic care to prevent caries, desensitization of hypersensitive teeth, and proper pulp protection by using cavity varnish or base before placement of restoration is recommended
- If pain persists despite of proper treatment, pulpal inflammation should be considered as irreversible and it should be treated by pulp extirpation

Irreversible Pulpitis

Definition

"It is a persistent inflammatory condition of the pulp, symptomatic or asymptomatic, caused by a noxious stimulus." It has both symptomatic and asymptomatic stages in pulp.

Etiology

Irreversible pulpal inflammation can result from
- Dental caries (most common cause)
- Chemical, thermal, mechanical injuries of pulp
- Untreated reversible pulpitis

Symptoms

- Rapid onset of pain, caused by sudden temperature change, sweet, or acidic food. Pain remains even after removal of stimulus
- Pain can be spontaneous in nature which is sharp, piercing, intermittent, or continuous in nature
- Pain exacerbated on bending down or lying down due to change in intrapulpal pressure from standard to supine
- Pain is so severe that it keeps the patient awake in night
- Presence of referred pain
- In later stages, pain is severe, boring, and throbbing in nature which increases with hot stimulus. Pain is relieved by using cold water. Sometimes pain is so severe that patient may report dental clinic with jar of ice cold water
- Apical periodontitis develops in later stages when inflammation extends to periodontal ligament

Histopathology

Pulp shows acute and chronic inflammatory changes such as
- Vascular dilatation and edema
- Granular cell infiltration
- Odontoblasts are destroyed
- Formation of minute abscess formation
- In later stages, pulp undergoes liquefaction and necrosis

Diagnosis

- *Visual examination and history:* One may find deep cavity involving pulp **(Fig. 3.12)** or secondary caries under restorations **(Fig. 3.13)**

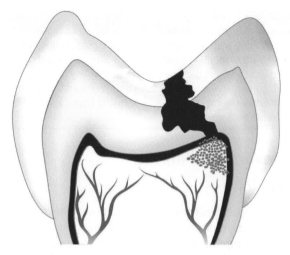

Fig. 3.12 Deep dental caries causing exposure of pulp.

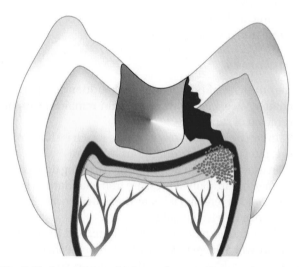

Fig. 3.13 Secondary caries beneath restoration causing pulpal exposure.

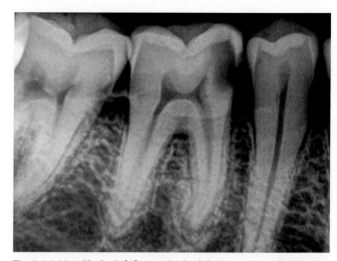

Fig. 3.14 Mandibular left first molar had deep mesio-occlusal caries. Patient complained of sensitivity to hot and cold liquids initially but later pain became spontaneous. EPT test showed lingering pain even after removal of the stimuli. Response to both percussion and palpation was normal. ***Diagnosis: symptomatic irreversible pulpitis.*** Treatment given was nonsurgical endodontic treatment followed by a permanent restoration.

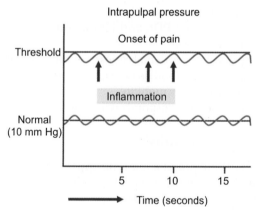

Fig. 3.15 Increased intrapulpal pressure causing pulpal pain.

❑ *Radiographic findings:*
- Shows depth and extent of caries **(Fig. 3.14)**
- Periapical area shows normal appearance but a slight widening may be evident in advanced stages of pulpitis
❑ *Percussion:* Sometimes tooth is tender on percussion because of increased intrapulpal pressure due to exudative inflammatory tissue **(Fig. 3.15)**
❑ *Vitality tests:*
- **Thermal test:** Hyperalgesic pulp responds more readily to cold stimulation than for normal tooth, pain may persist even after removal of irritant. As

pulpal inflammation progresses, heat intensifies the response because of its expansible effect on blood vessels. Cold tends to relieve pain because of its contractile effect on vessels, thereby reducing the intrapulpal pressure
- **Electric test:** Less current is required in initial stages. As tissue becomes more necrotic, more current is required to generate the response

Treatment

Pulpectomy, i.e., root canal treatment.

Chronic Hyperplastic Pulpitis

It is an inflammatory response of pulpal connective tissue due to extensive carious exposure of a young pulp. It shows overgrowth of granulomatous tissue into carious cavity (**Fig. 3.16**).

Etiology

Hyperplastic form of chronic pulpitis is commonly seen in teeth of children and adolescents because in these pulp tissue has high resistance and large carious lesion permits free proliferation of hyperplastic tissue.

Differential diagnosis of reversible and irreversible pulpitis		
Features	*Reversible pulpitis*	*Irreversible pulpitis*
Pain type	Sharp and momentary pain which ceases after stimulus is removed	Intense, continuous, and prolonged pain due to pressure of secondary irritants
Stimulus	External stimulus, for example, heat, cold, and sugar	• Spontaneous in nature • Heat acts as stimulant • Dead or injured pulp tissue acts as secondary stimulant
Pain at night/postural	No	Yes
Pain localization	Only with applied cold stimulus or PDL inflammation	Only with applied heat stimulus or PDL inflammation
Referred pain	Usually not found	Common finding
History	• History of recent dental procedure • Sometimes cervical erosion/abrasion	History of: • Deep caries • Trauma • Extensive restoration
Percussion/occlusion	If due to occlusion, percussion test is positive, otherwise normal	If PDL is involved, percussion test is positive, otherwise normal
Pulp tests • EPT • Cold • Heat	• Normal response • Exaggerated response • Normal—exaggerated response	• Normal to elevated response • Pain relieved by cold occasionally • Acute pain
Color change	No	Yes
Radiograph	Caries, defective restoration without pulp protection	Caries, defective restorations, PDL space enlargement
Treatment	Removal of decay, repair of defect, restoration, Zinc oxide eugenol (ZOE) dressing, occlusal adjustment	Endodontic treatment

Signs and Symptoms

- It is usually asymptomatic
- Fleshy pulpal tissue fills the pulp chamber. It is less sensitive than normal pulp but bleeds easily due to rich network of blood vessels
- Sometimes this pulpal growth interferes with chewing

Histopathology

- Tissue of pulp chamber is transferred into granulation tissue which projects out from pulp chamber
- Granulation tissue contains PMNs, lymphocytes, and plasma cells

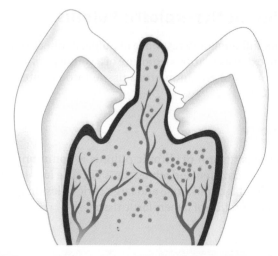

Fig. 3.16 Schematic representation of hyperplastic form of chronic pulpitis.

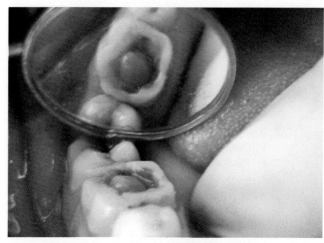

Fig. 3.17 Hyperplastic form of pulpitis showing fleshy reddish pulpal mass filling the pulp chamber.

- Surface of pulp polyp is usually covered by stratified squamous epithelium which may be derived from gingiva, desquamated epithelial cells of mucosa and tongue
- Nerve fibers may be present in the epithelial layer

Diagnosis

- *Pain:* It is usually absent
- Hyperplastic form shows a fleshy, reddish pulpal mass which fills most of pulp chamber or cavity (**Fig. 3.17**). It is less sensitive than normal pulp but bleeds easily when probed. When it is cut, it does not produce pain but pain can result due to pressure transmission to apical part

- *Vitality tests*
  - Tooth may respond feebly or not at all to thermal test, unless one uses extreme cold
  - More than normal current is required to elicit the response by electric pulp tester
- *Differential diagnosis:* Hyperplastic pulpitis should be differentiated from proliferating gingival tissue. It is done by raising and tracing the stalk of tissue back to its origin, that is, pulp chamber

Treatment

- In case of hyperplastic pulpitis, removal of polypoid tissue using periodontal curette or spoon excavator followed by root canal treatment
- If tooth is at nonrestorable stage, it should be extracted

Internal Resorption/Pink Tooth of Mummery

Internal resorption was first reported by Bell in 1830. It is known as Pink tooth of Mummery because of pink discoloration of the crown and named after the anatomist Mummery.

Internal resorption is an idiopathic slow or fast progressive resorption occurring in dentin of the pulp chamber or root canals of the teeth (**Fig. 3.18**).

Etiology

Exact etiology is unknown. Patient may present history of trauma or persistent chronic pulpitis, or history of pulpotomy.

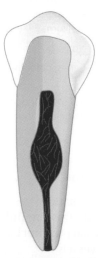

Fig. 3.18 Schematic representation of ballooning of pulpal cavity showing internal resorption of the tooth.

Mechanism of resorption
Pulp inflammation due to infection
↓
Alteration or loss of predentin and odontoblastic layer
↓
Undifferentiated mesenchymal cells come in contact with mineralized dentin
↓
Differentiate into dentinoclasts
↓
Resorption results

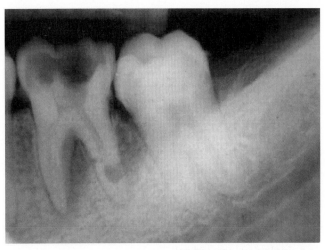
Fig. 3.20 Radiograph showing internal resorption in distal root of mandibular first molar.

Symptoms

❑ Usually asymptomatic, recognized clinically through routine radiograph
❑ Pain occurs if resorption perforates the root **(Fig. 3.19)**
❑ "Pink tooth" is the pathognomonic feature of internal root resorption
❑ Pulp shows either partial or complete necrosis. In actively progressive lesion, pulp is partially vital and may show symptoms of pulpitis
❑ In anterior teeth, it is typically seen in middle of the tooth in mesiodistal direction but in multirooted teeth, it can be present mesial, distal, or center

Diagnosis

❑ *Clinically:* "Pink tooth" appearance
❑ Radiographic changes **(Fig. 3.20)**:
  • Classical description of internal resorption, that is, clearly well-defined radiolucency of uniform density which balloons out of root canal was given by Gartner el al.

  • Original root canal outline distorted
  • Bone changes are seen only when root perforation into periodontal ligament takes place
❑ *Pulp tests:* Positive, though coronal portion of pulp is necrotic, apical pulp could be vital

Differential Diagnosis

It is difficult to differentiate internal resorption from external resorption when it progresses to periodontal space causing root perforation.

It can be differentiated by
❑ History: Giving history of trauma, pulpotomy, etc.
❑ Pink tooth appearance
❑ Taking radiographs at different angles; radiolucency does not move when radiograph is taken at different angle, whereas in external resorption, radiolucent lesion changes position on changing angle.
  • Uniform ballooning of root canal is seen in internal resorption, whereas irregular border with alteration of adjacent bone is seen in external resorption

Treatment

❑ Pulp extirpation stops internal root resorption
❑ Surgical treatment is indicated if conventional treatment fails

▌ Pulp Degeneration

Pulp degeneration is generally present in old age. In young age, it may result from persistent mild irritation. Common causes of pulp degeneration are attrition, abrasion, erosion, operative procedures, caries, pulp capping, and reversible pulpitis. Forms of pulp degeneration:

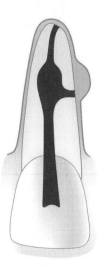
Fig. 3.19 Internal resorption of tooth causing perforation of root.

Calcific Degeneration

In calcific degeneration, part of pulp tissue is replaced by calcific material. Mainly three types of calcifications are seen in pulp:

1. Dystrophic calcifications
2. Diffuse calcifications
3. Denticles/pulp stones

Dystrophic Calcifications (Figs. 3.21 and 3.22)

❑ They occur by deposition of calcium salts in dead or degenerated tissue. Local alkalinity of destroyed tissues attracts the salts
❑ They occur in minute areas of young pulp affected by minor circulatory disturbances, in blood clot, or around a single degenerated cell
❑ They can also begin in the connective tissue walls of blood vessels and nerves and follow their course

Diffuse Calcifications

❑ They are generally observed in root canals
❑ The deposits become long, thin, and fibrillar on fusing

Denticles/Pulp Stones

These are usually seen in pulp chamber.

Classification of pulp stones:

According to Location (Fig. 3.23):
❑ Free
❑ Embedded
❑ Attached

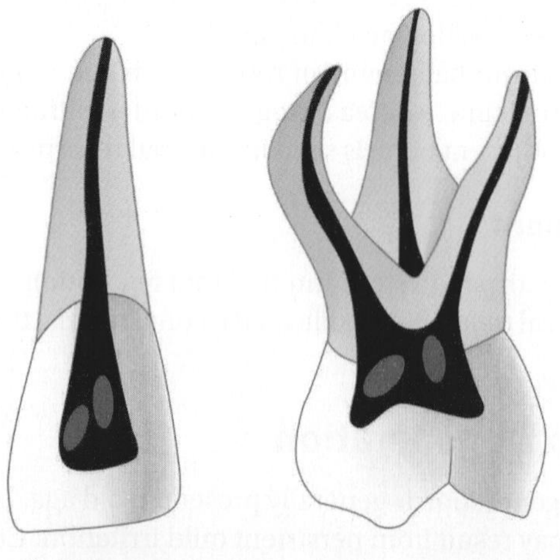

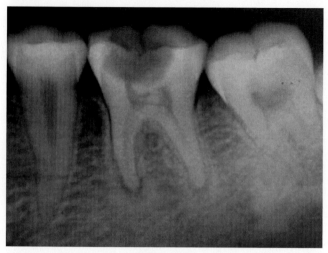

Fig. 3.22 Radiograph showing pulp stone in pulp chamber of mandibular first molar.

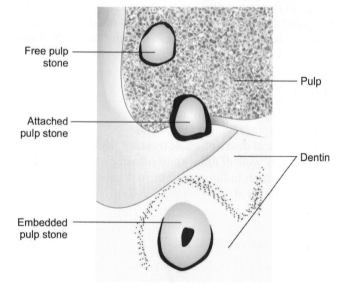

Free pulp stone

Pulp

Attached pulp stone

Dentin

Embedded pulp stone

Fig. 3.23 Types of pulp stones according to location.

According to Structure:
❑ True
❑ False

True denticle: It is composed of dentin formed from detached odontoblasts or fragments of Hertwig's enamel root sheath which stimulates the undifferentiated cells to assume dentinoblastic activity.

False denticle: Here degenerated tissue structures act as nidus for deposition of concentric layers of calcified tissues.

Multiple pulp stones present in pulp chamber

Fig. 3.21 Line diagram showing pulp stones present in pulp chamber of teeth

Atrophic Degeneration

❏ It is wasting away or decrease in size which occurs slowly as tooth grows old **(Fig. 3.24)**
❏ Here fewer stellate cells are found and pulp is less sensitive than normal

Fibrosis Degeneration

❏ There is gradual shift in ratio and quality of tissue elements. Here, the number of collagen fibers/unit area increases leading to fibrosis. Pulp has a characteristic leathery appearance
❏ Number and size of cells decrease so cells appear as "shrunken solid particles in a sea of dense fibers"
❏ Fibroblastic processes are lost, cells have round and pyknotic nuclei
❏ Dentinoblasts decrease in length, appear cuboidal or flattened

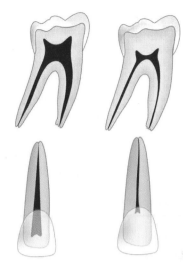

Fig. 3.24 Line diagram showing decrease in size of pulp cavity of anterior and posterior teeth due to secondary dentin deposition with age.

Features of different forms of pulpitis

Features	Reversible pulpitis	Symptomatic irreversible pulpitis	Asymptomatic irreversible pulpitis	Hyperplastic pulpitis	Pulp necrosis
Pain and stimulus	Mild pain lasting for a moment	Constant-to-severe pain caused by hot or cold stimuli	Mild and intermittent	Pain not present but bleeds due to presence of rich network of blood vessels in granulomatous tissue into carious cavity	Not present
Stimulus	Cold or sweet	• Hot or cold • Spontaneous	• Spontaneous • Dead/injured pulp tissue acts as secondary stimulus		
Pulp test					
• Thermal	Readily responds to cold	Acute pain to hot stimuli	No response	No response	No response
• Electric	Normal response	Normal to elevated response	More current is required	More current is required	• In cases of liquefaction necrosis, positive response is seen with electric tester
Radiograph	• Deep caries • Defective restoration	• Deep caries • Defective restoration	• Chronic apical periodontitis • Local condensing osteitis	• Chronic apical periodontitis • Local condensing osteitis	• Large restoration • Sometimes apical periodontitis or condensing osteitis
Treatment	• Removal of decay • Restoration with pulp protection and occlusal adjustment	• Root canal therapy	• RCT • Extraction of non-restorable tooth	• Removal of polypoid tissue with curette/spoon excavator followed by RCT	• RCT • Extraction of nonrestorable tooth

Symptoms of different forms of pulpitis			
	Symptoms	*X-ray findings*	*Pulp vitality tests*
Reversible pulpitis	Asymptomatic or slight symptoms to thermal stimulus	No changes	Gives response to vitality tests
Irreversible pulpitis	Asymptomatic or may have spontaneous or severe pain to thermal stimuli	No changes but condensing osteitis is seen in long cases	Gives response
Pulp necrosis	None	Depends on periapical status	No response
Acute apical periodontitis	Pain on biting or pressure	Not significant	Depending on status of pulp, response or no response
Chronic apical periodontitis	Mild or none or no response	Not significant	Depending on pulp status, response
Acute apical abscess	Pain and/or swelling	Radiolucency at apical end	No response
Chronic apical abscess	Draining sinus	Radiolucency	No response
Condensing osteitis	Varies according to status of pulp or periapex	Increased trabecular bone or no response	Depending on pulp status response

Pulp Necrosis

Pulp necrosis or death is a condition following untreated pulpitis. Pulpal tissue becomes nonvital and if the condition is not treated, noxious materials will leak from pulp space forming the lesion of endodontic origin **(Fig. 3.25)**.

Necrosis may be partial or total, depending on extent of pulp tissue involvement.

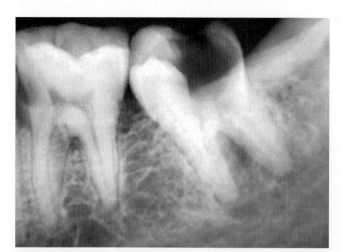

Fig. 3.25 Mandibular third molar was hypersensitive to cold and sweets over the past few months but the symptoms were subsided. Then there was no response to thermal testing but tenderness on biting and pain on percussion were present. Electrical pulp testing showed negative response. Radiographically, there was presence of large carious lesion involving the pulp, loss of lamina dura and periapical radiolucency. *Diagnosis: Pulp necrosis; symptomatic apical periodontitis.* Treatment: Nonsurgical endodontic treatment followed by coronal restoration.

Types of pulp necrosis:
1. *Coagulation necrosis:* In coagulation necrosis, protoplasm of all cells becomes fixed and opaque. Cell mass is recognizable histologically, intracellular details lost
2. *Liquefaction necrosis:* In liquefaction necrosis, the entire cell outline is lost. Liquefied area is surrounded by dense zone of PMNL (polymorphonuclear leukocytes) and chronic inflammatory cells

Etiology

Necrosis is caused by noxious insult and injuries to pulp by bacteria, trauma, and chemical irritation.

Symptoms

- Discoloration of tooth due to extravasation of pulpal blood into dentin as a result of trauma **(Fig. 3.26)**
- Lack of translucency/dull or opaque appearance
- History from patient
- Tooth might be asymptomatic

Diagnosis

- *Pain:* It is absent in complete necrosis
- *History of patient:* History reveals past trauma or past history of severe pain which may have lasted for some time followed by complete and sudden cessation of pain
- *Radiographic changes:* Radiograph shows a large cavity or restoration **(Fig. 3.27)** or normal appearance unless there is concomitant apical periodontitis or condensing osteitis
- *Vitality test:* Usually, vitality tests show negative response. But multirooted teeth may show mixed response because

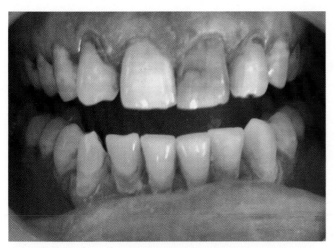

Fig. 3.26 Photograph showing discolored maxillary left central incisor due to pulpal necrosis.

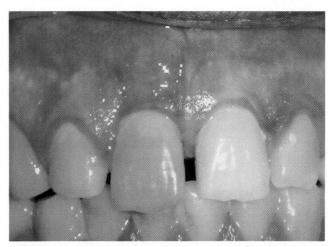

Fig. 3.28 Lack of normal translucency in nonvital maxillary right central incisor.

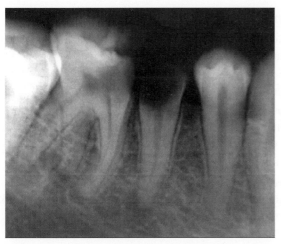

Fig. 3.27 Radiograph showing a large carious lesion in premolar resulting in pulp necrosis.

only one canal may have necrotic tissue. Sometimes teeth with liquefaction necrosis may show positive response to electric test when electric current is conducted through moisture present in a root canal

❑ *Visual examination:* Tooth shows color change like dull or opaque appearance due to lack of normal translucency **(Fig. 3.28)**

❑ *Histopathology:* Necrotic pulp tissue, cellular debris, and microorganisms are seen in pulp cavity. If there is concomitant periodontal involvement, there may be presence of slight evidence of inflammation

Treatment

Complete removal of pulp followed by restoration or extraction of nonrestorable tooth.

▌ Pathologies of Periradicular Tissues

Periradicular tissue contains apical root cementum, periodontal ligament, and alveolar bone.

Etiology

Bacterial

❑ Root canal is unique, stringent ecological niche for bacterial growth because of lack of oxygen. Primary nutrient source for root canal biotic is host tissues and tissue fluids

❑ Microorganisms in chronically infected root canals are mainly anaerobic and Gram-negative type

Most common microorganisms seen in periradicular diseases are
• *Streptococcus*
• *Peptostreptococcus*
• *Prevotella*
Black-pigmented microorganisms
• *Porphyromonas*
• *Enterococcus*
• *Campylobacter*
• *Fusobacterium*
• *Eubacterium*

Routes

❑ Untreated pulpal infection leads to total pulp necrosis and further periapical infection **(Fig. 3.29)**

❑ Anachoresis

❑ Invasion of microorganisms into pulp from periodontal pocket and accessory canals resulting in formation of lesion of endodontic origin

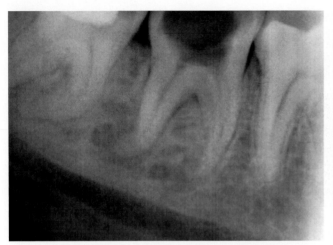

Fig. 3.29 Radiograph showing that untreated caries in mandibular second molar resulting in periapical pathology.

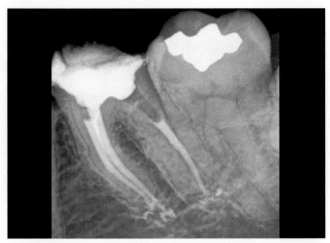

Fig. 3.30 Overextended obturating material may cause periradicular inflammation.

Trauma

☐ Physical trauma to tooth or operative procedures result in dental follicle desiccation or heat transfer causes sufficient damage to pulp and its blood supply

☐ Severe trauma to tooth and heat production during tooth preparation causes immediate interruption of blood supply resulting in pulp necrosis even though it is not infected

☐ Persistent periapical tissue compression from traumatic occlusion may lead to apical inflammatory response

Factors Related to Root Canal Procedures

☐ It is impossible to extirpate pulp without initiating an inflammatory response

☐ Using strong or excessive amounts of intracanal medicaments between appointments may induce periapical inflammation

☐ Improper manipulation of instruments within root canal or overinstrumentation can force dentinal debris, irrigating solution, and toxic components of necrotic tissue in the periapex

☐ Overextended endodontic filling material may induce periapical inflammation by directly inducing foreign body reaction which is characterized by presence of leukocyte infiltration, macrophages, and other chronic inflammatory cells **(Fig. 3.30)**

Diagnosis

Chief Complaint

Patient usually complains of pain on biting, pain with swelling, pus discharge, etc.

Dental History

Patient gives history of recurring episodes of pain and sometimes swelling with discharge.

Objective Examinations

Extraoral examination

General appearance, skin tone, facial asymmetry, swelling, extraoral sinus, sinus tract, tender or enlarged cervical lymph nodes.

Intraoral examination

It includes examination of soft tissues and teeth to look for discoloration, abrasion, caries, restoration, etc.

Clinical Periapical Tests

Percussion

Indicates inflammation of periodontium **(Fig. 3.31)**.

Palpation

Determines how far the inflammatory process has extended periapically.

Pulp vitality

☐ Thermal tests which can be heat or cold

☐ Electrical pulp testing

Periodontal examination

It is important because periapical and periodontal lesion may mimic each other and require differentiation.

☐ *Probing:* Determines the level of connective tissue attachment. Probe can penetrate into an inflammatory periapical lesion that extends cervically **(Fig. 3.32)**

☐ *Mobility:* Determines the status of periodontal ligament

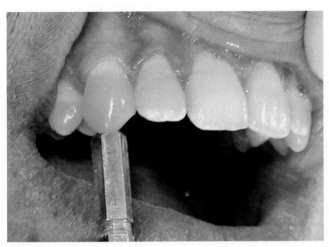

Fig. 3.31 Pain on percussion indicates inflamed periodontium.

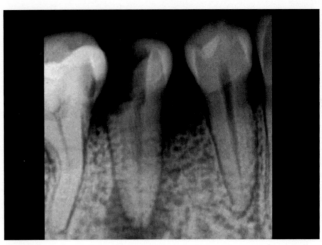

Fig. 3.33 Radiograph showing large disto-occlusal caries, loss of lamina dura and periapical radiolucency at apex of mandibular second premolar.

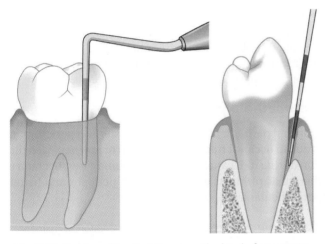

Fig. 3.32 Probing of tooth determines the level of connective tissue attachment.

Radiographic examination (Fig. 3.33)

Periradicular lesions of pulpal origin have four characteristics:
1. Loss of lamina dura apically
2. Radiolucency at apex regardless of cone angle
3. Radiolucency resembling a hanging drop
4. Cause of pulp necrosis is usually evident

Recent advances in radiography:
- Digital subtraction radiography
- Xeroradiography
- Digital radiometric analysis
- Computed tomography
- Radiovisiography
- Magnetic resonance imaging

Classification of Periradicular Pathologies

Grossman's Classification

1. Symptomatic periradicular diseases:
   a. Symptomatic apical periodontitis previously known as acute apical periodontitis (AAP):
      i. Vital
      ii. Nonvital
   b. Acute alveolar abscess
   c. Phoenix abscess
2. Asymptomatic periradicular diseases:
   a. Asymptomatic apical periodontitis (chronic apical periodontitis)
   b. Chronic alveolar abscess
   c. Radicular cyst
   d. Condensing osteitis
3. External root resorption
4. Persistent Apical periodontitis
5. Disease of the periradicular tissues of nonendodontic origin

WHO Classification

K 04.4 — Acute apical periodontitis
K 04.5 — Chronic apical periodontitis (apical granuloma)
K 04.6 — Periapical abscess with sinus
K 04.60 — Periapical abscess with sinus to maxillary antrum
K 04.61 — Periapical abscess with sinus to nasal cavity
K 04.62 — Periapical abscess with sinus to oral cavity
K 04.63 — Periapical abscess with sinus to skin
K 04.7 — Periapical abscess without sinus
K 04.8 — Radicular cyst (periapical cyst)
K 04.80 — Apical and lateral cyst

K 04.81 — Residual cyst
K04.82 — Inflammatory paradental cyst

Ingle's Classification of Pulpoperiapical Pathosis

1. *Painful pulpoperiapical pathosis:*
   a. Symptomatic Acute apical periodontitis
   b. Advanced apical periodontitis:
      i. Acute apical abscess
      ii. Phoenix abscess
      iii. Suppurative apical periodontitis (chronic apical abscess)
2. *Nonpainful pulpoperiapical pathosis*:
   a. Condensing osteitis
   b. Chronic apical periodontitis both incipient and advanced stages
   b. Chronic apical periodontitis:
      i. Periapical granuloma
      ii. Apical cyst
      iii. Suppurative apical periodontitis

Symptomatic Apical Periodontitis (Acute Apical Periodontitis)

Symptomatic apical periodontitis is defined as painful inflammation of the periodontium as a result of trauma, irritation, or infection through the root canal, regardless of whether the pulp is vital or nonvital (**Fig. 3.34**). It is an inflammation around the apex of a tooth.

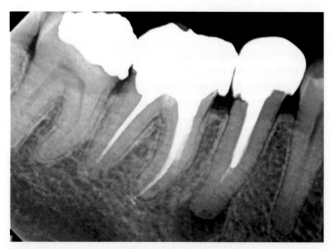

Fig. 3.34 Mandibular left second premolar was endodontically treated >5 years ago. The patient was complaining of pain on biting over past 2 months. There appeared to be apical radiolucency around the root. The tooth was tender to both percussion and biting. *Diagnosis: previously treated; symptomatic apical periodontitis.* Treatment done was nonsurgical endodontic retreatment followed by permanent restoration of the access cavity.

Etiology

- In vital tooth, it is associated with occlusal trauma, high points in restoration, wedging or forcing object between teeth
- In nonvital tooth, it is associated with sequelae to pulpal diseases
- Iatrogenic causes can be overinstrumentation of root canal, pushing debris and microorganisms beyond apex, overextended obturation, and root perforations

Signs and Symptoms

Apical periodontitis serves as protective function, confining the microorganisms extruded from root canal space and preventing them from spreading in adjacent bone marrow areas. But it can't eradicate the source of infection because defense mechanism of pulp can't come in to play due to lack of vascular supply, once the pulp is nonvital. This mechanism occurs at apical area but can't penetrate in fully matured tooth, so lack of proper treatment can result in chronic lesion.
- Tooth is tender on percussion
- Tooth may present mild-to-severe soreness
- Dull, throbbing, and constant pain
- Pain occurs over a short period of time
- Pain on mastication

Histopathology

Pulp and periradicular tissue may be sterile if periodontitis is due to occlusal trauma or chemical or mechanical irritation during root canal treatment. In some cases, bacteria or their toxic products extrude through periapex and irritate periradicular area.

Inflammatory reaction occur in apical periodontal ligament
↓
Dilatation of blood vessels
↓
Initiation of inflammatory response due to presence of polymorphonuclear leukocytes and round cells
↓
Accumulation of serous exudate
↓
Distention of periodontal ligament and extrusion of tooth, slight tenderness
↓
If irritation continues
↓
Loss of alveolar bone (unavoidable side effect of defensive process by host to provide necessary effective immune response to root canal infection)

Diagnosis

- Tooth is tender on percussion
- Radiographic picture of vital tooth may show no change, whereas in case of nonvital tooth, it may show widening of apical periodontal ligament space and loss of lamina dura

Differential Diagnosis

It should be differentiated from acute apical abscess on the basis of history, symptoms, and clinical tests.

Treatment

- ❑ If cause is irreversible pulpitis or necrotic pulp, initiate endodontic treatment
- ❑ If cause is hyperocclusion, adjust the occlusion for immediate relief
- ❑ To control postoperative pain following initial endodontic therapy, analgesics are prescribed
- ❑ Use of antibiotics, either alone or in conjunction with root canal therapy is not recommended
- ❑ For nonrestorable teeth, extraction is indicated

❙ Acute Apical Abscess

Synonyms: Acute Abscess, Acute Dentoalveolar, Abscess, Acute Periapical Abscess, Acute Radicular Abscess.

It is an inflammatory reaction to pulp infection and necrosis characterized by rapid onset, pus formation, spontaneous pain, tenderness on percussion, and eventual swelling of associated tissues **(Fig. 3.35)**.

Etiology

- ❑ Most common cause is invasion of bacteria from necrotic pulp tissue
- ❑ Trauma, chemical, or any mechanical injury resulting in pulp necrosis
- ❑ Irritation of periapical tissue by chemical or mechanical treatment during root canal treatment

Tissue at surface of swelling appears taut and inflamed and pus starts to form underneath it. Surface tissue may become inflated from the pressure of underlying pus and finally rupture from this pressure. Initially, the pus comes out in the form of a small opening but latter it may increase in size or number depending upon the amount of pressure of pus and softness of the tissue overlying it. This process is beginning of chronic abscess.

Pathophysiology of Apical Abscess Formation

Increase in pulpal pressure
↓
Collapse of venous circulation
↓
Hypoxia and anoxia of local tissue
↓
Localized destruction of pulp tissue
↓
Formation of pulpal abscess because of breakdown of PMNs, bacteria, and lysis of pulp remnants

Symptoms

- ❑ In early stage, there is tenderness of tooth which is relieved by continued slight pressure on extruded tooth to push it back into alveolus
- ❑ Later on, throbbing pain develops with diffuse swelling of overlying tissue
- ❑ Tooth becomes more painful, elongated, and mobile as infection increases in later stages
- ❑ Patient may have systemic symptoms like fever and increased WBC count
- ❑ Spread of lesion toward a surface may take place causing erosion of cortical bone or it may diffuse and spread widely leading to formation of cellulitis **(Fig. 3.36)**. Location of swelling is determined by relation of apex of involved tooth to adjacent muscle attachment **(Fig. 3.37)**

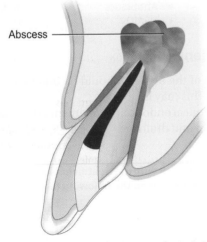

Fig. 3.35 Line diagram showing periapical abscess.

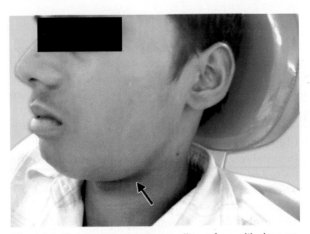

Fig. 3.36 Photograph showing swelling of mandibular area because of apical abscess.

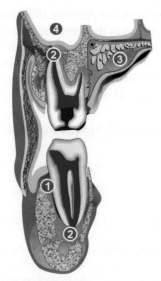

Fig. 3.37 Spread of apical abscess to surrounding tissues, if it is not treated: (1) vestibular abscess, (2) periapical abscess, (3) palatal abscess, and (4) maxillary sinus.

Histopathology

Polymorphonuclear leukocytes infiltrate and initiate inflammatory response
↓
Accumulation of inflammatory exudates in response to active infection
↓
Distention of periodontal ligament
↓
Extrusion of the tooth
↓
If the process continues, separation of periodontal ligament
↓
Tooth becomes mobile
↓
Bone resorption at apex
↓
Localized lesion of liquefaction necrosis containing polymorphonuclear leukocytes, debris, cell remnants, and purulent exudates

Diagnosis

- Clinical examination
- In initial stages, locating a tooth is difficult due to diffuse pain. Location of the offending tooth becomes easier when tooth gets slightly extruded from the socket
- Negative response to pulp vitality tests
- Tenderness on percussion and palpation
- Tooth may be slightly mobile and extruded from its socket

- Radiography helpful in determining the affected tooth as it may show caries or evidence of bone destruction at root apex

Viva voce	
Tooth involved	**Swelling present**
Maxillary anterior tooth	swelling of upper lip
Maxillary posterior tooth	swelling on check
Mandibular anterior teeth	swelling of lower lip, chin, and neck in severe cases
Mandibular posterior teeth	may involve cheek, ear, and lower border of mandible

Differential diagnosis of acute alveolar abscess and periodontal abscess		
Features	*Acute alveolar abscess*	*Periodontal abscess*
Pain type	Pulsating, pounding, continuous	Dull
Pain localization	Easily localized due to percussive tenderness	Upon probing
Pain at night/postural	Pain continuous	No
Mobility	Yes	Sometimes
Pulp tests • EPT • Cold • Heat	No response No response No response	Normal Normal Normal
Swelling	Yes, often to large size	Occasionally
Radiograph	Caries, defective restorations	Possible foreign body or vertical bone loss
Treatment	• Establish drainage (Incision and drainage) • Antibiotics • NSAIDs	• Removal of foreign body • Scaling • Curettage, if necessary

Management

- Drainage of the abscess should be initiated as early as possible. This may include
  - Nonsurgical endodontic treatment **(Figs. 3.38A to C)**
  - Incision and drainage
  - Extraction

Considerations regarding the treatment of a tooth with periapical abscess depend on the following factors:
- Prognosis of the tooth
- Patient preference
- Strategic value of the tooth
- Economic status of the patient

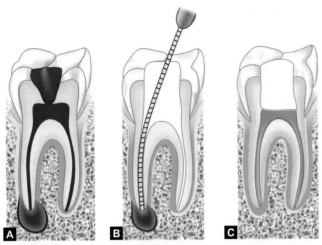

Figs. 3.38A to C Management of periapical abscess. (A) Deep caries causing pulp necrosis followed by periapical abscess; (B) Initiation of endodontic treatment; (C) Obturation of root canal system after proper cleaning and shaping of the canals.

- In case of localized infections, systemic antibiotics provide no additional benefit over drainage of abscess
- In the case of systemic complications such as fever, lymphadenopathy, cellulitis, or patient who is immunocompromised, antibiotics should be given in addition to drainage of the tooth
- Relieve the tooth out of occlusion in hyperocclusion cases
- To control postoperative pain following endodontic therapy, nonsteroidal anti-inflammatory drugs should be given

Phoenix Abscess/Recrudescent Abscess/Acute Exacerbation of Asymptomatic Apical Periodontitis

Phoenix abscess is defined as an acute inflammatory reaction superimposed on an existing asymptomatic apical periodontitis.

Etiology

Chronic periradicular lesions such as granulomas are in a state of equilibrium during which they can be completely asymptomatic. But sometimes, influx of necrotic products from diseased pulp or bacteria and their toxins can cause the dormant lesion to react. This leads to initiation of acute inflammatory response. Lowered body defenses also trigger an acute inflammatory response.

Symptoms

- Clinically, often indistinguishable from acute apical abscess

- At the onset, tenderness of tooth and extrusion of the tooth from socket
- Tenderness on palpating the apical soft tissue

Diagnosis

- Most commonly associated with initiation of root canal treatment
- History from patient
- Pulp tests show negative response
- Radiographs show large area of radiolucency in the apex created by inflammatory connective tissue which has replaced the alveolar bone at the root apex
- Histopathology of phoenix abscess shows areas of liquefaction necrosis with disintegrated polymorphonuclear leukocytes and cellular debris surrounded by macrophages, lymphocytes, plasma cells in periradicular tissues
- Phoenix abscess should be differentiated from acute alveolar abscess by patient's history, symptoms, and clinical tests results

Treatment

- Establishment of drainage
- Once symptoms subside—complete root canal treatment

Asymptomatic Apical Periodontits/ Chronic Apical Periodontitis

It is sequelae of symptomatic apical periodontitis resulting in inflammation and destruction of periradicular area due to extension of pulpal infection, characterized by asymptomatic periradicular radiolucency. It is seen as chronic low-grade defensive response of periradicular area to pulpal infection.

Etiology

Necrosis of pulp causing continued irritation and stimulation of periradicular area resulting in formation of granulation tissue.

Clinical features:
1. Tooth is nonvital
2. Usually asymptomatic but in acute phase, dull, throbbing pain may be present

Possible complications of chronic apical periodontitis
- Formation of periapical granuloma, radicular cyst, sinus tract, and acute exacerbation of the disease

Differential Diagnosis

Main characteristic feature is nonvital pulp with periapical lesion **(Fig. 3.39)**. If pulp is vital:

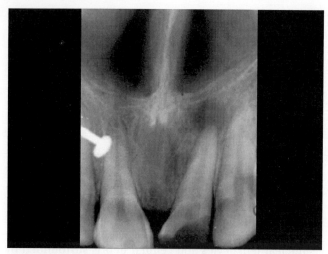

Fig. 3.39 Maxillary left lateral incisor showed an apical radiolucency. There was no history of pain and the tooth was asymptomatic. There was no response to EPT, whereas the adjacent teeth responded normally to vitality tests. There was no tenderness to percussion or palpation. ***Diagnosis: pulp necrosis; asymptomatic apical periodontitis.*** Treatment done was nonsurgical endodontic treatment followed by core build up and crown.

❑ Rule out lateral periodontal abscess, central giant cell granuloma, and cemental dysplasia
❑ Check medical history to rule out hyperparathyroidism or presence of malignant lesion

Treatment

❑ Endodontic therapy of affected tooth
❑ In acute phase, treatment is same as acute apical abscess, i.e. cleaning and shaping of canals followed by analgesics if required
❑ Extraction of nonrestorable teeth.

Chronic Alveolar Abscess

Chronic alveolar abscess is a long-standing low-grade infection of periradicular bone characterized by presence of an abscess draining through a sinus tract.

Synonyms: Chronic suppurative apical periodontitis, Chronic apical abscess, Suppurative periradicular periodontitis, Chronic periradicular/periapical abscess.

Etiology

It is similar to acute alveolar abscess. It also results from pulpal necrosis and is associated with chronic apical periodontitis that has formed an abscess.

Symptoms

❑ Generally asymptomatic
❑ Detected either by the presence of a sinus tract or on routine radiograph
❑ In case of open carious cavity, drainage through root canal sinus tract prevents swelling or exacerbation of lesion

Diagnosis

❑ Chronic apical abscess is associated with asymptomatic or slightly symptomatic tooth
❑ Patient may give history of sudden sharp pain which subsided and has not reoccurred
❑ Clinical examination may show a large carious exposure, discoloration of crown, or restoration
❑ Presence of sinus tract prevents exacerbation or swelling so usually asymptomatic but may show symptoms if sinus tract gets blocked
❑ Vitality tests show negative response because of presence of necrotic pulps
❑ Site of origin is diagnosed by radiograph after insertion of gutta-percha in sinus tract
❑ *Radiographic examination* shows diffuse area of rarefaction. The rarefied area is so diffuse that fades indistinctly into normal bone

Location of sinus tract according to tooth involved	
Involved tooth	**Location of sinus**
Maxillary teeth	Labial bone
Maxillary lateral incisor	Palatal surface
Palatal root of maxillary molar	Palatal surface
Mandibular anterior teeth	Buccal vestibule
Mandibular posterior teeth	Lingual bone

Differential Diagnosis

Chronic alveolar abscess must be differentially diagnosed from a granuloma or cyst by carrying histopathological examination. It should also be differentiated from cementoma which is associated with vital tooth.

Treatment

Removal of irritants from root canal and establishing drainage is the main objective of the treatment. Sinus tract resolves following endodontic treatment.

Draining sinus is active with pus discharge surrounded by reddish pink color mucosa. It can be detected by inserting gutta-percha **(Figs. 3.40A to D)**. Healed sinus shows absence of pus discharge and normal colored mucosa **(Figs. 3.41A and B)**.

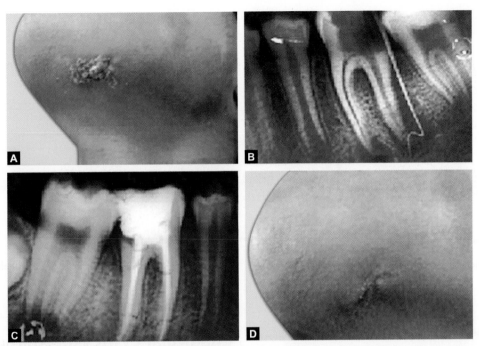

Figs. 3.40A to D Patient had draining sinus in submandibular region. Radiograph with gutta-percha in sinus tract revealed periapical radiolucency. There was no history of pain and the tooth is asymptomatic. There was no response to EPT, whereas the adjacent teeth respond normally to vitality tests. There was no tenderness to percussion or palpation. ***Diagnosis: chronic suppurative apical periodontitis.*** Treatment was nonsurgical endodontic treatment followed by core buildup and crown. (A) Extraoral sinus; (B) Source of sinus tracked using gutta-percha; (C) Postobturation radiograph; (D) Photograph showing healed sinus.

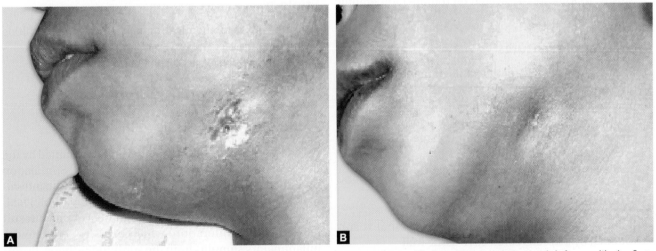

Figs. 3.41A and B Preoperative photograph showing: (A) Extraoral sinus in submandibular region in relation with left mandibular first molar; (B) Postoperative photograph after 3 months showing healed sinus.

Periapical Granuloma

Periapical granuloma is one of the most common sequelae of pulpitis. It is usually described as a mass of chronically inflamed granulation tissue found at the apex of nonvital tooth **(Fig. 3.42)**.

Etiology of Periapical Granuloma

Periapical granuloma is a cell-mediated response to pulpal bacterial products. Bacterial toxins cause mild irritation of periapical tissues. This leads to cellular proliferation and thus granuloma formation.

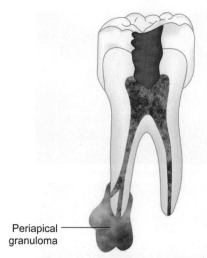

Fig. 3.42 Periapical granuloma present at the apex of nonvital tooth.

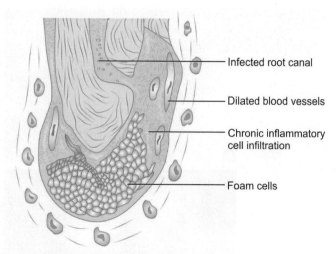

Fig. 3.43 Histopathology of periapical granuloma.

Clinical Features

- Most of the cases are asymptomatic but sometimes pain and sensitivity is seen when acute exacerbation occurs
- Tooth is not sensitive to percussion
- No mobility
- Soft tissue overlying the area may/may not be tender
- No response to thermal or electric pulp test
- Mostly, lesions are discovered on routine radiographic examination

Radiographic Features

- Mostly discovered on routine radiographic examination
- The earliest noticeable change seen is thickening of periodontal ligament at the root apex
- Lesion may be well circumscribed or poorly defined
- Size may vary from small lesion to large radiolucency exceeding >2 cm in diameter
- Presence of root resorption is also seen

Histopathologic Features (Fig. 3.43)

- It consists of inflamed granulation tissue that is surrounded by a fibrous connective tissue wall
- The granulation consists of dense lymphocytic infiltrate which further contains neutrophils, plasma cells, histiocytes and eosinophils
- Sometimes, Russell bodies may also be present

Treatment and Prognosis (Figs. 3.44A to E)

- In restorable tooth, endodontic treatment and in case of nonrestorable tooth, extraction followed by curettage of apical soft tissue is recommended

Radicular Cyst/Cystic Apical Periodontitis

The radicular cyst is an inflammatory cyst which results because of extension of infection from pulp into the surrounding periapical tissues.

Etiology

- Caries, physical, chemical, or mechanical injury resulting in pulp necrosis
- Irritating effects of restorative materials
- Trauma
- Pulpal death due to development defects

Pathogenesis

Periapical granulomas are initiated and maintained by the degradation products of necrotic pulp tissue. Stimulation of epithelial rests of Malassez occurs in response to inflammatory products.

According to Nair, cyst formation occurs as a result of epithelial proliferation, which helps to separate the inflammatory stimulus from the surrounding bone. By this mechanism, cyst is formed and it is explained by the following two hypotheses:

Nutritional Deficient Theory

It says that periapical inflammatory changes cause epithelium to proliferate and make center mass deprived of nutrition from peripheral tissues. It results in necrotic changes in the center lined by epithelial cells at the periphery.

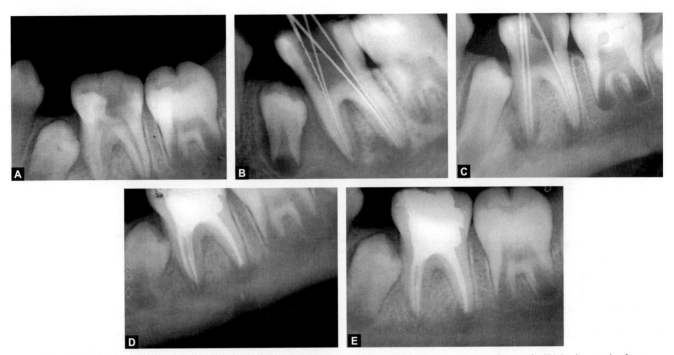

Figs. 3.44A to E (A) Preoperative radiograph; (B) Working length radiograph; (C) Master cone radiograph; (D) Radiograph after obturation; (E) Follow-up after 3 months
Courtesy: Manoj Hans.

Abscess Theory

It says when an abscess is formed in connective tissue, epithelial cells proliferate and form a wall around the cavity because of their inherent tendency to cover the exposed connective tissue.

Valderhaug (1972) explained the following stages of cyst formation:

1. Initial stage: Bacterial endotoxins cause inflammation in the apical region of a nonvital tooth which leads to the proliferation of epithelial cells of Malassez **(Fig. 3.45)**
2. Cyst development stage: Proliferative epithelial cells serve as building blocks for cyst wall development. This occurs due to simultaneous decomposition of epithelial and granulation tissue and convergence of multiple cavities, with subsequent epithelialization
3. Cyst growth stage: Due to the decomposition of epithelial cells, leukocytes and accumulation of plasma exudates, the osmolality of the cyst fluid becomes higher than that of the serum. As a result, hydrostatic internal pressure becomes greater than capillary pressure. Tissue fluid therefore diffuses into the cyst, making it increase in size. With osteoclastic bone resorption, the cyst expands. Other bone-resorbing factors, such as prostaglandins, interleukins, and

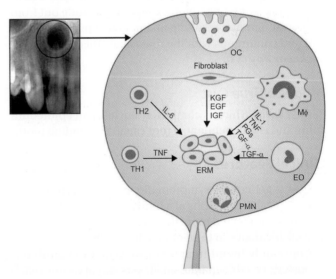

Fig. 3.45 A schematic illustration of the mechanism of epithelial rest cells proliferation. Growth factors (like EFG, IGF, and KGF released by stromal fibroblast, TGF-α by macrophages and lymphocytes) bind to their specific receptor of cell membrane and induce epithelial cell rests to divide and proliferate resulting in formation of apical cysts.

proteinases, from inflammatory cells and cells in the peripheral portion of the lesion permit additional cyst enlargement

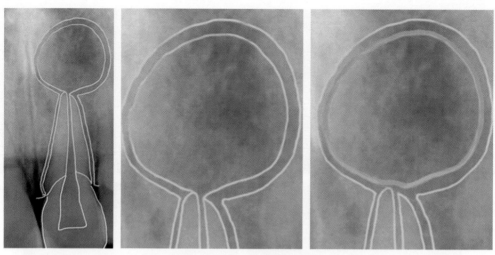

Fig. 3.46 Types of radicular cysts.

Types of Radicular Cysts

Nair gave the following two types of radicular cysts **(Fig. 3.46)**:

Periapical Pocket or Bay Cyst

When proliferation occurs within the body of the granuloma, it plugs the apical foramen which limits the egress of bacteria. Sometimes, epithelial plugs protrude out from the apical foramen resulting in a pouch connected to the root and continuous with the root canal. This is termed as *pocket or bay cyst*.

Periapical True Cyst

It is the cavity which is completely enclosed in epithelium lining and is independent of root canal of offending tooth.

Clinical Features

- Cyst is generally asymptomatic. It is discovered when periapical radiographs of a nonvital tooth is taken
- Males are affected more than females
- Peak incidence in third or fourth decades
- Commonly found in anterior maxilla. In mandibular posterior teeth, separate small cysts may arise from each apex of multirooted teeth
- Involved tooth is nonvital, discolored, fractured, or shows failed root canal
- It grows as slowly enlarging swelling. As cyst increases in size, the covering bone becomes thin and exhibits springiness due to fluctuation
- In maxilla, palatal expansion is commonly seen with maxillary lateral incisor

Radiographic Features

Radiographically, radicular cyst appears as round, pear, or ovoid-shaped radiolucency, outlined by a thin radiopaque margin **(Fig. 3.47)**.

Differential diagnosis

- Periapical granuloma: Histological and radiological features differentiate these lesions. Moreover cyst is usually larger than periapical granuloma
- Periapical cemento-osseous dysplasia: It is seen associated with vital teeth or in regions of extractions. Lesion tends to become more opaque internally with time and does not exhibit extensions into adjacent bone

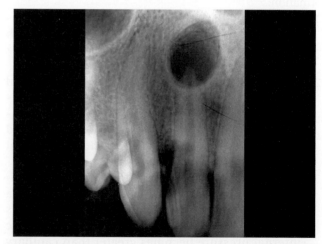

Fig. 3.47 Radicular cyst in relation to maxillary lateral incisor showing as round radiolucency, outlined by a thin radiopaque margin.

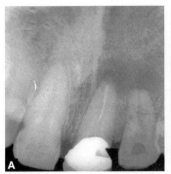 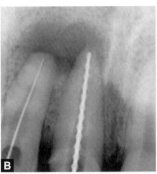 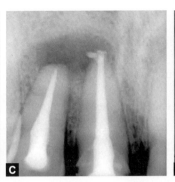 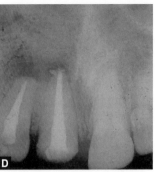

Figs. 3.48A to D (A) Preoperative radiograph showing periapical radiolucency in relation to maxillary central and lateral incisors; (B) Working length determination; (C) Postobturation radiograph; (D) 4 months recall radiograph showing decrease in size of radiolucency.

- Traumatic bone cyst: hollow cavity, not lined by epithelium but by fibrous tissue. Treated by aspiration of fluid from the cavity
- Globulomaxillary cyst: Fissural cyst, tooth may be vital and develops between maxillary lateral incisor and canine
- Lateral periodontal cyst: It is associated with periodontal signs and symptoms
- Normal bony cavity: It appears dissociated from root apex whereas residual cyst remains attached to the root apex
- Previously treated apical pathology/surgical defect or periapical scar
- Odontogenic tumors: Ossifying fibroma is commonly seen in posterior region of mandible, adenomatoid odontogenic tumor in anterior maxilla, calcifying cystic odontogenic tumor is associated with unerupted teeth. In these lesions, pulp is usually vital
- Giant cell lesion
- Metastatic lesion

Treatment (Figs. 3.48A to D)

Different options for management of residual cyst are
- Endodontic treatment
- Apicoectomy
- Extraction (severe bone loss)
- Enucleation with primary closure
- Marsupialization (in case of large cysts)

Condensing Osteitis

Condensing osteitis is a diffuse radiopaque lesion believed to form a localized bone reaction to a low-grade inflammatory stimulus, normally seen at an apex of a tooth in which there has been a long-standing pulp disease.

Clinical Features

- Usually asymptomatic, it is commonly seen around the apices of mandibular molars and premolars with chronic pulpitis
- Pulp can be vital and chronically inflamed or necrotic
- Tooth has radiopaque area due to overproduction of bone in the periapical area. Radiopacity may or may not disappear after endodontic treatment or tooth extraction

Diagnosis

Usually discovered on routine radiograph, it appears as localized area of radiopacity surrounding the offending tooth.

Histopathology

Dense bone around root apex shows less trabecular pattern and borders lined with osteoblasts along with presence of chronic inflammatory cells in bone marrow.

Treatment

- Endodontic treatment may result in complete resolution

External Root Resorption

Resorption is associated with either physiologic or a pathologic process that results in loss of tissues like dentin, cementum, or alveolar bone.

In external root resorption, root resorption affects the cementum or dentin of the root. It can be
- Apical root resorption
- Lateral root resorption
- Cervical root resorption

Etiology

Periradicular inflammation due to
- Infected necrotic pulp
- Over instrumentation during root canal treatment
- Trauma
- Granuloma/cyst applying excessive pressure on root
- Replantation of teeth
- Adjacent impacted tooth

Symptoms

- Asymptomatic during development
- When root is completely resorbed, tooth becomes mobile

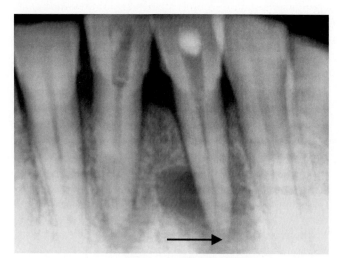

Fig. 3.49 Radiographic appearance of external root resorption of mandibular central incisor

- When external root resorption extends to crown, it gives "pink tooth" appearance
- When replacement resorption results in ankylosis, tooth becomes immobile with characteristic high percussion sound

Radiographic Features (Fig. 3.49)

- Radiolucency at root and adjacent bone
- Irregular shortening or thinning of root tip
- Loss of lamina dura

Differential Diagnosis

It should be differentiated from internal resorption which shows ballooning of pulpal space.

Treatment (Fig. 3.50)

- Removal of stimulus of underlying inflammation
- Nonsurgical endodontic treatment should be tried first before attempting surgical treatment

Persistent Apical Periodontitis

It is post treatment apical periodontitis in an endodontically treated tooth. *Enterococcus faecalis* is the most consistently reported organism in persistent apical periodontitis.

Etiology

- It may result because of incomplete cleaning of complex pulp space which is inaccessible to instrumentation, irrigation and thus obturation

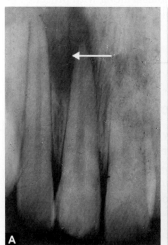
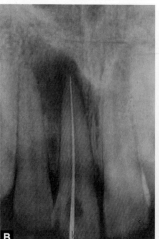
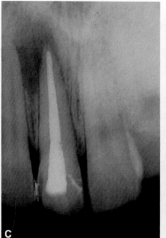
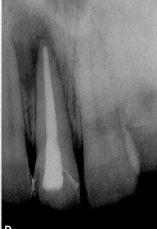

Figs. 3.50A to D Management of external root resorption of maxillary central incisor. (A) Preoperative radiograph showing external resorption; (B) Working length radiograph; (C) Radiograph after obturation; (D) Follow-up after 6 months.

- Nair listed the following extraradicular factors which contribute to persistent apical periodontitis:
  - Foreign body reaction to gutta-percha
  - Periapical biofilms
  - Cholesterol crystals
  - Periapical scar tissue
  - *Actinomyces* infection

Diseases of Periradicular Tissue of Nonendodontic Origin

Periradicular lesions may arise from the remnants of odontogenic epithelium.

Benign Lesions

- Early stages of periradicular cemental dysplasia
- Early stages of monostotic fibrous dysplasia
- Ossifying fibroma
- Primordial cyst
- Lateral periodontal cyst
- Dentigerous cyst
- Traumatic bone cyst
- Central giant cell granuloma
- Central hemangioma
- Hyperparathyroidism
- Myxoma
- Ameloblastoma

Radiographic Features of Lesions of Nonodontogenic Origin

- Presence of radiolucent areas
- Intact lamina dura

Diagnosis

Teeth associated with nonodontogenic lesions are usually vital. Final diagnosis is based on surgical biopsy and histopathological examination.

Malignant Lesions

They simulate endodontic periradicular lesions and are often metastatic in nature:
- Squamous cell carcinoma
- Osteogenic sarcoma
- Chondrosarcoma
- Multiple myeloma

Diagnosis

- *Vitality:* Involved tooth is vital but disruption of sensory nerves may show no response

- *Radiographic features:* Lesions are associated with rapid and extensive loss of hard tissue, that is, bone and tooth
- *Biopsy:* Histological evaluation of diagnosis

Conclusion

One of the most important clinical factor for pulpal pain is caries which affect pulp by bacteria or their byproducts. Once the pulp gets affected by bacteria or their by products, it's inflammation starts, which if not timely treated, might develop into pulp necrosis. Toxic byproducts formed as a result of pulp decomposition act as irritants on the periapical tissues and give rise to many forms of reactions and latter involve periradicular tissues. Some of these reactions occur for a short time accompanied by signs and symptoms, others develop slowly and are asymptomatic. To save a tooth from sacrificing, proper diagnosis based on clinical, radiographical and histological basis should be made so as to provide optimal treatment to the lesion. In suspicious cases, biopsy of the lesion, referral to the pathologist, and long-term follow-up is required.

Questions

1. Enumerate etiology of pulpal diseases. Write in detail about reversible pulpitis.
2. Classify pulpal pathologies. What are clinical features of irreversible pulpitis?
3. Explain the etiology and classification of periradicular pathologies.
4. Discuss differential diagnosis and treatment of pulp polyp (chronic hyperplastic pulpitis).
5. Classify diseases of pulp. How will you differentiate between hyperemia and acute pulpitis?
6. Describe diagnosis and treatment plan of reversible and irreversible pulpitis.
7. Write short notes on
   - Phoenix abscess
   - Radicular cyst
   - Differentiate acute abscess and chronic abscess
   - Chronic hyperplastic pulpitis/pulp polyp.

Bibliography

1. American Association of Endodontists (2003) Glossary of endodontic terms, 7th edition. Chicago, IL: American Association of Endodontists.
2. Baume LJ. Diagnosis of diseases of the pulp. Oral Surg Oral Med Oral Pathol 1970;29:102–16.
3. Bender IB. Pulpal pain diagnosis—a review. J Endod 2000;26:175–9.

4. Carrotte P. Current practice in endodontics 2: diagnosis and treatment planning. Dent Update 2000;27:388–91

5. Cohen's Pathway of the Pulp.Elsevier Mosby; 2011.

6. Dummer P, Hicks R, Huws D. Clinical signs and symptoms in pulp disease. Int Endod J 1980;13:27–35.

7. Hargreaves, KM. Goodis, HE. Seltzer and Bender's Dental Pulp. Quintessence, 2002.

8. Kuc I, Peters E, Pan J. Comparison of clinical and histologic diagnoses in periapical lesions. Oral Surg Oral Med Oral Pathol Oral Radiol Endod. 2000; 89(3): 333–7.

9. Ruddle CJ. Endodontic diagnosis. Dent Today. 2002;21(10): 90–2, 94, 96–101.

10. Seltzer S. Classification of pulpal pathosis. Oral Surg Oral Med Oral Pathol 1972;34:269–87.

11. Seltzer S. Pain. In: Seltzer S (Editor). Endodontology: biologic considerations in endodontic procedures. 2nd ed. Philadelphia: Lea & Febiger; 1998. p. 471–499.

12. Shafer WG, Hine MK, Levy BM. A textbook of Oral Pathology. Ed 4. Philadelphia, PA: Saunders, 1983.

13. Smulson MH. Classification and diagnosis of pulpal pathosis. Dent Clin North Am 1984;28:699–723.

14. Torabinejad, M. Walton, RE. Endodontics: Principles and Practice. 4th Edition. Elsevier Health Sciences, March 2008.

Endodontic Microbiology

Introduction

For many years, the interrelationship of microorganisms and root canal system has been proved. Leeuwenhoek observed infected root canal of a tooth and found "cavorting beasties." After this, it took 200 years for WD Miller to make the correlation between microorganisms and pulpal or periradicular pathologies.

In 1965, Kakehashi et al. found that bacteria are the main etiological factors in the development of pulpal and periradicular diseases. Kakehashi et al. proved that without bacterial involvement, only minor inflammation occurred in exposed pulp.

All the surfaces of human body are colonized by microorganisms. Colonization is the establishment of bacteria in a living host. It occurs if biochemical and physical conditions are available for growth. Permanent colonization in symbiotic relationship with host tissue results in establishment of normal flora.

Infection results if microorganisms damage the host and produce clinical signs and symptoms. Degree of pathogenicity produced by microorganisms is called **virulence**.

History of microbiology in association to endodontics
17th century: AV Leeuwenhoek first described oral microflora
1890: WD Miller (Father of oral microbiology) authorized book "Microorganisms of human mouth"
1904: F Billings described theory of focal infection as a circumscribed area of tissue with pathognomic microorganisms

1909: EC Rosenow described theory of focal infection as localized or generalized infection caused by bacteria traveling via bloodstream from distant focus of infection
1939: Fish observed four distinct zones of periapical reaction in response to infection
1965: Kakehashi et al. proved that bacteria are responsible for pulpal and periapical disease
1976: Sundqvist used different culturing techniques for identification of both aerobic and anaerobic organisms and concluded that root canal infections are multibacterial

Portals of Entry for Microorganisms

Microorganisms may gain entry into pulp through several routes.

Entry through Open Cavity

This is the most common way of entry of microorganisms into the dental pulp. When protective layers of a tooth (enamel and dentin) get destroyed by caries (**Fig. 4.1**), traumatic injuries, fractures, cracks, or restorative procedures, microorganisms can gain access to the pulp.

Through Open Dentinal Tubules

Microorganisms can pass into the dentinal tubules and subsequently to the pulp. Bacteria are preceded in course

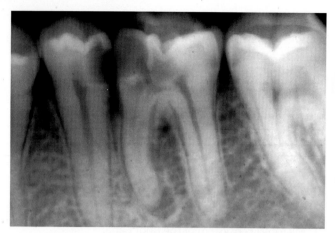

Fig. 4.1 Radiograph showing deep carious lesion in mandibular 2nd premolar and 1st molar involving the pulp.

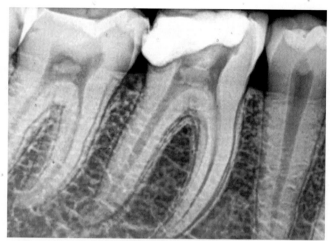

Fig. 4.3 Radiograph showing faulty restoration in mandibular 1st molar involving pulp.

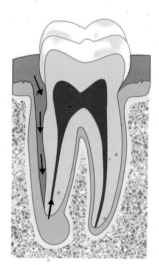

Fig. 4.2 Periodontal lesion causing inflammation of pulp.

of tubules by their breakdown products which may act as pulp irritants.

Through the Periodontal Ligament or the Gingival Sulcus

Periodontal pathology or treatment can remove cementum and exposes dentinal tubules to oral flora through which microorganisms gain entry into pulp via accessory and lateral canals **(Fig. 4.2)**.

Anachoresis

Anachoresis is a process by which microorganisms are transported in blood to an area of inflammation where they establish an infection.

Through Faulty Restoration

Faulty restoration with marginal leakage can result in contamination of the pulp space by bacteria **(Fig. 4.3)**.

Classification of Microorganisms

Microbial flora can be classified **(Fig. 4.4)** on the basis of **Gram-positive organisms,** for example, *Streptococcus, Enterococcus, Treponema, Candida, Actinomyces, Lactobacillus.*
   Gram-negative organisms, for example, *Fusobacterium, Campylobacter, Bacteroides, Veillonella, Neisseria.*
- ❏ ***Obligate aerobes:*** These organisms require oxygen for their growth because they can't ferment or respire anaerobically, for example, tubercle bacilli
- ❏ ***Facultative anaerobes:*** These organisms can grow in the presence or absence of oxygen, for example, *Staphylococcus*
- ❏ ***Microaerophilic:*** These organisms grow in an oxygen environment but derive their energy only from fermentative pathways that occur in absence of oxygen, for example, *Streptococcus*
- ❏ ***Obligate anaerobes:*** These bacteria can grow only in absence of oxygen, for example, *Bacteroides, Fusobacterium*

Microbial Virulence and Pathogenicity

- *Pathogenicity* is the ability of microorganisms to produce a disease
- *Virulence* is degree of pathogenicity of a microorganism

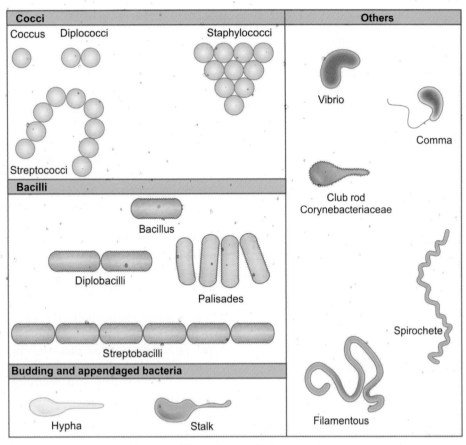

Fig. 4.4 Different types of microorganisms.

In 1965, Hobson gave an equation showing the relation of number of microorganisms, their virulence, resistance of host, and severity of the disease.

$$\frac{\text{Number of microorganisms} \times \text{virulence of microorganisms}}{\text{Resistance of host}} = \text{Severity of the disease}$$

Virulent factors
- Lipopolysaccharides (LPS)
- Extracellular vesicles
- Enzymes
- Fatty acids
- Polyamines
- Capsule
- Pilli

Lipopolysaccharides

❑ LPS are present on the surface of Gram-negative bacteria
❑ LPS have nonspecific antigens which are not neutralized by antibodies

❑ They exert numerous biologic functions when released from cells in the form of endotoxins. Endotoxins have capability to diffuse into dentin

Extracellular Vesicles

❑ Extracellular vesicles are produced by Gram-negative bacteria in form of endotoxins, outer membrane fragments, or blebs. Vesicles contain enzymes and toxic products which are responsible for hemagglutination, hemolysis, and bacterial adhesion
❑ These have trilaminar structure similar to outer membrane of the parent bacteria. Since they have antigenic properties similar to the parent bacteria, they may protect bacteria by neutralizing specific antibodies

Enzymes

❑ Enzymes produced by bacteria can result in spread of the infection, neutralization of immunoglobulin, and complement components
❑ PMN (Polymorphonucleocytes) leukocytes release hydrolytic enzymes which degenerate and lyse to form purulent exudates and have adverse effects on the surrounding tissues

Fatty Acids

❑ Various short chain fatty acids like propionic acid, butyric acid, etc. are produced by anaerobic bacteria. These cause neutrophil chemotaxis, degranulation, phagocytosis, and stimulate interleukin-1 production which further cause bone resorption and periradicular diseases

Polyamines

❑ These are biologically active chemicals found in the infected canals
❑ Some of polyamines such as cadaverine, putrescine, spermidine help in regulation of the cell growth, regeneration of tissues, and modulation of inflammation
❑ Other virulent factors, like **capsules** present in Gram-negative black-pigmented bacteria, enable them to resist phagocytosis. **Pilli** may play an important role in attachment of bacteria to surfaces and interaction with other bacteria

Factors Influencing the Growth and Colonization of Microorganisms

Influence of Oxygen

❑ A factor highly selective for the microbial flora of root canal is low availability of oxygen in infected root canals
❑ In the initial stages, there is predominance of facultative organisms, but later they are replaced by anaerobic bacteria

Nutritional Factors

❑ Bacteria obtain their nutrition from tissue fluid and the breakdown products of necrotic pulp tissue. Other source of nutrition for bacteria is inflammatory exudates containing serum and blood factors discharged from related inflammatory processes in the remaining pulp or the periapical tissues

Bacteriocins

Some bacteria produce bacteriocins, which are antibiotics like proteins produced by one species of bacteria to inhibit another species of bacteria.

Coaggregation

It is the existence of "symbiotic relationship" between some bacteria which may result in an increase in virulence by the organisms in that ecosystem.

Bacterial Interrelationships

Interrelationships between certain bacteria can be commensal or antagonistic which affect their survival.

Microbial Ecosystem of the Root Canal

❑ Microorganisms which can survive in environment of low oxygen tension and can survive the rigors of limited pabulums are found in root canals
❑ On an average, 10^3–10^8 bacteria are found in endodontic infections accounting >700 species
❑ Most commonly seen bacteria in root canals is streptococci (Gram-positive facultative anaerobic) especially in coronal part of root canal, others can be *Staphylococcus*, Gram-negative, and anaerobic bacteria
❑ A new nomenclature is given to species *Bacteroides*
❑ In necrotic pulp, there is a lack of circulation with compromised host defense mechanism; this makes pulp a reservoir for invading microbes

Here, tissue fluids and disintegrated cells from necrotic tissue, low oxygen tension, and bacterial interactions determine predominance of particular type of bacteria. Growth of one bacterial species is dependent on other bacterial species which supplies the essential nutrients. In the similar way, antagonistic relationship may occur in bacteria, that is, by-products of some bacterial species may kill or retard the growth of others species **(Fig. 4.5)**.

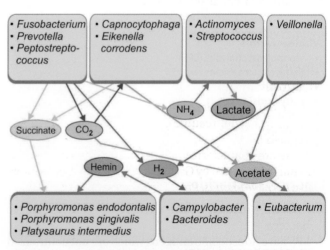

Fig. 4.5 Interrelationship of various root canal microorganisms.

New nomenclature of *Bacteroides* species
- *Porphyromonas*—Dark-pigmented (asaccharolytic *Bacteroides* species)
  - *Porphyromonas asaccharolytica*
  - *Porphyromonas gingivalis*
  - *Porphyromonas endodontalis*
- *Prevotella*—Dark-pigmented (saccharolytic *Bacteroides* species)
  - *Prevotella melaninogenica*
  - *Prevotella denticola*
  - *Prevotella intermedia*
  - *Prevotella nigrescens*
  - *Prevotella corporis*
  - *Prevotella tannerae*
- *Prevotella*—Nonpigmented (saccharolytic *Bacteroides* species)
  - *Prevotella buccae*
  - *Prevotella bivia*
  - *Prevotella oralis*

Naidorf summarized following generalizations in relation to organisms isolated from the root canals
- Mixed infections are more common than single organism
- Pulp contains flora almost similar to that of oral cavity
- Approximately 25% of isolated organisms are anaerobes
- Organisms isolated from flare-up as well as asymptomatic cases are almost similar
- Various researchers have identified wide variety of microorganisms in the root canals which is partially related to personal interest and culture techniques used by them

Types of Endodontic Infections

According to location of infection in relation to root canal, it can be classified as intraradicular and extraradicular.

Intraradicular Infections

In intraradicular infections, microorganisms are present within the root canal system. These can be primary, secondary, and persistent infections according to the time of organisms' entry into the canal.

Primary Intraradicular Infections (Virgin Infection)

- These are those microorganisms which initially invade the pulp tissue, resulting in inflammation and then necrosis
- These are characterized by presence of mixed habitat, mainly dominated by Gram-negative obligate anaerobes like *Porphyromonas, Prevotella, Fusobacterium, Dialister, Campylobacter,* and *Treponema*
- Gram-positive anaerobes like *Peptostreptococcus, Eubacterium, Actinomyces,* and *Streptococcus* are also seen in primary intraradicular infections

Secondary Intraradicular Infections

- These infections are introduced during or after the treatment
- In these infections, those organisms are present which were not prevalent during primary endodontic infections
  - Sources of microbes during treatment can be:
    - Remnants of caries, plaque or calculus
    - Leakage of rubber dam
    - Contamination of instruments and irrigation solutions
  - Sources of microbes between the appointments
    - Leakage of restorative materials
    - Tooth opened for drainage
    - Fracture of tooth/teeth
  - Sources of microbes after root canal treatment
    - Leakage of restorative materials
    - No use of rubber dam
    - Fracture of teeth
    - Secondary dental caries
  - Commonly found microorganisms in these infections can be *Pseudomonas aeruginosa, Staphylococcus, Escherichia coli, Enterococcus faecalis,* and *Candida* sp.

Persistent Intraradicular Infections

- These are those microorganisms which survive in root canal after intracanal antimicrobial procedures. Gram-positive are most common persistent bacteria
- In these infections, *E. faecalis* is the most commonly found organism
- *E. faecalis* is considered to be most common reason for failed root canals and in canals with persistent infection
- It is a Gram-positive cocci and is facultative anaerobe
- ***Because of following features, E. faecalis can survive in root canals even in adverse conditions:***
  - It can *persist in poor nutrient environment* of root canal treated teeth
  - It can *survive in presence of medicaments* like calcium hydroxide
  - It can *stay alive in presence of irrigants* like sodium hypochlorite
  - It can *convert into viable but noncultivable state (VBNC)*
  - It can *form biofilms* in medicated canals
  - It can penetrate and *utilize fluid present in dentinal tubules*
  - It can survive in *prolonged periods of starvation and utilize tissue fluid that flow from periodontal ligament*
  - It can *survive in low pH* and *high temperature*
  - It can *acquire gene encoding resistance* combined with natural resistance to antibiotics
  - It can *establish monoinfections* in medicated root canals
  - It's main virulent factors are hemolysin, gelatinase, aggregation substance, and extracellular superoxide

Extraradicular Infections

- These are characterized by microbial invasion and pro-liferation in the inflamed periradicular tissues as a result of intraradicular infections, for example, acute alveolar abscess
- Extraradicular infections can be caused by intraradicular bacteria or bacteria from outer side
- Commonly found microorganisms in extraradicular infections are *Actinomyces* sp., *Treponema* sp., *P. gingivalis*, *Fusobacterium nucleatum*, and *P. endodontalis*

Other microorganisms found in endodontic infections are

- Fungi
- HIV in vital pulp of HIV/AIDS patient
- Virus can't survive in necrotic pulp cases because they require living cells for their growth

Available nutrients utilized by bacteria in root canal:

- Necrotic pulp tissue
- Salivary components
- Proteins and glycol proteins from tissue fluid
- By-products of bacteria

Pathogenicity of Bacteroides is related to presence of LPS and peptidoglycans. These
- Induce cytokinins which play an important role in inflammation
- Stimulate B-lymphocytes
- Activate complement cascade
- Release various enzymes like collagenase
- Enhance production of various pain mediators like bradykinin, histamine, and prostaglandins
- LPS once released (as endotoxin) causes biological effects including inflammation and bone resorption

Microbiology of infected root canal

Obligate anaerobes	Facultative anaerobes
Gram-negative bacilli	**Gram-negative bacilli**
Porphyromonas*	Capnocytophaga
Prevotella†	Eikenella
Fusobacterium	
Campylobacter	
Bacteroides	
Gram-negative cocci	**Gram-negative cocci**
Veillonella	Neisseria
Gram-positive bacilli	**Gram-positive bacilli**
Actinomyces	Actinomyces
Lactobacillus	Lactobacillus
Propionibacterium	
Gram-positive cocci	**Gram-positive cocci**
Streptococcus	Streptococcus
Peptostreptococcus	Enterococcus
Spirochetes	**Fungi**
Treponema	Candida

*Dark pigmented bacteria.
†Dark pigmented bacteria and nonpigmenting bacteria.

Identification of the Bacteria

Following tests can be done to detect microorganisms and their sensitivity to particular antibiotic.

Gram's Stain

- It was developed by Christian Gram in 1884
- It helps in differentiating bacteria in Gram-positive and Gram-negative organisms

Culture

Culture taking method though done less these days still holds its importance because of wide range of bacteria found in the endodontic infections.

Principle of Culturing

Culturing of root canals is done for two main reasons:

1. In the cases of persistent infection, to grow and isolate the microbial flora for antibiotic sensitivity and resistance profiles
2. To assess the bacteriologic status of root canal system before obturation and determine the effectiveness of debridement procedure

Types of tissue cultures
- *Cell culture:* It is an in vitro growth of cells; although the cells proliferate, they do not organize into tissue
- *Anaerobic culture:* This culture is carried out in absence of air
- *Pure culture:* This culture consists of a single cell species, without presence of any contaminants
- *Primary culture:* Refers to cultures prepared from tissues taken directly from animals
- *Secondary culture:* It refers to a subculture derived from a primary culture
- *Plate culture:* This culture is grown on a medium, usually agar or gelatin, on a petri dish
- *Streak culture:* In this culture, medium is inoculated by drawing an infected wire across it
- *Suspension culture:* It refers to a culture in which cells multiply while suspended in a suitable medium
- *Slant culture:* This culture is made on the surface of solidified medium in a tube which has been tilted to provide a greater surface area for growth
- *Stab culture:* In this culture, medium is inoculated by thrusting a needle deep into its substance
- *Tissue culture:* It refers to the culture in which maintenance or growth of tissue, organ primordia, or whole or part of an organ in vitro is done so as to preserve its architecture and function

Types of Culture Medium

- Liquid (broth)
- Solid (agar)
- Semisolid

Liquid culture medium
- The original liquid media developed by Louis Pasteur contained wine or meat broth
- In liquid media, nutrients are dissolved in water, and bacterial growth is indicated by a change in the broth's appearance from clear to turbid
- Minimum of 10^6 bacteria per milliliter of broth are required for turbidity to be detected with unaided eye
- Formation of turbidity is directly proportional to the bacterial growth.

Solid media
- It was developed by Robert Koch in 1881. It contained pieces of potato, gelatin, and meat extract
- Since gelatin used to liquefy at 24°C, so he substituted it with agar

Bacteriological media
It consists of water, agar, growth-enriching constituents like yeast extract and blood.

Anaerobic Culture Method
- An anaerobic bacteria culture is a method used to grow anaerobes from a clinical specimen
- Anaerobic bacterial culture is performed to identify bacteria that grow only in absence of oxygen

Culture Technique
For culturing, samples can be obtained either from an infected root canal or from a periradicular abscess.

Sample from draining root canal
- Isolate the tooth with a rubber dam. Disinfect the surface of the tooth and surrounding area with betadine, chlorhexidine, or sodium hypochlorite
- Gain access in root canal using sterile burs and instruments
- If there is drainage, collect the sample using a sterile needle and syringe or sterile absorbent paper points. Place the aspirate in anaerobic transport media

Sample from dry canal
- To sample a dry canal, use a sterile syringe to place transport media into canal
- Take the sample using a syringe or paper points and place the aspirate in anaerobic media

Sample from the abscess
- Palpate the fluctuant abscess and determine the most dependent part of swelling
- Disinfect the surface of mucosa with alcohol or iodophor
- Penetrate a sterile 16–20 gauge needle in the surface and aspirate the exudates
- Inject this aspirate into anaerobic transport media

Culture Reversal
- Sometimes negative culture becomes positive after 24–48 hours
- So it is advised to allow >48 h between taking culture and obturation

Advantages of culturing method
- Culture helps to determine bacteriological status of root canal
- It helps to isolate microbial flora for resistant profiles and for antibiotic sensitivity
- Helps in identification of broad range of microorganisms

Disadvantages of culturing method
- Unable to grow several microorganisms which can give false negative results
- Strictly depend on mode of sample transport which must allow growth of anaerobic bacteria
- Low sensitivity and specificity
- Time-consuming
- Expensive and laborious

Molecular Diagnostic Methods

Advantages of molecular methods
- Helpful in detection of both cultivable and uncultivable microbial species
- Higher sensitivity
- Have greater specificity
- Less time-consuming
- Do not need special control for anaerobic bacteria
- Are useful when a large number of samples are needed to be analyzed for epidemiologic studies
- Do not require cultivation
- Can be identified even when they are viable
- Can be used during antimicrobial treatment
- Large number of samples can be stored at low temperature and surveyed at once

- To overcome disadvantages of culturing method, various molecular diagnostic methods have developed
- Molecular diagnostic methods identify the microorganisms using gene as a target which are unique for each species. These are classified into four categories:
  1. Hybridization
  2. Amplification
  3. Sequencing
  4. Enzyme digestion of nucleic acid

DNA–DNA Hybridization Method (Fig. 4.6)
- This method uses DNA probes which target genomic DNA or individual genes
- It helps in simultaneous determination of the presence of a multitude of bacterial species in single or multiple clinical samples and is especially useful for large scale epidemiologic research

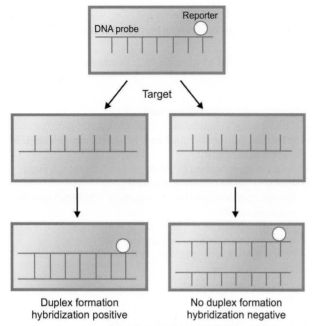

Fig. 4.6 Diagrammatic representation of DNA–DNA hybridization method.

- It employs use of DNA probes, single stranded DNA, labeled with an enzyme or radioactive isotope, which locates and binds to complementary nucleic acids sequence of known identity to form a double-stranded molecule or hybrid
- Since hybridization requires nucleic acid sequence homology, a positive hybridization reaction between two nucleic acid strands, each from a different source, indicates genetic relationship the between two organisms that were formed

Advantages of DNA–DNA hybridization method
- Can be used for large-scale epidemiological research
- Allows simultaneous detection of multiple species
- Microbial contaminants are not cultivated, and their DNA is not amplified

Disadvantages of DNA–DNA hybridization method
- Cross reaction can occur on nontarget microorganisms
- Identifies only cultivable microorganisms
- Does not detect unexpected
- Detects only target microorganisms

Amplification/Polymerase Chain Reaction Method (Fig. 4.7)

Though hybridization methods are highly specific for detection of microorganisms and identification, they have less sensitivity. So, if sufficient target nucleic acid in the reaction is not present, false-negative results occur. Hence, hybridization methods necessitate "amplification" of target nucleic acid by multiplying the target organisms to bigger numbers in culture.

The three strategies for molecular amplification are target nucleic acid amplification, nucleic acid probe amplification, and amplification of the probe "signal." Polymerase chain reaction (PCR) method involves in vitro replication of DNA; therefore, it is also called "genetic xeroxing" method. Here, multiple copies of specific region of DNA are made by repeated cycles or heating and cooling.

Then this amplified target formed is detected by different methods like:
- Electrophoresis in agarose gel
- Cloning and sequencing
- Microarray analysis
- Reverse capture checker board analysis
    DGGE (Denaturing Gradient Gel Electrophoresis)

Advantages of PCR method
- PCR has remarkable sensitivity and specificity because each distinct microbial species has unique DNA sequences
- PCR can be used to detect virtually all bacterial species in a sample
- It is also used to investigate microbial diversity in a given environment. Clonal analysis of microorganisms can also be done by PCR method

Disadvantages of PCR method
- Identify microorganisms qualitatively not quantitatively
- Detect only target microorganisms
- Difficult in microorganisms with thick wall like fungi
- Possibility of false positive and negative results

How to Combat Microbes in the Endodontic Therapy?

The microbial ecosystem of an infected root canal system and inflammatory response caused by it will persist until source of irritation is completely removed. The main factor which is needed for successful treatment of pulp and periradicular inflammation is complete removal of the source of infection such as microorganisms and their by-products.

Following measures should be taken to completely get rid of these irritants.

Thorough Cleaning and Shaping of the Root Canal System

Thorough cleaning and shaping followed by three-dimensional obturation of the root canals have shown to produce complete healing of periradicular tissue. Complete debridement of canal should be done with adjunctive use of irrigants like sodium hypochlorite which efficiently removes bacteria as well as their substrate from irregularities of canal system where instruments cannot reach such as fins, indentations, cul-de-sacs etc.

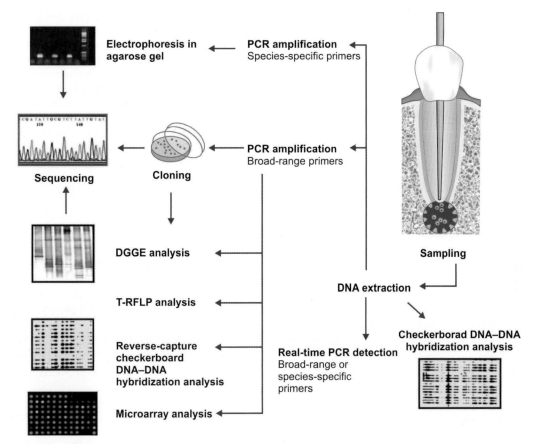

Fig. 4.7 Various molecular techniques used in endodontics.

Oxygenating a Canal

Oxygenating a canal simply by opening it is detrimental to anaerobes. Use of oxygenating agents as glyoxide can be of great help, but care should be taken to avoid inoculation of these oxygenating agents into periapical tissues.

Drain

A tooth with serous or purulent or hemorrhagic exudate should be allowed to drain with rubber dam in place for a time under supervision. An abscess, which is a potent irritant, has an elevated osmotic pressure. This attracts more tissue fluid and thus more edema and pain. Drainage by canal or by soft tissues decrease discomfort caused by inflammatory mediators.

Antibiotics

Antibiotics should also be considered as adjunctive in severe infections. The choice of antibiotic agent should be done on the knowledge of microorganisms associated with the endodontic infections.

Intracanal Medicaments

Intracanal medicaments play an important role in combating the microorganisms.

Use of Calcium Hydroxide in Canals

Use of calcium hydroxide in canals with necrotic pulps after instrumentation has shown to provide the beneficial results. Intracranial use of calcium hydroxide has shown to increase the efficiency of sodium hypochlorite and also the effectiveness of antimicrobial agent. Calcium hydroxide powder is mixed with water or glycerin to form a thick paste which is placed in pulp chamber with amalgam carrier or a syringe. This paste is covered with a sterile cotton pellet, and access is sealed with temporary restoration.

▌Conclusion

For successful endodontic outcome, one must have awareness of the close relationship between endodontic infections and microorganisms. The type of the microbial flora develop according to the surrounding environment.

Microorganisms which are present in the untreated root canal have plenty of nutritional diversity, whereas microbial flora of root canal treated tooth are in dry space devoid of nutrition, so as per the environment the type of flora changes. Therefore, we should obtain a better understanding of the characteristics and properties of bacteria along with environmental changes so as to increase the success of endodontic treatment.

Questions

1. What are different methods used for identification of bacteria. Write in detail about culture method?
2. Write short notes on:
   - Anachoresis.
   - Microbial virulence and pathogenicity.
   - Explain microbiology of infected root canals.

Bibliography

1. Costerton J, Stewart PS, Greenberg EP. Bacterial biofilm: A common cause of persistent infections. Science 1999;284:1318–22.
2. Dahle UR, Titterud Sunde P, Tronstad L. Treponemas and endodontic infections. Endod Top. 2003;6:160–70.
3. Gopikrishna AV, Kandaswamy D, Jeyavel RK. Comparative evaluation of the antimicrobial efficacy of five endodontic root canal sealers against Enterococcus faecalis and *Candida albicans*. J Conserv Dent 2006;9:2–12.
4. Hargreaves KM, Cohen S. Pathways of the pulp. 10th edition Mosby: Elsevier; 2012.
5. Ingle JI, Bakland LK, Decker BC. Endodontics. 6th edition Elsevier; 2008.
6. Kakehashi S, Stanley HR, Fitzgerald RJ. The effects of surgical exposures of dental pulps in germ-free and conventional laboratory rats. Oral Surg Oral Med Oral Pathol 1965;20:340–9.
7. Love RM. Enterococcus faecalis—a mechanism of its role in endodontic failure. Int Endod J 2001;34:399–405.
8. Nair PN. On the causes of persistent apical periodontitis, a review. Int Endod J 2006;39:249–81.
9. Siqueira JF, Jr. Aetiology of root canal treatment failure: Why well-treated teeth can fail. Int Endod J 2001;34:1–10.
10. Torabinejad M, Ung B, Kettering J. In vitro bacterial penetration of coronally unsealed endodontically treated teeth. J Endod 1990;16:566–9.
11. Tronstad L, Barnett F, Riso K, Slots J. Extraradicular endodontic infections. Endod Dent Traumatol 1987;3:86–90.

Biofilm and Smear Layer in Endodontics

Introduction

Persistence of microorganisms has shown to be the most important cause for endodontic failure. Root canal infections are biofilm mediated. The complexity and variability of the root canal system, along with multi-species nature of biofilms, make disinfection of this system extremely challenging. Due to increased concern about biofilms, endodontic research has focused on the characterization of root canal biofilms and the clinical methods to interrupt the biofilms along with killing microorganisms.

Biofilm in Endodontics

Endodontic infections are biofilm mediated. The complexity of root canal system, along with the multi-species nature of biofilms, makes the disinfection of this system extremely challenging. Microbial persistence is most important factor for root canal failure. Biofilm removal can be done by a chemo-mechanical process, using specific instruments and disinfecting chemicals in the form of irrigants and/or intracanal medicaments. Endodontic research has focused on the characterization of root canal biofilms and the clinical methods to disturb the biofilms along with killing microbes. The smear layer is a surface accumulation of debris formed on dentine during root canal instrumentation. It consists of organic and inorganic components and forms both a superficial and deeper layers. It can prevent the penetration of intracanal medicaments into dentinal tubules and influence the adaptation of filling materials to canal walls. Whether it should be removed or not is still a debatable issue.

Definition

Biofilm can be defined as a sessile multicellular microbial community characterized by cells that are firmly attached to a surface and enmeshed in a self-produced matrix of extracellular polymeric substances. Bacterial biofilms are very prevalent in the apical root canals of teeth with primary and post treatment apical periodontitis. These bacterial endodontic communities are often found adhered to or at least associated with the dentinal canal walls.

Characteristics of Biofilm

Microorganisms present in a biofilm must have the following four basic criteria to survive:

1. **Autopoiesis:** Ability to self-organize
2. **Homeostasis:** Resist environmental perturbations
3. **Synergy:** Effective in association than in isolation
4. **Communality:** Respond to environmental changes as a unit rather than single individuals

Quorum sensing: Cell-to-cell signaling is known as quorum sensing. In this, bacterial cells communicate with each other by releasing, sensing, and responding to small diffusible signal molecules. Ability of bacteria to communicate and behave as a group for interactions like a multicellular organism shows many benefits to bacteria in host colonization, formation of biofilms, defense against competitors and adaptation to changing environments **(Fig. 5.1)**. Microorganisms function less effectively as individuals compared to coherent groups. Quorum sensing allows bacteria to monitor the environment for other bacteria and allow alteration of one's behavior in a

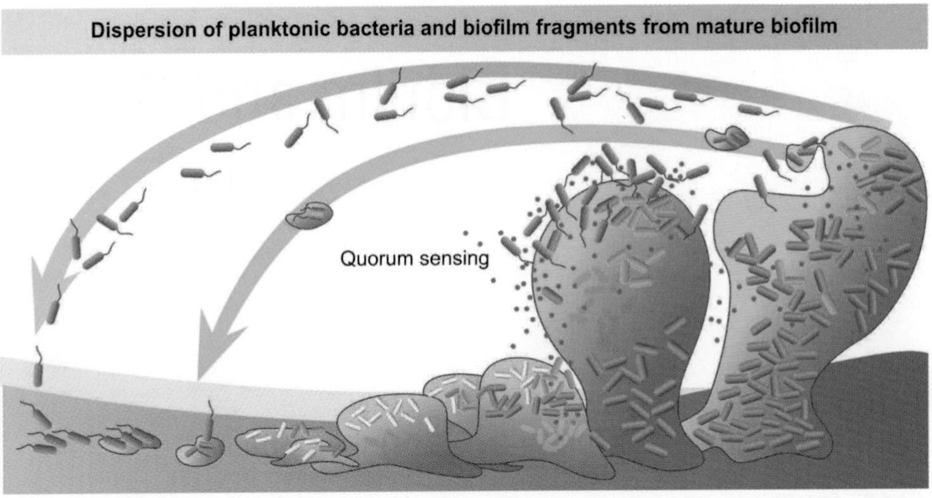

Fig. 5.1 Diagrammatic representation of Quorum Sensing showing release of chemical signal molecules by cells through which they communicate with each other.

population-wide scale. Pooling the activity of a quorum of cells can improve the successful persistence of bacteria.

Stages of Biofilm Formation (Fig. 5.2)

Formation of biofilm occurs in following developmental stages.
- *Attachment: It is the first stage* of biofilm formation which involves the adsorption of planktonic cells to the surface. Film on tooth surface consists of proteins, extracellular or DNA and glycoproteins from saliva and gingival crevicular fluid and microbial products
- *Growth: It is the second stage* which involves proliferation of microorganisms to form microcolonies. In this, cells start to secrete an extracellular matrix containing proteins and polysaccharides
- *Maturation: It is the third stage* which involves formation of a structurally organized mixed microbial community. Biofilm forms a mushroom-shaped structure with heterogeneous population
- *Dissemination: It is the fourth stage* which involves detachment of biofilm microorganisms. It is assumed that enzymes released from monolayers of bacteria result in their detachment. Detachment of microorganisms results in spreading and colonization to newer sites.

Types of Endodontic Biofilm

Types of endodontic biofilm
- Intracanal microbial biofilms
- Extraradicular microbial biofilms
- Periapical microbial biofilms
- Biomaterial-centered infections

Intracanal Microbial Biofilms

- This microbial biofilm formed on the root canal dentin of infected tooth
- First identification of biofilm was earlier reported by Nair in 1987 under transmission electron microscopy
- Mainly found bacteria in this biofilm are loose collections of cocci, rods, filaments, and spirochetes. Many other types of bacteria may also be found in these biofilms, but ability of *Enterococcus faecalis* to form calcified biofilm on root canal dentin can be a main factor that contributes to its persistence and resistance to the treatment.

Extraradicular Microbial Biofilms

- Also termed as *root surface biofilms*, formed on the root surface (cementum) adjacent to root apex of endodontically infected teeth
- Sites
  - Teeth with asymptomatic periapical periodontitis
  - Chronic periapical abscess associated with sinus tract
- In these biofilms, mainly found organisms are cocci and rods
- Filamentous and fibrillar forms have also been observed in these. In some cases, calcified biofilms have also been observed on the apical root surface of teeth with lesions refractory to root canal treatment.

Periapical Microbial Biofilms

- Periapical microbial biofilms are isolated biofilms found in the periapical region of an endodontically infected teeth, asymptomatic periapical lesions refractory to endodontic treatment

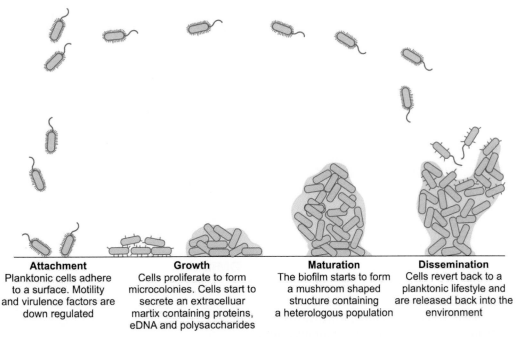

Attachment
Planktonic cells adhere
to a surface. Motility
and virulence factors are
down regulated

Growth
Cells proliferate to form
microcolonies. Cells start to
secrete an extracelluar
martix containing proteins,
eDNA and polysaccharides

Maturation
The biofilm starts to form
a mushroom shaped
structure containing
a heterologous population

Dissemination
Cells revert back to a
planktonic lifestyle and
are released back into the
environment

Fig. 5.2 Stages of biofilm formation.

- Microorganism involved are
  - *Actinomyces*
  - *Propionibacterium propionicum*

Fimbriae present on *Actinomyces* cells help them to adhere to the root canal wall and to dentinal debris pushed out in the periapical region during treatment and to adhere to other bacteria or host cells as they advance into periapical areas. This results in formation of aggregates of cohesive colonies of tangled filaments.

Biomaterial-Centered Infections

- Biomaterial-centered infection (BCI) occurs when bacteria adhere to an artificial biomaterial surface such as root canal obturating materials and form biofilms. It can be intraradicular or extraradicular depending on whether the obturating material is within the root canal space or it has extruded beyond the root apex
- Presence of biomaterial in close proximity to the host immune system can increase the susceptibility to BCI
- *Staphylococcus, Staphylococcus aureus,* enterocci, streptococci, *Pseudomonas aeruginosa,* and *E. faecalis* form biofilm on Gutta-Percha points where as *Fusobacterium nucleatum, Propionibacterium acnes, Porphyromonas gingivalis,* and *Prevotella intermedia* do not form biofilm on Gutta-Percha points.
- Bacterial adhesion to biomaterial surface can be explained in the following three phases:
  Phase 1: Transport of bacteria to biomaterial surface

Phase 2: Initial, nonspecific adhesion phase
Phase 3: Specific adhesion phase.

▌Ultrastructure of Biofilm (Fig. 5.3)

A fully formed biofilm is labeled as a heterogeneous arrangement of microbial cells on a solid surface.

Microcolonies

- Microcolonies or cell clusters form the basic structural unit of a biofilm. These are formed by adherence of bacterial cells on the surface
- These are isolated units of densely packed bacterial cell aggregates consisting of one or many species
- There is a 3-D distribution of bacterial cells of different physiological and metabolic states within a biofilm.

Glycocalyx Matrix

- A glycocalyx matrix, made up of EPS (extracellular polysaccharides), surrounds the microcolonies and holds the bacterial cell to substrate
- Biofilm consists of matrix material 85% and cells 15%
- A fresh biofilm matrix is made of biopolymers, such as polysaccharides, proteins, nucleic acids, and salts
- Structure and composition of mature biofilm gets modified according to environmental conditions like nutritional availability, nature of fluid movements, physicochemical properties of the substrate, etc.

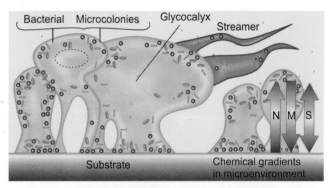

Fig. 5.3 Diagrammatic representation of the structure of a mature biofilm
Abbreviations: N: nutrients; M: metabolic products; S: signal molecules.

Water Channels

❑ Present in biofilms facilitate efficient exchange of materials between bacterial cells and fluid, which also helps to coordinate functions in a biofilm community. A fully hydrated biofilm appears as a tower- or mushroom-shaped structure adherent to a substrate.

▣ Microbes in Endodontic Biofilms

Methods to isolate microbes
- Culture
- Microscopy
- Immunological methods
- Molecular biology methods

Microorganisms involved in biofilm formation
- *E. faecalis*
- Coagulase–negative *Staphylococcus*
- Streptococci
- *Actinomyces* species
- *P. propionicum*
- Others: *P. aeruginosa*, fungi, *F. nucleatum*, *Porphyromonas gingivalis*, *Tannerella forsythensis*, *Actinomyces* species and *P. propionicum*

About 40%–55% of the endodontic *microbiota* in primary infections is composed of species still uncultivated.

▣ Methods to Eradicate Biofilms

Sodium Hypochlorite

It is effective against biofilms containing *P. intermedia*, *Peptostreptococcus micros*, *Streptococcus intermedius*, *F. nucleatum*, and *E. faecalis* as it disrupts oxidative phosphorylation and inhibits DNA synthesis of bacteria. Many studies have shown that NaOCl is the only irrigant that has a significant effect on biofilm viability and architecture.

Chlorhexidine Digluconate

It is effective against both Gram-positive and Gram-negative bacteria due to its ability to denature the bacterial cell wall while forming pores in the membrane. Williamson et al. showed that 2% of chlorhexidine was less effective against *E. faecalis* biofilm when compared to 6% NaOCl. Shen et al. showed that the combined use of chlorhexidine along with mechanical instrumentation showed more noticeable antimicrobial effect against the biofilms. It has been shown that bacteria in mature biofilms and nutrient-limited biofilms are more resistant to chlorhexidine than young biofilms.

QMix

QMix consists of EDTA, chlorhexidine, and detergent. It is as effective as 6% NaOCl in killing 1-day old *E. faecalis* but slightly less effective against bacteria in 3-week-old biofilm.

Iodine

It is bactericidal, fungicidal, tuberculocidal, virucidal, and sporicidal as it penetrates into microorganisms and attacks proteins, nucleotides, and fatty acids resulting in cell death. Studies have shown that iodine and NaOCl caused 100% bacteria elimination after 1 hour incubation for all used strains. However, 10% povidone iodine has shown to be less effective against *E. faecalis* biofilm as compared to NaOCl.

EDTA

It has little antibacterial activity. On direct exposure for extended time, EDTA extracts bacterial surface proteins by combining with metal ions from the cell envelope, which can eventually lead to bacterial death.

MTAD (*Mixture of a Tetracycline Isomer, an Acid, and a Detergent*)

It has been shown that that Biopure MTAD does not disintegrate and remove bacterial biofilms. It is not able to remove *E. faecalis* biofilm.

Tetraclean

It is a mixture of antibiotic, acid, and a detergent like MTAD but different concentration. Pappen et al. (2010) found that tetraclean is more effective than MTAD against *E. faecalis* in planktonic culture.

Calcium Hydroxide (CH)

A commonly used intracanal medicament has been shown to be ineffective in killing *E. faecalis* on its own, especially when a high pH is not maintained. However, combination of calcium hydroxide and camphorated paramonochlorophenol completely eliminates *E. faecalis*. 2% chlorhexidine gel when combined with calcium hydroxide achieves a pH of 12.8 and can completely eliminate *E. faecalis* within dentinal tubules.

Ultrasonically Activated Irrigation

Bhuva et al. (2010) found that use of ultrasonically activated irrigation using 1% sodium hypochlorite, followed by root canal cleaning and shaping improves canal and isthmus cleanliness in terms of necrotic debris/biofilm removal.

Ozone/Ozonated Water

Viera et al. (1999) reported that Ozone in 0.1 ppm concentration is able to completely kill bacteria after 15 or 30 min of contact time. But Hems et al. showed that NaOCl is superior to Ozonated water in killing *E. faecalis* in biofilm.

Lasers

Lasers induce thermal effect producing an alteration in the bacterial cell wall leading to changes in the osmotic gradients and cell death. Noiri et al. found that Er:YAG irradiation reduces the number of viable cells in most of the biofilms of *A. naeslundii*, *E. faecalis*, *Lactobacillus casei*, *P. acnes*, *F. nucleatum*, *P. gingivalis*, and *Prevotella nigrescens*.

Plasma Dental Probe

It is effective for tooth disinfection. Plasma emission spectroscopy identifies atomic oxygen as one of the likely active agents for the bactericidal effect.

Photoactivated Disinfection

It is a combination of a photosensitizer solution and low-power laser light. Photodynamic therapy/Light-activated therapy destroys an endodontic biofilm when a photosensitizer selectively accumulated in the target cell is activated by a visible light of appropriate wavelength.

Antibacterial Nanoparticles

Antibacterial nanoparticles bind to negatively charged surfaces and have excellent antimicrobial and antifungal activities. Studies have also shown that the treatment of root dentin with ZnO nanoparticles, chitosan-layer–ZnO nanoparticles, or chitosan nanoparticles produces an 80%–95% reduction in the adherence of *E. faecalis* to dentin.

Endoactivator System

It is able to debride lateral canals, remove the smear layer, and dislodge simulated biofilm clumps within the curved canals.

Herbal Irrigants

Herbs like green tea, Triphala, German chamomile, tea tree oil can be used as irrigants because of their anti-inflammatory antioxidant, and radical scavenging activity. But when compared, studies have shown 5% NaOCl to be more effective against biofilm.

Smear Layer in Endodontics

Smear layer in instrumented root canals was first researched by McComb and Smith. It contains remnants of odontoblastic processes, pulp tissue, bacteria, and dentin.

AAE (American Association of Endodontists) defined smear layer as "surface film of debris retained on dentin or other tooth surfaces like enamel, cementum after instrumentation with either rotary instruments or endodontic files."

Structure of Smear Layer

It consists of two separate layers, a superficial layer and a layer loosely, attached to underlying dentin. It is composed of organic and inorganic component. Organic component consists of heated coagulated proteins, necrotic or viable pulp tissues, odontoblastic processes, saliva, blood cells, and microorganisms. Inorganic component is made up of tooth structure and some nonspecific inorganic constituents.

Smear layer on deep dentin contains more organic material than superficial dentin. It is because of greater number of proteoglycans lining the tubules or the greater number of odontoblastic processes near the pulp. Dentin debris enters the tubules and forms smear plugs to occlude the ends of tubules. Smear layer is 2–5 µm thick with particles ranging in size from 0.5 to 1.5 µm. Depth entering the dentinal tubules varies from few micrometers to 40 µm. Its thickness depends upon the type and sharpness of cutting instruments, the amount and type of irrigating solution used and whether dentin is wet or dry when cut. There does not seem to be consensus on removing of smear layer. It has both advantages and disadvantages remain controversial.

- Motorized preparation with Gates Glidden or postdrills produce greater volume of smear layer as compared to hand filing due to increased centrifugal forces resulting from proximity of instrument to the dentin wall. Also, filing a canal without irrigation will produce a thicker smear layer
- Post space preparation results in thicker smear layer and also consists of fragments of sealer and gutta-percha. So when posts are cemented without removal of smear layer it will bond to loosely adherent smear layer and ultimately bond will break

Advantages

- ☐ It provides a natural barrier to bacteria/bacterial products into the dentinal tubules
- ☐ Removal of smear layer may lead to bacterial invasion of dentinal tubules if seal fails
- ☐ Reduction of dentin permeability to bacterial toxins and oral fluids
- ☐ Reduction of diffusion of fluids and prevents wetness of cut dentin surface.

Disadvantages

- ☐ It acts as a barrier against the action of irrigants and disinfectants during chemo-mechanical preparation of root canal
- ☐ It may harbor bacteria which multiply by taking nourishment from smear layer or dentinal fluid
- ☐ Bacteria may penetrate deeper into the dentinal tubules
- ☐ It is loosely adherent and so may lead to microleakage between root canal filling and dentinal wall
- ☐ It doesn't allow root canal sealer to penetrate into the dentinal tubules and hence jeopardize the fluid tight seal
- ☐ Smear layer when exposed to periapical exudate dissolves that leads to leakage and void between the dentin and obturating materials
- ☐ Smear layer itself is infected.

To Keep or Remove the Smear Layer?

Drake et al. showed that removal of smear layer opened the dentinal tubules allowing bacteria to colonize in the tubules to a much higher degree compared with roots with an intact smear layer. Removal of smear layer facilitates passive penetration of bacteria. It is not practical to remove smear layer completely due to anatomical complexity of root canal. Also, 95% success rate has been achieved in root canal treatment even without removal of smear layer.

On the other hand, removal of smear layer improved fluid tight seal of root canal system by opening up the tubules and exposing the surface collagen for covalent linkage while filing technique/sealer doesn't make much difference. After removing smear layer thermoplasticized gutta-percha adapts better with/without sealer.

Also, sealers/obturating material/cements for postcementation require removal of smear layer. Removal of smear layer results in sealer penetration from 40 to 60 μm which increases the interface between the obturating material and the dentin.

However, ZOE (Zinc oxide eugenol) sealers are the most commonly used. But their particle size is >1 μm. Diameter of dentinal tubules is <1 μm near the apex. So, after the removal of smear layer seal at the apex is questionable.

Agents Used for Removal of Smear Layer

- ☐ *Sodium hypochlorite:* Dissolves organic tissues. Hence, it will dissolve organic components of the smear layer. It's ability is increased with increased temperature
- ☐ *Chelating agents*
  - *EDTA:* It forms chelates with calcium of dentin. It decalcifies dentin to a depth of 20–30 μm in 5 min. However, effect was negligible in apical one-third of root canals. Paste type EDTA is less effective in removing smear layer than liquid. Some EDTA preparations contain wax which leave a residue on walls and prevents formation of fluid tight seal. Optimal working time of EDTAC in root canal is 15 min and no further chelating action occurs after that
  - *Salvizol:* 0.5% BDAC (bis-dequalinium-acetate) removes organic as well as inorganic smear layer throughout the root canal. It has better cleaning than EDTAC and removal of organic portion is comparable to 5.25% NaOCl
  - *EGTA [Ethylene glycol-bis (β-aminoethyl ether)-N,N,N-tetraacetic acid]:* EDTA was more effective in removing the smear layer than EGTA which was much less effective in apical third. But EDTA also leads to erosion of peritubular and intertubular dentin
  - *Tetracycline:* Tertracycline hydrochloride, minocycline, doxycycline
    They have low pH and can act as chelator. Barkhordar et al. reported that doxycycline hydrochloride was effective in removing the smear layer from instrumented canals and root end cavity preparations
  - *MTAD:* Removes smear layer and also leads to disinfection of root canal
  - *Citric acid:* 10%, 25%, 50% solution can be used. But 25% citric acid was less effective than 17% EDTA-NaOCl combination.
    Also, citric acid left precipitates on root canal wall which might be disadvantageous to root canal obturation.
  - 3% and 20% polyacrylic acid, lactic acid, and 25% tannic acid may be used. Berry et al. reported 40% polyacrylic acid to be very effective in removal of smear layer.
  - 5.2% NaOCl and 17% EDTA: Alternate use can remove both inorganic and organic portion of smear layer
- ☐ *Chlorhexidine:* Does not dissolve or remove the smear layer
- ☐ *Ultrasonics:* Final irrigation with ultrasonics for 3–5 min produced smear layer free canals. When used during instrumentation direct contact of file with canal walls decreases acoustic streaming. Acoustic streaming is maximized when small file as No. 15 is used which increases microstreaming for debris removal

  Other investigations have shown that it is not effective and it is unnecessary to combine 15% EDTAC with distilled water or 1% NaOCl to remove the smear layer.

- *Lasers:* Vaporize tissues in main root canal and remove smear layer
  - Nd:YAG laser, CO_2 laser, argon fluoride excimer laser: Have shown variable results from no effect, disruption of smear layer to actual melting and recrystallization of dentin
  - Er:YAG: Removal of smear layer without melting/ charring or recrystallization. But destruction of peritubular dentin has been observed
    However, lasers have large probes and hence cannot be used in small canals.
- *Micro endobrush:* Invented by Ruddle. They can be used with hand, rotary or sonic or ultrasonic handpieces. Brush is made of a braided/twisted wire base which is flexible to reach all irregularities of root canal. Bristles are made of nylon that radiate from wire base

	D_0	D_{16}
i. Fine	0.2 mm	1 mm
ii. Fine-Medium	0.35 mm	1.25 mm
iii. Medium	0.5 mm	1.5 mm
iv. Medium-Large	0.7 mm	2.0 mm

It can be used in slow speed handpiece at a speed of 150–300 rpm.

- **Endoactivator**
- *Maleic acid:* 5%–7% can be used
- *QMix:* Contains a mixture of bisguanide [antimicrobial agents, polyamino carboxylic acid (as calcium chelating agent)]. It removes smear layer and can be used as a final rinse instead of EDTA followed by CHX.

Modification of Smear Layer

A percentage of 4% of titanium fluoride and 30% potassium oxalate have been used to modify the smear layer. Titanium is a polyvalent metal and has remarkable capacity to bind to organic material of dentin forming a tenacious coating of titanium dioxide which is resistant to dissolution by KOH washing/HCl treatment.

Conclusion

The most common cause of endodontic infection is surface-associated growth of microorganisms. To understand pathogenesis and disinfection of root canal microflora, biofilm concept should be applied. One must understand formation and mechanism of resistant endodontic biofilms. Contrary to the vulnerable planktonic state, bacteria are protected from the antibacterial agents in biofilms. To date, with advent of scientific approaches along with coordination of newer clinical, laboratory, chemical, and

research methods, it is possible to imagine overcoming biofilm problems.

Problem of smear layer is still a controversy. However, growing evidence supports its removal. If it is to be removed 5% NaOCl followed by 10 mL of EDTA for 1 min should be used. NaOCl should not be used after EDTA as it leads to remarkable erosion of dentin. CHX can be used in the end to disinfect dentin. Alternatively, final rinse with MTAD/ QMix or ultrasonic may be used.

Sealers with bonding ability like AH Plus show greater bond strength when smear layer has been removed. However, some studies show decreased bond strength, but completely reversed by application of 10% ascorbic acid/10% sodium ascorbate. With the advent of adhesive dentistry for endodontics use of medicated and resin based sealers and obturating materials like Resilon and Active GP (Gutta percha) definitely mandates the removal of smear layer for producing secondary and tertiary monoblocks for adequate bonding and to obtain optimal bond strength for a fluid tight seal.

Questions

1. Define biofilm. What are different stages of biofilm formation?
2. What are different types of biofilms? Enumerate various methods to eradicate biofilms.
3. Write short notes on:
   - Ultrastructure of biofilm.
   - Microbiology of biofilms.
4. Explain significance of smear layer in endodontics.
5. Write in detail different ways to manage smear layer in endodontics.

Bibliography

1. Ajeti MSN, Hoxha SV, Elezi SX, et al. Demineralization of root canal dentine with EDTA and citric acid in different concentrations, pH and application times. ILIRIA Int Rev 2011;1(2).
2. Buyukyilmaz T, Ogaard B, Rolla G. The resistance of titanium tetrafluoride treated human enamel to strong hydrochloric acid. Eur J Oral Sci 1997;105:473–7.
3. Chavez de Paz LE. Redefining the persistent infection in root canals: Possible role of biofilm communities. J Endod 2007;33:652–62.
4. Chávez de Paz LE, Bergenholtz G, Svensäter G. The effects of antimicrobials on endodontic biofilm bacteria. J Endod 2010;36:70–7
5. Distel JW, Hatton JF, Gillespie MJ. Biofilm formation in medicated root canals. J Endod 2002;28:689–93.
6. Donlan RM, Costerton JW. Biofilms: survival mechanisms of clinically relevant microorganisms. Clin Microbiol Rev 2002;15:167–93.

7. Donlan RM, Costerton JW. Biofilms: Survival mechanisms of clinically relevant microorganisms. Clin Microbiol Rev 2002;15:167–93.

8. Galvan DA, Ciarlone AE, Pashley DH, et al. Effect of smear layer removal on the diffusion permeability of human roots. J Endod 1994;20(2):83–6.

9. Gencoglu N, Samani S, Gunday M. Dentinal wall adaptation of thermoplasticized gutta-percha in the absence or presence of smear layer: a scanning electron microscopic study. J Endod 1933;19:558–62.

10. Gencoglu N, Samani S, Gunday M. Evaluation of sealing properties of Thermafil and Ultrafil techniques in the absence or presence of smear layer. J Endod 1992;19:599–603.

11. Hargreaves KM, Cohen S. Pathways of the pulp. 10th ed. Mosby: Elsevier; 2012.

12. Ingle JI, Bakland LK, Decker BC. Endodontics. 6th ed. Elsevier; 2008.

13. Kishen A, Haapasalo M. Biofilm models and methods of biofilm assessment. Endod Topics 2010;22:58–78.

14. Kishen A. Advanced therapeutic options for endodontic biofilms. Endod Topics 2010;22:99–123.

15. Kishen A. Advanced therapeutic options for endodontic biofilms. Endo Topics 2012;22:99–123.

16. Lester KS, Boyde A. scanning electron microscopy of instrumented, irrigated, filled root canals. Brit Dent J 1977;43:359.

17. Mader CL, Baumgartener JC, Donald DP. Scanning electron microscope investigations of the smeared layer on root canal walls. J Endod 1984;10:477–83.

18. Sahar-Helft S, Stabholtz A. Rermoving smear layer during endodontic treatment by different techniques - a invitro study. A clinical case - Endodontic treatment with Er:YAG Laser. Stoma Edu J 2016;3(2):162–7.

19. Serper A, Calt S. The demineralizing effects of EDTA at different concentrations and pH. J Endod 2002;28(7):501–2.

20. Shahravan A, Haghdoost AA, Adl A, et al. Effect of smear layer on sealing ability of canal obturation: A systematic review and meta-analysis. J Endod 2007;33(2):96–105.

21. Shehadat SA. Smear layer in endodontics: role and management. J Clin Dent Oral Health 2017;1:1–2.

22. Siqueira JF, Jr, Rôças IN. Exploiting molecular methods to explore endodontic infections: Part 2-Redefining the endodontic microbiota. J Endod. 2005;31:488–98.

23. Svensater G, Bergerholtz G. Biofilms in endodontic infections. Endo Topics 2004;9:27–36.

24. Usha HL, Kaiwar A, Mehta D. Biofilm in endodontics: New understanding to an old problem. Int J Contem Dent 2010;1:44–51.

25. Vallabhaneni K, Kakarla P, Avula SSJ, et al. Comparative analyses of smear layer removal using four different irrigant solutions in the primary root canals–A scanning electron microscopic study. J Clin Diagn Res 2017;11(4):ZC64.

26. Violich DR, Chandler NP. The smear layer in endodontics - A review. Int Endod J 2010;43(1):2–15.

27. White RR, Goldman M, Lin RS. The influence of the smeared layer upon dentinal tubule penetration by plastic filling materials. J Endod 1984;10:558–62.

Rationale of Endodontic Treatment

Endodontic pathology is mainly caused by injury to the tooth which can be physical, chemical, or bacterial. Such injury can result in reversible or irreversible changes in the pulp and periradicular tissues. These resultant changes depend on the intensity, duration, pathogenicity of the stimulus, and the host defense mechanism. The changes that occur are mediated by a series of inflammatory and immunological reactions (in the vascular, lymphatic, and connective tissues). All these reactions take place to eliminate the irritant and repair any damage. However, certain conditions are beyond the reparative ability of the body and need to be treated endodontically to aid the survival of tooth. Rationale of endodontic therapy is complete debridement of root canal system followed by three-dimensional obturation.

Theories of Spread of Infection

Focus of infection
It refers to a circumscribed area of tissue, which is infected with exogenous pathogenic microorganisms and is usually located near a mucous or cutaneous surface.

Focal infection
It is localized or general infection caused by the dissemination of microorganisms or toxic products from a focus of infection.

Mechanism of Focal Infection

Two most accepted mechanisms considered responsible for initiation of focal infection are

1. Metastasis of microorganisms from infected focus by either hematogenous or lymphogenous spread
2. Carrying of toxins or toxic by-products through blood stream and lymphatic channel to site where they may initiate a hypersensitive reaction in tissues

For example, in scarlet fever, erythrogenic toxin liberated by infected streptococci is responsible for cutaneous features of this disease.

Oral Foci of Infection

Possible sources of infection in oral cavity which may later on set up distant metastasis are
- Infected periapical lesions such as
  - Periapical granuloma
  - Periapical abscess
  - Periapical cyst
- Teeth with infected root canals
- Periodontal diseases with special reference to tooth extraction

Culprit of Endodontic Pathology

Many studies have shown that root canal infections are multibacterial in nature. In 1965, Kakehashi found that when dental pulps of conventional and germ-free rats were exposed to their own oral microbial flora, the conventional rats showed pulpal and periapical lesions, whereas the germ-free rats did not show any development of lesion.

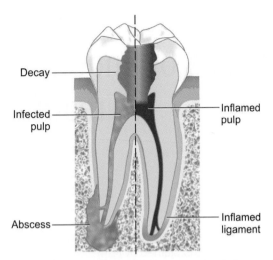

Fig. 6.1 Line diagram showing bacteria causing inflammation and infection of pulp.

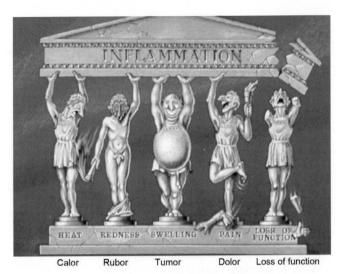

Fig. 6.2 Signs of inflammation.

So he described importance of microorganisms for the development of pulpal and periapical pathologies.

Portals for Entry of Microorganisms

❑ Dental caries (most common route) (**Fig. 6.1**)
❑ Open dentinal tubules
❑ Accessory and lateral canals which connect pulp and periodontium
❑ Through defective restorations with marginal leakage
❑ Anachoresis (microorganisms are transported in blood to an area of inflammation where they establish an infection).

▌Inflammation

Inflammation is defined as a local physiological response of living tissue to an irritant or injury. Objective of inflammation is to limit the spread or eliminate the irritant and repair damage to the tissues. Inflammation can result from
❑ Physical agents like cold, heat, mechanical trauma, or radiation
❑ Chemical agents like organic and inorganic poisons
❑ Infective agents like bacteria, viruses, and their toxins
❑ Immunological agents like antigen–antibody cell-mediated reactions.

Signs of Inflammation

Roman writer Celsus in 1st century AD gave the following four cardinal signs of inflammation (Celsus Tetrad):
1. Rubor (redness)
2. Tumor (swelling due to filtration of macromolecules and fluids in affected area)
3. Calor, i.e., Heat (due to vasodilatation and blood inflow in affected area)
4. Dolor (pain due to effect of cytotoxic agents on nerve endings)

Virchow later added the fifth sign function lasea (loss of function due to changes in affected tissue) (**Fig. 6.2**).

Types of Inflammation

❑ Acute inflammation (dominated by polymorphonuclear neutrophils and macrophages)
❑ Chronic inflammation (dominated by lymphocytes, macrophages, and plasma cells)

Tissue Changes Following Inflammation

Two types of tissue changes are seen following inflammation:
1. ***Degenerative changes*** in the pulp can be
   a. Fibrous
   b. Resorptive
   c. Calcific
      • Continuous degeneration of tissue can cause thrombosis of blood vessels resulting in necrosis
      • Suppuration is another form of degeneration which can occur due to injury to polymorphonuclear cells. This injury causes release of proteolytic enzymes, resulting in liquefaction of dead tissues leading to suppuration
      • Proteolytic enzymes digest not only leukocytes but also adjacent dead tissue. An abscess can result even in absence of microorganisms because of chemical or physical irritation. For example, sterile abscess is formed in absence of microorganisms
      • If irritant is weak and reaction is not great, serous exudate is formed consisting of serum, lymph, and fibrin

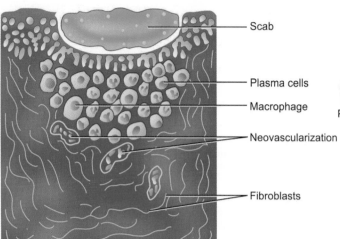

Fig. 6.3 Inflammatory cells present at the healing site. Note that in center of the inflamed area plasma cells and macrophages are seen, whereas at the periphery, proliferation or repair cells, i.e. fibroblasts are predominant.

Three requisites necessary for suppuration are
- Tissue necrosis
- Presence of polymorphonuclear leukocytes (PMNLs)
- Digestion of the necrotic material by proteolytic enzymes released by injured polymorphonuclear cells

2. ***Proliferative changes (Fig. 6.3)***
   - Proliferative changes are produced by irritants mild enough to act as stimulants. These irritants may act as both irritant and stimulant, for example, Calcium hydroxide
   - In center of the inflamed area, the irritant may be strong enough to produce degeneration or destruction, whereas at the periphery, irritant may be mild enough to stimulate proliferation
   - Principal cells of proliferation or repair are the fibroblasts, which lay down cellular fibrous tissues
   - In some cases, collagen fibers are substituted by a dense acellular tissue. In either case, it results in formation of fibrous tissue. Destroyed bone may also be replaced by formation of fibrous tissue

Inflammatory Cells (Figs. 6.4 and 6.5)

Neutrophils

- ❏ Along with basophils and eosinophils, polymorphonuclear (PMN) neutrophils are called granulocytes because of presence of granules in the cytoplasm
- ❏ These are the first cells to migrate from vessels to site of inflammation
- ❏ These are attracted to inflammatory site because of chemotactic factors produced by bacteria or by

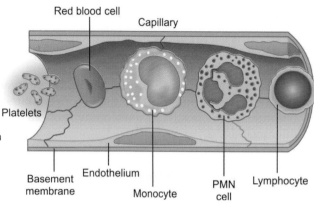

Fig. 6.4 Inflammatory cells
Abbreviation: PMN: polymorphonuclear.

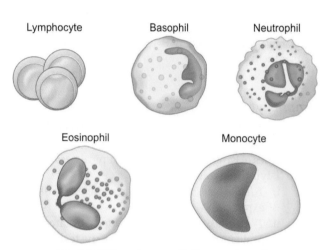

Fig. 6.5 Different types of inflammatory cells.

complement. For bacteria to be recognized, they must be coated in opsonins, and the process is called antibody opsonization
- ❏ Neutrophils engulf and kill bacteria by forming phagosome into which hydrolytic enzymes and reactive oxygen species are secreted
- ❏ Production of enzymes and lactic acid during phagocytosis lowers the tissue fluid pH to 6.5. It results in death of PMNs and thus release of proteolytic enzymes (pepsin and cathepsin), prostaglandins (PGs), and leukotrienes (LTs)
- ❏ All these changes result in breakdown of the tissue and, thus, formation of an abscess (dead PMNs and debris).

Eosinophils

Eosinophils have many functional and structural similarities with neutrophils like their formation in bone marrow, phagocytosis, presence of granules in the cytoplasm, bactericidal and toxic action against many parasites.

Macrophages

- ❑ When PMNs fail to remove bacteria, circulating mono-cytes reach the site of inflammation and change into macrophages
- ❑ These macrophages are slow moving and remain at site of inflammation for longer time (approximately 2 months). This results in development of chronic inflammation

Macrophages perform the following functions:
- Help in phagocytosis and pinocytosis
- Perform immunological function
- Secrete lysosomal enzymes
- Secrete complement protein and PGs
- Provide antigen to the immunocomplement cells
- Act as scavenger of dead cells, tissues, and foreign bodies
- Fuses with other macrophages to produce multinucleated giant cells like osteoclasts, dentinoclasts, and foreign body giant cells

Lymphocytes

- ❑ These are the most numerous cells (20%–45%) after neutrophils
- ❑ Two types of lymphocytes are seen in apical periodontitis:
    - a. **T-lymphocytes**
        - i. *T-helper cells:* Present in the acute phase of lesion expansion
        - ii. *T–suppressor cells:* Predominate in later stages preventing rapid expansion of the lesion
    - b. **B-lymphocytes:** On getting signals from antigens and T-helper cells, they transform into plasma cells and secrete antibodies. Their number increases in hypersensitivity state and prolonged infection with immunological response

Osteoclasts

- ❑ In physiologic state, preosteoclasts remain dormant as monocytes in periradicular bone. During apical periodontitis, they proliferate and fuse on stimulation by cytokines and other mediators to form osteoclasts
- ❑ These osteoclasts are responsible for demineralization of the bone and enzymatic dissolution of organic matrix at the osteoclast–bone interface. This results in bone resorption

Epithelial Cells

- ❑ Cytokines and other mediators stimulate the dormant cell rests of Malassez
- ❑ These cells undergo division and proliferation which results in inflammatory hyperplasia

Nonspecific Mediators of Periradicular Lesions (Flowchart 6.1)

Flowchart 6.1 Types of nonspecific mediators.

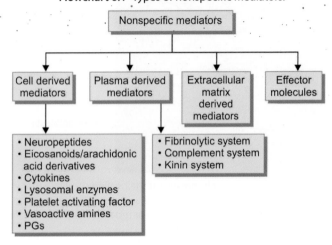

Cell-Derived Mediators (Flowchart 6.2)

Neuropeptides

- ❑ These are produced following tissue injury by the soma-tosensory and autonomic nerve fibers. These include:
    - **Substance P (SP):** Causes vasodilatation, increased vascular permeability and blood flow
    - **Calcitonin-gene-related peptide (CGRP):** Causes vasodilatation

Eicosanoids

Injury to cells releases membrane phospholipid, arachidonic acid which is metabolized by either cyclooxygenase pathway or lipo-oxygenase pathway to form PGs or LTs, respectively. These PGs and LTs involve in inflammatory process.
- ❑ *PGs* like PGE_2, PGD_2, PGF_{2a}, PGI_2 are commonly found in inflammatory lesions
- ❑ *LTs* like LTB4, LTC4, LTD4, and LTE4 are commonly found in periradicular lesions **(Flowchart 6.3)**

Cytokines

- ❑ These are low molecular weight polypeptides secreted by activated structural and hematopoietic cells. Different cytokines like interleukins and tumor necrosis factor (TNF) cause development and perpetuation of per-iradicular lesions
    - **Proinflammatory cytokines**
        - **IL1:** Effects of IL1 are
            - Enhance leukocyte adhesion to endothelial walls
            - Stimulate PMNLs and lymphocytes

Flowchart 6.2   Cell-derived mediators.

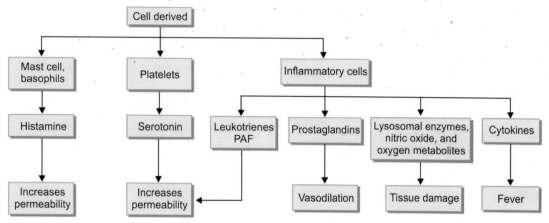

Abbreviation: PAF: platelet activating factor

Flowchart 6.3   Leukotrienes.

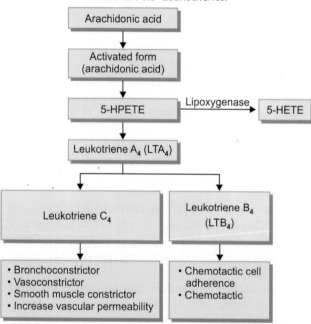

Abbreviations: 5-HPETE: 5-hydroperoxyeicosatetraenoic acid;
5-HETE: 5-hydroxyeicosatetraenoic acid

- ◆ Activate production of PGs and proteolytic enzymes
- ◆ Increase bone resorption
- ◆ Inhibit bone formation
- ◆ IL1β is predominant in cases of periapical pathology
- – **IL6:** It is secreted by lymphoid and nonlymphoid cells and causes inflammation under the influence of IL1, TNFα, and interferon γ (IFN). It is seen in periapical lesions

- – **IL8:** It is produced by macrophages and fibroblasts under the influence of IL1β and TNFα and is associated with acute apical periodontitis
- • **Chemotactic cytokines**
  - – **TNF:** It is seen in chronic lesions associated with cytotoxic and debilitating effect. TNFα is seen in chronic apical lesions and root canal exudates
  - – **Colony stimulating factor (CSF):** They are produced by osteoblasts and regulate the proliferation of PMNLs and preosteoclasts
  - – **Growth factors (GFs):** These are the proteins produced by normal and neoplastic cells that regulate the growth and differentiation of non-hematopoietic cells. They can transform a normal cells to neoplastic cells and are known as transforming GFs (TGF)

    Two types of GFs:

    i. TGFα (produced by malignant cells)—not seen in periapical lesions

    ii. TGFβ (produced by normal cells and platelets)

    They counter the adverse effects of inflammatory host response by
    - ◆ Activating macrophages
    - ◆ Proliferation of fibroblasts
    - ◆ Synthesis of connective tissue fibers and matrices

Lysosomal Enzymes

Lysosomal enzymes such as alkaline phosphatase, lysozyme, peroxidases, and collagenase cause increase in vascular permeability, leukocytic chemotaxis, bradykinin formation, and activation of complement system.

Platelet Activating Factor

❑ It is released from IgE sensitized basophils or mast cells
❑ It causes increase in vascular permeability, chemotaxis, adhesion of leukocytes to endothelium and bronchoconstriction

Vasoactive Amines

❑ Vasoactive amines such as histamine and serotonin are present in mast cells, basophils, and platelets
❑ They cause increase in tissue permeability, vasodilation, and vascular permeability

Prostaglandins

❑ These are produced by activation of cyclo-oxygenase pathway of arachidonic acid metabolism **(Flowchart 6.2)**
❑ Periradicular lesions show presence of high levels of PGE_2. Torbinejad et al. found that periradicular bone resorption can be inhibited by administration of indomethacin, an antagonist of PGs

Plasma Derived Mediators (Flowchart 6.4)

Fibrinolytic System

❑ Fibrinolytic system is activated by Hageman factor which causes activation of plasminogen
❑ This results in release of fibrinopeptides and fibrin degradation products which cause increase in vascular permeability and leukocytic chemotaxis

Complement System

Trauma to periapex can result in activation of kinin system which in turn activates complement system.

Kinin System

❑ These are produced by proteolytic cleavage of kininogen
❑ Release of kinins cause smooth muscle contraction, vasodilation and increase in vascular permeability **(Flowchart 6.5)**.

Flowchart 6.4 Plasma-derived mediators.

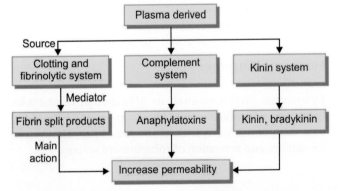

Flowchart 6.5 Kinin system.

Effector Molecules

Inflammatory process in periradicular pathosis causes destruction of cells and degradation of extracellular matrix by enzymatic effector molecules produced in the following pathways like:
❑ Osteoclast-regulated pathway
❑ Phagocyte-regulated pathway
❑ Plasminogen-regulated pathway
❑ Metalloenzyme-regulated pathway [matrix metalloproteinases (MMPs)]

Collagen (proteins) based matrices are degraded by MMPs.

Antibodies (Specific Mediators of Immune Reactions)

These are produced by plasma cells and are of two types:
1. **Polyclonal antibodies** are nonspecific like IgE mediated reactions which interact with antigen resulting in release of certain chemical mediators like histamine or serotonin
2. **Monoclonal antibodies**, like IgG and IgM, interact with bacteria and their by-products to form antigen–antibody complexes that bind to platelets resulting in release of vasoactive amines which increase vascular permeability and chemotaxis of PMNs. Monoclonal antibodies exhibit antimicrobial effect
   a. In acute abscess, the complex enters the systemic circulation. The concentration of these complexes return to normal levels after endodontic treatment
   b. In chronic lesions, the Ag–Ab complexes are confined within the lesion and do not enter into the systemic circulation

Role of Immunity in Endodontics

Immune system of human being is a complex system consisting of cells, tissues, organs as well as molecular mediators that act together to maintain the health and well-being of the individual. Cells and microbial irritants interact with each other through number of molecular mediators and cell surface receptors resulting in defense reactions.

Immunity is of two types:
1. Innate immunity
2. Acquired/adaptive immunity

Innate Immunity

❑ Innate immunity is responsible for the initial nonspecific reactions
❑ It consists of cells and molecular elements which act as barriers to prevent dissemination of bacteria and bacterial products into the underlying connective tissue
❑ Cells providing innate immunity are neutrophils, monocytes, eosinophils, basophils, NK cells, dendritic cells, and odontoblasts

Acquired/Adaptive Immunity

❑ It involves release of specific receptor molecules by lymphocytes which recognize and bind to foreign antigens
❑ Adaptive immunity is provided by
  • T lymphocytes that release T-cell antigen receptors
  • B lymphocytes that release B-cell antigen receptors or immunoglobulins

Histopathology of Periapical Tissue Response to Various Irritants (Fig. 6.6)

Root canal of teeth contains various irritants because of pathologic changes in pulp. Penetration of these irritants from infected root canals into periapical area can lead to formation and perpetuation of periradicular lesions. Periradicular tissue has unlimited source of undifferentiated cells which can participate in inflammation and repair. Depending upon severity and duration of irritant, host response to periradicular pathosis may range from slight inflammation to extensive tissue destruction. Reactions involved are highly complex and are usually mediated by nonspecific and specific mediators of inflammation.

Endodontic Implications (Pathogenesis of Apical Periodontitis as Explained by Fish) (Fig. 6.7)

Fish described reaction of periradicular tissues to bacterial products, noxious products of tissue necrosis, and antigenic agents from the root canal. He established an experimental focus of infection in the guinea pigs by drilling openings in the jaw bone and packing it with wool fibers saturated with a broth culture of microorganisms. Fish in 1939 said that the zones of infection are not an infection by themselves but the reaction of the body to infection. Thus he concluded that the removal of this nidus of infection will result in resolution of infection.

Four well-defined zones of reaction were found during the experiment (Fig. 6.7):
1. Zone of infection (PMN and microorganisms)
2. Zone of contamination (round cells, lymphocytes, and toxins)
3. Zone of irritation (macrophages, histiocytes and osteoclasts)
4. Zone of stimulation (fibroblasts, osteoblasts, and collagen fibers)

Zone of Infection

❑ In Fish's study, infection was confined to center of the lesion and microorganisms were confined to that area only

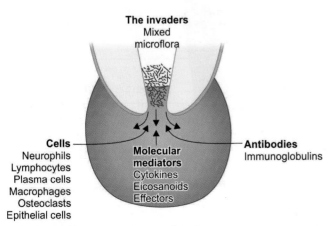

Fig. 6.6 Schematic representation of inflammatory response of periradicular area to root canal irritants.

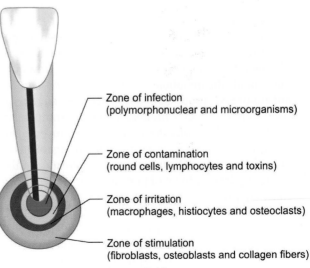

Fig. 6.7 Fish's zones.

❑ This zone is characterized by polymorphonuclear leukocytes and microorganisms along with the necrotic cells and destructive components released from phagocytes

❑ Microorganisms which are not destroyed by PMNs enter in Haversian canals or in bone matrix during drilling in bone.

Zone of Contamination

❑ Around the central zone, Fish observed the area of cellular destruction

❑ This zone was not invaded by bacteria, but destruction was due to toxins discharged from microorganisms in central zone

❑ Round cell infiltration, lymphocytes, osteocyte necrosis, and empty lacunae were found in this zone

Zone of Irritation

❑ It is found away from the central lesion because toxins get more diluted

❑ This zone is characterized by macrophage, histiocytes, and osteoclasts. Degradation of collagen framework by phagocytic cells and macrophages, osteoclasts attacking the bone tissue is found

❑ Histologic picture simulates body's attempt to repair

Zone of Stimulation

❑ It is found at the periphery, because toxins are mild enough to act as stimulant

❑ In response to this stimulation, fibroblasts and osteoblasts secrete collagen fibers

❑ These collagen fibers act as wall of defense around the zone of irritation and as a scaffolding on which the osteoblasts synthesize new bone

Knowledge gained from Fish study can be applied for better understanding of reaction of periradicular tissues to a nonvital tooth. Root canal is the main source of infection. Microorganisms present in root canal are rarely motile. Though they do not move from the root canal to the periapical tissues, they can proliferate sufficiently to grow out of the root canal. The metabolic by-products of these microorganisms or toxic products of tissue necrosis may also get diffused to periradicular tissues. As the microorganisms enter in the periradicular area, they are destroyed by the polymorphonuclear leukocytes. But if microorganisms are highly virulent, they overpower the defensive mechanism and result in development of periradicular lesion.

Toxic by-products of microorganisms and necrotic pulp in the root canal are irritating and destructive to the periradicular tissues. These irritants along with proteolytic enzymes (released by the dead polymorphonuclear leukocytes) result in the formation of pus. This results in development of chronic abscess.

At the periphery of the destroyed area of osseous tissue, toxic bacterial products get diluted sufficiently to act as stimulant. This results in formation of a granuloma.

After this, fibroblasts come in play and build fibrous tissue, osteoblasts restrict the area by formation of sclerotic bone. Along with these if epithelial rests of Malassez are also stimulated, it results in formation of a cyst.

Kronfeld's Mountain Pass Theory (1939) (Figs. 6.8 and 6.9)

Kronfeld gave mountain pass concept in 1939 to understand the close relationship between pulp and periodontium. He employed Fish concept to explain the tissue reaction in and around the granulomatous area.

Zone A

Kronfeld compared the bacteria in the infected root canal with the army of enemies embedded behind "high and inaccessible mountains." The apical foramen serves as mountain passes.

Zone B

Army tries to descend through mountain pass to invade into plains (periradicular tissue) beyond mountain pass.

Another army in plains takes care of the invaders. By forming trenches and reinforcement in form of acute and chronic inflammatory cells it tries to block advances of enemies. These defenders are white blood cells and other cells of granulomatous tissue. This corresponds to the accumulation of white blood cells near root apex.

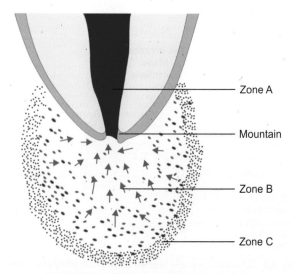

Fig. 6.8 Kronfeld's mountain pass theory.

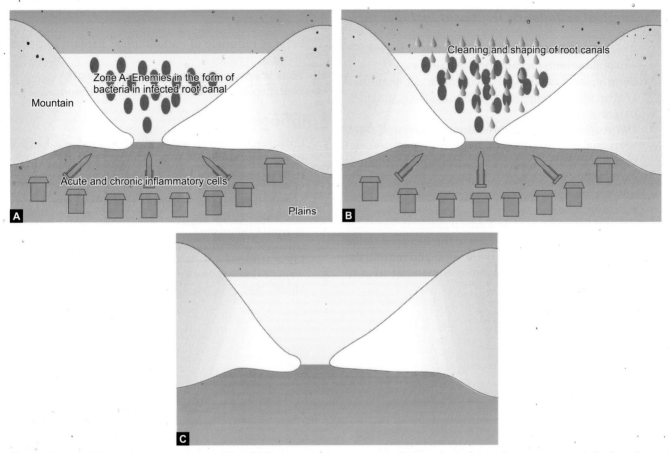

Figs. 6.9A to C Schematic representation of Kronfeld's mountain pass concept; (A) Enemies in form of microorganisms of infected root canals need pass to enter the plains which is guarded by soldiers in form of acute and chronic inflammatory cells; (B) Cleaning and shaping of root canals neutralize the enemies by attacking from behind; (C) If enemies are eliminated by the attack, soldiers are not required. But if mass attack of invaders occur, battle between invaders and soldiers result in acute inflammation. If few invaders enter the plain, they are destroyed by soldiers.

When a few invaders enter the plain through mountain pass, they are destroyed by the defenders (leukocytes). A mass attack of invaders results in a major battle, analogous to acute inflammation.

Zone C

Between the battle of invaders and defenders, if bacteria win and invade the plains, it results in septicemia or acute alveolar abscess or they may get destroyed by defenders. Only complete elimination of invaders from their mountainous entrenchment eliminates the need for a defense forces in "plains." Once this is accomplished, the defending army of leukocytes withdraws, local destruction created by battle is repaired (granulation tissue), and the environment returns to its normal pattern.

This explains the rationale for the nonsurgical endodontic treatment for teeth with periapical infection. Complete elimination of pathogenic irritants from canal followed by

three-dimensional fluid impervious obturation will result in complete healing of periapical area.

▌Rationale of Endodontic Therapy

Rationale of root canal treatment relies on the fact that nonvital pulp, being avascular, has no defense mechanisms. Affected tissues within root canal undergoes autolysis and resulting break down products diffuse into the surrounding tissues causing periapical irritation associated with the portals of exit even in absence of bacterial contamination. Therefore, endodontic therapy must seal the root canal system three-dimensionally so as to prevent tissue fluids from percolating in the root canal and toxic by-products from both necrotic tissue and microorganisms regressing into the periradicular tissues.

Endodontic therapy includes:
❑ Nonsurgical endodontic treatment
❑ Surgical endodontic treatment

Nonsurgical endodontic treatment includes three phases:

1. ***Access preparation:*** Rationale for this is to create a straight line path for canal orifice and apex
2. ***Shaping and cleaning:*** For complete elimination of vital or necrotic pulp tissue, microorganisms, and their by-products.
3. ***Obturation:*** To have a three-dimensional well-fitted root canal with fluid tight seal so as to prevent percolation and microleakage of periapical exudate into root canal space and to prevent infection by completely obliterating the apical foramen and other portals of communication.

Rationale of surgical endodontic treatment: Rationale of surgical endodontics is to remove the diseased tissue present in the canal and around the apex, and retrofill the root canal space with biologically inert material so as to achieve a fluid tight seal.

Questions

1. What is rationale of endodontics? Explain in detail about Fish zones.
2. What is Kronfeld's mountain pass concept?
3. Explain pathophysiology of periapical lesion.

Bibliography

1. Grossman LI, Oliet FS and DelRio CE. Endodontic Practice (11th Edition) Lea and Febiger; 1988.
2. Hargreaves KM, Cohen S. Pathways of the pulp. 10th edition Mosby: Elsevier; 2012.
3. Ingle JI, Bakland LK, Decker BC. Endodontics. 6th edition Elsevier; 2008.
4. Ricucci D, Langeland K. Apical limit of root canal instrumentation and obturation, part 2. A histological study. Int Endod J 1998;31(6):394-409.
5. Weine F. Endodontic Therapy. 3rd edition St. Louis: CV Mosby; 1982.

Diagnostic Procedures

Diagnosis is defined as utilization of scientific knowledge for identifying a diseased process and to differentiate from other disease process.

It is the procedure of accepting a patient, recognizing his/her problem, finding the cause, and planning the treatment which would solve the problem.

Diagnostic process actually consists of **four steps:**

1. **First step:** Assemble all the available facts gathered from chief complaint, medical and dental history, diagnostic tests, and investigations
2. **Second step:** Analyze and interpret the assembled clues to reach the tentative or provisional diagnosis
3. **Third step:** Make differential diagnosis of all possible diseases which are consistent with signs, symptoms, and test results collected
4. **Fourth step:** Select the closest possible choice

The importance of making an accurate diagnosis cannot be overlooked. To avoid irrelevant information and to prevent errors of omission in clinical tests, the clinician should establish a routine for examination, consisting of chief complaint, past medical and dental history, and any other relevant information in the form of case history.

Case History

The purpose of case history is to know whether patient has any general or local condition that might alter the treatment plan.

Chief Complaint

It consists of information which encourages the patient to visit a clinician. It should be noted in patient's own words. After recording chief complaint, history of present illness is recorded. History tells severity and urgency of the treatment.

Symptoms

Symptoms are defined as signs of deviation from the normal. Symptoms can be subjective and objective.

Subjective Symptoms

Subjective symptoms are perceived by the patient only and not evident to the examiner. Most common subjective symptom is pain. One should ask about following questions regarding pain:

- **Quality:** Dull, sharp, throbbing, constant
- **Location:** Localized, diffuse, referred, radiating
- **Duration:** Constant or intermittent lasting for seconds, minutes or hours
- **Onset:** Stimulation required, intermittent, spontaneous
- **Initiated:** Cold, heat, palpation, percussion
- **Relieved:** Cold, heat, any medications, sleep

If a chief complaint is toothache but symptoms are too vague to establish a diagnosis, then analgesics should be

	Type of pain	Reason for pain	Provisional diagnosis
Location	• Localized pain	Presence of proprioceptive A-β fibers present in periodontal ligament	• Periodontal pain
	• Diffuse pain	Lack of proprioceptive fibers in pulp	• Pulpal pain
Duration	• Momentary pain on stimulation		• Reversible pulpitis
	• Spontaneous pain for long duration		• Irreversible pulpitis
Nature	• Sharp shooting momentary pain on applying stimulus	Stimulation of Aδ fibers because of movement of dentinal fluid present in odontoblastic processes	• Dentinal pain • Reversible pulpitis
	• Sharp shooting pain on mastication		• Irreversible pulpitis • Fracture of tooth
	• Spontaneous dull, throbbing pain for long duration	Stimulation of C-fibers	• Irreversible pulpitis
Stimulus	• Sweet and sour	Due to stimulation of Aδ fibers present in odontoblastic processes	• Reversible pulpitis
	• Heat	Vasodilatation caused by heat stimulates C-fibers of pulp	• Irreversible pulpitis
	• Cold	Stimulation of Aδ fibers due to fluid movement in odontoblastic processes	• Dentin hypersensitivity
	• Heat and cold		• Early stages of irreversible pulpitis
	• Stimulated by heat and relieved by cold		• Late stages of irreversible pulpitis
	• On lying down or sleep		• Acute irreversible pulpitis

prescribed to help the patient in tolerating the pain until the toothache localizes. A history of pain which persists without exacerbation may indicate problem of nonodontogenic origins.

Pulpal pain can be sharp, piercing, and lancinating. It is due to stimulation of Aδ fibers. Dull, boring, excruciating, or throbbing pain occurs if there is stimulation of C-fibers. Pulp vitality tests are usually done to reach the most probable diagnosis. If pain is from periodontal ligament, the tooth will be sensitive to percussion, chewing, and palpation. Localization of pain also tells origin of pain since pulp does not contain proprioceptive fibers; it is difficult for patient to localize the pain unless it involves the periodontal ligament.

Medical History

There are no medical conditions which specifically contraindicate endodontic treatment, but there are several which require special care. **Scully and Cawson** have given a checklist of medical conditions which are needed to be taken a special care.

Checklist for medical history (Scully and Cawson)
- **A**nemia
- **B**leeding disorders
- **C**ardiorespiratory disorders
- **D**rug treatment and allergies
- **E**ndocrine disease
- **F**its and faints
- **G**astrointestinal disorders
- **H**ospital admissions and attendance
- **I**nfections
- **J**aundice
- **K**idney disease
- **L**ikelihood of pregnancy or pregnant itself

If there is any doubt regarding state of health of patient, consult medical practitioner before initiating endodontic treatment. Care should also be taken whether patient is on medication such as corticosteroids or anticoagulant therapy. According to standards of American Heart Association, patient should be given antibiotic prophylaxis if there is high risk of developing bacterial endocarditis for example, in patients with prosthetic cardiac valves, history of infective endocarditis, cardiac transplant, congenital heart disease, etc.

Objective Findings

Subjective findings are obtained by questioning and performing tests on the basis of patient's symptoms. Following examination and tests should be performed by clinician to get objective findings:

- Visual and tactile inspection
- Percussion test
- Palpation
- Periodontal examination
- Differential diagnosis
- Radiographs
- Pulp vitality tests

Visual and Tactile Inspection

Before conducting intraoral examination, check the degree of mouth opening. For a normal patient, it should be at least two fingers **(Fig. 7.1)**. During intraoral examination, look at the following structures systematically:

- Buccal, labial, and alveolar mucosa
- Hard and soft palate
- Floor of the mouth and tongue
- Retromolar region
- Posterior pharyngeal wall and faucial pillars
- Salivary glands

After examining this, general dental state should be recorded, which include

- Oral hygiene status
- Amount and quality of restorative work
- Prevalence of caries
- Missing tooth
- Presence of soft or hard swelling
- Periodontal status
- Presence of any sinus tracts
- Discolored teeth
- Tooth wear and facets **(Fig. 7.2)**

Percussion Test

Percussion test helps to evaluate the status of periodontium surrounding a tooth. Pain on percussion indicates inflammation in periodontal ligament which could be due to trauma, sinusitis, and/or periodontal (PDL) disease.

Percussion can be carried out by gentle tapping with gloved finger **(Fig. 7.3)** or blunt handle of mouth mirror **(Fig. 7.4)**. Each tooth should be percussed on all the surfaces of tooth until the patient is able to localize the tooth with pain.

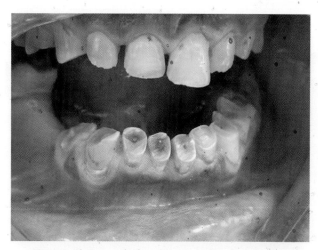

Fig. 7.2 Photograph showing generalized tooth wear.

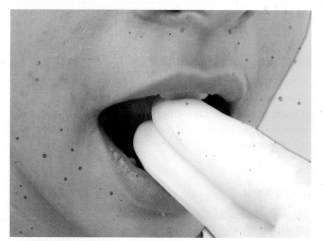

Fig. 7.1 Degree of mouth opening in a normal patient should be at least two fingers.

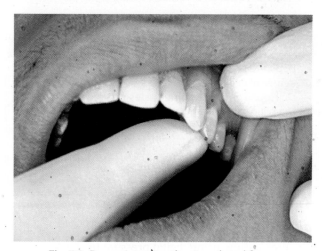

Fig. 7.3 Percussion of tooth using gloved finger.

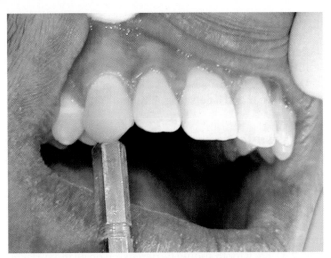

Fig. 7.4 Percussion of tooth using blunt handle of mouth mirror.

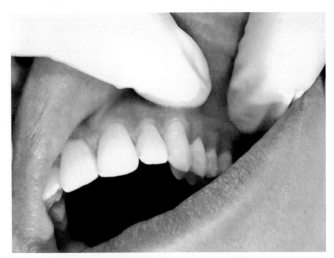

Fig. 7.5 Palpation of soft tissue using digital pressure.

POINTS TO REMEMBER

- Degree of response to percussion is directly proportional to degree of inflammation
- Dull sound on percussion indicates abscess formation while sharp indicates inflammation
- Pain on percussion is indicative of possibility of following conditions:
  - Periodontal abscess
  - Pulp necrosis (partial or total)
  - High points in restorations

Palpation

Palpation is done using digital pressure to check any tenderness in soft tissue overlying suspected tooth **(Fig. 7.5)**. Sensitivity may indicate inflammation in periodontal tissues surrounding the affected tooth. Further palpation can

tell any other information about fluctuation or fixation or induration of soft tissue, if any.

If any localized swelling is present, then look for
- Local rise in temperature
- Tenderness
- Extent of lesion
- Induration
- Fixation to underlying tissues, etc.

Provisional diagnosis after examination of lymph nodes	
Examination	*Provisional diagnosis*
Enlargement of submental lymph nodes	Infection of anterior teeth
Involvement of submandibular lymph nodes	Mandibular molar infection
Enlargement of lymph nodes at angle of mandible	May indicate tonsillar infection
Firm and tender palpable lymph nodes associated with fever and swelling	Acute infection
Palpable lymph node not associated with pain	Chronic infection
Hard-fixed lymph node with stone-like consistency	Malignancy
Matted, nontender lymph nodes	Tuberculosis

Periodontal Examination

It can be assessed from palpation, percussion, mobility of tooth, and probing. Mobility of a tooth is tested by placing a finger **(Fig. 7.6)** or blunt end of the instrument **(Fig. 7.7)** on either side of the crown and pushing it and assessing any movement with other finger.

Miller Tooth Mobility Index

☐ Grade I: Distinguishable sign of tooth movement more than normal
☐ Grade II: Horizontal tooth movement not >1 mm
☐ Grade III: Movement of tooth >1 mm or when tooth can be depressed.

Radiograph

A good radiograph helps in diagnosing and treatment planning. But it should be kept in mind that it is a two-dimensional picture of a three-dimensional object. Though it has many limitations, an appropriately taken and processed radiograph can give enough information to aid in diagnosis. A perfect periapical radiograph must have adequate contrast with minimal processing error. It should include

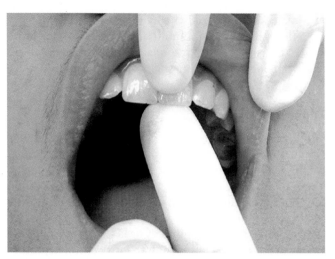

Fig. 7.6 Checking mobility of a tooth by palpating with fingers.

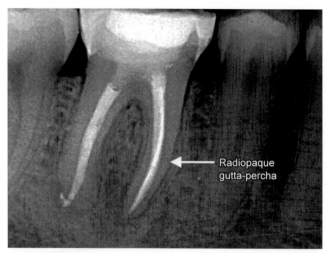

Radiopaque
gutta-percha

Fig. 7.8 Radiograph showing obturation in mandibular first molar.

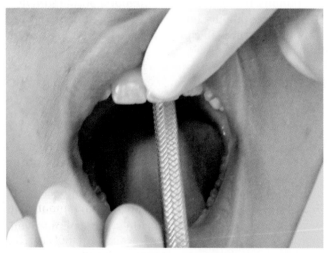

Fig. 7.7 Checking mobility of a tooth using blunt end of instrument.

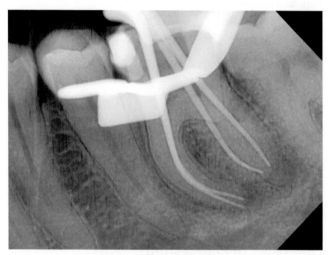

Fig. 7.9 Master cone radiograph.

minimum of 3 mm of adjacent periapical area so as to have accurate assessment of the target tooth.

Radiographs help us in following ways:

❑ Establishing diagnosis
❑ Determining the prognosis of tooth
❑ Disclosing the presence and extent of caries
❑ Check the thickness of periodontal ligament
❑ To see continuity of lamina dura
❑ To look for any periodontal lesion associated with tooth
❑ To see the number, shape, length, and pattern of the root canals
❑ To check any obstructions present in the pulp space
❑ To check any previous root canal treatment if done **(Fig. 7.8)**
❑ To look for presence of any intraradicular pins or posts
❑ To see the quality of previous root canal filling
❑ To see any resorption present in the tooth

❑ To check the presence of calcification in pulp space
❑ To see root end proximal structures
❑ Help in determining the working length, length of master gutta-percha cone, and quality of obturation **(Fig. 7.9)**
❑ During the course of treatment, radiographs help in knowing the level of instrumental errors like perforation, ledging, and instrumental separation

Characteristic features of periapical lesions of endodontic origin (Fig. 7.10):

❑ Loss of lamina dura in the apical region
❑ Apparent etiology of pulpal necrosis
❑ Radiolucency remains at the apex even if radiograph is taken by changing the angle

Following lesions should be differentiated from the lesions of endodontic origin while interpreting radiographs:

❑ Periodontal abscess
❑ Idiopathic osteosclerosis

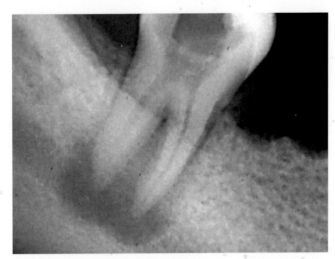

Fig. 7.10 Radiograph showing periapical lesion of endodontic origin. Note the large carious lesion involving the pulp, loss of lamina dura and radiolucency present at root apex.

❑ Cementomas
❑ Giant cell lesions
❑ Cysts
❑ Tumors.

▌ Pulp Vitality Tests

Pulp testing is often referred to as vitality testing. Pulp vitality tests play an important role in diagnosis because these tests not only determine the vitality of tooth but also the pathological status of pulp.

Objectives of Pulp Testing

❑ To assess health of pulp based on its qualitative sensory response prior to restorative, endodontic procedures
❑ To differentially diagnose periapical pathologies of pulpal or periodontal origin
❑ To assess status of pulp as a follow-up after trauma to teeth
❑ To check status of tooth especially that has past history of pulp capping or deep restoration
❑ To diagnose oral pain whether it is of pulpal or periodontal origin or because of other reason

Various types of pulp tests performed are:
• Thermal test
  – Cold test
  – Heat test
• Electrical pulp testing
• Test cavity
• Anesthesia testing
• Bite test

Most commonly used vitality testers evaluate integrity of Aδ fibers by applying stimulus to the outer surface of the tooth surface. A positive response means functional nerve fibers but does not indicate status of blood supply.

Thermal Test

In thermal test, the response of pulp to heat and cold is noted. The basic principle for pulp to respond to thermal stimuli is that patient reports sensation, but it disappears immediately. Any other type of response, that is, painful sensation even after removal of stimulus or no response is considered abnormal.

Cold test: It is the most commonly used test for assessing the vitality of pulp. Cold causes contraction of dentinal tubules resulting in outward flow of fluid from tubules and thereby pain. This test is used to differentiate reversible and irreversible pulpitis. If pain persists after removal of cold stimuli, it is irreversible pulpitis, but if pain disappears on removal of stimulus, it is reversible pulpitis. Cold test is more reliable than heat test.

Cold testing can be done in a number of ways.
❑ Wrap an ice piece in the wet gauge and apply to the tooth. Ice sticks can be prepared by filling the discarded anesthetic carpules with water and placing them in refrigerator
❑ Spray with cold air directed against the isolated tooth
❑ Use of ethyl chloride (boiling point −41°C) in the form of
  • Cotton pellet saturated with ethyl chloride **(Fig. 7.11)**
  • Spray of ethyl chloride: After isolation of tooth with rubber dam, ethyl chloride spray is employed.

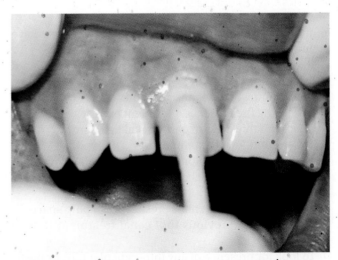

Fig. 7.11 Application of cotton pellet saturated with ethyl chloride.

The ethyl chloride evaporates so rapidly that it absorbs heat and thus cools the tooth
- Frozen carbon dioxide (dry ice) is available in the form of solid stick which is applied to facial surface of the tooth. Advantage of using dry ice is that it can penetrate

full coverage restoration and can elicit a pulpal reaction to the cold because of its very low temperature (–78°C)
- Dichlorodifluoromethane (Freon) (–21°C) and 1,1,1,2-tetrafluoroethane (–15 to –26°C) are also used as cold testing material.

Sites of localization of acute dental infections		
Teeth	Usual exit from bone	Site of localization
Mandibular incisors	Labial	Submental space, oral vestibule
Mandibular canine	Labial	Oral vestibule
Mandibular premolars	Buccal	Oral vestibule
Mandibular first molar	Buccal or lingual	Oral vestibule, buccal space, sublingual space
Mandibular second molar	Buccal or lingual	Oral vestibule, buccal space, sublingual space, submandibular space
Maxillary central incisor	Labial	Oral vestibule
Maxillary lateral incisor	Labial or palatal	Oral vestibule, palatal
Maxillary premolars	Buccal or palatal	Oral vestibule, palatal
Maxillary molars	Buccal or palatal	Oral vestibule, buccal space, palatal

Clinical Tips
- Use of rubber dam is specially recommended when performing the test using the ice-sticks because melting ice will run on to adjacent teeth and gingivae resulting in false-positive result
- While performing cold test, one should begin with the posterior tooth and then move toward anterior teeth. It will prevent melted ice water from dripping in posterior direction, thus giving false results

Heat test: It is most advantageous in the condition where patient's chief complaint is intense dental pain upon contact with any hot object or liquid. Preferred temperature for heat test is 150°F (65.5°C).

Different methods used for heat test are:
- Direct warm air to the exposed surface of tooth and note the patient response
- Apply heat to gutta-percha stick **(Fig. 7.12).** Tooth is coated with a lubricant such as petroleum jelly to prevent gutta-percha from adhering to tooth surface. The heated gutta-percha is applied at the junction of cervical and middle third of facial surface of tooth. Gutta-percha softens at 65°C and can deliver up to 150°C. Disadvantage of using gutta percha stick is that because of high temperature pulpal damage can occur. Heat test should not be done for >5 s because prolonged heat application causes biphasic stimulation of Aδ fibers followed by C fibers, which can result in persistent pain

- Application of hot burnisher, hot compound, or any other heated instrument **(Fig. 7.13)**
- Use of frictional heat produced by rotating polishing rubber disk against the tooth surface
- Use of warm water from a syringe on rubber dam isolated tooth
- Use of laser beam (Nd:YAG laser) is done to stimulate pulp

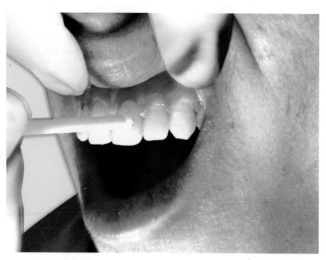
Fig. 7.12 Application of heated gutta-percha stick on tooth for heat test.

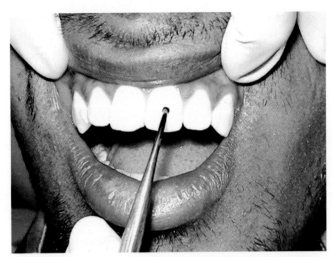

Fig. 7.13 Application of hot burnisher to check vitality of tooth.

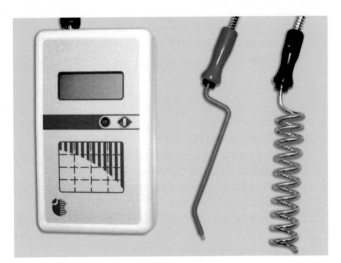

Fig. 7.14 Electric pulp tester.

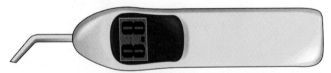

Fig. 7.15 Battery operated pulp tester.

Electric Pulp Testing

Electric pulp tester stimulates Aδ nerve fibers by applying electrical current. Pain occurs because of ionic shift in dentinal fluid resulting in depolarization of Aδ fibers. Pulp testers are battery operated or available with cord which plug into electric outlets for power source (Figs. 7.14 and 7.15). It acts by generating pulsatile electrical stimuli and stimulation of Aδ nerve fibers.

Procedure

❑ Before starting the procedure, patient must be explained about the method to reduce anxiety
❑ Isolate the teeth to avoid any type of false-positive response. This can be done by use of interproximal plastic strip, drying tooth surface and rubber dam application
❑ Apply an electrolyte on the tooth electrode and place it on the facial surface of tooth (Fig. 7.16). Commonly used electrolytes are Nichollas-colloidal graphite, Grossman toothpaste. To have fast response, electrode should be applied at the area of high neural density like incisal one third of anterior teeth (it's close to pulp horns) and middle third of posterior teeth.
❑ Precaution should be taken to avoid it contacting adjacent gingival tissue or metallic restorations to avoid false-positive response
❑ Confirm the complete circuit from electrode through the tooth to the body of the patient and then back to the electrode. If gloves are not used, the circuit gets completed when clinician's finger contact with electrode and patient's cheeks. But with gloved hands, it can be done by placing patient's finger on metal electrode handle or by clipping a ground attachment on to the patient's lip
❑ Once the circuit is complete, slowly increase the current and ask the patient to point out when the sensation occurs
❑ Each tooth should be tested two to three times, and the average reading is noted. If the vitality of a tooth is in question, the pulp tester should be used on the adjacent teeth and the contralateral tooth, as control

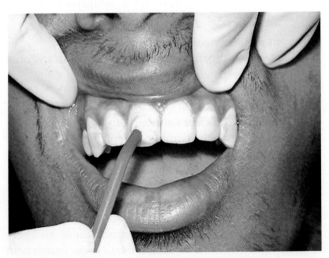

Fig. 7.16 Checking vitality of tooth using electric pulp tester.

Disadvantages of electric pulp testing

- False-positive response in
  - Teeth with acute alveolar abscess because gaseous or liquefied products within the pulp canal can transmit electric current
  - Electrode may contact gingival tissue, thus giving the false-positive response
  - In multirooted teeth, pulp may be vital in one or more root canals and necrosed in others, thus eliciting a false-positive response
- False-negative response in
  - Recently traumatized tooth
  - Recently erupted teeth with immature apex
  - Patients with high pain threshold
  - Calcified canals
  - Poor battery or electrical deficiency in plug in pulp testers
  - Teeth with extensive restorations or pulp protecting bases under restorations
  - Patients premedicated with analgesics or tranquilizers, etc.
  - Partial necrosis of pulp sometimes is indicated as totally necrosis by electric pulp tester

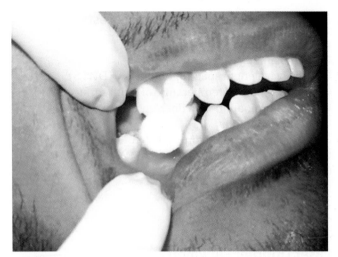

Fig. 7.17 Patient is asked to bite on cotton swab or hard object for bite test.

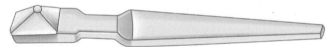

Fig. 7.18 Tooth slooth.

Test Cavity

This method should be used only when all other test methods are inconclusive in results. Here a test cavity is made with high speed number one or two round burs with appropriate air and water coolant. The patient is not anesthetized while performing this test. Patient is asked to respond if any painful sensation occurs during drilling. The sensitivity or the pain felt by the patient indicates pulp vitality. Here, the procedure is terminated by restoring the prepared cavity. If no pain is felt, cavity preparation may be continued until the pulp chamber is reached, and later on endodontic therapy may be carried out.

Anesthesia Testing

It is indicated when patient can't differentiate whether pain is in mandibular or maxillary arch. Main objective of this test is to anesthetize a single tooth at a time until the pain is eliminated. It should be accomplished by using intraligamentary injection. Injection is administered to the most posterior tooth in the suspected quadrant. If the pain persists, even after tooth has been fully anesthetized, then repeat the procedure to the next tooth mesial to it. It is continued until the pain disappears. If source of pain cannot be determined, repeat the same technique on the opposite arch. This test has advantage over test cavity because later results in iatrogenic damage.

Bite Test

Bite test helps in identifying a cracked or fractured tooth. This is done if patient complains of pain on mastication.

Tooth is sensitive to biting if pulpal necrosis has extended to the periodontal ligament space or if a crack is present in a tooth. In this, patient is asked to bite on a hard object such as cotton swab, tooth pick, or orange wood stick with suspected tooth and the contralateral tooth **(Fig. 7.17)**. Tooth slooth is another commercially available device for bite test. It has a small concave area on its top which is placed in contact with the cusp to be tested **(Fig. 7.18)**. Pain present on biting indicates apical periodontitis, and pain present on release of biting force indicates a cracked tooth.

Recent Advances in Pulp Vitality Testing

Assessment of pulp vitality is a crucial diagnostic procedure in dental practice. Commonly used methods (thermal, electrical, or direct dentine stimulation) rely on stimulation of Aδ nerve fibers and give no direct indication of blood flow within the pulp. These tests can give false-positive and negative results. Moreover, being subjective tests, result depends on patient's perceived response to the stimulus and dentist's interpretation of that response.

Recent studies have shown that blood circulation is the most accurate determinant in assessing pulp vitality as it provides an objective differentiation between necrotic and vital pulp tissue.

Recently Available Pulp Vitality Tests

- Laser Doppler flowmetry (LDF)
- Pulp oximetry
- Dual wavelength spectrophotometry (DWLS)
- Measurement of temperature of tooth surface
- Transillumination with fiber-optic light
- Plethysmography
- Detection of interleukin-1 (IL-1)β
- Xenon-133
- Hughes Probeye camera
- Gas desaturation
- Radiolabeled microspheres
- Electromagnetic flowmetry

Laser Doppler Flowmetry

LDF was first described by Gazelius in 1986. Technique depends on Doppler principle in which a low power light from a monochromatic laser beam of known wavelength along a fiber-optic cable is directed to the tooth surface. As light enters the tissue, it is scattered and adsorbed by stationary and moving tissues. Photons that contact with moving red blood cells are scattered and shifted, photon that interacts with stationary tissues is scattered but not shifted. Part of light is returned back to photon detector and signal is produced. Since RBCs represent main moving entity in pulp, Doppler shifted light is inferred as an index of pulpal blood flow (**Fig. 7.19**). Blood flow measured by laser Doppler technique is termed "flux," which is proportional to the product of average speed of blood cells and their concentration.

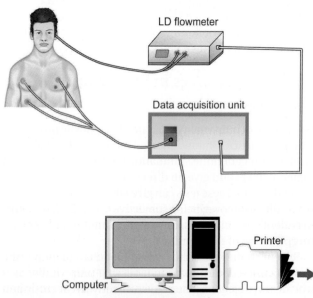

Fig. 7.19 Working of LDF.

Pulp is a highly vascular tissue, and cardiac cycle blood flow in the supplying artery is transmitted as pulsations. These pulsations are apparent on laser Doppler monitor of vital teeth and are absent in nonvital teeth. Blood flux level in vital teeth is much higher than for nonvital teeth. Currently available flowmeters display the signal on a screen, from which the clinician can interpret whether pulp is vital or nonvital.

Advantages
- An objective test
- Accurate to check vitality

Disadvantages
- Cannot be used in patients who cannot refrain from moving or if tooth to be tested cannot be stabilized
- Medications used in cardiovascular diseases can affect the blood flow to pulp
- Requires higher technical skills to achieve
- Use of nicotine affects blood flow to pulp
- Expensive

Pulse Oximetry

Pulse oximeter is a noninvasive oxygen saturation monitor widely used in medical practice for recording blood oxygen saturation levels during intravenous anesthesia. It was introduced in Aoyagi in the 1970s.

Principle of this technique is based on modification of Beer's law. It tells absorption of light by a solute to its concentration and optical properties at a given wavelength. Pulse oximeter sensor consists of two light emitting diodes, one to transmit red light (wavelength approximately 660 nm), other to transmit infrared light (wavelength 850 nm), and a photodetector on opposite side of vascular bed. When LED transmits light through vascular bed, different amount of light is absorbed by oxygenated and deoxygenated hemoglobin. Pulsatile change in blood volume causes change in the amount of light absorbed by vascular bed. This change is analyzed in pulse oximeter to evaluate saturation of arterial blood.

Advantages
- Effective and objective method to evaluate pulp vitality
- Useful in the cases of traumatic injuries where the blood supply remains intact but nerve supply is damaged
- Can detect pulpal circulation independent of gingival circulation
- Easy to reproduce pulp pulse readings

Disadvantages
- If arterial pulsatile blood flow is low, readings can't be obtained. For example, in peripheral vasoconstriction, hypovolemia, and hypothermia cases
- Background absorption associated with venous blood

- ☐ False-negative results in the cases of coronal calcification where radicular pulp is vital
- ☐ Low specificity in the cases of deep restorations or traumatic injuries

Dual Wavelength Spectrophotometry

DWLS is a method independent of a pulsatile circulation. Presence of arterioles rather than arteries in the pulp and its rigid encapsulation by surrounding dentine and enamel make it difficult to detect a pulse in the pulp space. This method measures oxygenation changes in the capillary bed rather than arteries.

Advantages of DWLS

- ☐ In the case of avulsed and replanted teeth with open apices where the blood supply is regained within first 20 days, but the nerve supply takes time. Repeated readings for 40 days in such teeth reveal the healing process
- ☐ It uses visible light which is filtered and guided to the tooth by fiber optics
- ☐ Noninvasive objective test
- ☐ Instrument is small, portable, and inexpensive

Measurement of Surface Temperature of Tooth

This method is based on the assumption that if pulp becomes nonvital, tooth no longer has internal blood supply, thus should exhibit a lower surface temperature than that of its vital counterparts.

Fanibunda in 1985 showed that it is possible to differentiate vital and nonvital teeth by means of crown surface temperature. He used a thermistor unit consisting of two matched thermistors connected back to back, one measuring the surface temperature of the crown (measuring thermistor) while other acting as a reference thermistor. Tooth to be tested was dried with gauze, and the thermistor unit was positioned so that measuring thermistor contacted center of the buccal surface of crown. Reference thermistor was suspended in air, close to it, but not touching either measuring thermistor or the enamel surface.

Equilibrium was then achieved between the temperatures of the thermistors, crown surface, and immediate environment by holding the measuring unit in the described position until a steady state was established for ≥20 s. Stimulation of crown surface was carried out by means of a rubber-polishing cup fitted to a dental contra-angle handpiece. The recordings were continued for a period of time following the stimulation period. It was found that a difference was obtained between the critical period for vital and nonvital teeth, and the difference corresponded with a specific temperature change.

Transillumination with Fiber-Optic Light

In this, light is passed through a fine glass or plastic fibers by a process known as total internal reflection.

Nonvital tooth which is not discolored may show difference in translucency when a shadow produced on a mirror is compared to that of adjacent vital teeth.

Detection of Interleukin-1β in Human Periapical Lesion

The inflammatory periapical lesions are common sequelae of infected pulp tissue. These areas contain PMN leukocytes, T and B lymphocytes, macrophages, plasma cells, etc. These inflammatory cells produce IL-1, which acts as a mediator of various immunologic and inflammatory responses. This lymphocyte-activating factor IL-1 is responsible for osteoclast activation which results in bone resorption which is frequently a feature of inflammatory response.

Plethysmography

In this, analysis of optical properties of selected tissue is done. It was introduced as a modification of pulp oximetry by adding a light of shorter wavelength.

Role of Ultrasound

Images produced by ultrasound are three dimensional and have high resolution. It does not expose patients to any radiation. It uses sound waves with frequency outside the audible range. Since different biological tissues have different acoustic and mechanical properties, ultrasound waves at edge two tissues of different acoustic impedance undergo reflection and refraction. Ultrasound wave which is reflected back from the tissues appears as echo. In healthy state, alveolar bone appears as white(total reflection), roots of teeth appear whiter (hyperechoic). A fluid-filled cavity appears dark (hypoechoic). Degree of reflection depends on the clarity of the fluid (hypoechoic). Ultrasound can compliment conventional radiographs since it can differentiate between cystic and non-cystic lesions.

Fiber-Optic Fluorescent Spectrometry

In this, ultraviolet light is projected toward dental tissues to produce fluorescence. Teeth with vital pulps fluoresce normally, but the teeth with necrotic nonvital pulp don't fluoresce when exposed to ultraviolet light. Differences in fluorescence is due to loss of mineralized tissue components and increased organic presence and water in carious when compared to healthy dentin.

Cholesteric Liquid Crystals

Cholesteric crystals are "liquid" crystals which are easily affected by change in temperature or pressure because of their fluidity. These crystals are thermochromic (color of crystals vary with change in pressure or temperature). Howell et al. and Lexington found when applied to tooth surface, crystals showed color change when compared with adjacent or contralateral teeth. This principle is used to detect pulp vitality because vital pulp has higher tooth-surface temperature due to presence of vascular supply, when compared with nonvital teeth that had no blood supply.

Ultrasound Doppler or Color Power Doppler

Color Power Doppler flowmetry detects presence and direction of the blood flow within the tissue. Intensity of Doppler signal is shown by changes on graph (Doppler). Positive Doppler shift (shown in red) is caused by blood moving toward the transducer, and negative Doppler shift (shown in blue) is caused by blood moving in the opposite direction. In vital teeth, Doppler tells a "pulsating" waveform and sound characteristic, and nonvital teeth show linear nonpulsed waveform without pulsating sound.

Thermographic Imaging

In this, color image is produced due to change in temperature in both superficial and deep areas. In 1989, Pogrel et al. found that Hughes Probeye 4300 Thermal Video System was sensitive to measure even 0.1°C of temperature differences. However, nowadays less cumbersome and easier methods are available to replace this.

Differential Diagnosis

Differential diagnosis is distinguishing a particular disease from others that present the similar clinical features. After differential diagnosis, to reach at definitive diagnosis, the clinician should get investigations done like laboratory investigations, radiographs, pulp vitality tests.

Diagnostic Perplexities

There are certain conditions in which it is difficult to reach proper diagnosis even after detailed history and examination. These conditions can be
- Idiopathic tooth resorption
- Treatment failures
- Cracked tooth syndrome
- Persistent discomfort
- Unusual radiographic appearances
- Paresthesia

Role of Radiographs in Endodontics

Radiographs play an important role in diagnosis of endodontic problems. Clinician should be familiar with normal radiographic landmarks.

Interpretation of radiograph according to appearance (Fig. 7.20)	
Appearance	*Tentative finding*
Black/gray area	a. Decay
	b. Pulp
	c. Gingiva or space between teeth
	d. Abscess
	e. Cyst
White area	a. Enamel
	b. Restoration (metal, gutta-percha, etc.)
Creamy white area	Dentin appears as creamy white area
White line around teeth	Lamina dura around teeth

It should be kept in mind that radiograph should be of good quality because a poor quality radiograph not only fails to yield diagnostic information but also causes unnecessary radiation to the patient.

In order to decrease radiation exposure, one should
- Use of faster F-speed film reduces exposure 25% compared to E-speed film and 60% compared to D-speed film
- Use rectangular collimation instead of round collimator
- Use thyroid collar and lead apron
- Use of aluminum filters
- Use digital radiographic techniques
- Use electronic apex locator in endodontic treatment

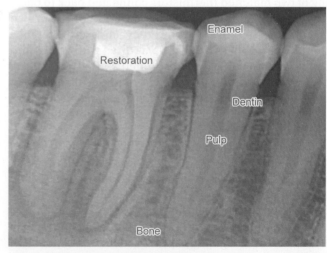

Fig. 7.20 Radiograph showing enamel, dentin, pulp, restoration and alveolar bone.

History of dental radiology

1895	WC Roentgen	Discovery of X-rays
1895	Otto Walkhoff	First dental radiograph of his own teeth
1899	Edmund Kells	Used radiograph to check working length
1900	Weston Price	Advocated radiograph to check quality of obturation
1901	WH Rollins	Presented first paper on dangers of X-rays
1904	WA Price	Introduction of Bisecting technique
1913	Eastman Kodak company	Introduction of prewrapped dental films
1920	Eastman Kodak company	Introduction of machine made film packets
1925	HR Raper	Introduction of Bitewing technique
1947	FG Fitzgerald	Introduction of Paralleling cone technique

Types of Radiographs

- ❏ Intraoral
  - • Intraoral periapical
  - • Occlusal
  - • Bitewing
- ❏ Extraoral
  - • Panaromic
  - • Lateral cephalograms
  - • Tomograms
  - • Computed tomography

Intraoral Periapical Radiographs

Intraoral Periapical (IOPA) radiographs are used to detect any abnormalities in relation to roots and surrounding bone structures.

Techniques for exposing teeth:

Bisecting Angle Technique (Fig. 7.21)

Here, X-ray beam is directed perpendicular to an imaginary plane which bisects the angle formed by recording plane of X-ray film and the long axis of the tooth.

Advantages
- ❏ Can be performed without using film holders
- ❏ More comfortable because film is placed at angle to long axis of teeth, so it doesn't impinge soft tissues
- ❏ Anatomical structures do not pose much problems because of angulated film placement
- ❏ Quick and comfortable for the patient when rubber dam is in place

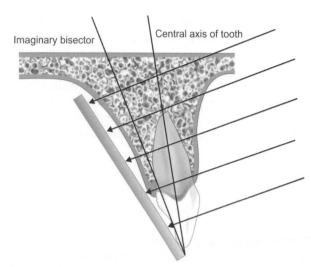

Fig. 7.21 In Bisecting angle technique, X-ray beam is directed perpendicular to an imaginary plane which bisects the angle formed by recording plane of X-ray film and the long axis of the tooth.

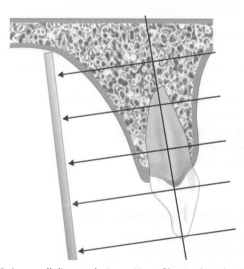

Fig. 7.22 In paralleling technique, X-ray film is placed parallel to long axis of the tooth and X-ray beam is directed perpendicular to film.

Disadvantages
- ❏ Cone cutting
- ❏ Image distortion
- ❏ Since film holder is not used, it's difficult to visualize where the X-ray beam should be directed
- ❏ Superimposition of anatomical structures
- ❏ Difficulty to reproduce the periapical films

Paralleling Technique (Fig. 7.22)

Here X-ray film is placed parallel to the long axis of the tooth to be exposed, and the X-ray beam is directed perpendicular to the film. If film is kept in upright position, patient won't be able to close on biteblock, and film will not be parallel. To aid film placement, film is tipped to 20° beyond parallel.

Since palate and floor of mouth are shallow, film should be placed away from the teeth to achieve parallelism. If film is placed at a distance, it results in increase in magnification (size) but decrease in sharpness. To compensate it, film-target distance should be increased. For this, **Walton** gave a modified paralleling technique in which central beam is oriented perpendicular to radiographic film but not to teeth. Modified paralleling technique covers the disadvantages of paralleling technique.

Advantages
- Better accuracy of image
- Reduced dose of radiation
- Reproducibility
- Because of paralleling instrument with aiming ring, X-ray beam is easy to align irrespective of position of head
- Better images of bone margins, interproximal regions, and maxillary molar region
- When using paralleling instrument with aiming ring, alignment of X-ray beam is simplified

Disadvantages
- Since film is more upright in paralleling technique, it impinges more on floor of mouth or palate so more uncomfortable
- Difficult to use in patients with Shallow vault
- Gag reflex
- When rubber dam is in place
- Extremely long roots
- Uncooperative patients
- Tori

Indications of IOPA Radiograph
- To see apical inflammation
- Check periodontal status
- Check alveolar bone
- See unerupted teeth
- Check status of tooth after trauma
- During and after endodontic treatment
- Evaluation of implants postoperatively

Bitewing Radiographs

Bitewing radiographs include the crowns of maxillary and mandibular teeth and alveolar crest in the same film **(Fig. 7.23)**.

Advantages
- Helps in detecting interproximal caries
- Evaluate periodontal conditions
- Evaluate secondary caries under restorations
- Help in assessing alveolar bone crest and changes in bone height by comparing it with adjacent teeth

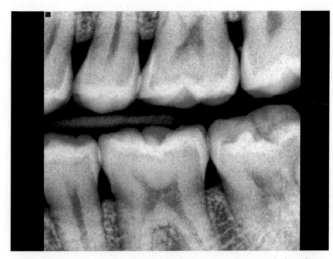
Fig. 7.23 Bitewing radiograph showing crowns and alveolar crest area.

Cone Image Shift Techique

A periapical film identifies the location of an object vertically and horizontal (mesiodistal) direction. However, buccolingual position cannot be determined because film is two dimensional. To locate buccolingual position, same lingual opposite buccal (SLOB) rule is used. Principle of technique is that as the vertical or horizontal angulations of X-ray tube head changes, object buccal or closest to the tube head moves to opposite side of radiograph when compared to lingual object **(Figs. 7.24 and 7.25)**. When two objects and film are in fixed position and the tube head is

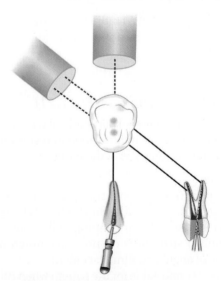
Fig. 7.24 Cone-shift technique.

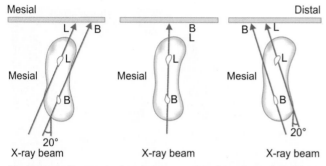

Mesial   Distal

Fig. 7.25 As X-ray tube head changes, the object buccal or closest to the tube head moves to opposite side of radiograph when compared to lingual object.

moved, images of both objects moving in opposite direction, resultant radiograph shows lingual object that moved in the same direction as the cone, and the buccal object moved in opposite direction. This is also known as "SLOB" rule. To simplify the understanding of SLOB rule, Walton gave an easy method. Place two fingers directly in front of open eyes so that one finger is superimposed on the other. By moving head from one side to another, the relative position of fingers changes. Same effect is produced with two superimposed roots when center beam is shifted.

Horizontal tube shift: When tubehead is moved mesially, beam should be moved distally(from the mesial side) and vice a versa.

Vertical tube shift: It says downward movement of tubehead requires beam to be directed upward, and when tubehead is moved upward, beam should be directed downwards.

Advantages of "SLOB" Rule
- Helps in separation and identification of overlapping canals, for example, in maxillary premolars and mesial canals of mandibular molars
- Working length radiographs are better traced from orifice to the apex by this technique
- Helps to locate the root resorption site in relation to tooth
- Helps in locating relationship of canal to radiopaque margin, for example, position of bur during access opening
- Helps in identification of anatomic landmarks and pathosis
- Increases visualization of apical anatomy by moving anatomic landmarks such as zygomatic process or the impacted tooth
- Helps to identify the angle at which particular radiograph was taken, even if information was not recorded
- Helps to identify missed or calcified canals and canal curvature

- Helps to locate foreign bodies and anatomical landmarks in relation to the root apex such as mandibular canal.

Disadvantages of "SLOB" Rule
- It results in blurring of the object. The clearest radiograph is achieved by parallel technique, so when central beam changes direction relative to object and the film, object becomes blurred
- It causes superimposition of the structures. Objects which have natural separation on parallel technique, with cone shift may move relative to each other and become superimposed. For example, in the case of maxillary molars, all three separate roots are visible on parallel radiographs, but an angled radiograph may move palatal root over the distobuccal or mesiobuccal root and thus decreasing the ability to distinguish apices clearly.

Synonyms of cone image shift technique
- BOR (buccal object rule)
- SLOB
- BOMM (buccal object moves most)
- Tube shift technique
- Clark's rule
- Walton projection

Advantages of Radiographs in Endodontics

In endodontics, the radiographs perform essential functions in three main areas, viz., diagnosis, treatment, and recall.

Diagnosis
- Help to know extent of caries, restoration, evidence of pulp capping or pulpotomy, etc. **(Fig. 7.26)**

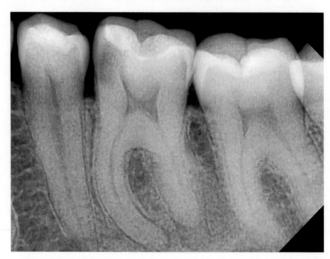

Fig. 7.26 Extent of caries can be seen on the radiograph.

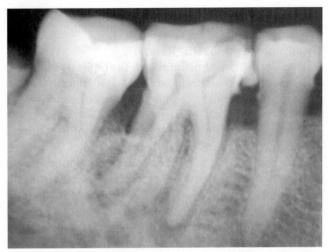

Fig. 7.27 Radiograph showing extra root in first molar.

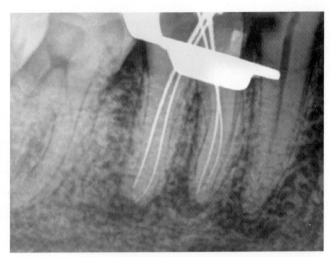

Fig. 7.29 Working length radiograph.

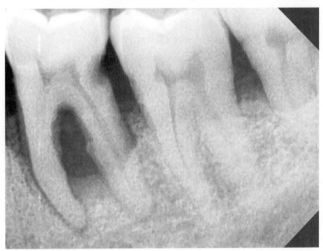

Fig. 7.28 Radiograph showing periodontal involvement of mandibular first molar.

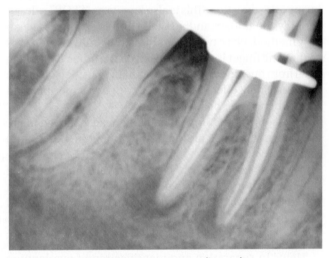

Fig. 7.30 Master cone radiograph.

❑ Useful to know anatomy of pulp cavity, curvature of canal, number of roots and canals, variation in root canal system, that is, presence of fused or extra roots and canals **(Fig. 7.27)**, bifurcation or trifurcation in the canal system if present

❑ Help to know pulp conditions present inside the tooth like pulp stones, calcification, internal resorption, etc.

❑ Provides information on orientation and depth of bur relative to pulp cavity

❑ Help in knowing external resorption, thickening of periodontal ligament, extent of periapical, and alveolar bone destruction **(Fig. 7.28)**

Treatment

❑ **Working length determination:** In this, radiograph is used to determine the distance from the reference point to apex **(Fig. 7.29)**. By using different cone angulations, superimposed structures can be moved to give clear image

❑ **Master cone radiographs:** Master cone radiograph is used to evaluate the length and fit of master gutta-percha cone **(Fig. 7.30)**

❑ **Obturation:** Radiographs help to know the length, density, configuration, and the quality of obturation **(Fig. 7.31)**

Recall

❑ Evaluate post-treatment periapical status **(Figs. 7.32A and B)**

❑ Presence and nature of lesion (periapical, periodontal, or non-endodontic) occurred after the treatment are best detected on radiographs

❑ Recall radiographs help to evaluate success of treatment

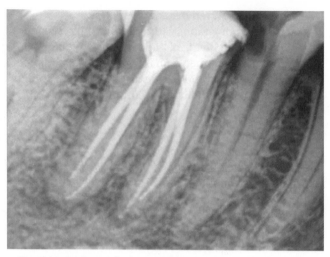

Fig. 7.31 Radiograph showing obturation of mandibular first molar.

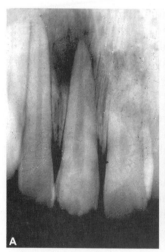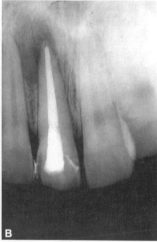

Figs. 7.32A and B Radiograph showing comparison of size of periapical radiolucency: (A) Preoperative; (B) 6 months post-treatment.

Disadvantages of Radiographs

- ❑ Radiograph represents two-dimensional picture of a three-dimensional object
- ❑ For a hard tissue lesion to be evident on a radiograph, there should be at least a mineral loss of 6.6%
- ❑ Pathological changes in pulp are not visible in radiograph
- ❑ Initial stages of periradicular disease produce no changes in radiograph
- ❑ Radiographs do not help in exact interpretation of the lesion, for example, radiographic picture of an abscess, inflammation, and granuloma is almost same
- ❑ Misinterpretation of radiographs can lead to inaccurate diagnosis
- ❑ Radiographs can misinterpret the anatomical structures like incisive and mental foramen with periapical lesions
- ❑ Chronic inflammatory lesion cannot be differentiated from healed fibrous scar tissue

- ❑ Buccolingual dimensions cannot be assessed from IOPA radiograph

To know the exact status of multirooted teeth, multiple radiographs are needed at different angles which further increase the radiation exposure.

Digital Radiography

Digital imaging: Digital imaging uses standard radiology technique in which film is used to record the image, and then final image is subjected to digital processing to produce the final result. Digital radiography is obtained by two methods:

1. Direct digital radiograph
2. Video recording and digitization of conventional radiograph

Digital Dental Radiography

Digital imaging systems require an electronic sensor or detector, an analog to digital converter, a computer, and a monitor or printer for image of the components of imaging system.

General Principles of Digital Imaging

- ❑ Chemically produced radiograph is represented by data that is acquired in a parallel and continuous fashion known as analogue
- ❑ Computers use binary (0 or 1) language, where information is usually handled in eight character words called bytes
- ❑ Each character can be either 0 or 1, this results in 28 possible combinations (words) that is 256 words. Thus, digital dental images are limited to 256 shades of gray
- ❑ Digital images are made-up of pixels (picture elements), each allocated a shade of gray
- ❑ Spatial resolution of a digital system is heavily dependent upon the number of pixels available per millimeter of image

CCD System

CCD is a solid state detector composed of array of X-ray or light sensitive phosphorus on a pure silicon chip. These phosphores convert incoming X-rays to a wavelength that matches the peak response of silicon.

Radiovisiography (RVG)

RVG is composed of three major parts:

1. Radio part consists of a conventional X-ray unit and a tiny sensor to record the image. Sensor transmits information via fiber-optic bundle to a miniature CCD **(Figs. 7.33 and 7.34)**
2. "Visio" portion of the system receives and stores incoming signals during exposure and converts them point by point

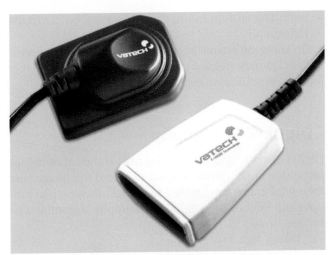

Fig. 7.33 Sensor used for RVG.

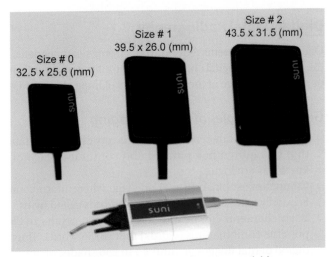

Size # 0
32.5 x 25.6 (mm)

Size # 1
39.5 x 26.0 (mm)

Size # 2
43.5 x 31.5 (mm)

Figs. 7.34 Different sizes of sensors available.

into one of 256 discrete gray levels. It consists of a video monitor and display processing unit **(Figs. 7.35 A to E)**

3. "Graphy" part of RVG unit consists of digital storage apparatus. It can be connected to various print out or mass storage devices for immediate or later viewing

Advantages
- Low radiation dose
- Darkroom is not required as instant image is viewed
- Image distortion from bent radiographic film is eliminated
- The quality of the image is consistent
- Greater exposure latitude
- Elimination of hazards of film development
- Diagnostic capability is increased through digital enhancement and enlargement of specific areas for closer examination
- Contrast and resolution can be altered, and images can be viewed as grey scale or colored

- Images are displayed instantly
- Full mouth radiographs can be made within seconds
- Storages and archiving of patient information
- Transfer of images between institutions (teleradiology)
- Infection control and toxic waste disposal problems associated with radiology are eliminated

Disadvantages
- Expensive
- Life expectancy of CCD is not fixed
- Solid state sensors when used for bitewing examination are small as compared to size-2 film
- Large disk space required to store images
- Bulky sensor with cable attachment, which can make placement in mouth difficult
- Soft tissue imaging is not very nice

Phosphor Imaging System

Imaging using a photostimulable phosphor can also be called as an indirect digital imaging technique. The image is captured on a phosphor plate as analogue information and is converted into a digital format when the plate is processed.

Advantages
- Low radiation dose (90% reduction)
- Almost instant image (20–30 s)
- Wide exposure latitude (almost impossible to burn out information)
- Same size receptor as films
- X-ray source can be remote from PC
- Image manipulation facilities

Disadvantages
- Cost
- Storage of images (same as with CCD systems)
- Slight inconvenience of plastic bags

Cone-Beam Computed Tomography

Successful endodontic treatment depends on diagnostic imaging techniques to provide the critical information about the teeth and their surrounding tissues. Though conventional radiography has been used since ages, modern techniques of imaging have also been successfully utilized. Introduction of maxillofacial cone-beam computed tomography (CBCT) in 1996 provided the first clinically practical technology demonstrating application of 3D imaging for endodontic considerations. CBCT has cone-shaped X-ray beam that captures a cylindrical or spherical volume of data, described as the field of view. Here, a 3D volume of data is achieved with a single sweep of the scanner, using a simple and direct relationship between beam source and sensor; the latter rotating 180–360°

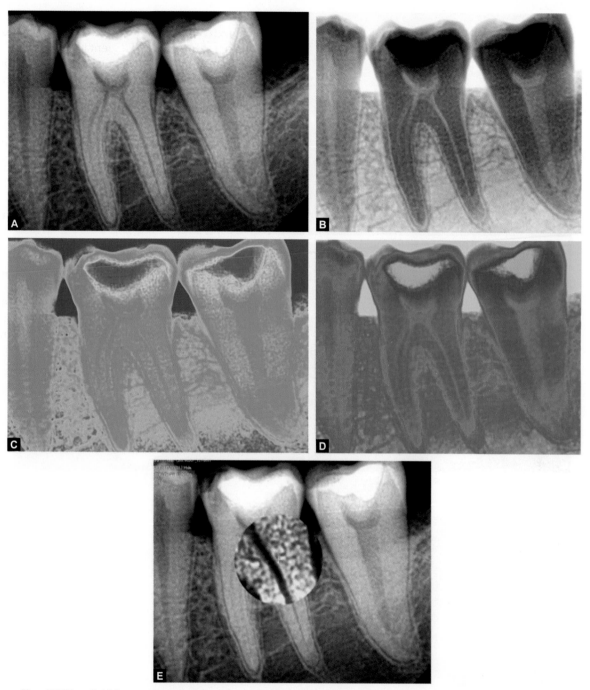

Figs. 7.35A to E Visio part displays the captured images. Diagnostic capability is increased by changing the color, contrast and magnification of the area.

around the patient's head. During the exposure sequence, hundreds of planar projection images are obtained from the field of view, in an arc of ≥180°. Thus, we get accurate and immediate 3D radiographic images **(Figs. 7.36A to E)**.

To have better resolution of images, radiation exposure is increased by two to threefolds but CBCT systems utilize a pulsatile X-ray beam, therefore, actual patient exposure time can be very low as 2–10 s.

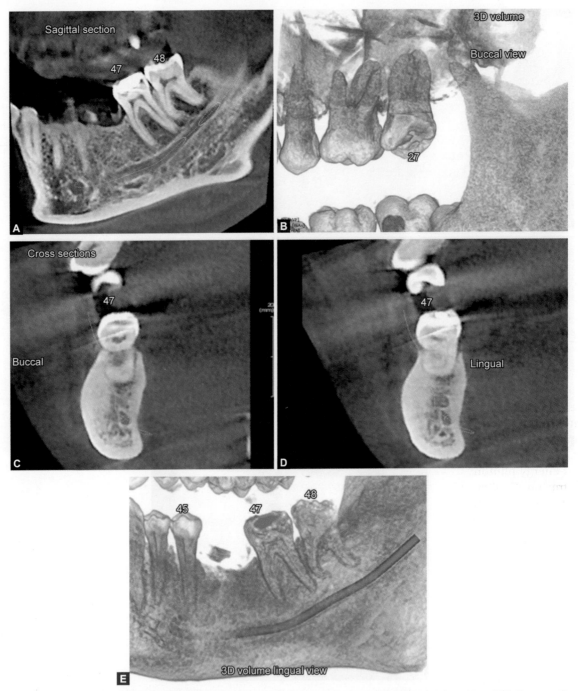

Figs. 7.36A to E CBCT showing: (A). Sagittal section of mandible; (B). 3D image of maxillary molars; (C and D). Cross section of mandibular molars; (E). 3D lingual view of mandibular teeth along with inferior alveolar nerve.

Radiation Dose Considerations

For a significant comparison of radiation risk, radiation exposures are converted to effective dose, measured in sieverts (Sv). The Sv is a large unit; so in maxillofacial imaging, milli-[10–3 mSv] or micro-[10–6 µSv] sieverts are used.

Advantages of CBCT

- ❑ CBCT overcomes the shortcomings of conventional radiography by producing 3D images that show accurate anatomy and spatial relationship of the pathosis and anatomical structures
- ❑ Clinician can choose and view slices of the volumetric data in all the planes, eliminating the anatomical noise
- ❑ CBCT voxels are isotropic, ensuring geometrical accuracy of the images
- ❑ Reduced patient exposure to ionizing radiation and superior image quality of dental hard tissues
- ❑ Since, X-ray source can be collimated so that the radiation is limited to the target area, further reducing the radiation exposure to the patient.

Limitations of CBCT

- ❑ Spatial resolution and the contrast resolution of CBCT is lower than that of intraoral radiography
- ❑ Chances of radiographic artifacts are more with CBCT, for example, when CBCT X-ray beam encounters a very high density object, like enamel or metallic restorations, lower energy photons in the beam are absorbed by the structure. By this, mean energy of the X-ray beam increases producing two types of artifacts that can reduce the diagnostic yield of the images
- ❑ Patient has to stay absolutely still, because movement can affect the sharpness of the final image during the scan.

Applications of CBCT in Endodontics

Though there are many advantages of CBCT, but, due to higher effective dose of ionizing radiation in comparison to conventional radiographs, in endodontics CBCT should be used for evaluation and management of complex endodontic conditions. It can be used for the following cases.

Preoperative Evaluation

- ❑ **Tooth morphology:** CBCT helps in detecting accurate degree of curvatures of roots of teeth, aberrations present in teeth, anomalies such as dens invaginatus or tooth fusion. It can detect MB2 better than 2D conventional radiography

- ❑ **Dental periapical pathosis and apical periodontitis:** CBCT gives more accurate images for identification of apical periodontitis. It can demonstrate bone defects of the cancellous bone and cortical bone separately. It can also tell invasion of lesion into the maxillary sinus, thickening of sinus membrane, and missed canals
- ❑ **Diagnosis of different types of root resorption:** CBCT helps in detection of small lesions, localizing and differentiation of the external root resorption from external cervical resorption, internal resorption, and other conditions
- ❑ **Root fracture:** CBCT provides accurate assessment of dentoalveolar trauma, especially root fractures as compared to conventional radiography
- ❑ **In surgical endodontics:** It tells accurate spatial relationship of the target tooth to adjacent anatomical structures like inferior alveolar nerve, mental foramen, and maxillary sinuses
- ❑ **Assessment of traumatic dental injuries:** It helps in accurate detection of horizontal root fractures, degree and direction of displacement related to luxation injuries than multiple periapical radiographs.

Postoperative Assessment

- ❑ It helps in monitoring the healing of apical lesions accurately as compared to conventional radiography
- ❑ CBCT is used to initial and subsequent monitoring of the integrity of root canal obturation
- ❑ CBCT helps in determining the precise nature of a perforation and healing on subsequent treatment.

▮ Questions

1. Define diagnosis. Enumerate various diagnostic techniques in endodontics. Describe in detail on electric pulp tester.
2. Enumerate the various diagnostic aids in endodontics, and describe in detail on thermal testing.
3. Describe the various pulp vitality tests. Add a note on the recent method to determine the vascularity of the tooth.
4. What are the various methods employed to detect the vitality of a tooth.
5. Discuss role of radiographs in endodontics.
6. CBCT in endodontics.
7. Write short notes on:
   - Pulp vitality tests
   - Thermal test for pulp vitality
   - Recent advances in pulp vitality testing
   - Role of radiograph in endodontics
   - Digital radiography
   - RVG/radiovisiography
   - Electric pulp testing

- Diagnostic aids in endodontics
- Test cavity
- Thermal testing
- RVG
- SLOB rule
- Electric pulp tester
- Interpretation of vitality tests
- False-positive and false-negative readings in electric pulp testing
- Laser Doppler flowmetry.

▌ Bibliography

1. Bastos JV, Goulart EM, de Souza Cortes MI. Pulpal response to sensibility tests after traumatic dental injuries in permanent teeth. Dent Traumatol. 2014;30:188–92.
2. Durack C, Patel S. Cone beam computed tomography in endodontics. Braz Dent J 2012;23(3):179–91.
3. Matherne RP, Angelopoulos C, Kulild JC, Tira D. Use of cone-beam computed tomography to identify root canal systems in vitro. J Endod 2008;34(1):87–9.
4. Mejare IA, Axelsson S, Davidson T, et al. Diagnosis of the condition of the dental pulp: a systematic review. Int Endod J. 2012;45:597–613.
5. Michaelson PL, Holland GR. Is pulpitis painful? Int Endod J. 2002;35:829–32.
6. Nance R, Tyndall D, Levin LG, Trope M. Identification of root canals in molars by tuned-aperture computed tomography. Int Endod J 2000;33(4):392–6.
7. Narhi MV. The characteristics of intradental sensory units and their responses to stimulation. J Dent Res. 1985;64:564–71.
8. Patel S, Dawood A, Ford TP, Whaites E. The potential applications of cone beam computed tomography in the management of endodontic problems. Int Endod J 2007;40(10):818–30.
9. Patel S, Ford TP. Is the resorption external or internal? Dent Update 2007;34(4):218–20, 222, 224–6, 229.
10. Patel S. New dimensions in endodontic imaging: Part 2 cone beam computed tomography. Int Endod J 2009;42(6):463–75.
11. Ricucci D, Loghin S, Siqueira Jr JF. Correlation between clinical and histologic pulp diagnosis. J Endod. 2014;40:1932–9.
12. Stavropoulos A, Wenzel A. Accuracy of cone beam dental CT, intraoral digital and conventional radiography for detection of periapical lesions. An ex vivo study in pig jaws. Clin Oral Invest. 2007;11:101–6.
13. Tyndall DA, Rathore S. Cone-beam CT diagnostic applications: caries, periodontal bone assessment, and endodontic applications. Dent Clin North Am 2008;52(4):825–41.
14. Villa-Chavez CE, et al. Predictive values of thermal and electrical dental pulp tests: a clinical study. J Endod. 2013;39(8):965–9.
15. Walton RE. Diagnostic imaging A. endodontic radiography. In: Ingle JI, Bakland LK, Baumgartner JC, editors. Ingles' Endodontics. 6th edition Hamilton, ON, Canada: BC Decker; 2008. p. 554.
16. Weisleder R, Yamauchi S, Caplan DJ, et al. The validity of pulp testing: a clinical study. J Am Dent Assoc. 2009;140(8):1013–7.

Differential Diagnosis
of Orofacial Pain

Pain is an unpleasant, subjective, sensational, and emotional experience associated with actual or potential tissue damage. Orofacial pain is the field of dentistry related to diagnosis and management of chronic, complex facial pain and orofacial disorders. Orofacial pain, like pain elsewhere in the body, is usually the result of tissue damage and the activation of nociceptors, which transmit a noxious stimulus to the brain. Orofacial disorders are complex and difficult to diagnose due to rich innervations in head, face and oral structures. In order to establish proper diagnosis, one should take detailed subjective description of pain including quality, intensity, duration, frequency, and periodicity of the pain.

▌Definition

Dorland's Medical Dictionary defines pain as "A more or less localized sensation of discomfort, distress or agony resulting from the stimulation of nerve endings." It indicates that pain is a protective mechanism against injury. ***International Association for Study of Pain (IASP) defined pain as*** "an unpleasant sensory and emotional experience associated with actual or potential tissue damage, or described in terms of such damage."

Basically, pain has the function of a warning to tissue damage and activation of defensive mechanism with the aim of prevention of further damage.

▌Diagnosis

For establishing the correct diagnosis, the clinician must record all relevant information regarding signs, symptoms,

history of present complaint and past medical and dental history.

History of Pain

History is an important part of diagnosis; it should assess the present nature and site of pain, along with its causative and aggravating factors. It includes:

Chief Complaint
❑ Location
❑ Onset
❑ Chronology
❑ Quality
❑ Intensity
❑ Aggravating factors
❑ Precipitating factors
❑ Past medical and dental history
❑ Psychological analysis
❑ Review of systems

Location

By knowing patient's description about location of pain, clinician should determine whether it is the true source of pain or referred pain.

Onset
One should know the conditions associated with initial onset of pain. It may facilitate in recognizing the etiology of pain.

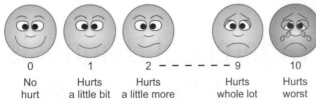

Fig. 8.1 VAS scale to check intensity of pain ranging from (0–10).

Chronology

Chronology of pain should be recorded in a following pattern:
- ❑ Initiation
- ❑ Clinical course:
  - • Mode
  - • Periodicity
  - • Frequency
  - • Duration

Quality

It tells how pain is felt to the patient, for example,
- ❑ Dull, gnawing, or aching
- ❑ Throbbing, pounding, or pulsating
- ❑ Sharp, recurrent, or stabbing
- ❑ Squeezing or crushing

Intensity

Intensity of pain is established by distinguishing mild, moderate, and severe pain. Visual analogue scale is used to assess the intensity of pain. Patient is given a line on which no pain is written at one end and severe at another end. Scale has markings from 0 to 10, where 0 indicates no pain and 10 as maximum pain.
- ❑ Pain index : 0–10 **(Fig. 8.1)**
- ❑ Pain classification : Mild
  Moderate
  Severe

Aggravating Factors

Aggravating factors can be local or conditional. Local factors can be irritants like heat, cold, sweets, sour and pain on biting, etc. Conditional factors can be change of posture, physical activities, and hormonal changes.

Orofacial Pain

Orofacial pain can be divided into odontogenic (dental pain) and nonodontogenic pain (nondental). Dental pain may originate from pulpal or periradicular tissue. Nondental pain can be in form of myofascial toothache, vascular headache, cluster headache, sinusitis, trigeminal neuralgia.

Sources of Odontogenic Pain

Dental Pain of Pulpal Origin

Pulpal pain is of threshold type, that is, no response occurs until threshold level is increased. Pulp may respond to chemical, mechanical, electrical, or thermal stimulation but not to ordinary masticatory functions. In healthy pulp, sensitivity produced by cold and warm stimuli lasts for 1–2 s.

POINTS TO REMEMBER

Stimulation of A-fibers produces a sharp, piercing, or stabbing sensation while C-fibers produce dull, burning, and aching sensation.

Since pulp does not contain proprioceptors, pulpal pain cannot be localized by the patient.

Dental Pain of Periodontal Origin

Periodontal pain is deep somatic pain of the musculoskeletal type. In periodontal ligament (PDL), proprioceptors are present which allow precise localization of pressure stimuli so that patient can localize pain of periodontal origin. This localization can be identified by applying pressure to tooth axially and laterally.

Sources of odontogenic pain

Pulpal pain
- • Dentinal sensitivity
- • Reversible pulpitis
- • Irreversible pulpitis
- • Necrotic pulp

Periodontal pain
- • Symptomatic apical periodontitis
- • Acute periapical abscess
- • Asymptomatic apical periodontitis
- • Periodontal abscess
- • Pericoronitis

Pulpal Pain

Dentinal Sensitivity

According to Holland et al., dentin hypersensitivity is characterized as a short, sharp pain arising from exposed dentin in response stimuli typically thermal, evaporative, tactile, osmotic, or chemical and which cannot be ascribed to any other form of dental pathology. It is caused by disturbance in fluid flow present in dentinal tubules which stretches or compresses the nerve endings that pass alongside the tubular extensions of odontoblasts.

Diagnosis

- Pain is the most common feature which can range from mild to severe
- Most commonly involved teeth are buccal surfaces of premolars and labial surfaces of incisors
- Stimuli causing pain can be thermal (hot and cold), mechanical (tooth brush), osmotic (sweet foods), and acidic (sour and citric juices) stimuli

Treatment

Main principles of treatment are to plug the dentinal tubules preventing the fluid flow and desensitize the nerve, making it less responsive to stimulation. It is done by application of dentifrices, in office products like varnishes and sealants, etc.

Reversible Pulpitis

In reversible pulpitis, short and sharp pain occurs that lasts only when stimuli is applied. On removal of stimuli, pain ceases within 1–2 s. Etiology can be caries, faulty restoration, trauma, or recent restorative procedures.

Diagnosis

Diagnosis is made by careful history and clinical examination. Short and sharp pain disappears on removal of stimuli. Pain is usually caused by cold, sweet, or sour things. Since pulp is especially sensitive to cold stimuli, cold test is best method to diagnose the case.

Differential Diagnosis

Reversible pulpitis can be differentiated from irreversible pulpitis by character of pain, thermal and electric pulp tests.

Treatment

- Removal of the cause if present (caries, fractured restoration, exposed dentinal tubules)
- If recent operative procedure or trauma has taken place, then postpone the additional treatment and observe the tooth
- If pulp exposure is detected, go for root canal treatment

Irreversible Pulpitis

Irreversible pulpitis develops if inflammatory process progresses to involve pulp. Patient may have history of spontaneous pain or exaggerated response to hot or cold that lingers even after the stimulus is removed. The involved tooth usually presents an extensive restoration and/or caries.

Diagnosis

Diagnosis is usually made after taking thorough history and clinical examination of the patient.

- Patient usually gives a history of spontaneous pain
- Tooth is hypersensitive to hot or cold that is prolonged in duration
- Pulp may be vital or partially vital
- In certain cases of irreversible pulpitis, the patient may arrive at the dental clinic with a glass of ice/cold water. In these cases, cold actually alleviates the patient's pain and, thus, can be used as a diagnostic test. Cooling of the dentin and the resultant contraction of the fluid in the tubules relieves the pressure on pulpal nerve fibers caused by edema and inflammation of the pulp

Differential Diagnosis

- Reversible pulpitis at early stage
- In case of symptomatic stage, it may resemble acute alveolar abscess

Treatment

Complete removal of pulpal tissue should be done, that is, endodontic therapy.

Necrotic Pulp

It results from continued degeneration of an acutely inflamed pulp. Literal meaning of necrosis is death, that is, pulpal tissue becomes dead because of untreated pulpal inflammation. In pulpal necrosis, there is progressive breakdown of cellular organization with no reparative function. It is frequently associated with apical radiolucent lesion. In case of multirooted teeth, one root may contain partially vital pulp, whereas other roots may be nonvital.

Diagnosis

- Tooth is usually asymptomatic, may give moderate to severe pain on biting pressure (it is not a symptom of necrotic pulp but it indicates inflammation)
- Pulp tests show negative response but in case of multi-rooted teeth, it can give false positive results.

Treatment

Complete removal of pulpal tissue that is root canal treatment.

Periodontal Pain

Symptomatic Apical Periodontitis

It is the inflammation of periodontal ligament which is caused by tissue damage, extension of pulpal pathology, or occlusal trauma. Tooth may be elevated out of the socket because of the built-up fluid pressure in the periodontal ligament. Pain remains until the bone is resorbed, fluid is drained, or irritants are removed.

Diagnosis

- ❑ Check for decay, fracture lines, swelling, hyperocclusion, or sinus tracts
- ❑ Patient has moderate to severe pain on percussion
- ❑ Mobility may or may not be present
- ❑ Pulp tests are essential and their results must be correlated with other diagnostic information in order to determine if inflammation is of pulpal origin or from occlusal trauma
- ❑ Radiographs may show no change or widening of periodontal ligament space in some cases

Differential Diagnosis

It should be differentiated from acute alveolar abscess. Patient's history, symptoms, clinical tests help in differentiating it from periodontal abscess

Treatment

- ❑ Complete removal of pulp
- ❑ Occlusal adjustment

Acute Periapical Abscess

Acute periapical abscess is an acute inflammation of periapical tissue characterized by localized accumulation of pus at the apex of a tooth. It is a painful condition that results from an advanced necrotic pulp. Patients usually relate previous painful episode from irreversible pulpitis or necrotic pulp. Swelling, tooth mobility, and fever are seen in advanced cases.

Diagnosis

- ❑ Spontaneous dull, throbbing, or persistent pain is present
- ❑ Tooth is extremely sensitive to percussion
- ❑ Mobility may be present
- ❑ On palpation, tooth may be sensitive
- ❑ Vestibular or facial swelling in seen in these patients
- ❑ Pulp tests show negative results

Differential Diagnosis

Pulp vitality tests help in reaching correct diagnosis

Treatment

- ❑ Drainage
- ❑ Complete extirpation of pulp
- ❑ Appropriate analgesics and antibiotics if necessary

Chronic Apical Periodontitis

It is caused by necrotic pulp which results from prolonged inflammation that erodes the cortical plate making a periapical lesion visible on the radiograph. The lesion contains granulation tissue consisting of fibroblasts and collagen.

Diagnosis

- ❑ It is usually asymptomatic but in acute phase may cause a dull, throbbing pain
- ❑ Pulp tests show nonvital pulp
- ❑ There is no pain on percussion
- ❑ Radiographically, it is usually associated with periradicular radiolucent changes

Differential Diagnosis

It can be differentiated on the basis of histopathological features

Periodontal Abscess

Acute periodontal abscess is a virulent infection of an existing periodontal pocket. It can also occur because of apical extension of infection from gingival pocket.

Diagnosis

- ❑ Tooth is tender to lateral percussion
- ❑ When sinus tract is traced using gutta-percha, it points toward the lateral aspect of the tooth

Treatment

Root planning and curettage.

Pericoronitis

It is inflammation of the periodontal tissues surrounding the erupting third molar.

Diagnosis

- ❑ Deep pain which radiates to ear and neck
- ❑ May be associated with trismus

Treatment

Operculectomy and surgical removal of tooth if required.

■ Sources of Nonodontogenic Pain

As dental pain is considered one of the most common causes of orofacial pain, the dentist can be easily drawn to diagnosis of pain of odontogenic origin. There are many structures in the head and neck region which can simulate the dental pain. Such types of pain are classified under heterotrophic pain. Heterotrophic pain can be defined as any pain felt in an area other than its true source.

There are three general types of pain:

1. Central pain
2. Projected pain
3. Referred pain

Referred Pain

Referred pain is a heterotrophic pain that is felt in an area innervated by a different nerve, from one that mediates the primary pain. Referred pain is wholly dependent upon the original source of pain. It cannot be provoked by stimulation where the pain is felt while it can be accentuated only by stimulation the area where primary source of pain is present. Referred pain can be of odontogenic or nonodontogenic origin.

Odontogenic Referred Pain

In this, pain originates from endodontically involved tooth and is referred to adjacent teeth/tooth or approximating deep and superficial structures **(Figs. 8.2 and 8.3)**. For example, pain from pulpal involvement of mandibular second or third molar is referred to ear. This pain is diagnosed by selective anesthesia technique.

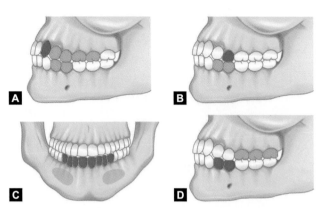

Figs. 8.2A to D Referred pain showing involved tooth (red color) and teeth affected (orange color) by this: (A). If maxillary canine is involved,it may refer pain to maxillary premolars,first and second molars,mandibular premolars; (B). Maxillary premolar refer pain to mandibular premolars; (C). Mandibular anterior and premolar teeth refer pain to mental area; (D). Mandibular premolars refer pain to maxillary molars.

Nonodontogenic Referred Pain

In this, pain originates from deep tissues, muscles, joints, ligaments, etc. and is perceived at a site away from its origin. Pain arising from musculoskeletal organs is deep, dull,

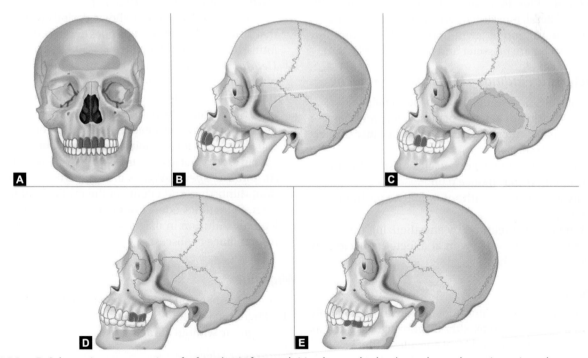

Figs. 8.3A to E Schematic representation of referred pain from pulpitis where red color shows the teeth causing pain and orange colored area shows the remote areas of referred pain: (A) Maxillary incisors refer pain to frontal area; (B) Maxillary canine and first premolar refer pain into the nasolabial area; (C) Maxillary second premolar and first molar refer pain to maxilla and back of temporal region; (D) Maxillary second and third molars refer pain to mandibular molar area and seldom in ear; (E) Mandibular first and second molars refer pain to ear and angle of the mandible.

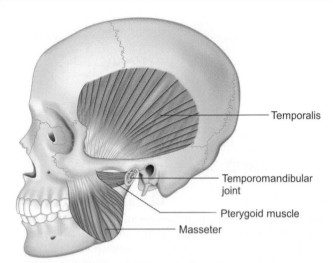

Fig. 8.4 Myofascial headache: myofascial headache occurs due to overstretching of mandible during dental procedures, parafunctional movements like bruxism.

aching and diffuse type. Pain form cutaneous origin is sharp, burning and localized (e.g., pain of maxillary sinusitis and may result pain in maxillary premolars).

Myofascial Pain

It is characterized by chronic pain which occurs during dental procedures, blow to the mandible. Characteristic of this pain are unilateral, muscle tenderness, presence of clicking sound and limitation of jaw functions. Most commonly affected muscles are masseter and temporalis (**Fig. 8.4**).

Characteristic Findings of Muscular Toothache

- Nonpulsatile, diffuse, dull, and constant pain
- Pain increases with function of masticatory muscles. For example, pain is increased on chewing because of effect on masseter muscle
- Palpation of the involved muscles at specific points (trigger points)* may induce pain
- Usually arise with or without pulpal or periradicular pathology
- Tooth pain is not relieved by anesthetizing the tooth; rather local anesthesia given at affected muscle may reduce the toothache

Diagnosis

These muscular pains as nonodontogenic tooth is purely based on lack of symptoms after diagnostic tests such as pulp testing, percussion and local anesthesia block.

Several therapeutic options used in the **management** of muscular pain are:

---

*Trigger points are hyperexcitable muscle tissues which may feel like taut bands or knots.

- Restriction of functional activities within painless limit
- Occlusal rearrangement
- Deep massage
- Spray and stretch technique
- Ultrasound therapy
- Local anesthesia at the site of trigger points
- Analgesics

Neurovascular Toothache (Fig. 8.5)

Most common neurovascular pain in the mouth and face is migraine. This category of pain includes three subdivisions of primary headache. These are:

1. Migraine
2. Tension type headache
3. Cluster headache

These neurovascular entities can produce relatively localized pains that match with the signs and symptoms with the toothache (Fig. 8.8). These accompanying toothaches are usually mistaken for true odontogenic pains and can be treated as separate entities.

Features of Neurovascular Toothache

- Pain is **deep, throbbing, spontaneous** in onset, variable in nature and pulsatile. These are characteristics which simulate pulpal pain
- **Pain** is predominantly **unilateral**
- Accompanying **toothache** shows periods of **remission** that imitates the pain-free episodes or temporal behavior found in neurovascular pain
- **Headache** is considered as the main symptom. It is most often accompanied by toothache
- **Recurrence** is characteristic finding in neurovascular pain. Sometimes, the pain may undergo remission after dental treatment has been performed in these teeth. It usually appears for a certain period of time and may even spread to adjacent teeth, opposing teeth, or the entire face
- **Autonomic effects** such as nasal congestion, lacrimation, rhinorrhea and edema of the eyelids and face are seen. Sometimes edema of the eyelids and face might lead to confusion in diagnosis as these features bear a resemblance to abscess

Migraine

Migraine has been divided into two main types:

1. Migraine with aura
2. Migraine without aura

Features of Migraine

- Commonly found between the age group **20–40 years**
- **Visual auras** are most common. These usually occur 10–30 min prior to the onset of headache pain (migraine with aura)

☐ Pain is usually unilateral, pulsatile, or throbbing in nature (**Fig. 8.5**)
☐ More common in *females*
☐ Patient usually experiences nausea, vomiting, photophobia
☐ Various drugs used in the *management* of migraine are sumatriptan, β-blockers, tricyclic antidepressants, and calcium channel blockers

Cluster Headache

☐ Commonly found in the age group 20–50 years
☐ Cluster headaches derive their name from the temporal behavior and usually occur in series, that is, one to eight attacks per day
☐ More common in males than females
☐ Pain is unilateral, excruciating and continuous in nature and usually found in orbital, supraorbital, or temporal region (**Fig. 8.6**)
☐ Autonomic symptoms such as nasal stuffiness, lacrimation, rhinorrhea, or edema of eyelids and face are usually found
☐ Standard treatment is inhalation of 100% oxygen

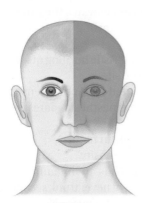

Migraine

Fig. 8.5 Throbbing pain with pulsating nature localized on one side of the head.

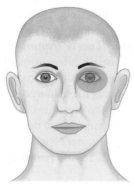

Cluster

Fig. 8.6 In cluster headache, pain is often around eyes.

Behavior of neurovascular variants should be well appreciated to avoid any unnecessary treatment and frustration felt by patient and clinician. Although the term neurovascular toothache is nondescriptive, it has given the dentist an important clinical entity that has been misdiagnosed and mistreated in the past.

Signs and symptoms of neurovascular headache that mimic the toothache are
• Periodic and recurrent nature
• Precise recognition of painful tooth
• Absence of local dental etiology

Cardiac Toothache

Excruciating referred pain felt in mandible and maxilla from area outside the head and neck region is most commonly from the heart. Cardiac pain is clinically characterized by heaviness, tightness, or throbbing pain in the substernal region which commonly radiates to left shoulder, arm, neck and mandible (**Fig. 8.7**).

Characteristics of cardiac toothache are:
☐ Pain is of sudden in onset, gradually increasing in intensity, diffuse with cyclic pattern that vary in intensity from mild to severe
☐ Tooth pain is increased with physical activities
☐ Chest pain is usually associated
☐ Pain is not relieved by anesthesia of lower jaw or by giving analgesics

Neuropathic Pain

Neuropathic pain is usually caused by abnormalities in the neural structures themselves. Neuropathic pain is

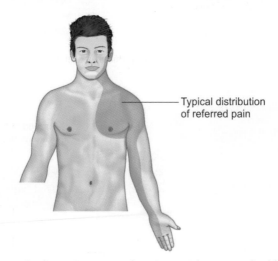

Typical distribution of referred pain

Fig. 8.7 Cardiac pain presents heaviness, tightness, or throbbing pain in the substernal region which commonly radiates to left shoulder, arm, neck, and mandible.

sometimes misdiagnosed as psychogenic pain because local factors cannot be visualized.

Neuropathic pain can be classified into different categories:

- Neuralgia
- Neuritis
- Neuropathy

Neuralgia

Paroxysmal, unilateral, severe, stabbing, or lancinating pains usually are the characteristics of all *paroxysmal neuralgias.* Pain is usually of short duration and lasts for few seconds.

Trigeminal neuralgia

- It is also known as **"tic douloureux"** which has literal meaning of *painful jerking*
- Usually characterized by paroxysmal, unilateral, sharp, lancinating pain typically confined to one or more branches of fifth cranial nerve **(Fig. 8.8)**
- Even slight stimulation of "trigger points" may elicit sharp, shooting pain **(Fig. 8.9)**. Sometimes trigger points are present intraorally. These are stimulated upon chewing which may lead to diagnosis of odontogenic pain. Intraoral trigger points always create confusion in diagnosis if not properly evaluated
- Local anesthesia given at the trigger point reduces the attacks
- It rarely crosses midline
- Commonly seen in patients over the age of 50 years
- Attacks generally do not occur at night
- Absence of dental etiology along with symptoms of paroxysmal, sharp, shooting pain always alert the dentist to include neuralgia in differential diagnosis
- *Treatment* includes surgical and medicinal. Usually medicinal approach is preferred. It includes administration of carbamazepine, baclofen, phenytoin sodium and gabapentin, etc.

Neuritis

Neuritis literally means inflammation of nerve. It is usually observed as heterotopic pain in the peripheral distribution of the affected nerve. It may be caused by traumatic, bacterial, and viral infection. In neuritis, the inflammatory process elevates the threshold for pricking pain but lowers it for burning pain. Characteristics of pain in neuritis are:

- Pain has a characteristic burning quality along with easy localization of the site
- It may be associated with other sensory effects such as hyperesthesia, hypoesthesia, paresthesia, dysesthesia, and anesthesia
- Pain is nonpulsatile in nature
- Pain may vary in intensity

Peripheral neuritis is an inflammatory process occurring along the course of never trunk secondary to traumatic, bacterial, thermal, or toxic causes. Neuritis of superior dental plexus has been reported when inflammation of sinus is present. Dental nerves frequently lie just below the lining mucosa or are separated by very thin osseous structure. These nerves are easily involved due to direct extension. Symptoms usually seen along with antral disease are pain, paresthesia and anesthesia of a tooth, gingiva, or area supplied by infraorbital nerve. *Mechanical nerve trauma* is more common in oral surgery cases. It usually arises from inflammation of the inferior dental nerve either due to trauma or infection.

Acute neuritis cases are always misdiagnosed and remain untreated. Most of the times, dental procedures are done to decrease the symptoms of neuritis as these are difficult to diagnose. These unnecessary dental procedures further act as aggravating factors for neuritis, making it chronic.

Treatment of neuritis

- Treatment is based on its etiology
- If bacterial source is present, antibiotics are indicated

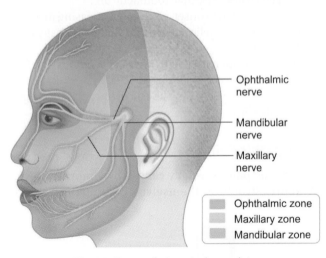

Fig. 8.8 Zones of trigeminal neuralgia.

Ophthalmic nerve
Mandibular nerve
Maxillary nerve

Ophthalmic zone
Maxillary zone
Mandibular zone

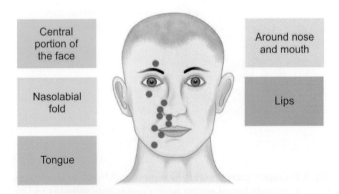

Fig. 8.9 Trigger zones for trigeminal neuralgia.

Central portion of the face

Nasolabial fold

Tongue

Around nose and mouth

Lips

- ❑ If viral infection is suspected, antiviral therapy should be started
- ❑ If there is no infection, steroids should be considered

Neuropathy

This is the term used for localized and sustained pain secondary to an injury or change in neural structure. Atypical odontalgia has been included in neuropathy. Atypical odontalgia means toothache of unknown cause. It is also known as ***"phantom tooth pain"*** or ***"dental migraine."*** Most patients who report with atypical odontalgia usually have multiple dental procedures completed before reaching a final diagnosis.

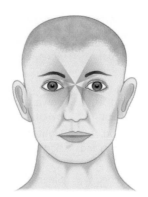

Fig. 8.10 In sinus headache, pain is behind the forehead and/or cheekbones.

Clinical characteristics of neuropathy
- ❑ Also called atypical odontalgia
- ❑ More common in women
- ❑ Frequently found in fourth or fifth decades of life
- ❑ Tooth pain remains constant or unchanged for weeks or months
- ❑ Constant source of pain in tooth with no local etiology
- ❑ Pain usually felt in these patients is dull, aching, and persistent
- ❑ Most commonly affected teeth are maxillary premolar and molar region
- ❑ Response to local anesthesia is equal in both pulpal toothache and atypical odontalgia

Sinus Toothache

Sinus and nasal mucosal pain is also another source which can mimic toothache. It is usually expressed as pain throughout the maxilla and maxillary teeth. Patient often complains of pain behind the forehead and/or cheeks (**Fig. 8.10**).

Clinical characteristics of sinus or nasal mucosal toothache are:
- ❑ Fullness or pressure below the eyes. Sinus pressure can cause tooth pain, especially in maxillary molars. Roots of maxillary molars lie next to maxillary sinus. Blood vessels and nerves which enter in apical foramina of molar may run right through the sinus to get into the tooth. Any pressure or inflammation in sinuses can irritate these nerves resulting in sinus toothache (**Fig. 8.11**)
- ❑ Increased pain sensation when head is placed lower than the heart
- ❑ Local anesthesia of referred tooth/teeth does not eliminated pain while topical anesthesia of nasal mucosa will eliminate the pain if etiology lies in nasal mucosa
- ❑ Different diagnostic aids used to diagnose sinus disease include paranasal sinus view, computed tomography imaging, and nasal ultrasound

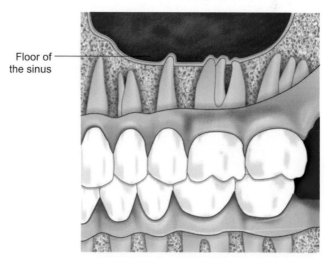

Floor of the sinus

Fig. 8.11 Sinus pressure can cause toothache especially in maxillary molars because roots of maxillary molars lie next to maxillary sinus.

Psychogenic Toothache

This is a category of mental disorders in which a patient may complain of physical condition without the presence of any physical signs. It must be noted that psychogenic pain is rare. So, all other possible diagnoses must be ruled out before making the diagnosis of psychogenic pain.

The following features are found in psychogenic toothache:
- ❑ Pain is observed in multiple teeth
- ❑ Precipitated by severe psychological stress
- ❑ Frequent changes in character, location, and intensity of pain
- ❑ Response to therapy varies which can include lack of response or unusual response
- ❑ Usually referred to a ***psychiatrist*** for further management

Different type of conditions along with nature of pain, aggravating factors, and duration			
Condition	Nature of pain	Aggravating factors	Duration
Odontalgia	Stabbing, throbbing intermittent	Hot, cold, lying down, tooth percussion	Hours to days
Trigeminal neuralgia	Lancinating, excruciating and episodic	Light touch on skin or mucosa	Second to minutes
Cluster headache	Severe ache, episodic retro-orbital component	Sleep, alcohol	Hours
Cardiogenic	Temporary pain in left side of mandible, episodic	Exertion	Minutes
Sinusitis	Severe ache, throbbing, nonepisodic involving multiple maxillary posterior teeth	Tooth percussion, lowering of head	Hours, days

Question

1. Write short notes on:
   • Dentin hypersensitivity
   • Enumerate sources of odontogenic pain
   • Acute periapical abscess
   • Enumerate sources of nonodontogenic pain
   • Trigeminal neuralgia
   • Referred pain

Bibliography

1. Hargreaves KM, Cohen S. Pathways of the pulp. 10th ed. Mosby: Elsevier; 2012.
2. Hargreaves KM, et al. Adrenergic regulation of capsaicinsensitive neurons in dental pulp. J Endod 2003;29:397–9.
3. Henry MA, Hargreaves KM. Peripheral mechanism of odontogenic pain. Dent Clin North Am 2007;51:19–44.
4. Ingle JI, Bakland LK, Decker BC. Endodontics. 6th ed. Elsevier; 2008
5. Merrill RL. Central mechanisms of orofacial pain. Dent Clin North Am 2007;51:45–59.
6. Merrill RL. Orofacial pain mechanisms and their clinical application. Dent Clin North Am 1997;41:167–88.

Case Selection and Treatment Planning

Every single tooth starting from central incisor to third molar can be a potential candidate for root canal therapy. According to treatment point of view, four factors determine the decision to do or not to do a root canal treatment. These factors are accessibility, restorability, strategic value of a tooth and general resistance of patient which ensures success. In this chapter, we will discuss indications, contraindications, and treatment planning regarding endodontic therapy.

Indications of Endodontic Treatment

Actual Reason for Endodontic Therapy

If pulp is involved due to caries, trauma, fracture, etc., tooth should be saved by endodontic treatment **(Figs. 9.1 and 9.2)**.

Elective Endodontics

In teeth with crack or large restoration, elective endodontics is done to prevent premature loss of cusp during their restoration because in these cases elective endodontics allows more predictable and successful results **(Fig. 9.3)**.

Inadequate Restorations

Sometimes when attempt is made to repair the teeth with cracks or inadequate crown margins, high degree of restorative failure is seen. In such cases, endodontic treatment followed by postendodontic restoration provide high success rate.

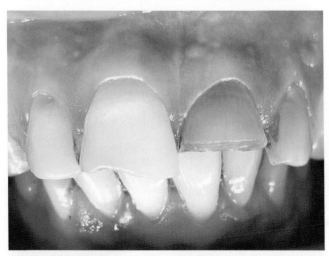

Fig. 9.1 Fractured and discolored maxillary left central incisor requires endodontic treatment followed by crown.

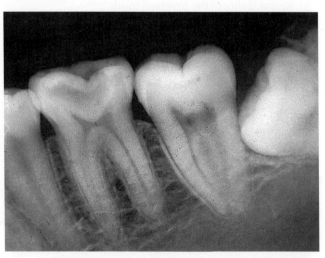

Fig. 9.2 Endodontic treatment is required to manage mandibular first molar with deep dental caries.

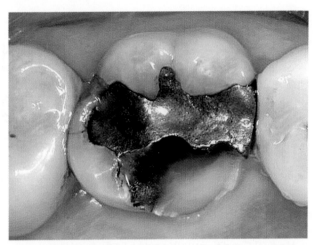

Fig. 9.3 Endodontic treatment and full coverage crown is indicated to manage fractured restoration of mandibular first molar.

Desensitization of Tooth

Sometimes teeth with attrition, abrasion, or erosion defects need endodontic treatment to get rid of the sensitivity of the patient.

Endodontic Emergency

If patient presents acute dental pain/swelling, endodontic treatment is indicated before complete examination and treatment plan.

Contraindications of Endodontic Therapy

The following four factors influence the decision of endodontic treatment:

1. Accessibility of apical foramen
2. Restorability of the involved tooth
3. Strategic importance of the involved tooth
4. General resistance of the patient

Though, there are only few absolute contraindications of the endodontic therapy, the following cases are considered *Poor candidates for endodontic treatment*:

❏ Teeth with extensive root caries, furcation caries, poor crown/root ratio and fractured root are contraindicated for endodontic treatment **(Fig. 9.4)**

❏ Teeth in which instrumentation is not possible like roots with dilacerations, calcifications, dentinal sclerosis, etc.

❏ Trismus or scarring from surgical procedures or trauma, etc. may limit the accessibility due to limited mouth opening

❏ Teeth with large, multiple external root resorptive lesions **(Figs. 9.5 and 9.6)**

❏ Teeth with vertical root fractures

❏ ***Teeth with no strategic value:*** Two main factors which determine status of a tooth are restorability and

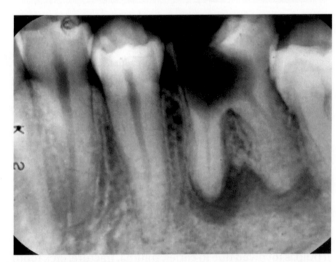

Fig. 9.5 Mandibular first molar with extensive caries and periapical radiolucency is poor candidate for endodontic treatment.

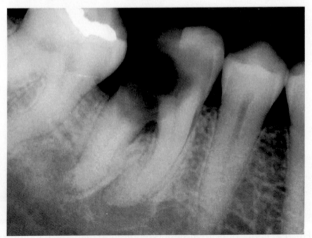

Fig. 9.4 Mandibular first molar with extensive root and furcation caries is poor candidate for endodontic treatment.

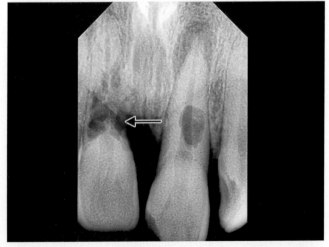

Fig. 9.6 Radiograph showing extensive external resorption of maxillary right central incisor; not indicated for endodontic treatment.

periodontal support. Tooth which cannot be restored or that has inadequate, amenable periodontal support has hopeless prognosis. Evaluation of the oral cavity can decide whether tooth is strategic or not, for example, if a person has multiple missing teeth, root canal of third molar may be needed. But in case of well-maintained oral hygiene with full dentition, an exposed third molar can be considered for extraction

❑ **Evaluation of the clinician:** Clinician should be honest to evaluate his/her efficiency to do the patient

❑ **Systemic conditions:** Most of the medical conditions do not contraindicate the endodontic treatment, but patient should be thoroughly evaluated in order to manage the case optimally

Treatment Planning

Treatment planning signifies the planning of management of the patient's dental problems in systematic and ordered way which assures complete knowledge of patient's needs, nature

Condition	Symptoms	Clinical tests	Radiographic experience	Treatment
Normal pulp	• No symptoms	• Response to cold testing and effect lasts only for 1–2 sec, then disappear • Response normally to electrical pulp testing	Normal PDL space and intact lamina dura	No treatment
Reversible pulpitis	• Discomfort or pain on **sweet/cold** food and beverages • It last for a **few seconds**, then relieved • Pain **never** spontaneous	• Cold test: response positive, enough for diagnosis • Electrical pulp test: response positive	• Intact lamina dura • Normal PDL space • Normal periapical area	• Prevention • Remove the offending stimulus and place sedative dressing
Irreversible pulpitis	• Spontaneous sharp pain • Pain lasts for minutes to hours • Poorly localized referred pain • Pain increases on bending and during sleep • Aggravated by hot, relieved by cold • Over-the-counter analgesics ineffective	• Responsive to heat test • EPT test gives positive response	• Intact lamina dura • Slight widening of PDL space • If infection is persistent, periapical radiolucency can be seen	Endodontic treatment
Necrotic pulp	• Asymptomatic • History of pulpitis or trauma • Lack of normal translucent enamel or discoloration of tooth	• Nonresponsive to heat test • EPT test gives negative response • If apical infection is present, tenderness on percussion is there	• Intact lamina dura • Slight widening of PDL space • If infection is persistent, periapical radiolucency can be seen	Endodontic treatment
Apical periodontitis	• Pain on biting and mastication	• Positive response to palpation and percussion	• Slight widening of PDL space may or may not be present • Periapical radiolucency may or may not be seen	Endodontic treatment
Acute apical abscess	• Spontaneous pain • Pain on biting • Swelling of apical area • Fever, malaise, and lymphadenopathy may be seen	• Positive response to palpation and percussion	• Slight widening of PDL space may or may not be present • Periapical radiolucency may or may not be seen	• RCT • Establish drainage
Chronic apical abscess	• Little or no pain • Tenderness of tooth to pressure • Swelling of apical area • Fever, malaise, and lymphadenopathy may be seen	• Positive response to palpation and percussion	• Slight widening of PDL space may or may not be present • Periapical radiolucency present	• RCT • Establish drainage

Abbreviations: PDL, periodontal ligament; EPT, electrical pulp test; RCT: root canal treatment.

of problem and prognosis of the treatment. Thus the stage of assessment of a complete picture overlaps with the stages of decision-making, treatment planning, and treatment phase.

Factors Affecting Treatment Planning

❑ Chief complaint regarding pain and swelling requires urgent treatment and planning for definitive solution
❑ Previous history of dental treatment (solve the residual problems of previous dental treatment)
❑ Medical history (identify factors which affect prognosis of the treatment)
❑ Intraoral examination (to know the general oral condition first before focusing on site of complaint so as not to miss the cause)
❑ Extraoral examination (to differentially diagnose the chief complaint)
❑ Oral hygiene
❑ Periodontal status (to see the periodontal foundation for long-term prognosis of involved tooth)
❑ Teeth and restorative status (to identify replacement of missing teeth, status of the remaining dentition)
❑ Occlusion (to check functional relationship between opposing teeth, parafunctional habits, etc.)
❑ Special tests (to explore the unseen tissues)
❑ Diagnosis (repeat the series of conclusion)
❑ Treatment options (evaluate various options to decide the best choice for long-term benefit of the patient)

Medical Conditions Influencing Endodontic Treatment Planning

Medical condition	Modifications in treatment planning
Patients with valvular disease and murmurs	
• Patients are susceptible to bacterial endocarditis secondary to dental treatment	• Prophylactic antibiotics are advocated before initiation of the endodontic therapy
Hypertensive condition	
• In these patients, stress and anxiety may further increase chances of myocardial infarction or cerebrovascular accidents	• Give premedication • Plan short appointments
• Sometimes antihypertensive drugs may cause postural hypotension	• Use local anesthetic with minimum amount of vasoconstrictors
Myocardial infarction	
• Stress and anxiety can precipitate myocardial infarction or angina	• Elective endodontic treatment is postponed if recent myocardial infarction is present, i.e., <6 months
• Some degree of congestive heart failure may be present • Chances of excessive bleeding when patient is on aspirin • If pacemaker is present, apex locators can cause electrical interferences	• Reduce the level of stress and anxiety while treating patient • Keep the appointments short and comfortable • Use local anesthetics without epinephrine • Antibiotic prophylaxis is given before initiation of the treatment
Prosthetic valve or implants	
• Patients are at high risk for bacterial endocarditis • Tendency for increased bleeding because of prolonged use of anticoagulant therapy	• Prophylactic antibiotic coverage before initiation of the treatment • Consult a physician for any suggestion regarding patient treatment
Leukemia	
Patient has increased tendency for • Opportunistic infections • Prolonged bleeding • Poor and delayed wound healing	• Consult the physician • Avoid treatment during acute stages • Avoid long-duration appointment • Strict oral hygiene instructions • Evaluate the bleeding time and platelet status • Use of antibiotic prophylaxis
Cancer	
• These patients suffer from xerostomia, mucositis, trismus, and excessive bleeding due to radiotherapy and chemotherapy regime • Prone to infections because of bone marrow suppression	• Consult the physician prior to treatment • Perform only emergency treatment if possible • Symptomatic treatment of mucositis, trismus, and xerostomia • Optimal antibiotic coverage prior to treatment • Strict oral hygiene regimen
Bleeding disorders	
Patients with hemophilia, thrombocytopenia, prolonged bleeding due to liver disease, on anticoagulant therapy have increased tendency for • Spontaneous bleeding • Prolonged bleeding • Petechiae, ecchymosis, and hematoma	• Take careful history of the patient • Consult the physician for suggestions regarding the patient • Avoid aspirin containing compounds and NSAIDs • In thrombocytopenia cases, replacement of platelets is done before procedure • Prophylactic antibiotic coverage to be given • In case of liver disease, avoid drugs metabolized by liver

Contd...

Contd...

Renal disease

• In this, patient usually has hypertension and anemia • Intolerance to nephrotoxic drugs • Increased susceptibility to opportunistic infections • Increased tendency for bleeding	• Prior consultation with a physician • Check the blood pressure before initiation of treatment • Antibiotic prophylaxis – Screen the bleeding time • Avoid drugs metabolized and excreted by kidney

Diabetes mellitus

• Patient has increased tendency for infections and poor wound healing • Patient may be suffering from diseases related to cardiovascular system, kidneys, and nervous system like myocardial infarction, hypertension, congestive heart failure, renal failure, and peripheral neuropathy	• Take careful history of the patient • Consult with a physician prior to treatment • Note the blood glucose levels • Patient should have normal meals before appointment • If a patient is on insulin therapy, he/she should have his/her regular dose of insulin before appointment • Schedule the appointment early in the morning • Antibiotics may be needed • Have instant source of sugar available in clinic • Patient should be evaluated for the presence of hypertension, myocardial infarction, or renal failure

Pregnancy

• In such patients, the harm to patient can occur via radiation exposure, medications, and increased level of stress and anxiety • In the third trimester, chances of development of supine hypotension are increased	• Do the elective procedure in second trimester • Use the principles of ALARA while exposing patients to the radiation • Avoid any drugs which can cause harm to the fetus • Consult the physician to verify the physical status of the patient and any precautions if required for the patient • Reduce the number of oral microorganism (by chlorhexidine mouthwash) • In third trimester, don't place patient in supine position for prolonged periods

Contd...

Anaphylaxis

Patient gives history of severe allergic reaction on administration of:
• Local anesthetics
• Certain drugs such as penicillin and its related drugs
• Latex gloves and rubber dam sheets
	• Take careful history of the patient
	• Avoid use of agents to which patient is allergic
	• Always keep the emergency kit available
	• In case the reaction develops:
	  – Identify the reaction
	  – Call the physician
	  – Place patient in supine position
	  – Check vital signs
	  – Provide CPR if needed
	  – Admit the patient

Abbreviation: ALARA, as low as reasonably achievable.

Summary

Efficient and successful endodontics begins with proper case selection. The clinician must know his/her limitations and select cases accordingly. Since success of endodontic treatment depends upon many factors which can be modified to get better before initiating the treatment. Therefore accurate and thorough preparation of both patient as well as tooth to be treated should be carried out to achieve the successful treatment results.

Questions

1. Discuss different factors affecting case selection for endodontic treatment.
2. Discuss indications and contraindications for root canal treatment.
3. Write short notes on:
   • Treatment planning in endodontics
   • Role of medical history in endodontics.

Bibliography

1. Hogan J, Radhakrishnan J. The assessment and importance of hypertension in the dental setting. Dent Clin North Am 2012;56:731–45
2. Malamed SF. Medical Emergencies in the Dental Office. 4th ed. St. Louis: CV Mosby Co; 1993; pp. 194–207.
3. Pototski M, Amenábar JM. Dental management of patients receiving anticoagulation or antiplatelet treatment. J Oral Sci 2007;49:253–8
4. Schwartz RS, Robbins JW. Post placement and restoration of endodontically treated teeth: a literature review. J Endod 2004;30:289–301.
5. Tomás Carmona I, Diz Dios P, Scully C. Efficacy of antibiotic prophylactic regimens for the prevention of bacterial endocarditis of oral origin. J Dent Res 2007;86:1142–59

Contd...

Asepsis in Endodontics

Dental professionals are exposed to wide variety of microorganisms in the blood and saliva of patients, making infection control procedures important. Common goal of infection control is to eliminate or reduce the number of microbes from being transferred from one person to another.

Rationale for Infection Control

Deposition of organisms in the tissues and their growth resulting in a host reaction is called an infection. Number of organisms required to cause an infection is termed as *the infective dose.*

Factors affecting infective dose are
- ❑ Virulence of the organism
- ❑ Susceptibility of the host
- ❑ Age, drug therapy, or pre-existing disease, etc.

Microorganisms can spread from one person to another via *direct contact (*by touching soft tissues or teeth of patients), *indirect contact* (injuries with contaminated sharp instruments, needlestick injuries, or contact with contaminated equipment and surfaces), and *droplet infection (*by large particle droplets spatter which is transmitted by close contact).

POINTS TO REMEMBER

- Aerosols are invisible particles ranging 5–50 μm in size. These microorganisms remain airborne for hours and can cause infection when inhaled

- Mists are droplets approximately 50 μm in size. These tend to settle from air after 10–15 min. Both aerosols and mists can transmit pulmonary infections
- Spatter are particles >50 μm in size. It has the potential of causing infection of dental personnel by blood-borne pathogens

Cross Infection

Cross infection is the transmission of infectious agents among patients and staff within a clinical environment **(Flowchart 10.1)**.

Different Routes of Spread of Infection

- ❑ Patient to dental health care worker
- ❑ Dental health care worker to the patient
- ❑ Patient-to-patient
- ❑ Dental office to the community
- ❑ Community to the patient (community to patient infection occurs through water supply of dental unit. These microorganisms colonize inside the water lines, and thereby form a biofilm which is responsible for causing infection)

Modes of Transmission

- ❑ Direct contact through break in skin or direct contact with mucous membrane
- ❑ Indirect contact via sharp cutting instruments and needlestick injuries
- ❑ Droplet infection by *spatter* produced during dental procedures

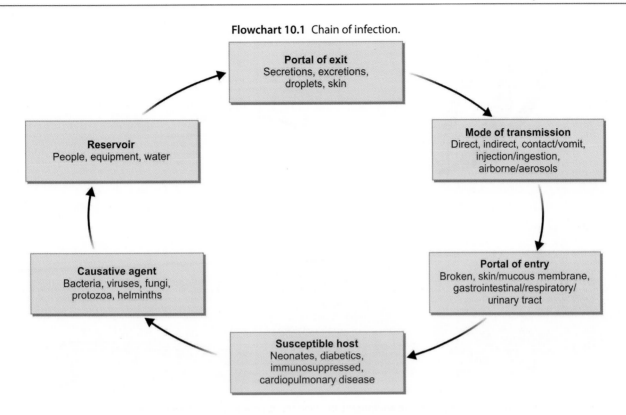

Flowchart 10.1 Chain of infection.

Objective of Infection Control

The main objective of infection control is elimination or reduction in spread of infection from all types of microorganisms.

Universal Precautions

It is always recommended to follow some basic infection control procedures for all patients, termed "universal precautions."

These are as follows:

- **Immunization:** All members of the dental team (who are exposed to blood or blood-contaminated articles) should be vaccinated against hepatitis B
- Use of **personal protective barrier techniques,** that is, use of protective gown, face mask, protective eyewear, gloves, etc. These reduce the risk of exposure to infectious material and injury from sharp instruments
- Maintaining **hand hygiene**

Personal Protection Equipment

Barrier Technique

Use of barrier technique is very important, which includes gown, face mask, protective eyewear, and gloves (**Fig. 10.1**).

Protective clothing should be made of fluid-resistant material and should not be worn out of the office for any reason. These should be washed in hot water (70–158°F) or cool water containing 50–150 ppm of chlorine.

Protective gown: Protective gown should be worn to prevent contamination of normal clothing and protect the skin of the clinician from exposure to blood and body substances.

- Gown can be reusable or disposable for use. It should have a high neck and long sleeves to protect the arms from splash and spatter
- Protective clothing must be removed before leaving the workplace

Facemask: A surgical mask that covers both the nose and mouth should be worn by the clinician during procedures. Though facemasks do not provide complete microbiological protection, they prevent the splatter from contaminating the face. Mask with 95% filtration efficiency for particles 3–5 μm in diameter should be worn.

- Outer surface of the mask can get contaminated with infectious droplets from spray or from touching the mask with contaminated fingers, so should not be reused
- Maximum time for wearing masks should not be more than one hour since it becomes dampened from respiration, resulting in its degradation
- To remove the mask, grasp it only by its strings not by the mask itself (**Fig. 10.2**)

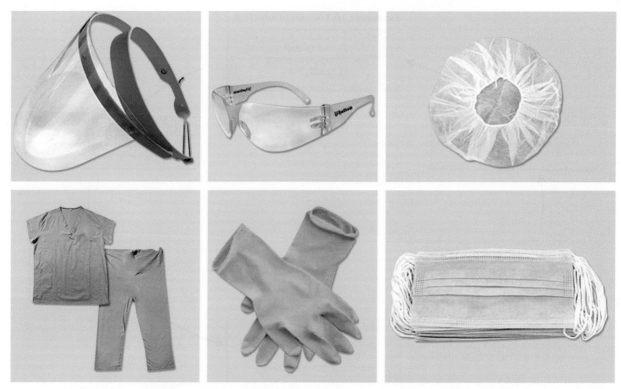

Fig. 10.1 Personal protective equipment showing mouth mask, gloves, eyewear, head cap.

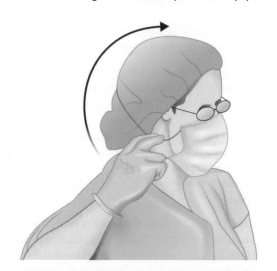

Fig. 10.2 Removal of facemask should be done by grasping it only by its strings, not by mask itself.

Head cap: Hairs should be properly tied and covered with a head cap.

Protective eyewear: Eyewear protects the eyes from injury and from microbes such as hepatitis B virus, which can be transmitted through conjunctiva. Eyewear should be clear, antifog, distortion free, close fitting and shielded. Face shield: chin length plastic face shield can be worn as alternate to protective eyewear

Gloves: Gloves should be worn to prevent contamination of hands when touching mucous membranes, blood, saliva, and to reduce the chances of transmission of infected micro-organisms from clinician to patient. Gloves should be of good quality and well-fitted. Gloves should be disposed after the activity for which they were used. Some persons can show allergic reactions to gloves due to latex (polyisoprene) or antioxidants such as mercaptobenzothiazole. Ensure that latex-free equipment and nonlatex gloves (polyurethane or vinyl gloves) are used on patients who have a latex allergy. Overgloves or paper towels should be used for opening drawers, cabinets, etc.

Hand Hygiene

Hand hygiene significantly reduces potential pathogens on the hands and is considered the single most critical measure for reducing the risk of transmitting organisms to patients and dentists. Flora present on the skin can be:

Transient flora, which colonize the superficial layers of the skin, are easier to remove by routine handwashing. These are acquired by direct contact with patients or contaminated environmental surfaces

Resident flora, attached to deeper layers of the skin, is more resistant to removal and less likely to be associated with such infections

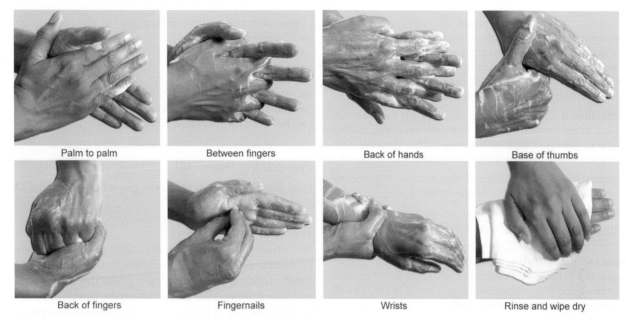

| Palm to palm | Between fingers | Back of hands | Base of thumbs |
| Back of fingers | Fingernails | Wrists | Rinse and wipe dry |

Fig. 10.3 Showing the technique of hand washing.

Purpose of surgical hand antisepsis is to eliminate transient flora and reduce resident flora for the duration of a procedure to prevent introduction of organisms in the operative wound if gloves become punctured or torn. Hand cleansers containing mild antiseptic like 3% PCMX (parachlorometaxylenol), triclosan, or chlorhexidine control transient pathogens and suppress overgrowth of skin bacteria.

Hand washing instructions (Fig. 10.3)

❑ Wet hands with warm water.
❑ Apply adequate amount of soap to achieve lather.
❑ Rub vigorously for a minimum of 15 seconds, covering all surfaces of hands and fingers. Pay particular attention to finger tips, between fingers, backs of hands, and base of thumbs, which are the most commonly missed areas.
❑ Rinse well with running water.
❑ Dry thoroughly with a disposable paper towel.

Indications for hand hygiene

❑ At the beginning and after completion of case.
❑ Before putting on and after removal of gloves.
❑ Before touching eyes, nose, face, or mouth
❑ Before eating and drinking
❑ After barehanded contact with contaminated equipment or surfaces and before leaving treatment areas
❑ At the end of the day

Classification of Instruments

Centers for Disease Control and Prevention (CDC) classified the instrument into critical, semicritical, and noncritical depending on the potential risk of infection during the use of these instruments. These categories are also referred to as **Spaulding classification** *(given by Spaulding in 1968).*

Classification of instrument sterilization			
Category	*Definition*	*Examples*	*Method of sterilization*
Critical	Where instruments enter or penetrate into sterile tissue, cavity, or blood stream	• Surgical blades and instruments • Surgical dental bur	Heat sterilization
Semicritical	Which contact intact mucosa or nonintact skin	• Amalgam condenser • Dental hand-pieces • Mouth mirror • Saliva ejectors	Heat sterilization
Noncritical	Which contact intact skin	• Pulse oximeter • Stethoscope • Light switches • Dental chair	High-level disinfectant after cleaning

Definitions

Cleaning: It is the process that physically removes contamination but does not necessarily destroy microorganisms. It is a prerequisite before decontamination by disinfection or sterilization of instruments since organic material prevents contact with microbes inactivates disinfectants.

Disinfection: It is the process of using an agent that destroys germs or other harmful microbes or inactivates them, usually referred to chemicals that kill the growing forms (vegetative forms) but not the resistant spores of bacteria.

Antisepsis: It is the destruction of pathogenic microorganisms existing in their vegetative state on living tissue.

Sterilization: Sterilization involves any process, physical, or chemical that will destroy all forms of life, including bacterial, fungi, spores, and viruses.

Aseptic technique: It is the method that prevents contamination of wounds and other sites by ensuring that only sterile objects and fluids come into contact with them, and that the risks of airborne contamination are minimized.

Antiseptic: It is a chemical applied to living tissues, such as skin or mucous membrane to reduce the number of microorganisms present, by inhibiting their activity or by destruction.

Disinfectant: It is a chemical substance that causes disinfection. It is used on nonvital objects to kill surface vegetative pathogenic organisms, but not necessarily spore forms or viruses.

Instrument Processing Procedures/ Decontamination Cycle

Instrument processing is the collection of procedures which prepare the contaminated instruments for reuse. For complete sterilization process, instruments should be processed correctly and carefully **(Flowchart 10.2)**.

Steps of instrument processing
- Presoaking (holding)
- Cleaning
- Corrosion control
- Packaging
- Sterilization
- Monitoring of sterilization
- Handling the processed instrument

Presoaking (Holding)

It facilitates cleaning process by preventing the debris from drying.

Procedure

Wear puncture-resistant heavy utility gloves and personnel protective equipment. Place loose instruments in a perforated cleaning basket and then place the basket into the holding solution. Perforated cleaning basket reduces the direct handling of instruments. So, chances of contamination are decreased. Holding solution for instruments can be neutral pH detergents, water, etc.

Cleaning

Cleaning reduces the bioburden, that is, microorganisms, blood, saliva, and other materials. Methods used for cleaning:
- *Manual scrubbing:* It is one of the most effective methods for removing debris, if performed properly. Brush delicately all the surfaces of instruments while submerged in cleaning solution using long-handled stiff nylon brush to keep the scrubbing hand away from sharp instrument surfaces. Use neutral pH detergents while cleaning.
- *Ultrasonic cleaning (Fig. 10.4):* It is an excellent cleaning method as it reduces direct handling of instruments

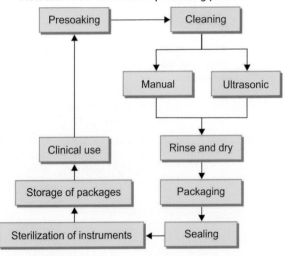

Flowchart 10.2 Instrument processing procedure.

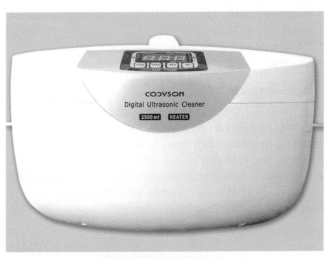

Fig. 10.4 Ultrasonic cleaner.

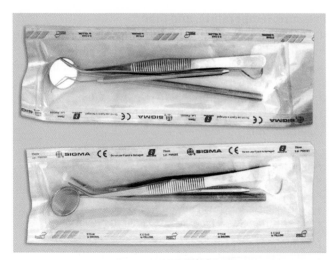

Fig. 10.5 Peel-pouches for packing instruments.

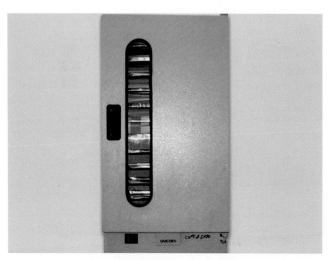

Fig. 10.6 Ultraviolet chamber for storage of sterile instruments.

❑ *Mechanism of action:* Ultrasonic energy generated in the ultrasonic cleaner produces billions of tiny bubbles which, further collapse and create high turbulence at the surface of the instrument. This turbulence dislodges the debris.

❑ Usually the time ranges vary from 4 to 16 min but time for cleaning vary due to
  • Nature of instrument
  • Amount of debris
  • Efficiency of ultrasonic unit

❑ *Mechanical–instrument washer:* These are designed to clean instruments in a hospital setup. Instrument washer also has the advantage that it reduces the direct handling of the instrument.

Control of Corrosion by Lubrication

For rust-prone instruments, use dry hot air oven/chemical vapor sterilization instead of autoclave. Use *rust inhibitor (sodium nitrite)* spray on the instruments.

Packaging

It maintains the sterility of instruments after the sterilization. Packaging materials can be self-sealing, paper–plastic, and peel-pouches. Instruments are kept wrapped until ready for use and sterilized packs should be allowed to cool before storage **(Fig. 10.5)**; otherwise condensation will occur inside the packs. Sterile packs should be stored in ultraviolet (UV) chamber **(Fig. 10.6)** or drums which can be locked.

Methods of Sterilization

Sterilization is the process by which an object, surface, or medium is freed of all microorganisms either in the vegetative or spore state **(Table 10.1)**.

Table 10.1: Sterilization method and type of packaging material

Sterilization method	Packaging material
Autoclave Wrapped cassettes	• Paper or plastic peel-pouches • Plastic tubing (made-up of nylon) • Thin clothes (thick clothes are not advised as they absorb too much heat) • Sterilization paper (paper wrap)
Chemical vapor	• Paper or plastic pouches • Sterilization paper
Dry heat	• Sterilization paper (paper wrap) • Nylon plastic tubing (indicated for dry heat) • Wrapped cassettes

Though there are many ways of sterilization, the following four methods are accepted methods in dental practice:
1. Moist/steam heat sterilization
2. Dry heat sterilization
3. Chemical vapor pressure sterilization
4. Ethylene oxide (ETOX) sterilization

Moist/Steam Heat Sterilization

Autoclave

❑ Autoclave provides the most efficient and reliable method of sterilization for all dental instruments

❑ It involves heating water to generate steam in a closed chamber resulting in moist heat that rapidly kills microorganisms **(Fig. 10.7)**

Saturated steam under pressure is the most efficient, quickest, safest, and effective method of sterilization because

❑ It has high penetrating power

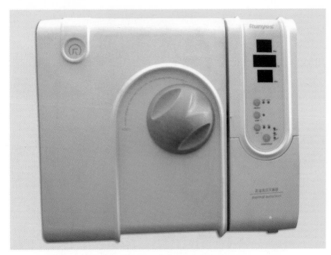

Fig. 10.7 Autoclave for moist heat sterilization.

☐ It gives up a large amount of heat (latent heat) to the surface with which it comes into contact and on which it condenses as water

Packaging of Instruments for Autoclaving

☐ For wrapping, closed containers such as closed metal trays, glass vials, and aluminum foils should not be used since they stop the steam from reaching the inner part of the packs

☐ For packaging of autoclaving instruments, one should use porous covering to permit steam to penetrate through and reach the instruments

☐ Materials used for packaging can be fabric or sealed paper or cloth pouches **(Fig. 10.8)** and paper-wrapped cassettes

☐ If instruments are to be stored and not used shortly after sterilization, the autoclave cycle should end with a drying phase to avoid tarnish or corrosion of the instruments

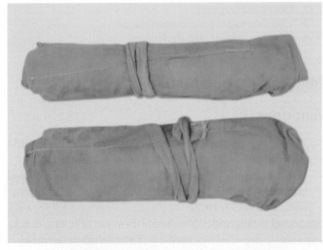

Fig. 10.8 Cloth pouches for instrument wrapping.

Pressure, temperature, and time

☐ Higher the temperature and pressure, shorter is the time required for sterilization

☐ At 15 psi pressure and temperature of 121°C, the time required is 15 min

☐ At 126°C, time required is 10 min

☐ At 132°C, time required is 3 min at 27–28 lbs—Flash sterilization

Advantages of autoclaving
- Time efficient
- Good penetration
- The results are consistently good and reliable
- The instruments can be wrapped prior to sterilization

Disadvantages of autoclaving
- Blunting and corrosion of sharp instruments
- Damage to rubber goods

Dry Heat Sterilization

Dry heat utilizes the hot air which has very little or no water vapors in it to sterilize the instruments.

Conventional Hot Air Oven

Hot air oven utilizes radiating dry heat for sterilization as this type of energy does not penetrate materials easily. So, long periods of exposure to high temperature are usually required. In conventional type of hot air oven, air circulates by gravity flow, thus it is also known as *Gravity convection*.

Packaging of Instruments for Dry Heat

Dry heat ovens usually achieve *temperature above 320°F (160°C)*. The packaging or wrapping material used should be able to withstand high temperature; otherwise, it may get charred. Acceptable materials for packaging are paper and plastic bags, wrapped cassettes, and aluminum foil. Unacceptable materials are plastic and paper bags which are not able to withstand dry heat temperature. Packs of instruments should be placed ≥1 cm apart for air to circulate in the chamber.

Recommended temperature and duration of hot oven				
Hot air oven				
Temperature (°C) 141	149	160	170	180
Time 3 h	2.5 h	2 h	1 h	30 min

Mechanism of Action

☐ Dry heat kills microorganisms by protein denaturation, coagulation, and oxidation

☐ Instruments that can be sterilized in dry hot oven are glassware such as pipettes, flasks, scissors, glass syringes, carbon steel instruments, and burs. Dry heat does not corrode sharp instrument surfaces. Also, it does not erode glassware surfaces

❑ Before placing in the oven, the glassware must be dried. The oven must be allowed to cool slowly for about 2 h as the glassware may crack due to sudden or uneven cooling.

Rapid heat transfer (forced air type): In this type of sterilizer, a fan or blower circulates the heated air throughout the chamber at a high velocity which, in turn, permits a more rapid transfer of heat energy from the air to instruments, thereby reducing the time.

Temperature/cycle recommended
370–375°F—12 min for wrapped instruments
370–375°F—16 min for unwrapped instruments

Advantages of dry heat sterilization
❑ No corrosion is seen in carbon steel instruments and burs
❑ Maintains the sharpness of cutting instruments
❑ Effective and safe for sterilization of metal instrument and mirrors
❑ Low cost of equipment
❑ Instruments are dry after cycle
❑ Industrial forced draft types usually provide a larger capacity at reasonable price
❑ Rapid cycles are possible at higher temperatures

Disadvantages of dry heat sterilization
❑ Poor penetrating capacity of dry heat
❑ A long cycle is required because of poor heat conduction and poor penetrating capacity
❑ High temperature may damage heat sensitive items such as rubber or plastic goods
❑ Instruments must be thoroughly dried before placing them for sterilization
❑ Inaccurate calibration and lack of attention to proper settings often lead to errors in sterilization
❑ Generally not suitable for handpieces
❑ Cannot sterilize liquids
❑ May discolor and char fabric

Chemical Vapor Sterilization/Chemiclave

Sterilization by chemical vapor under pressure is known as chemical vapor sterilization. Here, formaldehyde and alcohol formulation is heated in a closed chamber, producing hot vapors that kill microorganisms. Temperature, pressure, and time required for completion of one cycle is 270°F (132°C) at 20 lb for 30 min.

Chemical solution contents
❑ Active ingredient—0.23% formaldehyde
❑ Other ingredient—72.38% ethanol + acetone + water and other alcohols

Mechanism of Action
❑ Coagulation of protein
❑ Cell membrane disruption
❑ Removal of free sulfhydryl groups
❑ Substrate competition

Advantage
Eliminates corrosion of carbon steel instruments, burs and pliers.

Disadvantages
• The instruments or items which are sensitive to elevated temperature are damaged
• Sterilization of linen, textiles, fabric, or paper towels is not recommended
• Dry instruments should be loaded in the chamber

Ethylene Oxide (ETOX) Sterilization

This sterilization method is best used for sterilizing complex instruments and delicate materials. ETOX is a highly penetrative, noncorrosive gas above 10.8°C with a cidal action against bacteria, spores, and viruses.

Mechanism of Action

It destroys microorganisms by alkylation and causes denaturation of nucleic acids of microorganisms. The duration that the gas should be in contact with the material to be sterilized depends on temperature, humidity, pressure, and the amount of material.

Advantages
• It leaves no residue
• It is a deodorizer
• Good penetration power
• Can be used at a low temperature
• Suited for heat sensitive articles, for example, plastic, rubber

Disadvantages
• High cost of the equipment
• Toxicity of the gas
• Explosive and inflammable

Irradiation

Ionizing Radiation (X-rays, γ-rays, and High-speed Electrons)

Ionizing radiations are effective for heat labile items. They are commonly used by the industry to sterilize disposable materials such as needles, syringes, culture plates, suture material, cannulas, and pharmaceuticals sensitive to heat. High-energy γ-rays from cobalt-60 are used to sterilize such articles.

Nonionizing Radiation (Ultraviolet Light and Infrared Light)

- ❑ *Ultraviolet rays:*
  - UV rays are absorbed by proteins and nucleic acids and kill microorganisms by the chemical reactions
  - Their main application is air purification in operating rooms to reduce the bacteria in air, water, and on the contaminated surfaces
- ❑ *Infrared:*
  - It is used for sterilizing a large number of syringes sealed in metal container in a short period of time It is used to purify air in the operating room

Glass Bead Sterilizer

It is rapid method of sterilization which is used for sterilization of instruments **(Fig. 10.9)**. It uses table salt which consists approximately of 1% sodium silicoaluminate, sodium carbonate, or magnesium carbonate. So it can be poured more readily and does not fuse under heat. Salt can be replaced by glass beads provided the beads are smaller than 1 mm in diameter because larger beads are not efficient in transferring the heat to endodontic instruments due to presence of large air spaces between the beads.

Instruments can be sterilized in 5–15 seconds at a temperature of 437–465°F (260°C) even when inoculated with spores.

Advantages
- ❑ Commonly used salt is table salt which is easily available and cheap
- ❑ Salt does not clog the root canal. If it is carried into the canal, it can be readily removed by irrigation

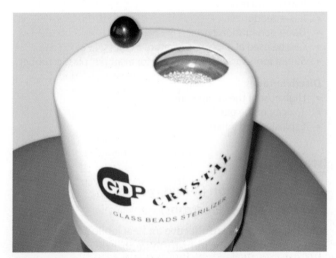

Fig. 10.9 Glass bead sterilizer.

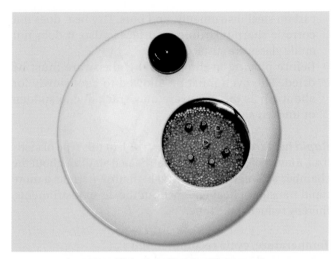

Fig. 10.10 Files placed in glass bead sterilizer.

Disadvantage
Handle portion is not sterilized, therefore instruments are not entirely "sterile" **(Fig. 10.10)**

Monitoring of Sterilization

Monitoring of instruments must be conducted through a combination of mechanical, chemical, and biological means, which evaluate both the sterilizing conditions and the procedure's effectiveness.

1. Mechanical indicators are the gauges on the sterilizer for cycle time, temperature, and pressure. Mechanical indicators must be checked and recorded for each load.
2. Chemical indicators use sensitive chemicals to assess physical conditions during the sterilization process. For example, when a heat-sensitive tape is applied to the outside of a package, rapid change in color indicates that the package has undergone a sterilization cycle, although it does not guarantee that sterilization has been achieved.
3. Biological indicators are the most accepted means for monitoring of sterilization because they assess the effectiveness of sterilization in killing the most resistant micro-organisms. In these, an inactivated BI signifies that other potential pathogens in the load have been killed.

Storage of Processed Instruments

After sterilization, instruments should be stored in an enclosed space like closed or covered cabinets. Date should be mentioned on storage packets because dating helps in assessing shelf life of sterilization. Packages containing sterile instruments should be inspected before use to verify barrier integrity and dryness. If packaging is compromised, the instruments should be cleaned, packaged, and sterilized again.

Disinfection

It is the term used for destruction of all pathogenic organisms, such as vegetative forms of bacteria, mycobacteria, fungi, and viruses, but not bacterial endospores.

Methods of Disinfection

Disinfection by Cleaning

Cleaning with a detergent and clean hot water removes almost all pathogens including bacterial spores.

Disinfection by Heat

Heat is a simple and reliable disinfectant for almost anything except living tissues. Mechanical cleaning with hot water provides an excellent quality of disinfection for a wide variety of purposes.

Low-Temperature Steam

Most vegetative microorganisms and viruses are killed when exposed to steam at a temperature of 73°C for 20 min below atmospheric pressure. This makes it a useful procedure to leave spoiled instruments safe to handle prior to sterilization.

Disinfection by Chemical Agents

They are used to disinfect the skin of a patient prior to surgery and to disinfect the hands of the operator.

Disadvantages of using chemicals
❑ No chemical solution sterilizes the instruments immersed in it
❑ There is a risk of producing tissue damage if residual solution is carried into the wound

Levels of Disinfectant

Alcohols—Low-Level Disinfectant
❑ Ethanol and isopropyl alcohols are commonly used as antiseptics
❑ Possess some antibacterial activity, but they are not effective against spores and viruses
❑ Act by denaturing proteins
❑ To have maximum effectiveness, alcohol must have a 10-min contact with the organisms
❑ Instruments made of carbon steel should not be soaked in alcoholic solutions, as they are corrosive to carbon steel
❑ Rubber instruments absorb alcohol, thus their prolonged soaking can cause a reaction when material comes in contact with living tissue

Phenolic Compounds—Intermediate Level, Broad-Spectrum Disinfectant
❑ The phenolic compounds were developed to reduce their side effects but are still toxic to living tissues
❑ At high concentration, these compounds are protoplasmic poison and act by precipitating the proteins and destroy the cell wall

	Method of sterilization	Sterilizing conditions	Advantages	Disadvantages
Dry heat	• Hot air oven • Rapid heat transfer	• 160°C for 60–120 min • 190°C for 6–12 min	• No corrosion • Instruments are dry after cycle • Low cost of equipment	• Poor penetration of dry heat • Long cycle of sterilization • Damage to rubber and plastic • Higher temperature may damage the instruments
Moist heat	• Autoclaving • Flash autoclaving	• 121°C at 15 psi for 15 min • 132°C at 27-28lb for 3–10 min	• Better penetration of moist heat • Rapid and effective method of sterilization • Does not destroy cotton or cloth products • Used for most of instruments	• Dulling and corrosion of sharp instruments • Damage to plastic and rubber • Instruments need to be air dried at the end of cycle
Chemical	• Chemical vapor pressure sterilization	• 127–131°C at 20 psi for 20 min	• Short sterilization cycle • Lack of corrosion of instrument • Effective method	• Requires adequate ventilation • Instruments should be dried before sterilization • May emit offensive vapor smell • Chemical vapors can damage sensitive instruments
Chemical	• Ethylene oxide sterilization		• Good penetration • Nontoxic • Heat sensitive articles can be sterilized	• Expensive • Explosive and inflammable • Toxicity of gas

- These compounds are used for disinfection of inanimate objects such as walls, floors and furniture
- They may cause damage to some plastics and they do not corrode certain metals such as brass, aluminum, and carbon steel

Aldehyde Compounds—High-Level Disinfectant

Formaldehyde
- Broad-spectrum antimicrobial agent
- Flammable and irritant to the eye, skin, and respiratory tract
- Has limited sporicidal activity
- Used for large heat sensitive equipment such as ventilators and suction pumps excluding rubber and some plastics
- Not preferred due to its pungent odor and because 18–30 h of contact is necessary for cidal action

Glutaraldehyde
- Toxic, irritant, and allergenic
- A high-level disinfectant
- Active against most vegetative bacteria, fungi, and bacterial spores
- Frequently used for heat sensitive material
- A solution of 2% glutaraldehyde (Cidex) requires immersion of 20 min for disinfection and 6–10 h of immersion for sterilization
- Safely used on metal instruments, rubber, plastics, and porcelain
- Activated by addition of sodium bicarbonate, but in its activated form, it remains potent only for 14 days

▌Antiseptics (Fig. 10.11)

Antiseptic is a chemical disinfectant that can be diluted sufficiently to be safe for application to living tissues like intact skin, mucous membranes, and wounds.

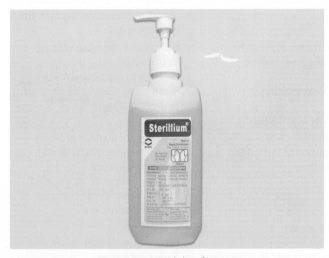

Fig. 10.11 Hand disinfectant.

Alcohols
- Two types of alcohols are used—ethyl alcohol and isopropyl alcohol
- Used for skin antisepsis
- Their benefit is derived primarily in their cleansing action
- The alcohols must have a prolonged contact with the organisms to have an antibacterial effect
- Ethyl alcohol is used in the concentration of 70% as a skin antiseptic
- Isopropyl alcohol is used in concentration of 60%–70% for disinfection of skin

Aqueous Quaternary Ammonium Compounds
- Benzalkonium chloride (Zephiran) is the most commonly used antiseptic
- It is well tolerated by living tissues

Iodophor Compounds
- Used for surgical scrub, soaps and surface antisepsis
- Usually effective within 5–10 min
- Discolor surfaces and clothes
- Iodine is complexed with organic surface-active agents such as polyvinylpyrrolidine (Betadine, Isodine). Their activity is dependent on the release of iodine from the complex
- Concentrated solutions have less free iodine. Iodine is released as the solution is diluted
- These compounds are effective against most bacteria, spores, viruses, and fungi

Chloride Compounds
- Commonly used are sodium hypochlorite and chlorine dioxide
- Sodium hypochlorite has rapid action
- A solution of one part of 5% sodium hypochlorite with nine parts of water is used
- Chlorous acid and chlorine dioxide provides disinfection in 3 min

Diguanides
- Chlorhexidine is active against many bacteria
- Gets inactivated in the presence of soap, pus, plastics, etc.
- Mainly used for cleaning skin and mucous membrane
- As a 0.2% aqueous solution or 1% gel, it can be used for suppression of plaque and postoperative infection

Disinfection of dental material		
Material	*Disinfectant*	*Technique*
Cast	Iodophor	Soaking for 10 min
Wax records	Iodophor, NaOCl	Immersion
Alginate impression	Iodophors, NaOCl Phenolic compound	Soaking for <10 min

Sterilization of the endodontic equipment	
Instrument	*Method*
Mouth mirror, probes, explorer	Autoclave
Endodontic instruments—files, reamers, broaches	Autoclave
Steel, burs	Disposable
Carbide and diamond burs	Autoclave
Local anesthetic cartridges	Presterilized/disposable
Needles	Disposable
Rubber dam equipment • Carbon steel clamps and metal frames • Punch	Dry heat, ethylene oxide, autoclave Dry heat, ethylene oxide
Gutta-percha points	Dip in 5.2% sodium hypochlorite for 1 min and then rinse with ethyl alcohol
Glass slab	Swabbing with tincture of thimerosal followed by double swabbing with alcohol
Silver cones	Passing them through flame 3–4 times or by immersion in glass bead sterilizer for 5 sec
Dental cements	γ-Radiations

Infection Control Checklist

Infection Control During the Pretreatment Period

- Use disposable items whenever possible
- Ensure before treatment that all equipment have been sterilized properly
- Remove avoidable items from the operatory area to facilitate a thorough cleaning following each patient
- Identify those items that will become contaminated during treatment, for example, light handles, X-ray unit heads, tray tables. Disinfect them when the procedure is complete
- Review patient records before initiating treatment
- Preplan the materials needed during treatment to avoid opening of the cabinets and drawers once the work is started
- Use separate sterilized bur blocks for each procedure to eliminate the contamination of other, unneeded burs
- Always keep rubber dam kit ready in the tray
- Follow manufacturer's directions for care of dental unit water lines (DUWL)
- Clinician should be prepared before initiating the procedure; this includes the use of personal protective equipment (gown, eyewear, masks, and gloves) and hand hygiene
- Update patient's medical history

Chairside Infection Control

- Treat all patients as potentially infectious
- Take special precautions while handling syringes and needles
- Use a rubber dam whenever possible
- Use high-volume aspiration
- Ensure good ventilation of the operatory area
- Be careful while receiving, handling, or passing sharp instruments
- Do not touch unprotected switches, handles and other equipment once gloves have been contaminated
- Avoid touching drawers or cabinets, once gloves have been contaminated. When it becomes necessary to do so, ask your assistant to do this or use another barrier, such as overglove to grasp the handle or remove the contaminated gloves and wash hands before touching the drawer and then reglove for patient treatment

Infection Control during the Post-treatment Period

- Remove the contaminated gloves used during treatment, wash hands and put on a pair of utility gloves before beginning the cleanup
- Continue to wear protective eyewear, mask, and gown during cleanup
- Dispose blood and suctioned fluids which have been collected in the collection bottles during treatment
- After disposing of blood and suctioned fluids, use 0.5% chlorine solution to disinfect the dental unit collection bottle. Keep the solution in the bottle for ≥10 min
- Clean the operatory area and disinfect all the items not protected by barriers
- Remove the tray with all instruments to sterilization area separate from the operatory area
- Never pick up instruments in bulk because this increases the risk of cuts or punctures. Clean the instruments manually or in an ultrasonic cleaner
- Sterilize the handpieces whenever possible. In general, handpiece should be autoclaved, but the handpiece that cannot be heat sterilized should be disinfected by the use of chemicals. Clean the handpiece with a detergent and water to remove any debris and sterilize it
- Waste that is contaminated with blood or saliva should be placed in sturdy leak proof bags
- Handle sharps items carefully
- Remove personal protective equipment after cleanup. Utility gloves should be washed with soap before removal
- At the end, thoroughly wash hands

Waste Disposal

Biomedical waste: Waste generated during the diagnosis, treatment, or immunization of human beings or animals or

Option	Waste category	Treatment and disposal
Category 1	Human anatomical waste	Incineration/deep burial
Category 2	Animal waste	Incineration/deep burial
Category 3	Microbiology and biotechnology waste	Incineration/deep burial
Category 4	Sharps	Incineration/disinfection/chemical treatment/mutilation
Category 5	Medicines and cytotoxic drugs	Incineration/destruction and disposal in secured landfill
Category 6	Solid waste (blood and body fluids)	Autoclave/chemical treatment/burial
Category 7	Solid waste (disposable items)	Autoclave/chemical treatment/burial
Category 8	Liquid waste (blood and body fluids)	Disinfection by chemicals/discharge into drains
Category 9	Incineration ash	Disposal in municipal landfill
Category 10	Chemical waste	Chemical treatment/secure landfill

research activities pertaining to, or production or testing of biological or in health camps.

Types of waste

Human Anatomical Waste

Human tissues, organs, body parts, etc.

Animal Anatomical Waste

Experimental animal carcasses, body parts, organs, tissues, including the waste generated from animals used in experiments.

Soiled Waste

Items contaminated with blood, body fluids like dressings, plaster casts, cotton swabs, and bags containing residual or discarded blood and blood components.

Expired or Discarded Medicines

Pharmaceutical waste like antibiotics and cytotoxic drugs including all items contaminated with cytotoxic drugs along with glass or plastic ampoules, vials, etc.

Chemical Waste

Chemicals used in production of biological and used or discarded disinfectants.

Chemical Liquid Waste

Liquid waste generated due to use of chemicals in production of biological and used or discarded disinfectants.

Microbiology, Biotechnology and Other Clinical Laboratory Waste

It include blood bags, cultures, specimens of microorganisms, vaccines, human and animal cell cultures used in research and industrial sectors.

Color coding	Type of container	Waste category	Treatment options as per schedule 1
Yellow	Plastic bag	Cat. 1, Cat. 2 and Cat. 3, Cat. 6	Incineration/deep burial
Red	Disinfected container/ plastic bag	Cat. 3, Cat. 6, Cat. 7	Autoclaving/ microwaving/ chemical treatment
Blue/ white translu- cent	Plastic bag/ puncture proof container	Cat. 4, Cat. 7.	Autoclaving/ microwaving/ chemical treatment and destruction/ shredding
Black	Plastic bag	Cat. 5 and Cat. 9 and Cat. 10 (solid)	Disposal in secured landfill

▌Questions

1. What is rationale of infection control? Mention different routes of infection transmission?
2. Define sterilization and disinfection. Describe the various methods to achieve sterilization of endodontic armamentarium.
3. Write short notes on:
   - Glass bead sterilizer.
   - Autoclave.
   - Asepsis in endodontics.

- Infection control during endodontic procedures.
- Sterilization of rotary equipment.
- Different routes of infection transmission.
- Sterilization of endodontic instruments.

▌Bibliography

1. Association reports: current status of sterilization instruments devices, and methods for the dental office. LADA 1981;102:683–9.

2. Miller CH. Cleaning, sterilization and disinfection. JADA 1993;24:48–56.
3. Miller CH. Sterilization and disinfection. JADA 1992; 123:46–54.
4. Stuart CH. *Enterococcus faecalis:* its role in root canal treatment failure and current concepts in retreatment. J Endod 2006;32:93–8.

Isolation of Teeth

An effective isolation of the teeth from tongue, soft tissues, gingival fluid, and saliva can prove crucial to have safe and successful endodontic therapy. Though many means of isolation are present, according to the American Association of Endodontists, rubber dam isolation is considered standard of care during endodontic treatment. This is because it acts as barrier to prevent oral pathogens to enter into accessed tooth, protects patient from irrigants and aspiration of instruments. It represents the indispensable "Gold Standard of Care" in endodontic practice.

Following components of oral environment need to be controlled during operative procedures:
- Saliva
- Moving organs
  - Tongue
  - Mandible
- Lips and cheek
- Gingival tissue
- Buccal and lingual vestibular spaces

Advantages of moisture control

Patient-related factors:
- Provides comfort to patient
- Protects patients from aspiration of foreign bodies
- Protects patient's soft tissues like tongue and cheeks by retracting them from operating field

Operator-related factors:
- A dry and clean operating field
- Infection control by minimizing aerosol production
- Increased accessibility to operative site
- Improved properties of dental materials, hence better results are obtained
- Protection of the patient and operator

- Improved visibility of the working field
- Less fogging of the dental mirror
- Prevents contamination of tooth preparation
- Hemorrhage from gingiva does not enter operative site

Isolation with Rubber Dam

Rubber dam was introduced by Sanford Christie Barnum, a New York dentist, in 1864. Rubber dam can be defined as a flat thin sheet of latex/non-latex that is held by a clamp and frame which is perforated to show the tooth/teeth to protrude through the perforations while all other teeth are covered and protected by sheet **(Fig. 11.1)**. Rubber dam is mandatory while doing root canal treatment in few parts of the world from medico legal point of view.

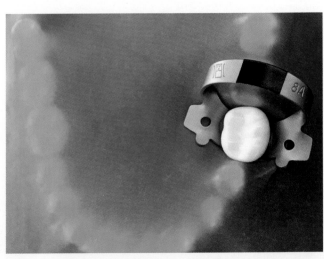

Fig. 11.1 Tooth isolation with rubber dam.

Advantages of using a rubber dam
- It helps in improving accessibility and visibility of the working area
- It gives a clean and dry aseptic field while working
- It protects the lips, cheeks and tongue by keeping them out of the way
- It acts as raincoat for the teeth
- It helps to avoid unnecessary contamination, thereby infection control
- It protects the patient from aspiration of instruments and medicaments
- It helps in keeping teeth saliva free while performing endodontic treatment so tooth does not get contaminated by bacteria present in saliva
- It improves the efficiency of the treatment
- It potentially improves the properties of dental materials
- It provides protection to patient and dentist

Disadvantages of using a rubber dam
- Incorrect use may damage porcelain crowns/crown margins or may traumatize gingival tissues
- Insecure clamps can be swallowed or aspirated
- Careless placing and removal of rubber dam can damage oral mucosa
- Time consuming and expensive
- There are chances of perforation during preparation of access cavity if tooth is abnormally positioned
- There are chances of incorrect shade while selecting shade for composite restoration due to bright colored dam
- Some patient may find it as claustrophobic
- Since it blocks off oral airway, it is difficult to use in patient with temporary nasal congestion

Contraindications of use of rubber dam
- Asthmatic patients
- Mouth breathers
- Extremely malpositioned tooth

Single tooth isolation	Multiple teeth isolation
Class I and V restoration of tooth	Bleaching
Direct and indirect pulp capping	Class II restoration
Pulpotomy	Multiple restorations
Pulpectomy/endodontic procedure	Quadrant dentistry

Rubber dam equipment
- Rubber dam sheet
- Rubber dam clamps
- Rubber dam forceps
- Rubber dam frame
- Rubber dam punch

Rubber dam accessories
- Lubricant/petroleum jelly
- Dental floss
- Rubber dam napkin

Rubber Dam Sheet

□ Rubber dam sheet is normally available in size 5 × 5 or 6 × 6 sq inches in light and dark colors (**Fig. 11.2**). Dark colors are preferred (green or black) for good contrast
□ Sheet has dry and shiny sides. Dull side faces the occlusal surface of isolated teeth because it is less reflective than shiny surface
□ It is available in three thicknesses, that is, light, medium, and heavy. Thicker dam is effective in retracting the tissues and is more resistant to tearing. These are preferred for isolating class V cavities with cervical retainer. Thinner dam can easily pass through the contacts easier, so specially helpful in cases of tight contacts. Middle grade is usually preferred as thin is more prone to tearing and heavier one is more difficult to apply
□ Latex-free dam is necessary as the number of patients is increasing with latex allergy
□ *Flexi dam* is latex-free dam of standard thickness with no rubber smell.

Thickness of rubber dam sheet
Thin	- 0.15 mm
Medium	- 0.20 mm
Heavy	- 0.25 mm
Extra heavy	- 0.30 mm
Special heavy	- 0.35 mm

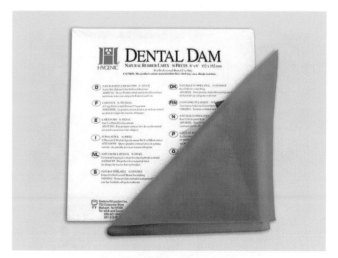

Fig. 11.2 Rubber dam sheet.

Rubber Dam Clamps

- ❑ Rubber dam clamps to hold the rubber dam onto the tooth are available in different shapes and sizes **(Fig. 11.3)**
- ❑ Clamps mainly serve two functions:
    1. They anchor the rubber dam to the tooth
    2. Help in retracting the gingiva.

Classification of Rubber Dam Clamps

On the Basis of Jaw Design
- ❑ Bland
- ❑ Retentive

Bland Clamps
- ❑ Bland clamps are usually identified by the jaws, which are flat and point directly toward each other
- ❑ In these clamps, flat jaws usually grasp the tooth at or above the gingival margin
- ❑ They can be used in fully erupted tooth where cervical constriction prevents clamp from slipping off the tooth

Retentive Clamps
- ❑ These clamps have jaws which are directed gingivally and grasp the teeth more gingivally
- ❑ Jaws of clamps should have a four-point contact and should not extend beyond mesial and distal line angles of the tooth. If not placed properly, it results in rocking and tilting of the clamp

Both bland and retentive can be divided into winged and wingless type **(Figs. 11.4A and B)**.

- ❑ **Winged:** These have anterior and lateral wings which provide extra retention of rubber dam. But these interfere with placement of matrix band retainers and wedges

- ❑ **Wingless:** They have no wings. Here retainer is first placed on the tooth and then dam is stretched over the clamp onto the tooth

On the Basis of Material Used
- ❑ Metallic
- ❑ Nonmetallic/plastic

Metallic: Traditionally, clamps have been made from tempered carbon steel and stainless steel. Problem with using metallic clamps is that they appear radiopaque on radiograph, thereby overlapping the structures **(Fig. 11.5)**.

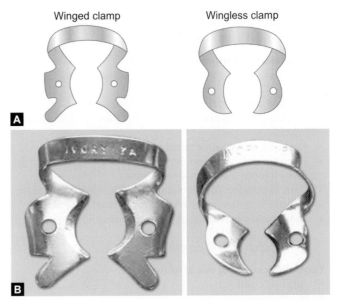

Figs. 11.4A and B Rubber dam clamps: (A) Schematic presentation of winged and wingless clamp; (B) Photograph showing winged and wingless clamp.

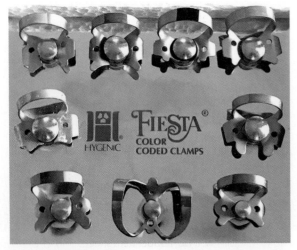

Figs. 11.3 Different shapes and sizes of rubber dam clamps.

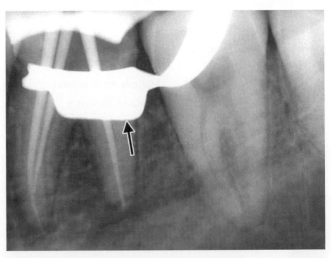

Fig. 11.5 Radiograph showing radiopaque metallic clamp (arrow).

Nonmetallic/plastic: Nonmetallic are made from polycarbonate plastic **(Fig. 11.6)**. These are radiolucent but they are bulky so don't easily fit the teeth.

Retainer number and their applications	
Retainer no.	**Application**
W2:	Small premolars
W4:	Most of premolars
W56:	Most of molars
W7:	Mandibular molars
W8:	Maxillary molars
W27:	Terminal Mandibular molar

Rubber Dam Forcep

- Rubber dam forcep is used to carry the clamp to the tooth
- When the handles of forcep are compressed together, it's two working ends move apart **(Fig. 11.7)**

- Working end has small projections that fit into two corresponding holes of the rubber dam clamp
- Area between working end and the handle has a sliding lock device which locks the handles in positions while the clinician moves the clamp around the tooth
- It should be taken care that forceps do not have deep grooves at their tips or they become very difficult to remove once the clamp is in place.

Rubber Dam Frame

- Rubber dam frame supports the edges of rubber dam **(Figs. 11.8A to C)**
- Frames have been improved dramatically since their old style with the huge "butterflies"
- Modern frames have sharp pins which easily grip the dam. These are mainly designed with the pins that slope backwards
- Rubber dam frames are available in either metal or plastic
- Plastic frames have advantage of being radiolucent.

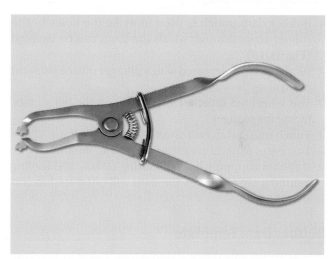

Fig. 11.6 Plastic rubber dam clamp.

Fig. 11.7 Rubber dam forceps.

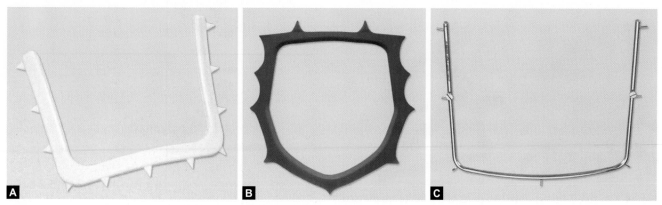

Figs. 11.8A to C Different types of Rubber dam frames (A) Ash pattern–most suitable for children; (B) Swenska N-O frame; (C) Young's holder–U-shaped metal frame with small metal projections for securing borders of the rubber dam.

❑ When taut, rubber dam sheet exerts too much pull on the rubber dam clamps, causing them to come loose, especially clamps attached to molars

❑ To overcome this problem, a new easy-to-use rubber dam frame, *Safe-T-Frame*, has been developed that offers a secure fit without stretching the rubber dam sheet **(Fig. 11.9)**. Instead, its "snap-shut" design takes advantage of the clamping effect on the sheet, which is caused when its two mated frame members are firmly pressed together. In this way, the sheet is securely attached, but without being stretched. Held in this manner, the dam sheet is under less tension, and hence, exerts less tugging on clamps especially on those attached to molars.

> **Rubber dam frames serve following purposes:**
> • Support the edges of rubber dam
> • Retract the soft tissues
> • Improve accessibility to the isolated teeth

Rubber Dam Punch

❑ Rubber dam punch is used to make the holes in the rubber sheet through which the teeth can be isolated **(Fig. 11.10)**

❑ Working end is designed with a plunger on one side and a wheel on the other side

❑ This wheel has different sized holes on the flat surface facing the plunger

❑ Punch must produce a clean cut hole every time

❑ Two types of holes are made, single and multihole

❑ If rubber dam punch is not cutting cleanly and leaving behind a tag of rubber, the dam will often split as it is stretched out.

Rubber Dam Template

❑ It is an inked rubber stamp which helps in marking the dots on the sheet according to position of the tooth **(Figs. 11.11 and 11.12)**

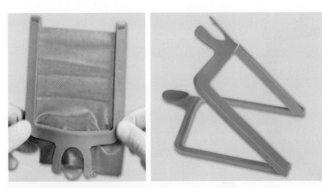

Fig. 11.9 In *Safe-T-Frame*, when two parts of the frame are pressed together, due to it's "snap-shut" design, sheet is secured, but without being stretched.

❑ Holes should be punched according to arch and missing teeth.

Rubber Dam Accessories

Lubricant

❑ It is applied on the under surface of dam in the area of punched holes to facilitate the passing of the dam through the proximal contacts

❑ Petroleum-based *lubricant* should be avoided because it is difficult to remove and can interfere bonding procedures. Thus, water-soluble lubricant like soap slurry should be preferred as a lubricant

❑ Petroleum jelly is often used at corner of mouth to prevent irritation.

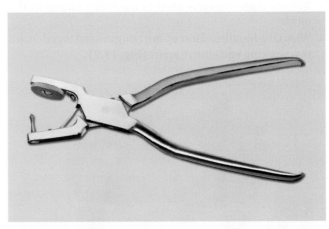

Fig. 11.10 Working end of rubber dam punch has plunger on one side and wheel with different sized holes on the other side.

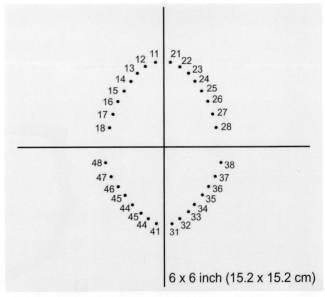

Fig. 11.11 Rubber dam template with position of teeth marked on it for punching holes on rubber dam sheet accordingly.

Dental Floss

- It is usually required for testing interdental contacts
- Floss is tied to the clamp to prevent its accidental aspiration **(Fig. 11.13)**

Wedjets

Wedjet cord is made up of natural latex to stabilize the dam with little chances of tissue trauma **(Figs. 11.14 and 11.15)**.

Modeling Compound

It is used to secure and stabilize the retainer to the tooth. In some cases, they can be used as retainer instead of clamps.

Rubber Dam Napkin

- This is a sheet of absorbent materials usually placed between the rubber sheet and soft tissues **(Fig. 11.16)**
- It absorbs saliva from corner of patient's mouth

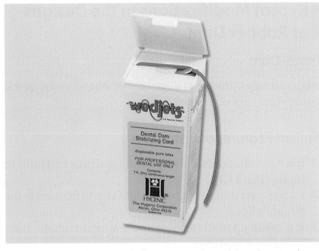

Fig. 11.14 Photograph showing wedjet rubber dam cord.

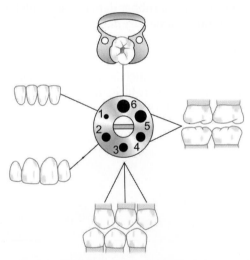

Fig. 11.12 Schematic representation of rubber dam punch holes; smaller holes for anterior teeth, medium for premolars, and larger ones for molars.

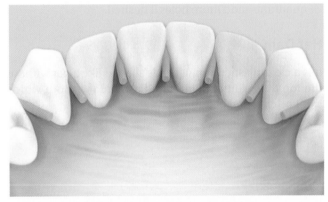

Fig. 11.15 Wedjets applied on teeth.

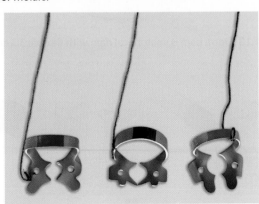

Fig. 11.13 Floss prevents accidental aspiration of the rubber dam clamp.

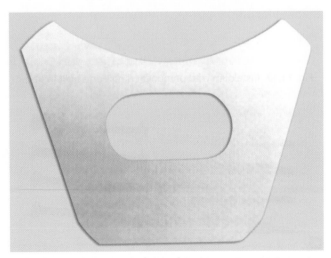

Fig. 11.16 Photograph showing rubber dam Napkin.

Recent Modifications in the Designs of Rubber Dam

Insta-Dam

It is a recently introduced disposable rubber dam for quick, convenient rubber dam isolation.

Salient Features of Insta-dam

❑ It is natural latex dam with prepunched hole and built-in frame (**Fig. 11.17**)
❑ Its compact design is just the right size to fit outside the patient's lips
❑ It is made up of stretchable and tear-resistant, medium gauge latex material
❑ Radiographs may be taken without removing the dam
❑ Built-in flexible nylon frame eliminates bulky frames and sterilization
❑ Off-center, prepunched hole customizes fit to any quadrant—add more holes if desired.

Hat Dam

It is a clear plastic form which is shaped like a hat without the top. It is trimmed and fitted around the tooth which can't be clamped.

Handi Dam

❑ Another recently introduced dam is *handi dam*
❑ This is preframed rubber dam eliminates the need for traditional frame
❑ Handi dam is easy to place and saves time of both patient and doctor
❑ It allows an easy access to oral cavity during the procedure

Optra Dam

It is an anatomically shaped rubber dam for isolation. It is made up of flexible latex. For use, intraoral ring is positioned in gingivobuccal fold and outer ring remains outside the mouth (**Fig. 11.18**). Dam is secured around the teeth by fitting septum of dam interproximally and in the sulcus using dental floss.

Dry Dam

Another newer type of rubber dam is also available which does not require a frame "*dry dam.*"

Liquid Dam

It is a resinous material which is applied on gingival aspect of the teeth specially before bleaching, microbrasion, sandblasting, etc. (**Figs. 11.19A to C**).

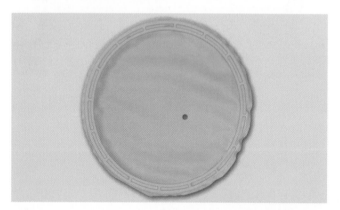

Fig. 11.17 Insta dam with prepunched hole and built in frame.

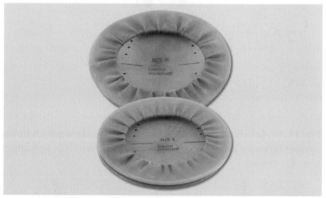

Fig. 11.18 Optra dam is anatomical dam with flexible 3D design.

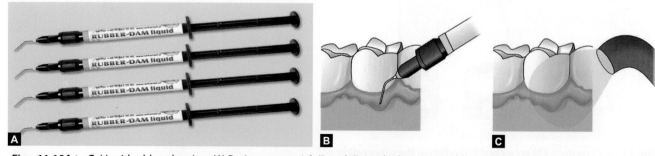

Figs. 11.19A to C Liquid rubber dam is a: (A) Resinous material; (B and C) Applied on gingival aspect of the teeth and cured to protect gingiva specially before bleaching, microbrasion, sandblasting, etc.

Placement of Rubber Dam

Before placement of rubber dam, the following procedures should be done:
- ❑ Thorough prophylaxis of the oral cavity
- ❑ Check contacts with dental floss
- ❑ Check for any rough contact areas
- ❑ Anesthetize the gingiva if required
- ❑ Rinse and dry the operated field.

Methods of Rubber Dam Placement

Method I: Clamp placed before rubber dam (Figs. 11.20A to C)

- ❑ Select an appropriate clamp according to the tooth size
- ❑ Tie a floss to clamp bow and place clamp onto the tooth
- ❑ Larger holes are required in this technique as rubber dam has to be stretched over the clamp. Usually two or three overlapping holes are made

- ❑ Stretching of the rubber dam over the clamps can be done in the following sequence:
  - Stretch the rubber dam sheet over the clamp
  - Then stretch the sheet over the buccal surface and allow to settle into place beneath buccal contour
  - Finally, the sheet is carried to palatal/lingual side and released

This method is mainly used in posterior teeth in both adults and children except third molar.

Method II: Placement of rubber dam and clamp together (Figs. 11.21A to C)

- ❑ Select an appropriate clamp according to tooth anatomy
- ❑ Tie a floss around the clamp and check the stability
- ❑ Punch the hole in rubber dam sheet
- ❑ Clamp is held with clamp forceps and its wings are inserted into punched hole
- ❑ Both clamp and rubber dam are carried to the oral cavity and clamp is tensed to stretch the hole

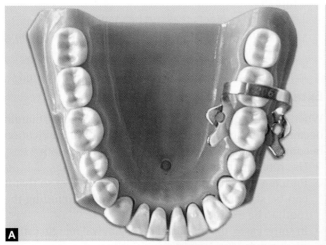
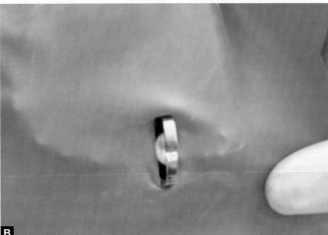
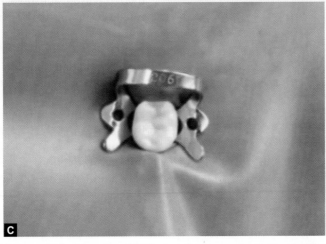

Figs. 11.20A to C Placement of rubber dam: (A) Placing clamp on selected tooth; (B) Stretching rubber dam sheet over clamp; (C) After complete stretching, tooth is isolated.

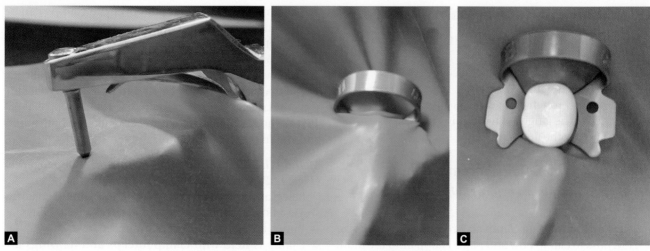

Figs. 11.21A to C (A) Punch hole in the rubber dam sheet according to selected tooth; (B) Clamp and its wings are inserted in the punched hole; (C) Carry both clamp and rubber dam over the crown and seat it.

❑ Both clamp and rubber dam is advanced over the crown. First, jaw of clamp is tilted to the lingual side to lie on the gingival margin of lingual side
❑ After this, jaw of the clamp is positioned on buccal side
❑ After seating the clamp, again check stability of clamp
❑ Remove the forceps from the clamp
❑ Now release the rubber sheet from wings to lie around the cervical margin of the tooth.

Method III: Split dam technique
This method is split dam technique in which rubber dam is placed to isolate the tooth without the use of rubber dam clamp. In this technique, two overlapping holes are punched in the dam. The dam is stretched over the tooth to be treated and over the adjacent tooth on each side. Edge of rubber dam is carefully teased through the contacts of distal side of adjacent teeth.

Split dam technique is indicated:
• To isolate anterior teeth
• When there is insufficient crown structure
• When isolation of teeth with porcelain crown is required. In such cases, placement of rubber dam clamp over the crown margins can damage the cervical porcelain
• Dam is placed without using clamp
• Here two overlapping holes are punched and dam is stretched over the tooth to be treated and adjacent tooth on each side

Management of Difficult Cases

Malpositioned Teeth

To manage these cases, the following *modifications* are done:
❑ Adjust the spacing of the holes
❑ In tilted teeth, estimate the position of root center at gingival margin rather than the tip of the crown

❑ Another approach is to make a customized cardboard template
❑ Tight broad contact areas can be managed by:
• Wedging the contact open temporarily for passing the rubber sheet
• Use of lubricant.

Extensive Loss of Coronal Tissue

When sound tooth margin is at or below the gingival margin because of decay or fracture, the rubber dam application becomes difficult. In such cases, to isolate the tooth
❑ Use retentive clamps
❑ Punch a bigger hole in the rubber dam sheet so that it can be stretched to involve more teeth, including the tooth to be treated
❑ In some cases, the modification of gingival margin can be tried so as to provide supragingival preparation margin. This can be accomplished by gingivectomy or the flap surgery.

Crown with Poor Retentive Shape

Sometimes anatomy of teeth limits the placement of rubber dam (lack of undercuts and retentive areas). In such cases, the following can be done:
❑ Placing clamp on another tooth
❑ By using clamp which engages interdental spaces below the contact point
❑ By building retentive shape on the crown with composite resin bonded to acid etched tooth surface.

Teeth with Porcelain Crowns

In such cases, placing a rubber dam may cause damage to porcelain crown. To avoid this
❑ Clamp should be placed on another tooth
❑ Clamp should engage below the crown margin

Table 11.1: Commonly encountered problems during application of rubber dam.

Problem	Consequences	Correction
1. Improper distance between holes		
a. Excessive distance between holes	i. Wrinkling of dam ii. Interference in accessibility	Proper placement of holes by accurate use of rubber dam punch and template
b. Too short distance between holes	i. Overstretching of dam ii. Tearing of dam iii. Poor fit	
2. Off-center arch form	i. Obstructs breathing ii. Makes patient uncomfortable	Folding of extradam material under the nose and proper punching of holes
3. Torn rubber dam	i. Leakage ii. Improper isolation	• Replacement of dam • Use of cavit, periodontal packs or liquid rubber dam

- Do not place clamp on the porcelain edges
- Place a layer of rubber dam sheet between the clamp and the porcelain crown which acts as a cushion and thus minimizes localized pressure on the porcelain.

Leakage

- Sometimes leakage is seen through the rubber dam because of the accidental tears or holes. Such leaking gaps can be sealed using cavit, periodontal packs, liquid rubber dam, rubber dam adhesives, or oraseal
- For sealing the larger gaps, the rubber dam adhesives in combination with orabase can be tried
- If leakage persists despite of these efforts, the rubber dam sheet should be replaced with new one
  - Depending upon the clinical condition, isolation of single or multiple teeth can be done with the help of rubber dam. **Table 11.1** entails problems commonly encountered during application of rubber dam.

Removal of Rubber Dam

- Before the rubber dam is removed, use the water syringe and high volume evacuator to flush out all debris that collected during the procedure
- Cut away tied thread from the neck of the teeth. Stretch the rubber dam facially and pull the septal rubber away from the gingival tissue and the tooth
- Protect the underlying soft tissue by placing a fingertip beneath the septum
- Free the dam from the interproximal space, but leave the rubber dam over the anterior and posterior anchor teeth
- Use the clamp forceps to remove the clamp

- Once the retainer is removed, release the dam from the anchor tooth and remove the dam and frame simultaneously
- Wipe the patient's mouth, lips and chin with a tissue or gauze to prevent saliva from getting on the patient's face
- Check for any missing fragment after procedure
- If a fragment of the rubber dam is found missing, inspect interproximal area because pieces of the rubber dam left under the free gingiva can result in gingival irritation.

Questions

1. Write in detail about rubber dam isolation.
2. Write short notes on
   - Rubber dam application in teeth with porcelain crowns.
   - Insta-dam.

Bibliography

1. Cohen S, Schwartz S. Endodontic complications and the law. J Endod 1987;13:191–7.
2. Govila CP. Accident swallowing of an endodontic instrument: a report of two cases. Oral Surg Oral Med Oral Pathol Oval Radiol Endod 1979;48:269–71.
3. Kosti E, Lambrianidis T. Endodontic treatment in cases of allergic reaction to rubber dam. J Endod 2002;28:787–9.
4. Miller CH. Infection control. Dent Clin North Am 1996; 40:437–56.
5. Lambrianidis T, Beltes P. Accident swallowing of endodontic instruments. Endod Dent Tramatol 1996:12:301–4.
6. Weisman MI. Remedy for dental dam leakage problems. J Endod 1991;17:88–9.

Pharmacology in Endodontics

Pain and periapical infections are the most common problems seen in patients with endodontic problems. Consequently, pain control and infection management are the foremost aim while performing the endodontic therapy. Therefore, use of analgesics and antibiotics has become an essential part of dental procedures for treating infections and providing pain-free procedures.

■ Pain Control

Though pain control in endodontics is not very difficult, sometimes it becomes almost impossible to control pain. Clinicians must be able to diagnose the source of pain and have strategies for its management. The "3-D" principle—diagnosis, dental treatment and drugs—should be applied to manage pain. Correct diagnosis of the etiological factors of pain and proper treatment of the problem relieves pain in many cases. Drugs should only be used as an adjunct to the dental treatment. While performing a dental procedure, it is necessary to maintain profound anesthesia that can be achieved using local anesthetics. Pain-management drugs include nonopioids [i.e., non-steroidal anti-inflammatory drugs (NSAIDs) and paracetamol] or opioids (i.e., narcotics). NSAIDs provide excellent pain relief due to their anti-inflammatory and analgesic action. The opioids are strong analgesics but have significant side effects, and therefore they should be reserved for severe pain only.

Pain control can be achieved through
- Local anesthesia
- Nonopioid drugs
- Opioid drugs.

Local Anesthesia

Definition

It is defined as a loss of sensation in a circumscribed area of the body caused by depression of excitation in nerve endings or an inhibition of the conduction process in peripheral nerves.

Purpose of Local Anesthetic

- To stop generation and conduction of nerve impulses
- To abort impulses from stimuli-like extraction or endodontic treatment.

Classification of Local Anesthetic Agents

1. *Based on chemical structure*

Ester group	Amide group
• Cocaine	• Lidocaine
• Benzocaine	• Mepivacaine
• Procaine	• Prilocaine
• Tetracaine	• Etidocaine
	• Bupivacaine

2. *Based on duration of action*

Short acting	Intermediate acting	Long acting
Procaine	Lignocaine	Bupivacaine

Mechanism of Action

The primary action of the local anesthetics agent is to decrease the nerve permeability to sodium (Na^+) ions, thus preventing the inflow of Na⁺ ions into the nerve. This interferes with sodium conductance and inhibits the propagation of impulse along the nerve fibers.

In tissues with lower pH, local anesthetics show slower onset of anesthesia than in tissues with higher pH because at alkaline pH, local anesthetic is present in an undissociated base form that penetrates the axon.

Composition of a local anesthetic agent
- Local anesthetic—salt form of lidocaine hydrochloride
- Vasoconstrictor—epinephrine
- Preservative for vasoconstrictor—sodium bisulfite
- Isotonic solution—sodium chloride
- Preservative—methylparaben
- Sterile water to make the rest of the volume

Techniques used for maxillary teeth and tissues	Techniques used for mandibular teeth and tissues
<ul><li>Supraperiosteal technique</li><li>Anterior and middle superior alveolar nerve block</li><li>Posterior superior alveolar nerve block</li><li>Greater palatine nerve block</li><li>Nasopalatine nerve block</li><li>Maxillary nerve block</li></ul>	<ul><li>Inferior alveolar nerve block</li><li>Buccal nerve block</li><li>Lingual nerve block</li><li>Mental nerve block</li><li>Vazirani-Akinosi closed mouth technique</li><li>Extraoral approach</li></ul>

Intrapulpal Injection

Adequate pulpal anesthesia is required for the treatment of pulpally involved tooth. Mandibular teeth usually offer some problems in obtaining profound anesthesia. This injection controls pain, by both applying pressure and utilizing the pharmacologic action of local anesthetic agent.

Indications: Lack of obtaining profound anesthesia in pulpally involved teeth by other techniques.

Nerves anesthetized: Terminal nerve endings at the site of injection.

Technique

- Insert 25 or 27 gauge needle firmly into the pulp chamber **(Fig. 12.1)**
- Before inserting the needle, patient must be informed that he/she may experience a brief period of sensitivity (mild to very painful) after giving the injection
- Always deposit local anesthetic solution under pressure as back pressure is shown to be the major factor in producing anesthesia
  - For creating back pressure, block the access with stoppers (cotton pellet). To prevent backflow, other

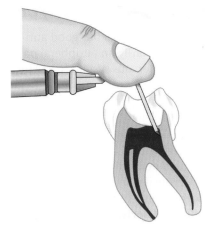

Fig. 12.1 For intrapulpal injection, needle is bent to gain access into the canal.
(Modified from Cohen S, Burns RC; Pathways of pulp, Ed 8, St. Louis 2001, Mosby)

stoppers that can be used are gutta-percha, waxes or pieces of rubber
- Deposit a very small amount of solution (0.2–0.3 mL) under pressure (5–10 s)
- Sometimes, bending of needle is done for gaining access to the canal.

Mechanism of Action

Success of intrapulpal injection depends on the fact that it has to be administrated under pressure. Monheim suggested that prolonged pressure may lead to degeneration of nerve fibers in many instances leading to profound anesthesia for endodontic procedures.

Advantages
- Requires less volume
- Early onset
- Easy to learn.

Disadvantages
- Results are not predictable as it may vary (it should always be given under pressure).
- Taste of local anesthetic drug is not accepted by patients as it may spill during administration of intrapulpal injection.
- Brief pain during or after insertion of solution (not tolerated by some patients).

Analgesics

The main purpose of using analgesics is to eliminate the source of pain. But, at first, one must consider adjusting regimens according to the patient's needs and response. Analgesics can be opioids or nonopioids.

Nonsteroidal Anti-inflammatory Drugs

These are weaker analgesics but good anti-inflammatory drugs. These act primarily on peripheral pain mechanism and also in central nervous system (CNS) to increase pain threshold.

Classification

Nonselective COX (cyclooxygenase) inhibitors
- **Salicylates:** Aspirin
- **Propionic acid derivatives:** Ibuprofen, naproxen
- **Pyrrolo-pyrrole derivative®:** Ketorolac
- **Indole derivatives®:** Indomethacin
- **Anthranilic acid derivatives®:** Mefenamic acid
- **Oxicam derivatives®:** Piroxicam, meloxicam
- **Perferential COX-2 inhibitors:** Diclofenac, aceclofenac, nimesulide, meloxicam
- **Highly selective COX-2 inhibitors:** Etoricoxib, parecoxib
- **Analgesics and antipyretics with poor anti-inflammatory effect:** Paracetamol (Acetaminophen).

Aspirin

- Rapidly converted in the body to salicylic acid that is responsible for most of the actions
- Aspirin inhibits COX (Cyclooxygenase) irreversibly. Return of COX activity depends on synthesis of fresh enzymes
- Analgesic action is mainly due to obtunding of peripheral pain receptors and prevention of prostaglandin-mediated sensitization of nerve endings
- Absorbed from stomach and small intestines
- **Analgesic dose and antipyretic effect:** 600 mg three times a day
- **Anti-inflammatory dose:** 3–6 g/day or 100 mg/kg/day

Side effects
- Gastric upset
- Irreversibly inhibits TXA_2 synthesis by platelets; thus, it interferes with platelet aggregation and prolong bleeding time
- Hypersensitivity.

Contraindications
- Peptic ulcer
- Bleeding disorders
- Chronic liver disease
- Pregnancy.

Ibuprofen

- Better tolerated alternative to aspirin
- Side effects are milder than aspirin

- Gastric discomfort, nausea and vomiting are less than aspirin
- **Dose:** 400–600 mg three times a day.

Diclofenac Sodium

- Most extensively used
- Epigastric pain, nausea, headache, dizziness and rashes are side effects
- Gastric ulceration and bleeding are less common
- **Dose:** 50 mg three times a day or 100 mg sustained release once a day.

Paracetamol

- Potent antipyretic and analgesic effects with poor anti-inflammatory activity
- Poor ability to inhibit COX in the presence of peroxides that are generated at the site of inflammation
- Well absorbed orally
- Plasma $t\frac{1}{2}$ is 2 to 3 h
- Should be used cautiously in patients with liver disease or chronic alcoholics
- Preferred analgesic and antipyretic in patients having peptic ulcer and bronchial asthma
- **Dose:** 0.5 to 1 g three times a day.

Choice of NSAIDs in Dentistry

- Mild-to-moderate pain with a little inflammation: paracetamol or low-dose ibuprofen
- Patients with history of asthma: Paracetamol or Nimesulide
- Postextraction or similar acute but short-lasting pain: Ketorolac, ibuprofen, diclofenac
- Gastric intolerance to conventional NSAIDs: Etoricoxib or paracetamol
- Pregnancy: paracetamol
- Hypertensive, diabetic, ischaemic heart disease, epileptic and other patients receiving long term regular medication: consult physician and consider interaction of drugs with NSAIDs.

Opioid Analgesic Drugs

Opioids analgesics are used to relieve acute, moderate-to-severe pain. The opioid receptors are located at several important sites in brain, and their activation inhibits the transmission of nociceptive signals from trigeminal nucleus to higher brain regions. Opioids also activate peripheral opioid receptors.

Classification

Natural	Semisynthetic	Synthetic
• Morphine • Codeine	• Diacetylmorphine (heroin) • Pholcodine	• Pethidine (Meperidine) • Tramadol • Fentanyl • Methadone • Dextropropoxyphene

Codeine

❑ It is a methylmorphine.
❑ Occurs naturally in opium, partly converted into morphine in body
❑ It is less potent than morphine. Codeine is 1/6–1/10 as analgesic to morphine.
❑ When compared to aspirin, it is more potent 60 mg codeine–600 mg aspirin.

Morphine

❑ It has site-specific depressant and stimulant actions in CNS.
❑ Degree of analgesia increases with dose
❑ Depresses respiratory center, death in morphine poisoning is due to respiratory failure
❑ Oral bioavailability averages one fourth of parenterally administered drug
❑ About 30% bound to plasma protein, and high first pass metabolism
❑ Plasma $t\frac{1}{2}$ = 2 to 3 h
❑ Morphine is noncumulative
❑ **Doses:** 10–15 mg intramuscular or subcutaneous (SC).

Side effects
Sedation, constipation, respiratory depression, nausea and vomiting

Antidote
Naloxone 0.4 to 0.8 mg IV repeated every 2 to 3 min till respiration picks up; used in acute morphine poisoning.

Dextropropoxyphene

❑ Half as potent as codeine
❑ Plasma $t\frac{1}{2}$ is 4–12 h
❑ **Doses:** 60–120 mg three times a day.

Tramadol

❑ Centrally acting analgesic; relieves pain by opioid as well as additional mechanism
❑ Injected IV 100 mg tramadol is equianalgesic to 10 mg morphine

❑ Plasma $t\frac{1}{2}$ is 3–5 h, effects last 4–6 h
  • Indicated for mild to medium intensity pain due to dental or surgical procedures.

Side effects: Dizziness, nausea, sleepiness, dry mouth, sweating.

∎ Infection Control

In general, pulpal invasion begins with the mixed infection of aerobes and anaerobes. As the infection increases, flora changes to obligate anaerobes and facultative organisms because of oxygen depletion. One of the primary goals of endodontic therapy is to eliminate a habitat of microorganisms in canal space. Thus, thorough sterilization is needed starting from the pulpal debridement up to the step of obturation. When drainage from root-canal system becomes difficult to obtain or when host resistance is low or when virulence of attacker is high, antibiotics are needed.

Antibiotics are substances that are produced by microorganisms, which suppress or kill other microorganisms at very low concentrations. Nowadays, oral and systemic antibiotics are most frequently used; hence, a thorough understanding about their pharmacologic profile is necessary. In this topic, we will discuss the indications, uses and side effects of the most commonly used antibiotics.

What are the principles of prescribing antibiotics?
❑ Use only when there is an indication.
❑ Choose the narrowest spectrum drug that will be effective.
❑ Consider the risk/benefit equation.
❑ Prescribe an adequate dose and with required duration.

Conditions requiring antibiotics	Conditions not requiring antibiotics
• Systemic involvement with symptoms like fever, malaise and lymphadenopathy • Presence of persistent infections • Indications of progressive infection like increasing swelling, cellulitis or osteomyelitis	• Localized fluctuant swelling • Chronic apical abscess • Teeth with sinus tract and necrotic pulp • Irreversible pulpitis without signs and symptoms of infection • Apical periodontitis without signs and symptoms of infection

Reasons for failure of endodontic therapy
❑ Improper drug or dose
❑ Bacterial resistance
❑ Compromised host defense
❑ Poor compliance.

Classification of Antimicrobial drugs

1. *Based on spectrum of activity*
   - a. Narrow spectrum
     - I. Penicillin G
     - II. Streptomycin
     - III. Erythromycin
   - b. Broad spectrum
     - I. Tetracyclines
     - II. Chloramphenicol
2. *Types of action*
   - a. Bactericidal
     - I. Penicillin and cephalosporins
     - II. Metronidazole
     - III. Fluoroquinolone
       - I. Ciprofloxacin
       - II. Ofloxacin
     - IV. Aminoglycosides
       - I. Streptomycin
       - II. Amikacin
   - b. Bacteriostatic
     - I. Sulfonamides
     - II. Tetracycline
     - III. Clindamycin
     - IV. Erythromycin.

Mechanism of action of antimicrobial agents	
Action	Antimicrobial agents
• Inhibition of cell-wall synthesis	• Penicillins, cephalosporins, vancomycin
• Inhibition of protein synthesis	• Aminoglycosides, tetracycline, chloramphenicol, lincomycin
• Interference in transcription/ translation of genetic information	• Ciprofloxacin, ofloxacin, gatifloxacin, metronidazole
• Antimetabolite actions	• Sulfonamides, trimethoprim

Penicillins

- ❑ It was the first antibiotic developed and used clinically in 1941.
- ❑ Aminopencillins i.e. Ampicillin and Amoxicillin are broad-spectrum drug effective against Gram-positive and Gram-negative bacteria.
- ❑ Amoxicillin is one of the most frequently used antibiotics for treatment of dental infections
- ❑ Dose of Amoxicillin - 250–500 mg t.i.d
- ❑ Amoxicillin is one of the most frequently used antibiotics for treatment of dental infections
- ❑ Dose of Amoxicillin - 250–500 mg t.i.d

Clindamycin

- ❑ An alternative for penicillin-allergic or penicillin-resistant patients
- ❑ Active against Gram-positive and Gram-negative anaerobes and facultative/aerobic bacteria
- ❑ Dose is 150–300 mg 6 hourly.

Tetracyclines

- ❑ This group includes tetracycline, doxycycline and minocycline which are broad-spectrum bacteriostatic antibiotics. These drugs inhibit bacterial protein synthesis
- ❑ These are useful in treatment of periodontal disease.

Macrolides

- ❑ This group includes erythromycin, clarithromycin and azithromycin.
  - • Erythromycin was the former drug of choice for penicillin-allergic/penicillin-resistant patients, but it showed gastrointestinal adverse effects.
- ❑ It is active against Gram-positive aerobic/facultative Staphylococci, Streptococci and Gram-negative anaerobes.

Metronidazole

- ❑ It is highly effective in most anaerobic infections.
- ❑ Patient should avoid alcohol during treatment with metronidazole.
- ❑ Dose is 200 to 400 mg thrice a day for orodental infections.

Antibiotic Prophylaxis Guidelines

Antibiotic prophylaxis is indicated in	Antibiotic prophylaxis is not indicated in
• Dental extraction • Periodontal procedures including surgery, scaling and root planning, probing • Dental implant placement • Root canal instrumentation beyond apex • Intraligamentary local anesthetic injections	• Restorative dentistry with or without retraction cord • Local anesthetic injections (nonintraligamentary) • Intracanal endodontic treatment; postplacement and core buildup • Placement of rubber dam • Postoperative suture removal

Standard antibiotic prophylaxis regimen **Table 12.1.**

Table 12.1: Antibiotic prophylactic regimens for certain dental procedures*.

Situation	Antibiotic[†]	Regimen[‡]
Standard prophylaxis	Amoxicillin	Adults, 2.0 g; children, 50 mg/kg orally 1 h before procedure
Cannot use oral medications	Ampicillin	Adults, 2.0 g IM[§] or IV[§]; children, 50 mg/kg IM or IV within 30 min before procedure
Allergic to penicillin	Clindamycin	Adults, 600 mg; children, 20 mg/kg orally 1 h before procedure
	Cephalexin or cefadroxil	Adult, 2.0 g; children, 50 mg/kg orally 1 h before procedure
	Azithromycin or clarithromycin	Adults, 500 mg; children, 15 mg/kg orally 1 h before procedure
Allergic to penicillin and unable to take oral medications	Clindamycin	Adult, 600 mg; children, 15 mg/kg IV 1 h before procedure
	Cefazolin	Adult, 1.0 g; children, 25 mg/kg IM or IV within 30 min before procedure

*Reprinted with permission of the Journal of the American Medical Association from Dajani et al.
[†]Cephalosporins should not be used in patients with immediate-type hypersensitivity reaction (urticaria, angioedema or anaphylaxis) to penicillins.
[‡]Total children's dose should not exceed adult dose.
[§]IM: intramuscular; IV: intravenous.

Bibliography

1. Cohen S, Hargreaves K. Pathways of the pulp. 9th edition St. Louis, MO: Mosby; 2006.
2. Kohn WG, Harte JA, Malvitz DM, et al. Guidelines for infection control in dental health care settings—2003. J Am Dent Assoc 2004;135:33–47.
3. Mickel AK, Wright AP, Chogle S, et al. An analysis of current analgesic preferences for endodontic pain management. J Endod 2006;32:1146–54.
4. Tong DC, Rothwell BR. Antibiotic prophylaxis in dentistry: a review and practice recommendations. J Am Dent Assoc 2000;131:366–74.
5. Tripathi KD. Essentials of pharmacology. 6th edition. New Delhi: Jaypee Brothers Medical Publishers; 2008.
6. Weber DJ, Tolkoff-Rubin NE, Rubin RH. Amoxicillin and potassium clavulanate: an antibiotic combination. Mechanism of action, pharmacokinetics, antimicrobial spectrum, clinical efficacy and adverse effects. Pharmacotherapy 1984;4:122–36.

Endodontic Instruments

Although a variety of instruments used in general dentistry are applicable in endodontics, some special instruments are unique to endodontic purpose.

The first endodontic file was made in mid 1800s by Edward Maynard by notching round wires (earlier got from watch spring and then from piano wires). In early 1900s, variety of tools like pathfinders, barbed broaches, reamers, files, etc. were available but there was little uniformity in quality control, taper of canal or instrument, and filling materials in terms of size and shape. 1958 was the hallmark year in the history of endodontic instruments. The manufacturers came together and a consensus was made on instruments and obturation materials.

Then in 1959, the following standardization for instruments and obturating materials was made:
- ❑ Formula for diameter and taper for each instrument introduced
- ❑ Formulae for graduated increment in size from one instrument to another was developed

In 1968, Jack Jacklich of Loyola University formed a group with other dentists and performed endodontic therapy. Over a period of time, he found endodontic treatment using hand instruments a tedious process and development of *"the scourge of digital hyperkeratosis."* All these problems led to many innovations in techniques and instruments. In 1989, American National Standards Institute (ANSI) granted the approval of American Dental Association (ADA) specification No. 28 for endodontic instruments.

Standardization of Instruments given by Ingle and Levine

Ingle and Levine using an electronic microcomparator found variation in the diameter and taper for same size of instrument. They suggested the following guidelines for instruments for having uniformity in instrument diameter and taper **(Figs. 13.1A to E):**
- ❑ Size: Instruments are numbered from 10 to 100. Each number should represent diameter of instrument in 100th of millimeter at the tip. For example, a No. 25 reamer shall have 0.25 mm at D1 and 0.57 mm (0.25 + 0.32) at D2. These sizes ensure a constant increase in taper, that is, 0.02 mm/mm of the instrument regardless of the size.
- ❑ There is increase in 5 units up to size 60 and in 10 units till they are size 100. This has been revised to include numbers from 6 to 140
- ❑ Length: Instruments are available in the following lengths: 21, 25, 28, 30, and 40 mm. 21 mm length is commonly used for molars, 25 mm for anteriors, 28 and 30 mm for canines and 40 mm for endodontic implants
- ❑ Tip angle: Tip angle of an instrument should be 75 ± 15°

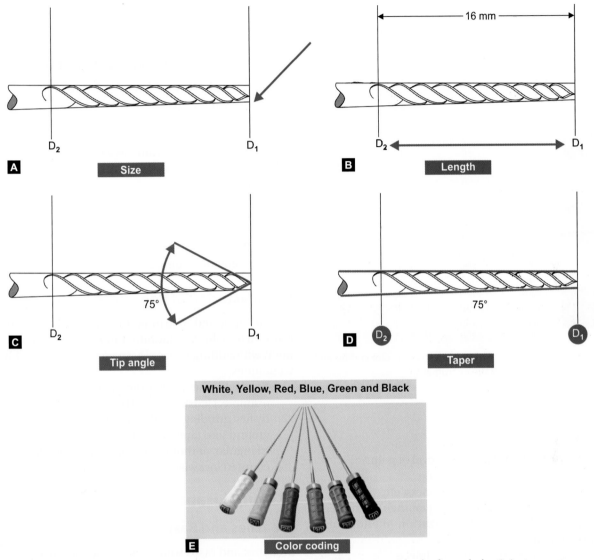

Figs. 13.1A to E Ingle Levine specifications of size, length, tip angle, taper and color for endodontic instruments.

- Taper: Working blade shall begin at tip (D1) and extend 16 mm up the shaft (D2). D2 should be 0.32 mm greater than D1, ensuring that there is constant increase in taper, that is, 0.02 mm/mm of instrument
- Color coding: Instrument handles should be color coded for their easier recognition **(Fig. 13.2)** (Pink, gray, purple, white, yellow, red, blue, green, black, white, etc.)

Modifications from Ingle's Standardization

- An additional diameter measurement point at D_3 is 3 mm from the tip of the cutting end of the instrument at D_0 (earlier it was D_1) and D_2 was designated as D_{16}
- Greater taper (GT) instruments (0.04, 0.06, 0.08, 0.10, 0.12) have also been made available.

To maintain these standards, American Association of Endodontists (AAE) recommended ADA and United States Bureau of Standards to form a committee for standardization of endodontic instruments.

ANSI and ISO/Federation Dentaire International (FDI) Numbering of endodontic instruments		
Instrument	*ANSI*	*FDI/ISO*
K files	28	3630/1
H files	58	3630/1
Barbed broaches and rasps	63	3630/1
Spreaders, pluggers	71	3630/2
Obturating points	78	6877
Absorbent points	73	7551
Root canal sealers	57	6876

Color	Color code	New number	Diameter	
			At tip	At 16 mm
	Pink	6	0.06	0.38
	Gray	8	0.08	0.40
	Purple	10	0.10	0.42
	White	15	0.15	0.47
	Yellow	20	0.20	0.52
	Red	25	0.25	0.57
	Blue	30	0.30	0.62
	Green	35	0.35	0.67
	Black	40	0.40	0.72
	White	45	0.45	0.77
	Yellow	50	0.50	0.82
	Red	55	0.55	0.87
	Blue	60	0.60	0.92
	Green	70	0.70	1.02
	Black	80	0.80	1.12
	White	90	0.90	1.22
	Yellow	100	1.00	1.32
	Red	110	1.10	1.42
	Blue	120	1.20	1.52
	Green	130	1.30	1.62
	Black	140	1.40	1.72
	White	150	1.50	1.82

Fig. 13.2 Table showing relationship between color coding and size of the instrument.

History

1750: Fauchard recommended removal of pulp.

1850: Wooden pegs for debriding pulp.

Early 1900: Introduction of files, reamers, etc.

1915: Kerr company obtained patent for their instruments.

1958: Ingle and Levine standardization of endodontic instruments.

1964: Introduction of giromatic handpiece.

1975: First potential application of NiTi alloys.

1976: First approved specification for root canal instruments.

1988: First use of NiTi in endodontics.

1989: ANSI approved specification No. 28 for endodontic reamers and files.

▌ Classification of Endodontic Instruments

Grossman's Classification
According to Function

Exploring: Smooth broaches and endodontic explorers (To locate canal orifices and determine patency of root canal)

Debriding or extirpating: Barbed broaches (To extirpate the pulp and other foreign materials from the root canal)

Cleaning and shaping: Reamers and files (Used to shape the canal space)

Obturating: Pluggers, spreaders and lentulospirals (To pack gutta-percha points into the root canal space).

Classification Based on Method of Use

Group I: Hand-operated endodontic instruments
- ❑ Broaches and rasps
- ❑ K-type reamers and files
- ❑ Hedstroem files

Group II: Low speed instruments with latch type attachment
- ❑ Gates-Glidden drills
- ❑ Peeso reamers

Group III: Engine-driven instruments
- ❑ Rotary NiTi instruments
- ❑ Reciprocating instruments

Group IV
- ❑ Sonics and ultrasonics.

Manufacturing of Hand Instruments

A hand-operated instrument reamer or file begins as a round wire which is modified to form a tapered instrument with cutting edges. These are manufactured by two techniques:

1. By machining the instrument directly on the lathe, for example, Hedstroem file (H-file), and NiTi instruments

2. By first grinding and then twisting. Here, the raw wire is ground into tapered geometric blanks, that is, square, triangular, or rhomboid. These blanks are then twisted counterclockwise to produce cutting edges.

▌ Group I Hand-Operated Instruments

Broaches and Rasps

Broaches and rasps were earliest endodontic instruments used to extirpate pulp and debris from the canal.

Broach

Broach is of two types:

1. *Barbed broach* (**Fig. 13.3**)
   - It is one of the oldest intracanal instruments with specifications by ANSI No. 63 and ISO No. 3630/1
   - It has ADA specification No. 6
   - Broach is short handled instrument meant for single use only
   - It is made from round steel wire. The smooth surface of wire is notched to from barbs bent at an angle from its long axis
   - Broaches are available in a variety of sizes, from triple extrafine to extra coarse
   - Broach does not cut the dentin but can effectively be used to remove cotton or paper points which might have lodged in the canal

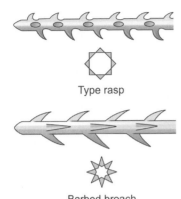

Type rasp

Barbed broach

Fig. 13.3 Schematic representation of rasp and barbed broach. Note longer and finer barbs in broach when compared to rasp.

K-Type Reamers and Files

Reamers and files are canal enlarging instruments, traditionally made from stainless steel and comprise of two basic designs, K-type instruments (K-files and K reamers) and the Hedstroem files. Since Kerr manufacturing company was first to produce them, so these were also called K-type instruments. These are made from rectangular or triangular blanks wires which are twisted to give the working end of the instruments a spiral form (**Fig. 13.4**). These instruments may have different spirals, cutting flutes.

Reamer

- Reamer is used to ream the canals. It cuts by inserting into the canal, twisting clockwise one quarter to half turn and then withdrawing, that is, penetration, rotation, and retraction (**Fig. 13.5**)
- Reamer has triangular blank and lesser number of flutes than file. Numbers of flutes in reamer are 0.5–1/mm (**Fig. 13.6**)
- Though reamer has fewer numbers of flutes than file, cutting efficiency is the same as that of files because more space between flutes causes better removal of debris
- Reamer tends to remain self-centered in the canal resulting in less chances of canal transportation.

Clinical Tips

- Broach should not be inserted into the root canal unless the canal has been enlarged to a size No. 25 reamer/file
- Broach should not be forced apically into the canal, as its barbs get compressed by the canal wall. While removing, the barbs get embedded into dentin resulting in fracture of the instrument on applying pressure
- If selected broach used is too narrow, it will not engage pulp tissue effectively
- If broach is too wide, it may bind to canal walls and thus may fracture

Uses of barbed broach

- Extirpation of entire pulp tissue
- Removal of cotton or paper points lodged in the canal
- Removal of necrotic debris and foreign material from canal.
  2. *Smooth broach:* It is free of barbs. Previously it was used as pathfinder, but at present flexible files are used for this.

Rasp/Rat Tail Files

- It has ADA specification No. 63
- Rasp has similar design to barbed broach except in taper and barb size. Barb size is larger in broach than rasp
- It is used to extirpate pulp tissue from canal space.

Broach	Rasp
• Barb extends to half of its core diameter, making it a weaker instrument	• Barbs extend to one third of the core, so it is not as weak as barbed broach
• Less taper (0.007–0.010 taper/mm)	• More taper (0.015–0.020 taper/mm)
• Barbs are very fine and longer (about 40 in no.)	• Barbs are blunt, shorter and shallower (50–60 in no.)

Difference between files and reamers		
	Files	*Reamers*
• Cross section	Square	Triangular
• Area of cross section	More	Less
• Flutes	More (1.5–2/mm)	Less (0.5–1/mm)
• Flexibility	Less	More (because of less work hardening)
• Cutting motion	Rasping and penetration (push and pull)	Rotation and retraction
• Preparation shape	Usually ovoid	Round
• Transport of debris	Poor because of tighter flutes	Better because of space present in flutes

Files

K-File

- It is triangular, square, or rhomboidal in cross section, manufactured from stainless steel wire, which is grounded into desired shape
- K-file has 1.5–2.5 cutting blades per mm of their working end.

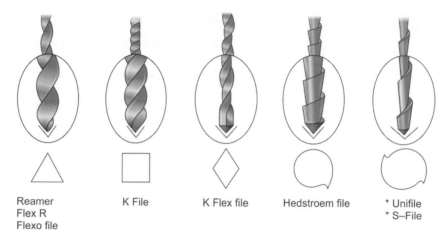

Fig. 13.4 Schematic representation of cross section of different files.

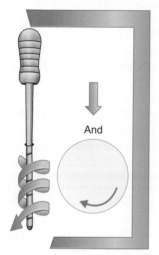

Fig. 13.5 Schematic representation of working of reamer-penetration, rotation and retraction.

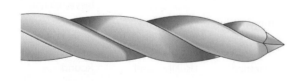

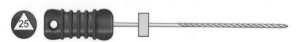

Fig. 13.6 Triangular cross section and lesser number of flutes in reamer.

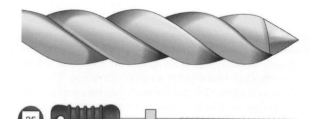

Fig. 13.7 Line diagram showing square cross section and more number of flutes in file.

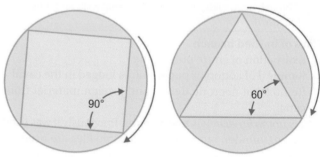

Fig. 13.8 Schematic representation showing that three point contact of file has more flexibility and more space for debris removal when compared to four point contact which has more cutting efficiency but less space for debris removal.

❑ File is predominantly used with filing or rasping action in which there is little or no rotation in the root canal. It is placed in root canal and pressure is exerted against the canal wall and instrument is withdrawn while maintaining the pressure **(Fig. 13.9).**

K-Flex File

❑ It was seen that square blank of file results in total decrease in the instrument flexibility. To maintain shape and flexibility of this file, K-flex file was introduced **(Fig. 13.10)**

❑ Tighter twisting of the file spirals increases the number of flutes in files (more than reamer) **(Fig. 13.7)**
❑ Triangular cross-sectioned file shows superior cutting and increased flexibility than the file or reamer with square blank **(Fig. 13.8)**

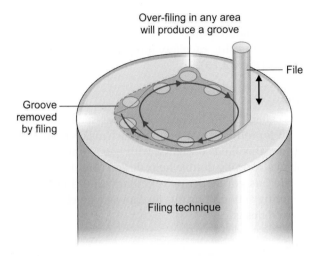

Fig. 13.9 File is worked along the canal wall in rasping action.

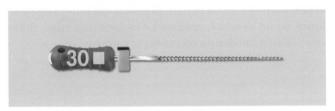

Fig. 13.10 Photograph showing K-flex file.

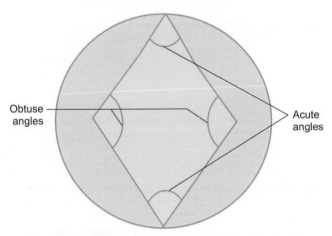

Fig. 13.11 Schematic representation of K-flex file showing rhomboidal cross section.

- K-flex file is rhombus in cross section having two acute angles and two obtuse angles **(Fig. 13.11)**
- Two acute angles increase sharpness and cutting efficiency of the instrument
- Two obtuse angles provide more space for debris removal
- Decrease in contact of instrument with canal walls provide more space for irrigation
- It is used with filing and rasping motion

Flexo File

- It is similar to the K-flex file except that it has triangular cross section **(Fig. 13.12)**. This feature provides more flexibility and an ability to resist fracture
- Tip of file is modified to noncutting type
- It is more flexible but has lesser cutting efficiency.

Triple Flex File

- It is made up of stainless steel and has triangular cross section
- It has more flutes then reamer but lesser than K-file
- Triangular cross section provides better flexibility and cutting efficiency.

Flex-R File/Roane File

- Flex-R file is made by removing the sharp cutting edges from the tip of the instrument **(Figs. 13.13)**. Noncutting tip enables the instrument to traverse along the canal rather than gouge into it
- This design reduces the ledge formation, canal transportation, and other procedural accidents when used with balanced force technique
- Another feature of flex-R file is presence of triangular cross section which provides it flexibility to be used in curved canals
- It is made up of NiTi and cuts during anticlockwise rotary motion.

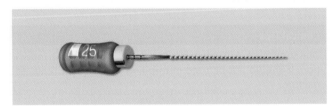

Fig. 13.12 Photograph showing flexo file.

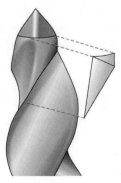

Fig. 13.13 Schematic representation showing non cutting tip of Flex R file.

Hedstroem File (H-File)

❑ H-file has flutes that resemble successively triangles set one on another **(Fig. 13.14)**
❑ It is made by cutting spiral grooves into round, tapered steel wire in the same manner as wood screws are made. This results in the formation of a sharp edge which cuts on removing strokes only
❑ H-file cuts only when instrument is withdrawn because its edges face handle of the instrument
❑ When used in torquing motion, its edges can engage in the dentin of root canal wall, causing H-files to fracture
❑ Rake angle and distance between the flutes are two main features which determine working of the file. H-file has positive rake angle, that is, its cutting edge is turned in the same direction in which force is applied which makes it to dig the dentin, thus more aggressive in cutting
❑ H-file should be used to machine the straight canal because it is strong and aggressive cutter. Since it lacks the flexibility and is fragile in nature, the H-file tends to fracture when used in torquing action

Advantages of H-files
❑ Better cutting efficiency
❑ Push debris coronally

Disadvantages of H-files
❑ Lack flexibility
❑ Tend to fracture
❑ Aggressive cutter

Clinical Tips

One should use Hedstroem files in only one direction, i.e., retraction. It should not be used in torquing motion as it tends to fracture.

Modifications in H-Files

Safety Hedstroem File
❑ This file has noncutting safety side along the length of the blade which reduces the chances of perforations

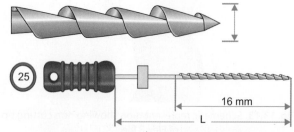

Fig. 13.14 H file resembles successive triangles set on one another.

❑ Noncutting side is directed to the side of canal where cutting is not required
❑ Noncutting side of safety file prevents lodging of the canals **(Fig. 13.15).**

S-File
❑ It is called "S" file because of its cross-sectional shape
❑ S-file is produced by grinding, which makes it stiffer than H-file. This file is designed with two spirals for cutting blades, forming double helix design **(Fig. 13.16)**
❑ S-file has good cutting efficiency in either filling or reaming action, thus this file can also be classified as a hybrid design.

A-File
❑ It's a variant of H-file
❑ Its cutting edges are at an acute angle to long axis of the file When used in curved canals, flutes on the inner edge collapse, so no dentin is removed. On the outer edge, flutes open, filling the dentin on outer curvature.

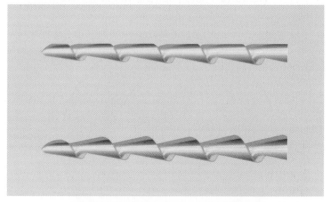

Fig. 13.15 Schematic representation of safety Hedstroem file.

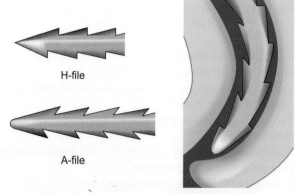

H-file

A-file

Fig. 13.16 Schematic representation of H and A- file.

Unifile

- It is machined from round stainless steel wire by cutting two superficial grooves to produce flutes in double helix design
- It resembles H-file in appearance
- It is less efficient
- Less prone to fracture.

C+ File

- C + file is made from specially treated stainless steel so have amazing stiffness and strength to be used for difficult and calcified canals. It has better buckling resistance than K-file (**Fig. 13.17**)
- Twisted file design provides greater strength
- It is available in size 8, 10, and 15 and in length 18, 21, and 25 mm.

Golden Medium File

- Golden medium file was described by Weine. It comes under intermediate files provided with half sizes between conventional instruments
- It is available in sizes from 12 to 37 like 12, 17, 22, 27, 32, and 37
- It is used for narrow canals since it provides more gradual increase in size than conventional files
- It is formed by cutting 1 mm from the tip of instrument. In this way No. 10 file can be converted to No. 12 and Nos. 15–17 and so on.

Group II Low Speed Instruments with Latch-Type Design

Gates-Glidden Drills

- Traditional engine-driven instruments include Gates-Glidden drills which have flame-shaped cutting point

mounted on long thin shaft attached to a latch-type shank (**Fig. 13.18**)
- Flame head cuts laterally, therefore used with gentle, apically directed pressure. It has safe tip to guard against perforations
- Gates-Glidden drills are available in a set from 1 to 6 with the diameters from 0.5 to 1.5 mm (**Fig. 13.19**)
- Due to their design, Gates-Glidden drills are side cutting instruments with safety tips
- They should be used in brushing strokes at the speed of 750–1,500 rpm
- Safety design of Gates-Glidden drills is that its weakest part lies at the junction of shank and shaft of the instrument (**Fig. 13.20**). If its cutting tip jams against the canal wall, fracture occurs at the junction of shank and the shaft but not at the tip. This makes removal of fractured drill from the canal by grasping with pliers easy
- GG drills can be used both in crown down as well as step back fashion.

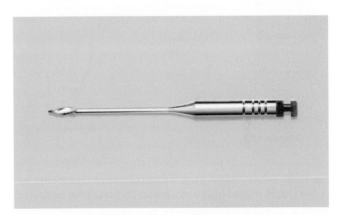

Fig. 13.18 Photograph showing Gates Glidden drill. Note the flame shaped head with latch type shank.

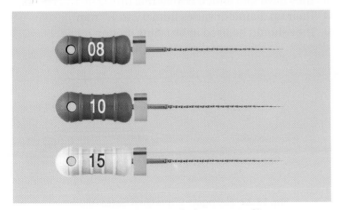

Fig. 13.17 Photograph showing C+ files
Courtesy: Dentsply India.

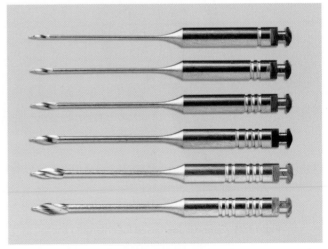

Fig. 13.19 Gates Glidden drills are numbered from 1 to 6 with diameter ranging from 0.5 to 1.5.

Number	Diameter at cutting tip (mm)
1	0.50
2	0.70
3	0.90
4	1.1
5	1.3
6	1.5

Uses of Gates-Glidden Drills

❑ For enlargement of root canal orifices (**Fig. 13.21**)
❑ For coronal flaring during root canal preparation

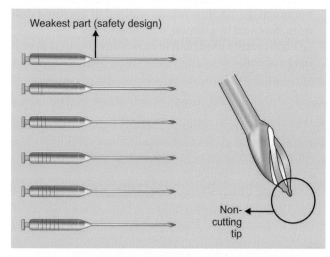

Fig. 13.20 Safety design feature of Gates Glidden drills showing non cutting flame shaped head and weakest portion at the junction of shank and shaft of the instrument.

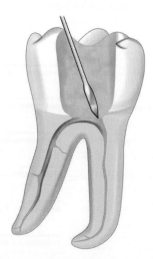

Fig. 13.21 Gates Glidden used for enlarging the root canal orifices.

❑ For removal of lingual shoulder during access preparation of anterior teeth
❑ During retreatment cases or postspace preparation for removal of gutta-percha
❑ For preparing space while removal of separated instrument
❑ If used incorrectly, for example, using at high rpm, incorrect angle of insertion, forceful drilling, GG drills can result in procedural accidents like perforations, instrument separation, etc.

Flexogates

❑ Flexogates are modified Gates-Glidden drills. They are made up of NiTi and have noncutting tip (**Fig. 13.22**)
❑ They are more flexible and used for apical preparation
❑ Flexogates can be rotated continuously in a handpiece through 360°
❑ These instruments have many advantages over traditional instruments in that they allow better debris removal because of continuous rotation and smoother and faster canal preparation with less clinician fatigue

---

Advantages of flexogates
- Safe noncutting guiding tip
- Safety design, i.e., its breakage point is 16 mm from the tip, so once fractured, it can be easily retrieved
- Flexible so used in curved canals

Peeso Reamers (Fig. 13.23)

❑ Peeso reamers are also stainless steel instruments like Gates-Glidden drills but they differ in that blades spread over a wide surface and their shape is cylindrical (**Fig. 13.24**)
❑ These are rotary instruments mainly used for postspace preparation
❑ They have safe ended noncutting tip
❑ Their tip diameter varies from 0.7 to 1.7 mm
❑ They should be used in brushing motion.

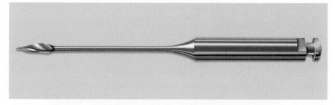

Fig. 13.22 Flexogate is modified Gates Glidden.

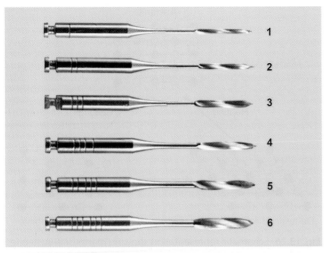

Fig. 13.23 Photograph showing 1 to 6 numbers Peeso reamers from tip diameter of 0.7 to 1.7 mm.

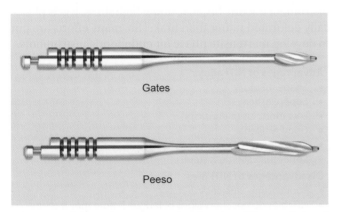

Fig. 13.24 Schematic representation showing difference in head design of Gates Glidden and Peesso reamer.

Number	Diameter at cutting tip (mm)
1	0.70
2	0.90
3	1.1
4	1.3
5	1.5
6	1.7

Uses

Peeso reamer is primarily used for postspace preparation when gutta-percha has to be removed from obturated root canal **(Fig. 13.25)**.

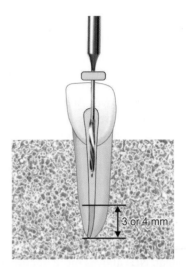

Fig. 13.25 Peeso reamer is used for removal of gutta-percha during post-space preparation.

Disadvantages

- They do not follow the canal curvature and may cause perforation by cutting laterally
- They are stiff instruments
- They have to be used very carefully to avoid iatrogenic errors.

Clinical Tips

Gates-Glidden drills and Peeso reamers are inflexible and aggressive cutting instrument. They should be used at slow speed with contra-angled handpiece with extreme caution to prevent perforations and overinstrumentation.

Group III Engine-Driven Instruments

NiTi Rotary Instruments

NiTi was developed by Buchler 60 years ago. NiTi is also known as the NiTinol (NiTi Navol Ordinance Laboratory in US). In endodontics, commonly used NiTi alloys are 55 NiTinol (55% weight Ni and 45% Ti) and 60 NiTinol (60% weight of Ni, 40% Ti). It was also called equiatomic NiTi alloy due to 1:1 atomic ratio of nickel to titanium. NiTi alloys with equiatomic ratio possess superelasticity and shape memory effect due to narrow solubility range of NiTi phase at 500° or below.

First use of NiTi in endodontics was reported in 1988 by Walia et al. when a 15 No. NiTi file was made from orthodontic wire and it showed superior flexibility and resistance to torsional fracture. This suggested the use of NiTi files in curved canals.

Superelasticity and shape memory of NiTi alloys is because of reversible stress induced martensitic transformation, that is, ability of NiTi alloy to undergo deformation at one temperature and then recover its original. Since this occurs at a narrow temperature change, no heating is necessary to cause undeformed shape to recover. At high temperature, lattice of NiTi alloy is simple, referred as austenite or parent phase.

On cooling, transformation induced in alloy occurs by shear type of process to a phase called martensitic phase. This causes change in physical properties of alloy, giving rise to shape memory effect. It has structure of a closely packed hexagonal lattice (**Fig. 13.26**). At this stage, unless external stress is applied, no macroscopic changes are seen. This martensite shape can be deformed easily to single orientation by process called detwinning when there is flipping over type of shear. NiTi alloy is more ductile in martensite phase than austenitic phase. This deformation can be reversed by heating the alloy. By heating, alloy resumes the original structure/austenite phase.

This transition from austenitic to martensitic phase can also occur by application of stress which occurs during root canal preparation. In response to external stress, austenitic phase changes to martensite phase. The deformation which occur below transformation temperature range is reversible.

R-phase

It is an intermediate phase with rhomboidal structure R phase possesses lower shear modulus than austenite or martensite phase, thus transformation strain for R phase . Transformation is less than other phases.

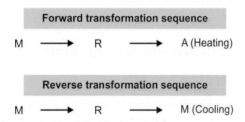

M-Wire

It is produced by thermomechanical processing . It contains all three crystalline phases including deformed, microtwinned martensite, R-phase and austenite. M-wire endodontic instruments like Profile GT-X, Profile Vortex, and Controlled Memory files like Hyflex CM files are used in martensitic state and possess shape memory effects. These files return to their original shape on autoclaving. Martensitic phase occurs at low temperature and has lower Young's modulus (20–50 GPa) than austenitic phase (40–90 GPa). This means that martensite gets easily deformed at lower stress than austenite. So martensitic phase is more flexible than austenitic phase and reduces the risk of

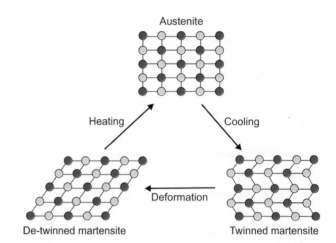

Fig. 13.26 Schematic representation showing martensite-austenite phase. Transition of Ni-Ti files for shape memory effect at atomic level.

instrument fracture because under high stress, it gets plastically deformed rather than brake. So, many efforts are put to develop martensite phase for endodontic instruments.

Advantages of NiTi alloys
- Shape memory
- Superelasticity
- Low modulus of elasticity
- Good resilience
- Corrosion resistance
- Softer than stainless steel

Disadvantages of NiTi files
- Poor cutting efficiency
- NiTi files do not show signs of fatigue before they fracture
- Poor resistance to fracture as compared to stainless steel

Generations of motors
- First generation: Motor without torque control
- Second generation: Motor with torque limit
- Third generation: Motor with simple torque control
- Fourth generation: Motor with apex locator and torque control

Characteristics/Properties of Rotary Instruments (Fig. 13.27)

❑ **Tip Design** (Fig. 13.28)
- Rotary file can have cutting (shaping Protaper files) or noncutting tip (ProFile, GT K3, Hero 642, RaCe, and finishing Protaper files)
- Cutting tip makes the file aggressive. Its advantage is that it can enter in narrow canals. If goes beyond apex, file with cutting tip results in elliptical tear at apex which is difficult to seal, whereas file with noncutting tip form concentric circle which can be sealed with gutta-percha

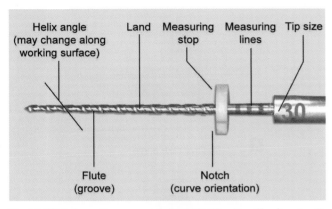

Fig. 13.27 Schematic representation of NiTi rotary file showing its different characteristics.

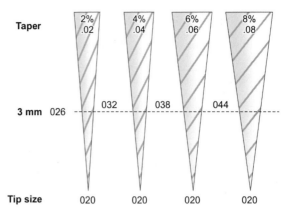

Fig. 13.29 Taper indicates increase in diameter of file from tip towards handle. Note in this figure, tip size is same but increase in taper proportionately increases the diameter towards handle.

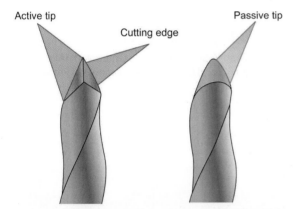

Fig. 13.28 Schematic representation of cutting and noncutting tip.

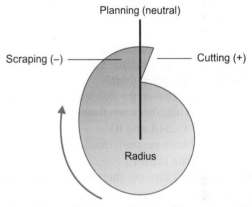

Fig. 13.30 Rake angle is the angle formed by cutting edge and cross section taken perpendicular to long axis of the tooth.

❑ *Taper*
  • It signifies per millimeter increase in file diameter from the tip toward handle of file **(Fig. 13.29)**. Difference in minimum and maximum diameter can be reduced so that torque required for rotating larger instruments does not exceed the plastic limit of smaller instrument
  • Traditional instrument used to have 2% taper but rotary endodontic files have 4%, 6%, 8%, 10%, or 12% taper. A zero taper or nearly parallel file can be used to enlarge the curved canals without undue file stress and pressing debris.
  • File can be of constant taper but with varying tip diameter or constant tip size with graduating taper from 0.04 to 0.12. With graduating taper, only minimal part of the file engages the canal wall resulting in reduced resistance and thus less torque to run the file
  • Protaper system has progressive taper which claims reduced torsional loading. GT series consists of GT 20, GT 30 and GT 40 with 10%, 8%, 6%, 4%. RaCe files

are available from 15 to 60 sizes with taper of 10%, 8%, 6%, 4%, and 2%. Hero 642 consists of 12 files with varying tip sizes, tapers

❑ *Blade*
  • It is the working area of file
  • It is the surface with the greatest diameter which follows the flute as it rotates.

❑ *Rake angle:*
  • It is the angle formed by cutting edge and cross section taken perpendicular to long axis of the tooth. Cutting angle is angle formed by cutting edge and radius when file is sectioned perpendicular to the cutting edge **(Fig. 13.30)**. It can be positive, neutral, or negative **(Fig. 13.31)**
  • If angle formed by leading edge and surface to be cut is obtuse, rake angle is *positive or cutting*
  • If angle formed by leading edge and surface to be cut is acute, rake angle is *negative or scrapping*
  • Positive rake angle cuts more efficiently than negative; it scrapes the canal wall. File with overly positive angle

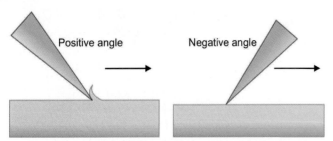

Fig. 13.31 Positive and negative rake angles. Positive angle results in cutting action; Negative angle results in scrapping action.

digs and gauges the canal and can result in instrument separation **(Figs. 13.32A and B)**

❑ *Flute:*
• It is a groove present on the working area of file to collect soft tissue and dentin chips removed from canal wall **(Fig. 13.33)**
• Effectiveness of flute depends upon depth, width, configuration, and surface finish

❑ *Radial land/marginal width:*
• It is the area between the flutes which projects axially from central axis, between flutes as far as the cutting edge **(Figs. 13.34A and B)**
• It acts as a blade support, that is, amount of material supporting the blades
• Most of rotary files get their strength from material mass of core
• Peripheral strength is gained by increasing the width of radial land
• Profile and K3 have full radial lands, so they show superior peripheral strength. Increase in peripheral mass prevents propagation of cracks, reducing chances of separation. Protaper, Hero 642, RaCe do not have radial lands.

❑ *Relief*
• Surface area of land which is reduced to a certain extent to reduce frictional resistance.

❑ *Helical angle:*
• It is the angle formed by cutting edge with the long axis of the file. File with constant helical angle results in inefficient removal of debris and is susceptible to "screwing in" forces **(Fig. 13.35)**
• This angle is important for determining which file technique to use
• Variable helix angle causes better removal of debris and reduces the chances of screwing into the wall
• In K3 file, there is increase in helical angle from tip to handle, resulting in better debris removal
• RaCe has alternating helical design which reduces rotational torque

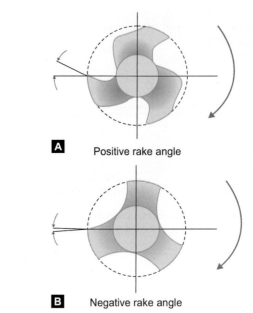

A   Positive rake angle

B   Negative rake angle

Figs. 13.32A and B Schematic representation of (A) positive rake of K3 file and (B) negative rake angle of Profile.

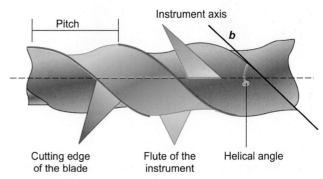

Pitch   Instrument axis   *b*

Cutting edge of the blade   Flute of the instrument   Helical angle

Fig. 13.33 Schematic representation of flute, cutting edge, helix angle and pitch of a rotary file.

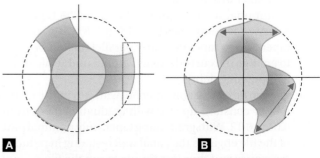

A   **B**

Figs. 13.34A and B Cross section: (A) Cross section of profile showing radial land; (B) K3 showing reduced radial land with wide blade support which adds peripheral strength to the file.

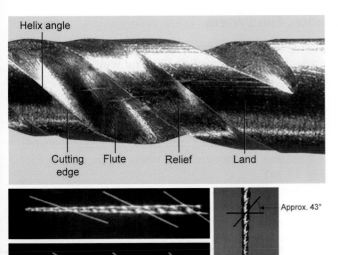

Fig. 13.35 Schematic representation of different helical angles.

- Pitch:
  - It is the distance between point on leading edge and corresponding point on leading edge
  - It shows number of threads per unit length. File with constant helical angles and pitch tend to screw in the file, whereas file with variable pitch and helical angle reduces the sense of being screwing into the canal.

Generations of NiTi Rotary Files

Generation	Characteristic feature	Example
1st	Passive cutting radial lands, fixed tapers of 4% and 6% over the length and negative rake angles for scraping	Profile, GT Rotary files, Quantec, HERO 642, Light speed
2nd	Active cutting edges, variable taper, fewer instruments needed to prepare the canal	Protaper Universal, K3, Protaper Gold, Hero shapers
3rd	Improvements in NiTi metallurgy, reduce cyclic fatigue and file separation	K3XF, Twisted files, Profile GT X series, Hyflex CM
4th	Reciprocation movement (bidirectional movement, single file concept.	Wave one, SAF, Reciproc
5th	Offset center of mass, mechanical wave of motion travelling along the length of the file, swaggering effect of file.	REVO-S, Protaper Next, One shape

First Generation NiTi Rotary Files

Profile System

Profile system made by Tulsa Dental was one of the first NiTi commercially available instruments. This system was introduced by Dr. Johnson in 1944. Profile NiTi line includes Series 29, orifice shapers, Profile 0.02, 0.04 and 0.06, GT files and ProTaper instruments **Series 29 instruments,** instead of increasing each file by 0.05 between sizes, it was increased by 29%. This system works well in small sizes, but in bigger instruments. This much increase is not possible.

Profile 0.02, 0.04 and 0.06

- These have safe ended noncutting tips with negative rake angle (−20°) which makes them to cut dentin in scrapping motion. Profile instrument tends to pull debris out of the canal because of presence of 20° helical angle **(Fig. 13.36)** Recommended rotational speed for profiles is 150–300 rpm.
- Cross section of profile shows three U-shaped grooves with radial lands **(Fig. 13.37).**

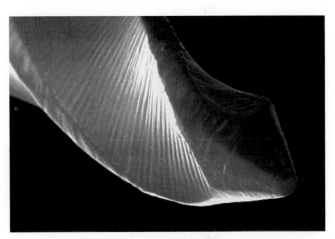

Fig. 13.36 Photograph showing noncutting tip of profile.

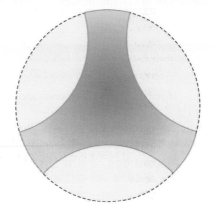

Fig. 13.37 Cross section of file showing three U-shaped grooves with radial land.

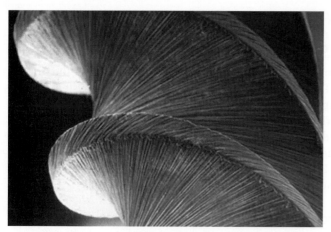

Fig. 13.38 Central parallel core of file increases flexibility of file.

❑ Central parallel core present in profile increases its flexibility **(Fig. 13.38)**.

Orifice Openers

❑ These extend 19 mm below the head of the handpiece and have 10 mm of cutting blade
❑ Series consists of six instruments which are safe ended with increasing D0 diameters
❑ Used to prepare coronal two third of root canal system

Greater Taper Files (Steve Buchanan in 1994)

❑ GT files possess U-shaped file design with ISO tip sizes of 20, 30 and 40 and tapers of 0.04, 0.06, 0.08, 0.010 and 0.12
❑ Accessory GT files for use as orifice openers of 0.12 taper in ISO sizes of 35, 50, 70 and 90 are also available
❑ Maximum diameter of GT file is 1 mm
❑ Recommended rotational speed for GT file is 300 rpm
❑ Negative rake angle of GT file makes it to scrape the dentin rather than cutting it.

Difference between profile and Protaper GT		
	Profile	Protaper GT
Working length	16 mm	Depends upon the taper
Number of spirals	Same throughout its length	More at the tip than near handle
Taper	0.02, 0.04, 0.06, 0.08, and 0.10	0.04, 0.06, 0.08, 0.10, 0.12 with three primary sizes 20, 30, and 40

Quantec File System

❑ Quantec file series were introduced in 1996 and are available in both safe cutting and noncutting tips with standard size of 25 No. in 0.12, 0.10, 0.08, 0.06, 0.05, 0.04, 0.03, and 0.02 tapers. 0.02 tapered. Axes handles are 30% shorter than other files. Recommended speed is 340 rpm
❑ Files have reduced radial land which decreases the surface tension, contact area and stress on the instrument **(Fig. 13.39)**
❑ Files have two flutes which increases the flute depth as compared to three flute design. This unique design minimizes its contact with the canal, thereby reducing the torque, providing greater space for debris removal, and reducing file separation
❑ Quantec system utilizes the "graduated taper technique" to prepare a canal. It is thought that using a series of files of single taper results in decreases in efficiency as the larger instruments are used. This happens because more of file comes in contact with the dentinal wall which makes it more difficult to remove dentin. But in graduated taper technique, restricted contact of area increases the efficiency of the instrument because now forces are concentrated on smaller area.

HERO 642

HERO	–	High elasticity in rotation
642	–	0.06, 0.04 and 0.02 tapers

❑ It was introduced by Daryl-Green
❑ HERO 642 (high elasticity in rotation, 0.06, 0.04 and 0.02 tapers) is used in at 300–600 rpm
❑ It has trihelical Hedstrom design with positive rake angle and sharp flutes **(Fig. 13.40)**. Cross section of HERO show geometrics similar to H file without radial lands.

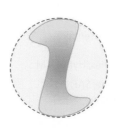 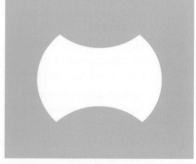

Fig. 13.39 Reduced radial land decreases the contact area and stress on the instrument.

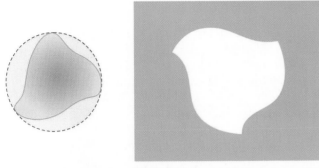

Fig. 13.40 Cross section of HERO 642 shows trihelical design with positive rake angle without radail lands.

☐ Due to progressively increasing distance between the flutes, there is reduced risk of binding the instrument in root canal

☐ Larger central core provides extra strength and resistance to fracture.

Light Speed System (Fig. 13.41)

☐ This system was introduced by Steve and Willian Wildely in 1990, now known as LS1

☐ Light speed system is engine-driven endodontic instrument manufactured from nickel–titanium. This is so named because a "light" touch is needed as "speed" of instrumentation is increased

☐ Light speed instrument is slender with thin parallel shaft and has noncutting tip with Gates-Glidden in configuration

☐ Recommended speed for use is 1,500–2,000 rpm

☐ These are available in sizes Nos. 20–140 including the half sizes, namely, 22.5, 27.5, 32.5. The half sizes are also color coded as full ones with only difference in that half size instruments have white or black rings on their handles

☐ Cutting head of light speed system has three different geometric shapes:

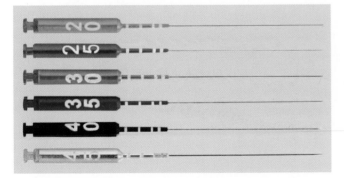

Fig. 13.41 Photograph showing light speed system.

• Size 20–30 short noncutting tips at 75° cutting angle
• Size 32.5 longer noncutting tip at 33° cutting angle
• Size 35–140 longer noncutting tip with 21° cutting angle

☐ Cutting heads basically have three radial lands with spiral-shaped grooves in between.

Difference between traditional hand files and light speed instruments	
Traditional hand files	*Light speed instruments*
• Made up of stainless steel • Intermediate sizes not available • Smallest size is 06 No. • Length of cutting head is 16 mm • Noncutting pilot tip is absent	• Made up of NiTi • Intermediate sizes available • Smallest size is 20 No. • Length of cutting head is 0.25–2.25 mm • Noncutting pilot tip is present

▌ Second Generation

Protaper Universal

These were designed by Dr. Cliff Ruddle, Dr. John West, and Dr. Pierre Machtou.

Features

Progressive tapers: This improves flexibility, cutting efficiency, and reduces the number of recapitulations needed to achieve length. One of the benefits of a progressively tapered Shaping file is that each instrument engages a smaller zone of dentin which reduces torsional loads, file fatigue and the potential for breakage.

Convex triangular cross section: This feature reduces the contact area between the blade and dentin, increases the cutting action, and improves safety by decreasing the torsional load (**Fig. 13.42**).

Helical angle and pitch: Continuously changing helical angle and pitch optimizes its cutting action, clears the debris out of the canal, and prevents screwing in of instrument in the canal.

Variable tip diameters: Variable D_0 diameter allows file to safely and efficiently follow the canal.

Modified guiding tip: This allows each instrument to better follow the canal without damaging the root canal walls.

Short handles
☐ Short 12.5 mm handle improves access in posterior regions.

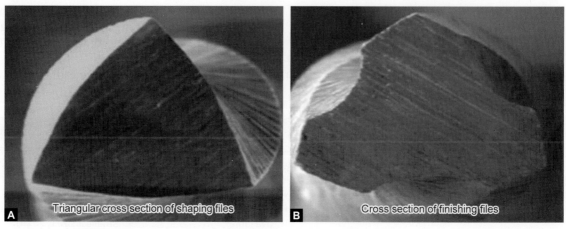

Fig. 13.42 Schematic representation of cross section of: (A) Shaping files; (B) Finishing files.

Shaping Files (Fig. 13.43)

File	S_x	S_1	S_2
Features	• No identification ring on its gold-colored handle • Shorter length of 19 mm • D_0 diameter is 0.19 mm • There is increase in taper up to D_9 and then taper drops off up to D_{14} which increases its flexibility • Use is similar to Gates-Glidden drills or orifice shapers	• Purple identification ring on its handle • D_0 diameter is 0.17 mm • Used to prepare coronal part of the root	• White identification ring on its handle • D_0 diameter is 0.20 mm • Used to prepare middle third of the canal

Finishing Files (Figs. 13.44 and 13.45)

File no.	F_1	F_2	F_3	F_4	F_5
D_0 diameter	20	25	30	40	50

ProTaper Gold

Developed with improved metallurgy, ProTaper Gold rotary files show the following features **(Fig. 13.46)**:

❑ Convex triangular cross section and progressive taper
❑ Increased flexibility due to advanced metallurgy process
❑ Greater resistance to cyclic fatigue so lesser chances of file separation

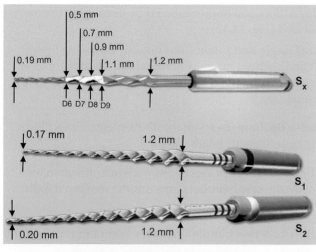

Fig. 13.43 Shaping files Sx, S1 and S2
Courtesy: Dentsply India.

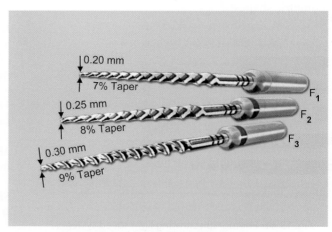

Fig. 13.44 Protaper finishing files F_1, F_2 and F_3.

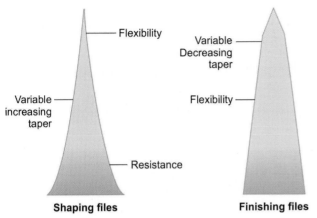

Fig. 13.45 Schematic representation showing differences in shaping and finishing files. Variable tapers of file improve flexibility of file.

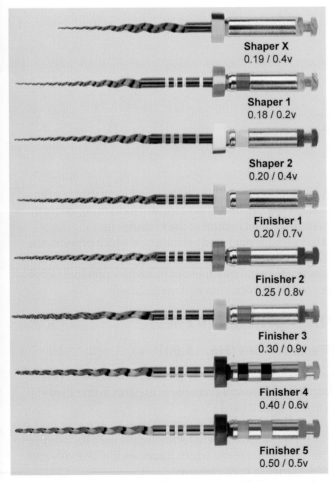

Fig. 13.46 Photograph showing Protaper Gold shaping and finishing files.
Courtesy: Dentsply India.

- Shorter 11 mm handle
- Noncutting tip design allows each instrument to safely follow the canal while the small flat area on the tip enhances its ability to find its way through soft tissue and debris.

K₃ Rotary File System

Dr. John McSpadden in 2002 in North America introduced K₃ system.

- K₃ files are available in taper of 0.02, 0.04, or 0.06 with ISO tip sizes. An Axxess handle design shortens the file by 5 mm without affecting its working length **(Fig. 13.47)**
- These files are flexible because of presence of variable core diameter
- Cutting head shows three radial lands with relief behind two radial lands. Asymmetrically placed flutes make the K₃ system with superior canal tracking ability, add peripheral strength to K₃ system, and prevent screwing into the canal **(Fig. 13.48)**
- Positive rake angle makes effective cutting surface
- K₃ files are color coded to differentiate various tip sizes and tapers
- Body shapers available in taper 0.08, 0.10, and 0.12, all with tip size 25 are used to prepare the coronal third of the canal.

Race Files (Reamers with Alternating Cutting Edges)

- Race has safety tip and triangular cross section. This file has two cutting edges, first alternates with a second which has been placed at different angle **(Fig. 13.49)**.

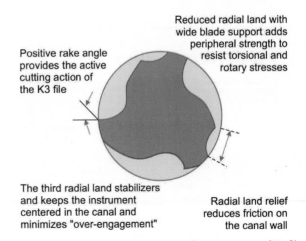

Fig. 13.47 Schematic representation of cross section of K3 file.

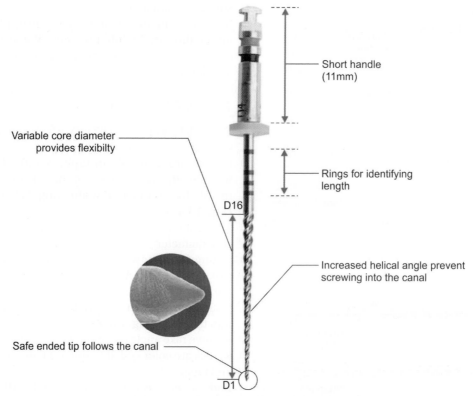

Fig. 13.48 Characteristic feature of K3 file.
Courtesy: SybronEndo.

Variable core diameter provides flexibilty

Safe ended tip follows the canal

Short handle (11mm)

Rings for identifying length

D16

Increased helical angle prevent screwing into the canal

D1

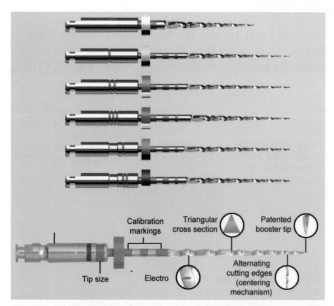

Calibration markings   Triangular cross section   Patented booster tip

Tip size   Electro   Alternating cutting edges (centering mechanism)

Fig. 13.49 Photograph showing characteristic features of Race file.
Courtesy: FKG Dentaire.

Alternating cutting edges help in reducing working time and decreasing operation torque. Noncutting safety tip helps in perfect control of the instrument

❑ It has variable pitch and helical angle which prevents the file from screwing into the canal

❑ Electrochemical treatment of these files provides better resistance to corrosion and metal fatigue.

Third Generation Files

TF Twisted Files (Fig. 13.50)

These are the first fluted NiTi files manufactured by plastic deformation. these are available in tip sizes from #25 to #50 and tapers from 0.04-.12.

Three unique features of these files are:

1. R-phase heat treatment technology is used to optimize the molecular phase which increases file flexibility and resistance to cyclic fatigue.

2. Twisted design, not ground; twisting helps preserve grain structure and reduces formation of

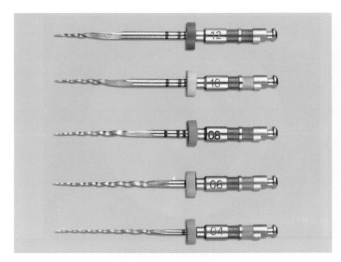

Fig. 13.50 Twisted files.
Courtesy: SybronEndo.

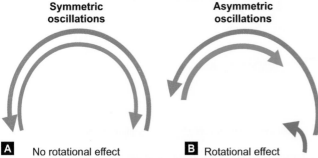

Symmetric oscillations

Asymmetric oscillations

A No rotational effect   **B** Rotational effect

Figs. 13.51A and B Reciprocating motion for endodontic instrumentation: (A) Complete reciprocation with horizontal rotational oscillations; (B) Partial reciprocation with rotational effect.

microfractures, making the file even more durable. Grinding weakens the metal's structure at the molecular level and creates microfractures on the metal's surface.

3. A proprietary surface conditioning treatment of the file.

Fourth-Generation Reciprocating Instruments

Reciprocation is defined as repetitive back and forth motion and it has been clinically utilized to use stainless steel files since 1958. In rotation, NiTi files require less inward pressure and take debris out of the canal, whereas reciprocation mimics the manual filing. These instruments result in less debris removal because of pecking motion and can result in debris extrusion **(Figs. 13.51A and B)**.

Advantages of reciprocating motion
- Less binding of the instrument leads to canals so less torsional stress.
- Decreased risk of instrument separation

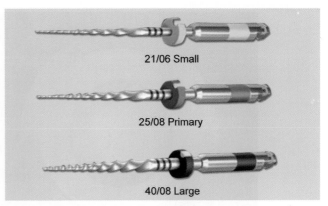

21/06 Small

25/08 Primary

40/08 Large

Fig. 13.52 WaveOne NiTi File System.
Courtesy: Dentsply India.

- Less flexural stress due to reduction in number of cycles with in the root canal.

Disadvantages
- Increased amount of debris extrusion during instrumentation procedure.
- Causes cracks in dentin due to reciprocating instrumentation technique.

WaveOne NiTi File System

It is a single-use, single-file system to shape the root canal completely from start to finish. It works in a similar but reverse "balanced force" action moving in a back and forth "reciprocal motion." There are three files in the WaveOne single-file reciprocating system, available in lengths of 21, 25 and 31 mm **(Fig. 13.52)**. These are used at speed of 300 rpm with torque of 5 N cm. These work with a reverse cutting action. They have modified convex triangular cross section **(Fig. 13.53)** at the tip end.

These work with a reverse cutting action. They have modified convex triangular cross section **(Fig. 13.53)** at the tip end.
- WaveOne small file has tip size of ISO 21 with taper of 6%. It is used in fine canals
- WaveOne primary file has tip size of ISO 25 with taper of 8% that reduces toward the coronal end
- WaveOne large file tip size of ISO 40 with taper of 8%. It is used in large canals

WaveOne Gold

WaveOne Gold incorporates the metallurgical advancements of Gold wire, improving flexibility by 80% over of WaveOne. It has parallelogram-shaped cross section, which helps in improving cutting efficiency and debris removal within the canal. It's variable taper helps it to perform better in smaller and narrower canal anatomy. Tip sizes match ISO Numbers 020, 025, 035 and 045 **(Figs. 13.54 and 13.55)**.

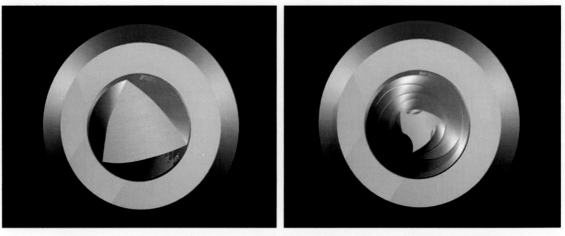

Fig. 13.53 Cross section of WaveOne NiTi File. Characteristic features of WaveOne Gold file.

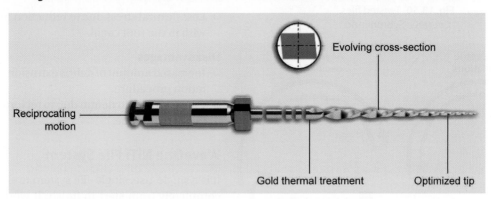

Fig. 13.54 Photograph showing characteristic features of WaveOne Gold file.
Courtesy: Dentsply India.

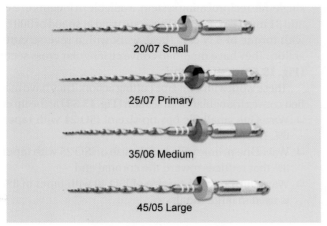

Fig. 13.55 WaveOne Gold files.
Courtesy: Dentsply India.

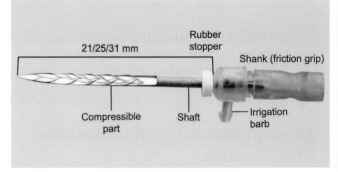

Fig. 13.56 Self adjusting file.
Courtesy: Redent NOVA.

Self-Adjusting File

The Self-Adjusting File is a hollow Nickel–Titanium lattice-like cylinder that scrubs the canal walls by vertical vibrations. Its hollow shape allows for the continuous flow of irrigant through its lumen to achieve superior disinfection

(Fig. 13.56). It is available in lengths 21, 25, and 31 mm and two diameters 1.5 and 2.0 mm.

It is used at 5,000 vertical vibrations per minute. Its abrasive surface acts similarly as sandpaper by scrubbing uniformly and gradually enlarging the root canal circumferentially. Slow, low-torque rotation occurs when the SAF is not engaged with the canal walls, allowing circular repositioning throughout the process.

TF Adaptive file system

TF adaptive file works as rotary under normal conditions but changes to reciprocation when stress is increased on file. these features allow better resistance to cyclic fatigue with higher durability.

Available in different sizes; for small canals as 20/0.04, 25/0.06, and 35/0.04 and for medium to large sized canals as 25/0.08, 36/0.06, and 50/0.04 **(Fig. 13.57)**.

▌ Fifth Generation Instruments

Revo-S

Revo-S has snake-like movement inside the canal. It has an asymmetrical cross section which provides more flexibility and less stress on the instrument **(Fig. 13.58)**. It works in a cyclic way (3C concept); cutting, clearance, and cleaning at rotation speed ranging between 250 and 400 rpm. It consists of three instruments: SC1, SC2, SU **(Fig. 13.59)**.

Protaper Next

Features

Shortens the shaping time; high cutting efficiency reduces the shaping time.

Swaggering Effect: Protaper Next's innovative off-centered rectangular cross section gives the file a snake like "swaggering" movement as it moves through the root canal. This helps in better removal of debris and canal tracking **(Figs. 13.60 and 13.61)**.

M-WIRE NiTi improves file flexibility, greater resistance to cyclic fatigue and cutting efficiency.

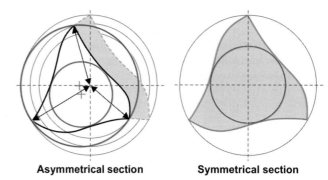

Asymmetrical section   **Symmetrical section**

Fig. 13.58 Asymmetrical cross section of Revo-S file provides more flexibility and reduces stress concentration.

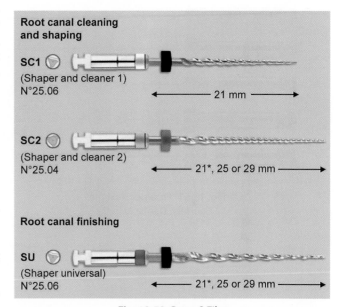

Root canal cleaning and shaping

SC1
(Shaper and cleaner 1)
N°25.06
◄——— 21 mm ———►

SC2
(Shaper and cleaner 2)
N°25.04
◄——— 21*, 25 or 29 mm ———►

Root canal finishing

SU
(Shaper universal)
N°25.06
◄——— 21*, 25 or 29 mm ———►

Fig. 13.59 Revo-S Files
Courtesy: Micro Mega.

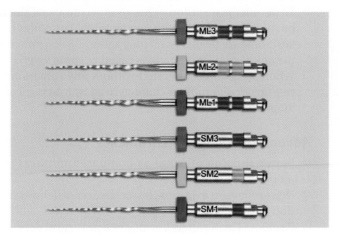

Fig. 13.57 Twisted adaptive files for small and large canals.

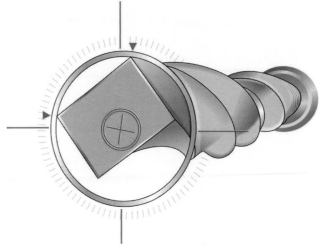

Fig. 13.60 Schematic representation showing swaggering movements of Protaper Next File.

ScoutRace Files

❏ ScoutRace is a sequence of three instruments with .02 taper and with ISO sizes of 10, 15 and 20 **(Fig. 13.62)**
❏ These are used at 600–800 rpm
❏ These have extreme flexibility due to 0.02 taper, rounded safety tip for precise guiding, alternating cutting edges to avoid screwing-in effect, sharp edges for best cutting efficiency and electrochemical polishing for better resistance to torsion and fatigue

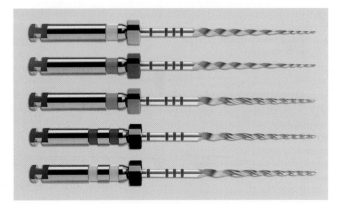

Fig. 13.61 Protaper Next files.
Courtesy: Dentsply India.

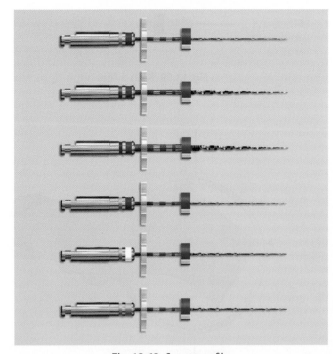

Fig. 13.62 Scoutrace file.
Courtesy: FKG Dentaire.

Group IV Sonics and Ultrasonics in Endodontics

Ultrasonic instrument was first used in dentistry for tooth preparation with abrasive slurry. Though it showed low cutting efficiency, it had many advantages like improved visualization, conservative approach, and selective cutting. Concept of using ultrasonics in endodontics was suggested by Richman in 1957. The pioneer research on endosonics was done by Cunningham and Martin in early 1980. Endosonics is a device which imparts sinusoidal vibration of high intensity to a root canal instrument.

Sonic Handpiece

❏ Sonic instruments rely on a passage of pressurized air through the instrument handpiece for use operating at 3–6 kHz. Its handpiece is attached to normal airline, so it uses compressed airline at a pressure of 0.4 MPa (already available in dental unit setup as its source of power)
❏ It has an adjustable ring to give oscillating range of 1,500–3,000 cps
❏ There are two options for irrigating the root canal while using sonic handpieces. Either the waterline of the dental units can be attached to the sonic handpiece or the water can be cut off and the dental assistant can introduce sodium hypochlorite from a syringe
❏ Sonic handpiece uses the following types of files:
  • Helio sonic (Trio sonic)
  • Shaper sonic
  • Rispi sonic
❏ All these instruments have safe ended noncutting tip 1.5–2 mm in length. The sizes for these instruments range from 15 to 40
❏ Instrument oscillates outside the canal which is converted into vibrational up and down movement in root canal. Sonic instruments are used in step down technique
❏ To permit the insertion of No. 15 sonic file, canal should be initially prepared with conventional hand files (No. 20). Sonic file begins its rasping action 1.5–2.0 mm from the apical stop. This length is called as *sonic length*
❏ When sonic file is operated without any constraint, it sets up circular motion characterized by true vertical or longitudinal movement.

Advantages of Sonic Instruments

❏ Better shaping of canal as compared to ultrasonic preparation
❏ Due to constant irrigation, lesser chances of debris extrusion beyond the apex
❏ Produces clean canals free of smear layer and debris

Disadvantages

❏ Walls of prepared canals are rough
❏ Chances of transportation are more in curved canals.

Ultrasonic Handpiece

❏ Ultrasonic endodontics is based on a system in which sound as an energy source (20–42 kHz) causes three-dimensional activation of a file in the surrounding medium. Ultrasound energy can be produced by magnetostriction; it converts electromagnetic energy into mechanical energy or piezoelectricity principle. In this, crystal is used which changes dimension when an electric charge is applied, therefore, electric current generate a wave in the crystals. This crystal deformation is converted to mechanical oscillation with no production of heat
❏ Ultrasonic systems involve a power source to which an endodontic file (K file) is attached with a holder and an adapter (**Fig. 13.63**). Before a size 15 can be freely used with ultrasonics, canal must be enlarged with hand instruments to a size Nos. 30–40 file

Irrigants are emitted from cords on the power source and travel down the file into the canal to be energized by the vibrations.

Advantages of Ultrasonics

❏ Clean canals free of smear layer and debris
❏ Enhanced action of NaOCl because of increased temperature and ultrasonic energy.

Disadvantage

Causes transportation of root canal if used carelessly.

Mechanism of Action/Biophysics

Cavitation

Cavitation is defined as the growth and subsequent violent collapse of a small gas filled pre-existing in homogeneity in the bulk fluid. When a vibrating object is immersed in a fluid, oscillations cause local increase (compression) or decrease (rarefaction) in fluid pressure. During rarefaction phase, at certain pressure amplitude, the liquid fail under acoustic stress and form cavitation bubbles. During next positive pressure phase, these vapor filled cavities implosively collapse resulting in shock waves (**Fig. 13.64**). Cavitation has been shown useful in removal of deposits in scaling procedure, but during its use in root canal regarding cavitation phenomenon, the following points are to be considered:

❏ Threshold power setting at which this phenomenon occurs is beyond the range that is normally used for endodontic purpose
❏ Cavitation depends on free displacement amplitude of the file. During root canal therapy, when file movement is restricted, this phenomenon is impossible to achieve.

Acoustic streaming

Acoustic streaming is defined as generation of time independent, steady, unidirectional circulation of fluid in vicinity of a small vibrating object. This flow of liquid has a small velocity, of the order of a few centimeters per second, but because of the small dimensions involved the rate of change of velocity is high. This results in the production of large hydrodynamic shear stresses around the file, which are more than capable of disrupting most biological material.

Uses of Endosonics

Access enhancement: Use of round or tapered ultrasonically activated diamond coated tips has shown to produce smoother shapes of access cavity (**Fig. 13.65**).

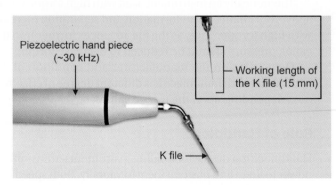

Fig. 13.63 Ultrasonic handpiece with attached K-File.

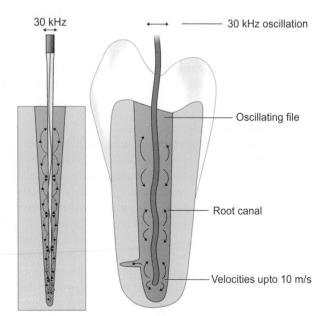

Fig. 13.64 Schematic representation of oscillating ultrasonic file and fluid movement in the canal.

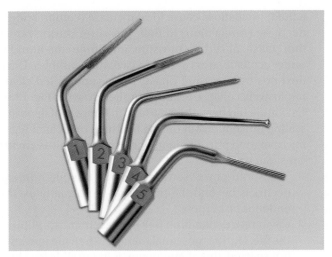

Fig. 13.65 Photograph showing different shapes of ultrasonic tips.

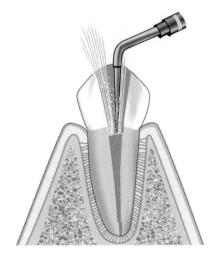

Fig. 13.66 Continuous irrigation using endosonics produce cleaner canals.

Orifice location: Ultrasonic instruments are very useful for removal of chamber calcifications, troughing for canals in isthmus and locating the canal orifices.

Irrigation: Endosonics results in activation of the irrigating solution in the canal by cavitation and acoustic streaming. This combined with oscillation of the instrument results in cleaner canals **(Fig. 13.66)**.

Sealer placement: Sealer is placed using an ultrasonic file which runs without fluid coolant.

Gutta-percha obturation: Moreno first suggested the technique of plasticizing gutta-percha in the canal with endosonics. Gutta-percha gets plasticized due to friction being generated. Final vertical compaction is done with hand or finger pluggers.

MTA (Mineral Trioxide Aggregate) placement: Low powered ultrasonics can be used to vibrate the material into position with no voids.

Endodontic retreatment
- *Intraradicular postremoval:* Ultrasonic help in removal of post by activating tip of ultrasonic instrument against metal post. The ultrasound energy transfers to the post and breaks down the luting cement resulting in loosening of the post
- *Gutta-percha removal:* Endosonics alone or with solvent helps in removing gutta-percha from canals
- *Silver point removal:* Krell introduced a conservative approach for removal of silver point. In this, a fine H-file is placed into the canal alongside the silver point. File is then activated by ultrasonic tip and slowly withdrawn. Ultrasonics with copious irrigation along with gentle up and down strokes is quite effective in removal of silver points, separated files, burs tips, etc.

Instrument Deformation and Breakage

An unfortunate thing about NiTi instruments is that their breakage can occur without any visible sign of unwinding or permanent deformation, that is, visual examination is not a reliable method for evaluation of any NiTi instrument.

There are two modes of rotary instrument separation, namely, torsional fracture and flexural fracture.

Torsional Fracture

Torsional fracture occurs when torque limit is exceeded. Term torque is used for forces which act in rotational manner. According to Marzouk, torque is ability of the handpiece to withstand lateral pressure on revolving tool without reducing its speed or cutting efficiency. Amount of torque is related to mass of the instrument, canal radius, and apical force when worked in the canal. As the instrument moves apically, the torque increases because of increased contact area between the file and canal wall.

Theoretically an instrument used with high torque is very active, but chances of deformation and separation increase with high torque. Thus, as the file advances further into the canal, pressure should be reduced to decrease torque.

Depending on the manufacturer and condition of the handpiece, each handpiece has different degree of effectiveness depending upon the torque values.

Role of Handpiece

Handpiece is a device for holding instruments, transmitting power to them and position them intraorally. Both speed and torque in a handpiece can be modified by incorporation of gear system. Various types of gear systems can be incorporated in handpiece but gearing is limited by the need to maintain the drive concentrically through handpiece and the head.

Torque control motors allow the setting of torque produced by the motor **(Fig. 13.67)**. In low torque control motors, torque values set on the motor are less than the value of torque at deformation and separation of the instruments. Whereas in high torque motors, torque value is higher as compared to torque at deformation and separation of the rotary instruments. During root canal preparation, all the instruments are subjected to different levels of torque. If torque level is equal or greater than torque at deformation, the instrument will deform or separate. Thus, with low torque control motors, motor will stop rotating and may even reverse the direction of rotation when instrument is subjected to torque level equal to torque value set at the motor. By this, instrument failure can be avoided. In high torque motors, instruments may deform or separate before the torque value of motor is achieved. So, we can say that torque control is an important factor to reduce NiTi fracture.

Flexural Fracture

When an instrument rotates in a curve, it gets compressed on the inner side of a curve and stretched on outer side of the curve. With every 180° of rotation, instrument flexes and stretches again and again resulting in the cyclic fatigue and subsequent fracture of the instrument.

In large size files because of more metal mass, more of tensile and compressive forces occur resulting in early fatigue of the instrument.

Elastic and fracture limit of NiTi rotary instruments are dependent on design, size and taper of the instrument. Thus to prevent instrument deformation and fracture, right torque value for each instrument should be calculated.

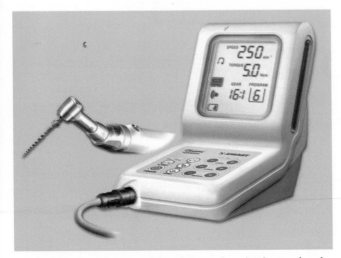

Fig. 13.67 Endomotor with handpiece where both speed and torque can be changed.

Sotokowa's classification of instrument damage (Fig. 13.68):
- Type I: Bent instrument
- Type II: Straightening of twisted flutes
- Type III: Peeling of metal at blade edges
- Type IV: Clockwise twist (partial)
- Type V: Cracking of instrument along its long axis
- Type VI: Full fracture of instrument

Prevention of Breakage of Instruments when using Nickel–Titanium Rotary Instruments

- Use only torque controlled electric handpiece for rotary instruments
- Proper glide path must be established before using rotary files, that is, getting the canal to at least size 15 before using them
- Use crown down method for canal preparation. By this apical curves can be negotiated safely
- Frequent cleaning of flutes should be done as it reduce the chances that debris will enter the microfractures and resulting in propagation of original fracture and finally the separation
- Do not force the file apically against resistance. File should be moved smoothly with 1–2 mm deep increments relative to the previous instrument
- Canals should be well lubricated and irrigated to reduce friction between instrument and dentinal walls
- Dentin mud collected in the canal increases the risk of fracture, it should be cleared off by frequent irrigation

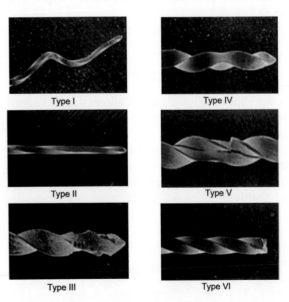

Fig. 13.68 Sotokawa's classification of instrument damage
Courtesy: Sotokawa T. : Intracanal Breakage of Root Cannal Instruments, The journal of japan endodomtic association, 1989;10:20–27.

- ❏ Discard a file if it is bent, stretched, or has a shiny spot
- ❏ Do not use rotary nickel–titanium files to true working length especially in teeth with S-shaped canals, canals with multiple and sharp curves and if there is difficult access of orifice because it can place stresses on the instrument which will cross the breaking torque value. In such cases, apical portion of canal should be prepared by hand files
- ❏ A file should be considered disposable when
  - It has been used in curved canals
  - Despite excellent glide path, it does not cut dentin properly

Two things can be done to reduce the risk of NiTi fracture:
1. Examine the file every time before placing it into the canal
2. Bend the file to at least 80° angle, every time before placing into the canal, to see if it will fracture

Instruments Used for Filling Root Canals

Spreaders and pluggers are used to compact the gutta-percha into root canal during obturation. In 1990, ISO/ADA Endodontic Standardization Committee recommended the size of 15–45 for spreaders and 15–140 for pluggers.

Hand Spreader (Fig. 13.69)

- ❏ It is made from stainless steel and is designed to facilitate the placement of accessory gutta-percha points around the master cone during lateral compaction technique
- ❏ Hand spreader does not have standardized size and shape
- ❏ It is not used routinely because excessive pressure may cause fracture of root.

Finger Spreader (Fig. 13.70)

- ❏ These are shorter in length which allows them to afford a great degree of tactile sense and allow them to rotate freely around their axis
- ❏ They are standardized and color coded to match the size of gutta-percha points
- ❏ They can be manufactured from stainless steel or nickel–titanium

- ❏ Stainless steel spreaders may pose difficulty in penetration in curved canals and may cause wedging and root fracture if forced during compaction. They also produce great stresses while compaction
- ❏ NiTi spreaders are recently introduced spreaders which can penetrate the curved canals and produce less stresses during compaction. But they may bend under pressure during compaction. So, we can say that combination of both types of spreaders, that is, stainless steel and NiTi, is recommended for compaction of gutta-percha, NiTi spreaders in apical area and stainless steel in coronal part of the root canal

Hand Plugger (Fig. 13.71)

- ❏ Hand plugger has diameter larger than spreader and have blunt end **(Fig. 13.70)**
- ❏ It is used to compact the warm gutta-percha vertically and laterally into the root canal
- ❏ It is also be used to carry small segments of gutta-percha into the canal during sectional filling technique
- ❏ Calcium hydroxide or MTA like materials may also be packed into the canals using hand plugger

Finger Pluggers (Fig. 13.72)

They are used for vertical compaction of gutta-percha. They apply controlled pressure while compaction and have more tactile sensitivity than hand plugger.

Care should be taken with spreaders and pluggers while compacting the gutta-percha in canals. They should be cleaned prior to their insertion in to the canal; otherwise, the set sealer from previous insertion may roughen their

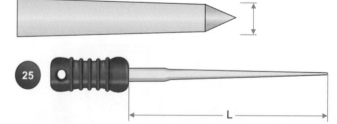

Fig. 13.70 Schematic representation showing finger spreader.

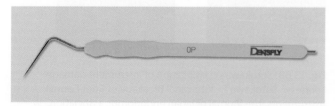

Fig. 13.69 Photograph showing hand spreader.

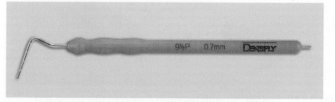

Fig. 13.71 Photograph showing hand plugger.

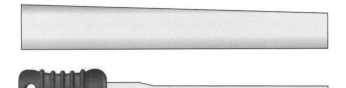

Fig. 13.72 Schematic representation showing finger plugger.

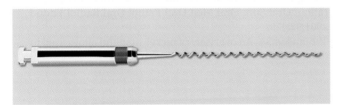

Fig. 13.73 Photograph showing Lentulo-spiral.

surface and may pull the cone outside the canal rather than packing it. Also, one should discard the instrument when it has become bent or screwed to avoid instrument separation while compaction.

Lentulo Spiral (Fig. 13.73)

❑ Lentulo spirals are used for applying sealer to the root canal walls before obturation
❑ Available in lengths of 17, 21 and 25 mm
❑ It has left-handed screw threading so that sealer flows down to the tip when rotated in low speed.

▌Conclusion

Since ages many areas offer many exciting research possibilities to further increase the performance of endodontic instruments by increasing flexibility, bending, torsional strength of files without compromising the cutting efficiency. In case of rotary NiTi instruments, use of right speed and torque are stressed for controlled instrumentation. One should not use rotary NiTi files overenthusiastically without complete understanding of physical and mechanical properties of NiTi instruments.

▌Questions

1. Classify endodontic instruments.
2. What are guidelines given for standardization of endodontic instruments?
3. Role of ultrasonics in endodontics.
4. Classify endodontic instruments. Describe the standardization of endodontic instruments.
5. Describe the standardization of endodontic instruments. What is endosonics? Add a note on NiTi instruments.
6. Compare reamers versus files. Add a note on their standardization.
7. Classify root canal instruments. Write on their standardization. Add a note on automated root canal instruments.
8. Classify and describe in details the instruments used for root canal preparation.
9. Enumerate instruments for root canal preparation. Describe in details on sonics and ultrasonics in endodontics.
10. Write short notes on
    • Broaches
    • Difference between files and reamers
    • K-files
    • H-files/Hedstroem files
    • ProTaper files
    • Profiles
    • Endosonics
    • NiTi instruments
    • Design of an endodontic instrument
    • Barbed broaches
    • ISO size No. 25 endodontic hand instrument
    • Physical characteristics of endodontic instruments
    • Broaches versus rasps
    • Classify endodontic instruments
    • Gates-Glidden drills
    • NiTi rotary instruments
    • Stainless steel versus NiTi–endo instruments
    • Standardization of endodontic instruments
    • Acoustic microstreaming and cavitation
    • Spreaders and pluggers
    • Peeso reamers and Gates-Glidden drills
    • Diagrammatically illustrate an endodontic instrument
    • Sotokowa's classification of instrument damage
    • Reamers
    • Rasps
    • Reciprocating handpieces.
    • Instruments for obturation
    • Instruments for radicular preparation.

▌Bibliography

1. Bergmans L, Van Cleynenbreugel J, Beullens M, Wevers M, Van Meerbeek B, Lambrechts P. Progressive versus constant tapered shaft design using NiTi rotary instruments. Int Endod J 2003;36:288-95.

2. Glickman GN, Koch KA, DMD. 21st Century Endodontics. Journal of the American Dental Association 2000;131:39–46.

3. Hargreaves KM, Cohen S. Pathways of the pulp, 10th edition St. Louis: Mosby Elsevier; 2011.

4. Hulsmann M, Schade M, Schafer's F. A comparative study of root canal preparation using Profile 0.04 and Light Speed NiTi instruments. Int Endod J 2001;34:538-46.

5. Lam TV, Lewis DJ, Atkins DR, et al. Changes in root canal morphology in simulated curved canals over-instrumented with a variety of stainless steel and nickel titanium files. Aust Dent J 1999;44:12–9.

6. McSpadden JT. Mastering endodontic instrumentation. Chattanooga, TN: Cloudland Institute; 2007.pp.51–2.

7. Patel S. Barnes J. The Principles of Endodontics. 2nd edition Oxford: Oxford University Press. 69–72.

8. Peter P, Gordon I, Messer HH. Factors influencing defects of rotary nickel-titanium endodontic instruments after clinical use. Journal of Endodontics 2004;30(10):722–5.

9. Plotino, G, Grande NM, Cordaro M, Testarelli L, Gambarini G. A review of cyclic fatigue testing of nickel-titanium rotary instruments. Journal of endodontics, 2009;35(11),1469–76.

10. Sotokawa T. Intracanal Breakage of Root Cannal Instruments, The Journal of Japan Endodomtic Association, 1989;10:20–7.

11. Spangberg L. The wonderful world of rotary root canal preparation. Oral Surg Oral Med Oral Pathol Oral Radiol Endod 2001;92:479.

12. Thompson SA. An overview of nickel-titanium alloys used in dentistry. Int Endod J 2000;33:297–310.

Internal Anatomy

Introduction

For the success of endodontic therapy, it is essential to have knowledge of normal configuration of pulp cavity. In addition to general morphology, variations in canal system must be kept in mind while performing the root canal therapy.

Pulp Cavity

Pulp cavity is the central cavity of a tooth containing dental pulp and consists of root canal and pulp chamber. It is enclosed by dentin all around, except at the apical foramen.

Pulp Chamber

- It occupies the coronal portion of pulp cavity and acquires the shape according to the external form of the crown of a tooth **(Figs. 14.1A and B)**
- Roof consists of dentin covering the pulp chamber occlusally or incisally
- Floor of pulp chamber merges into the root canal at orifices.

Pulp Horns

- Pulp horns are landmarks present occlusal to pulp chamber. These may vary in height and location. Occlusal

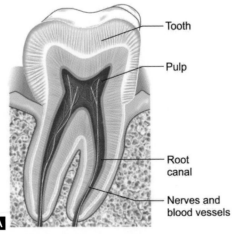

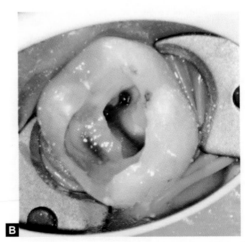

Tooth

Pulp

Root canal

Nerves and blood vessels

A

B

Figs. 14.1A and B (A) Line diagram showing pulp chamber and root canal in a tooth; (B) Access cavity of maxillary first molar showing roof and floor of chamber.

extent of pulp horn corresponds to the height of contour in young permanent teeth **(Fig. 14.2)**

- ❑ Pulp horn tends to be a single horn associated with each cusp of posterior teeth and mesial and distal in anterior teeth.

Canal Orifice

Canal orifices are openings in the floor of pulp chamber leading into root canals **(Fig. 14.3)**.

Root Canal

- ❑ Root canal extends from canal orifice to apical foramen
- ❑ In anterior teeth, the pulp chamber merges into the root canal **(Fig. 14.4)**, but in multirooted posterior teeth, this division becomes quite obvious **(Fig. 14.5)**
- ❑ Usually a root canal has curvature or constriction before terminating at the apex
- ❑ Curvature in root canal can be smooth or sharp, single or double in form of letter "S"

Apical Root Anatomy

Following anatomic and histological landmarks are seen in the apical part of root canal:

Apical Constriction (Minor Diameter) (Fig. 14.6)

- ❑ It is an apical part of root canal with the narrowest diameter short of apical foramina or radiographic apex
- ❑ Apical constriction is mostly located within the dentin or at CDJ and rarely in cementum. So, it may or may not coincide with CDJ

Apical Foramen (Major Diameter)

- ❑ It is the main apical opening on the surface of root canal through which blood vessels enter the canal

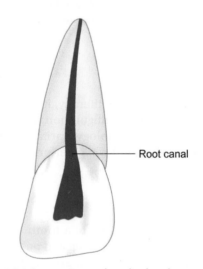

Fig. 14.4 In anterior teeth, pulp chamber merges into the root canal.

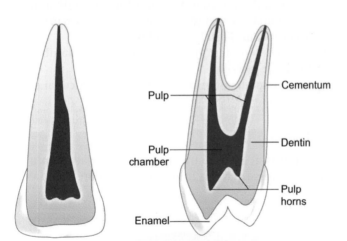

Fig. 14.2 Line diagram showing pulp horns of anterior and posterior teeth.

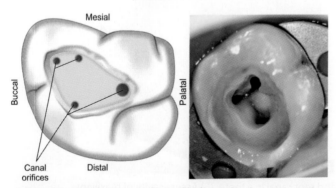

Fig. 14.3 Line diagram and mandibular molar showing canal orifices.

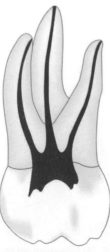

Fig. 14.5 In multirooted teeth, distinction between pulp chamber and root canal is remarkable.

❑ Its diameter is almost double the apical constriction giving it a funnel shape appearance, which has been described as ***morning glory or hyperbolic***

❑ Apical foramen may not always be located at center of the apex. It may exit mesial, distal, buccal, or lingual

---

POINTS TO REMEMBER

Average distance between minor and major diameter in young person is 0.5 mm and in older person, it is 0.67 mm.

Cementodentinal Junction

❑ Cementodentinal junction is the point in the canal, where cementum meets dentin

❑ Position of CDJ varies but usually it lies 0.5-1 mm from the apical foramen (**Fig. 14.7**)

❑ According to Kutler study, the average distance between minor and major diameter in young person is 0.5 mm and in older person, it is 0.67 mm.

Apical Delta

It is a triangular area of root surrounded by main canal, accessory canals and periradicular tissue (**Figs. 14.8 and 14.9**).

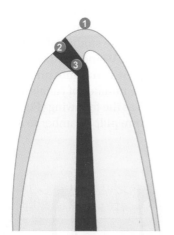

1. Tooth apex (radiographic apex)
2. Apical foramen (major foramen)
3. Apical constriction (minor foramen)

Fig. 14.6 Line diagram showing root apex

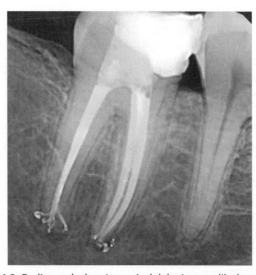

Fig. 14.8 Radiograph showing apical delta in mandibular second molar

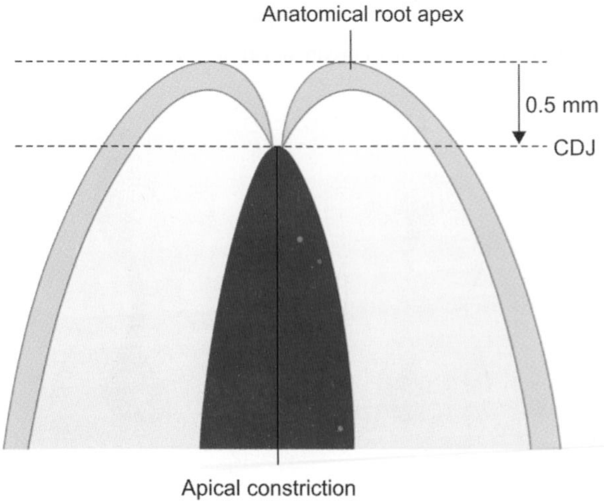

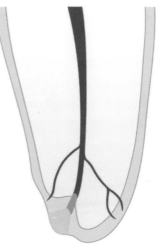

Fig. 14.9 Line diagram showing apical delta

Anatomical root apex

0.5 mm

CDJ

Apical constriction

Fig. 14.7 Position of CDJ usually lies 0.5-1 mm from apical foramen

Significance of Apical Third

❑ Apical constriction acts as a natural stop for filling materials. Root canal treatment of apical part is difficult because of presence of accessory and lateral canals, pulp stones, varying amounts of irregular secondary dentin and areas of resorption

❑ Most of the curvatures occur in apical third, so one has to be very careful during canal preparation

❑ Size and shape of foramen should always be maintained. Apical 3 mm of root is generally resected during endodontic surgery in order to eliminate canal aberrations

Isthmus

Isthmus is defined as narrow, ribbon-shaped communication between two root canals encompassing the pulp tissue. It can be seen in any two canals of the same root. It is a part of the root canal system and it is not a separate entity, so it should be cleaned, shaped and obturated as other root canals.

Identification

An isthmus can be identified by using methylene blue dye.

Classification

Hsu and Kin in 1997 classified isthmus (**Fig. 14.10**) as

Type I: Two or three canals with no visible communication (incomplete isthmus)

Type II: Two canals showing definite connection between them

Type III: Three canals showing definite connection between them

Type IV: It is similar to Type II or Type III with canals extending to isthmus area.

Type V: It is true connection throughout the section of root.

Clinical significance of isthmus
- Commonly isthmus is found between two canals present in one root like mesial root of mandibular molars
- Isthmus has shown to be main causative agent responsible for root canal failures. So, it is always mandatory to clean, shape and fill the isthmus area by orthograde or retrograde filling of root canals

▌Root Canal Classification

Various researches have been conducted to study normal and variations in anatomy of pulp cavity, but an exhaustive work on canal anatomy was done by *Hess*. He studied branching, anastomoses, intricate curvatures, shape, size and number of root canals in different teeth. Others who have contributed to the studies of pulp anatomy are Wheeler, Rankine-Wilson, Weine, Perth, etc.

Weine classified root canal morphology based on number of canal orifice, number of canals and number of foramina in each tooth as the following (**Fig. 14.11**):

Type I: Single canal from pulp chamber to apex.

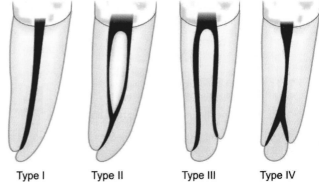

Type I   Type II   Type III   Type IV

Fig. 14.11 Weine's classification of root canals.

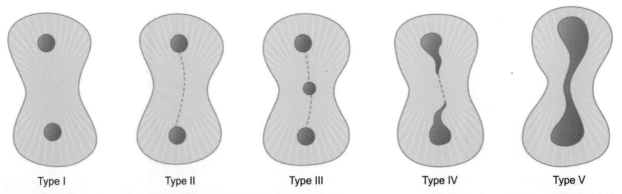

Type I   Type II   Type III   Type IV   Type V

Fig. 14.10 Hsu and Kin Classification of isthmus. Type I: Canals with no visible communication; incomplete isthmus; Type II: Two canals showing connection via a canal; Type III: Three canals showing connection between them; Type IV: Similar to Type II or III with canals extending to isthmus area; Type V: True connection throughout section of root.

Type II: Two separate canals leaving the chamber but exiting as one canal.

Type III: Two separate canals leaving the chamber and exiting as two separate foramina.

Type IV: One canal leaving the chamber but dividing into two separate canals and exiting in two separate foramina.

Vertucci gave eight different forms of pulp anatomy rather than four **(Fig. 14.12)**. It does not consider possible positions of auxilliary canals or exit position of apical foramen. Vertucci's classification:

Type I: A single canal extends from the pulp chamber to the apex (1).

Type II: Two separate canals leave the pulp chamber and join short of the apex to form one canal (2-1).

Type III: One canal leaves the pulp chamber and divides into two in the root; the two then merge to exit as one canal (1-2-1).

Type IV: Two separate, distinct canals extend from the pulp chamber to the apex (2).

Type V: One canal leaves the pulp chamber and divides short of the apex into two separate, distinct canals with separate apical foramina (1-2).

Type VI: Two separate canals leave the pulp chamber, merge in the body of the root and redivide short of the apex to exit as two distinct canals (2-1-2).

Type VII: One canal leaves the pulp chamber, divides and then rejoins in the body of the root and finally redivides into two distinct canals short of the apex (1-2-1-2).

Type VIII: Three separate, distinct canals extend from the pulp chamber to the apex (3).

Vertucci classification		
One canal at apex	Type I	1→1
	Type II	2→1
	Type III	1→2→1
Two canals at apex	Type IV	2→2
	Type V	1→2
	Type VI	2→1→2
	Type VII	1→2→1→2
Three canals at apex	Type VIII	3→3

Methods of Determining Pulp Anatomy

The following two methods are employed for determining pulp anatomy of teeth:
1. Clinical methods
   - Anatomic studies
   - Radiographs
   - Exploration
   - High-resolution computed tomography
   - Visualization endogram
   - Fiber-optic endoscope
   - MRI
2. In vitro methods
   - Sectioning of teeth
   - Use of dyes
   - Clearing of teeth
   - Contrasting media
   - Scanning electron microscopic analysis

Clinical Methods

Anatomic Studies

Knowledge of anatomy gained from various studies and textbooks is a commonly used method.

Radiographs

Good quality radiographs are useful in assessing the root canal anatomy **(Fig. 14.13)**. Since radiograph is a two-dimensional picture of a three-dimensional object, one has to analyze the radiograph carefully.

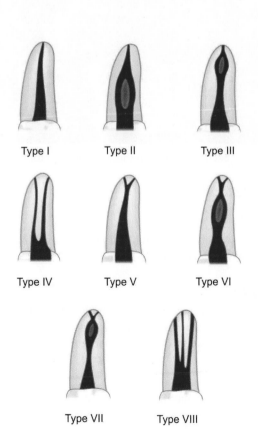

Type I   Type II   Type III

Type IV   Type V   Type VI

Type VII   Type VIII

Fig. 14.12 Vertucci's classification of root canals.

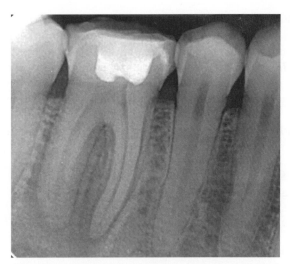

Fig. 14.13 Radiograph showing root canal anatomy of mandibular molar and premolars.

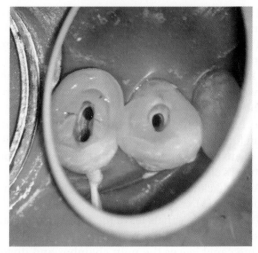

Fig. 14.14 Dentinal map of maxillary first premolar showing anatomic dark line connecting canal orifices.

High-Resolution Computed Tomography

It shows a three-dimensional picture of root canal system using computer image processing.

Fiber-Optic Endoscope

It is used to visualize canal anatomy.

Visualization Endogram

In this technique, an irrigant, called Ruddle's solution, is injected into canals to visualize them on radiograph. Ruddle's solution consists of

5% NaOCL + 17% EDTA + Hypaque = Ruddles solution

- *Sodium hypochlorite:* To dissolve organic tissues
- *17% EDTA:* To dissolve inorganic tissue
- *Hypaque:* It is an iodine containing radiopaque contrast media

Composition of Ruddle solution provides solvent action of sodium hypochlorite, visualization as it is radiopaque and improved penetration because EDTA lowers the surface tension.

MRI

It produces data on computer which helps in knowing canal morphology.

Exploration

On reaching pulpal floor, one finds the grooves and anatomic dark lines which connect the canal orifices called dentinal map. The map should be examined and explored using an endodontic explorer (**Fig. 14.14**).

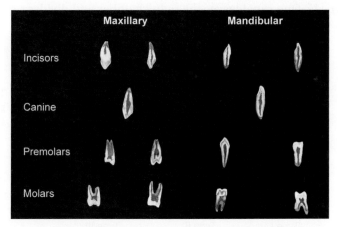

Fig. 14.15 Sectioning of teeth showing canal anatomy.

In Vitro Methods

Sectioning

In this, teeth are sectioned longitudinally for visualization of root canal system (**Fig. 14.15**).

Use of Dyes

Methylene blue or fluorescein sodium dyes help in locating pulp tissue preset in pulp chamber because dyes stain any vital tissue present in pulp chamber or root canals.

Clearing of Teeth

For clearing process, teeth are initially stored in 5% nitric acid for 5 days. Then these are rinsed, dried and dehydrated using increasing concentrations of ethanol (70%, 80% and 95%) successively for 1 day. Then teeth are rendered

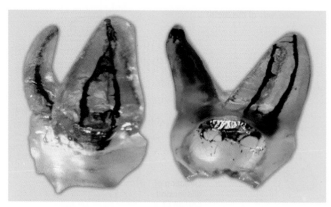

Fig. 14.16 Visualization of canal anatomy by making teeth transparent (clearing technique) and dye penetration.

transparent by immersing in methyl salicylate, into which dye is injected to visualize the anatomy **(Fig. 14.16)**.

Hypaque/Contrasting Media

It is an iodine containing media which is injected into root canal space and visualized on radiograph.

Scanning Electron Microscopic Analysis

Scanning electron microscopic (SEM) uses a focused beam of high energy electrons to generate a variety of signals at the surface of solid specimens. These signals reveal information about morphology, chemical composition and structure of that material. This is how SEM helps in evaluating root canal anatomy.

Variations in the Internal Anatomy of Teeth

Canal configuration can vary in some cases because of developmental anomalies, hereditary factors, trauma, etc. Usually the variations in root morphologies tend to be bilateral.

Variations of pulp space
1. Variations in development
   - Gemination
   - Fusion
   - Concrescence
   - Taurodontism
   - Talon's cusp
   - Dilacerations
   - Dentinogenesis imperfecta
   - Dentin dysplasia
   - Lingual groove
   - Extra root canal
   - Missing root
   - Dens evaginatus
   - Dens invaginatus

2. Variations in shape of pulp cavity
   - Gradual curve
   - Apical curve
   - C-shaped
   - Bayonet-shaped
   - Dilaceration
   - Sickle shaped
3. Variations in pulp cavity due to pathology
   - Pulp stones
   - Calcifications
   - Internal resorption
   - External resorption
4. Variations in apical third
   - Different locations of apex
   - Accessory and lateral canals
   - Open apex
5. Variations in size of tooth
   - Macrodontia
   - Microdontia

Variations in Development

Gemination

Gemination literally means twinning. It arises from an attempt at division of a single tooth germ by an invagination resulting in incomplete formation of two teeth **(Fig. 14.17A)**. It gives the appearance of completely or incompletely separated crowns having a single root canal.

Fusion

Fusion results in union of two normally separated tooth germ. Fused teeth may show separate or fused pulp space **(Fig. 14.17B)**.

Concrescence

In this, fusion occurs after the root formation has completed. Teeth are only joined by cementum.

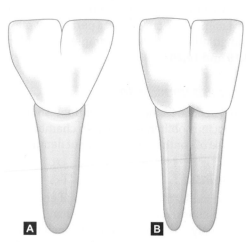

Figs. 14.17A and B Line diagram showing:
(A) Gemination; (B) Fusion.

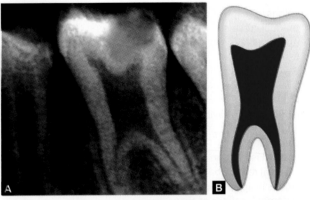

Figs. 14.18A and B Taurodontism showing large pulp chamber with greater apico-occlusal height in; (A) Radiograph of mandibular 1st molar; (B) Schematic representation.

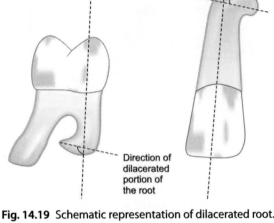

Fig. 14.19 Schematic representation of dilacerated root.

Taurodontism

In this, body of tooth is enlarged at the expense of roots (also called bull-like teeth). Pulp chamber of this tooth is extremely large with a greater apico-occlusal height **(Figs. 14.18A and B)**. Bifurcation/trifurcation may be present only few millimeters above the root apex. Pulp lacks the normal constriction at cervical level of tooth. This condition is commonly seen associated with syndromes like *Klinefelter syndrome* and *Down syndrome*.

Talon's Cusp

It resembles an eagle's talon. In this, an anomalous structure projects lingually from the cingulum area of maxillary or mandibular incisor. This structure blends smoothly with the tooth except that there is a deep developmental groove where that structure blends with the lingual surface of the tooth.

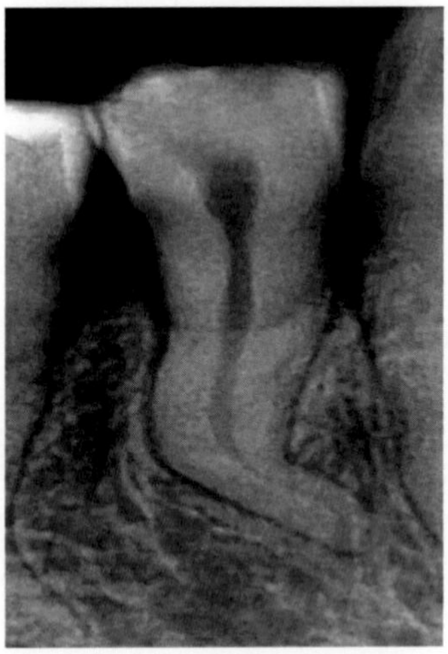

Dilaceration

Dilaceration is an extraordinary curvature in the roots. It can result from trauma during root development in which movement of the crown and a part of root may result in sharp angulation after tooth completes development **(Figs. 14.19 and 14.20)**.

Dentinogenesis Imperfecta

It results in defective formation of dentin. It shows partial or total precocious obliteration of pulp chamber and root canals because of continued formation of dentin.

Dentin Dysplasia

It is characterized by formation of normal enamel, atypical dentin and abnormal pulpal morphology. In this, root canals are usually obliterated so need special care while instrumentation.

Fig. 14.20 Radiograph showing dilacerated root of mandibular premolar.

Lingual Groove

It is a surface in the folding of dentin directed from the cervical portion toward apical direction. It is frequently seen in maxillary lateral incisors **(Fig. 14.21)**. Deep lingual groove is usually associated with deep narrow periodontal pocket which often communicates with pulp causing endodontic–periodontal relationship. Prognosis of such teeth is poor and treatment is difficult.

Presence of Extracanals

More than 90% of maxillary first molar show the occurrence of second mesiobuccal canal (MB2). Location of orifice can be made by visualizing a point at the intersection between a line running from mesiobuccal to palatal canal and a perpendicular line from the distobuccal canal **(Figs. 14.22A to F)**.

In mandibular molars, extracanals are found in 38% of the cases. A second distal canal is suspected when it does not lie in the midline of the tooth.

Two canals in mandibular incisors are reported in 41% of the cases, and among mandibular premolars, more than 11% of teeth show the presence of two canals.

Extra Root or the Missing Root

It is a rare condition which affects less than 2% of permanent teeth. *Radix entomolaris* was first described by Carabelli.

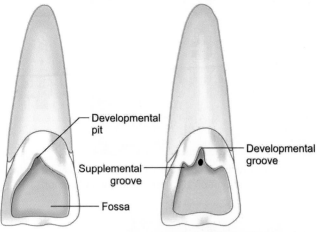

Fig. 14.21 Line diagram showing lingual groove

It is commonly seen in mandibular molars and is characterized by presence of an additional root, typically found distolingually (**Figs. 14.23 and 14.24**).

Dens in Dente or Dens Invaginatus

This condition represents an exaggeration of the lingual pit (**Fig. 14.25**). Most commonly seen in permanent maxillary lateral incisors, this condition may range from being superficial, that is, involving only the crown part to a pit in which both crown and root are involved. Tooth with dens invaginatus has a tendency of plaque accumulation which predisposes it to early decay and pulpitis.

Types of dens invaginatus (according to Oehlers) (Fig. 14.26):
Type I: Here, minor invagination occurs within crown and does not extend beyond CEJ.
Type II: Here invagination invades the roof as a blind sac and may or may not communicate with pulp.
Type III: Here invagination extends through the root and open in apical region without connection with pulp.

Dens Evaginatus

In this condition, an anomalous tubercle or cusp is located on the occlusal surface (**Fig. 14.27**). Because of occlusal

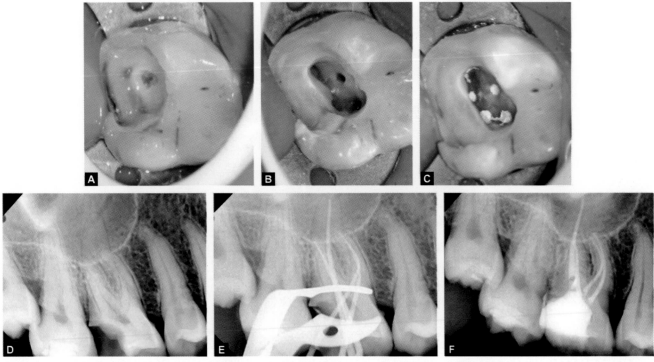

Figs. 14.22A to F Management of maxillary first molar with four canals; (A) Preoperative photograph; (B) Pulp chamber showing four canals viz; MB1, MB2, distal and palatal; (C) Post obturation photograph; (D) Preoperative radiograph showing deep caries in maxillary first molar with pulp involvement; (E) master cone radiograph; (F) Obturation radiograph

Courtsey: Punit Jindal

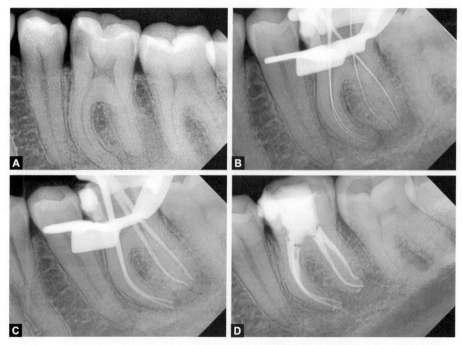

Figs. 14.23A to D Management of irreversible pulpitis in Mandibular 1st molar with Radix entomolaris; (A) Mandibular 1st molar with irreversible pulpitis; (B) Working length radiograph; (C) Master cone radiograph; (D) Post obturation radiograph.

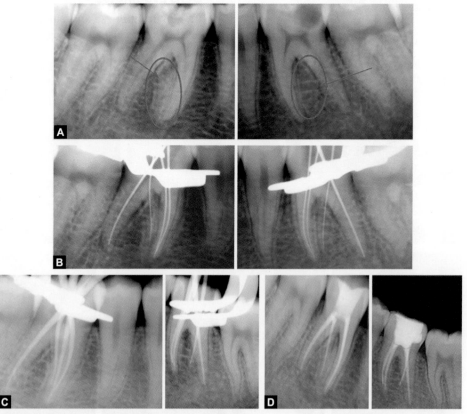

Figs. 14.24A to D Management of irreversible pulpitis in Mandibular Left   and right first molars (36 and 46) with radix entomolaris. (A) Preoperative radiograph 36 and 46; (B) Working length radiograph of 36 and 46; (C) Master cone radiograph of 36 and 46; (D) Post-obturation radiograph of 36 and 46.
Courtesy: Anil Dhingra.

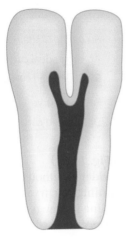

Fig. 14.25 Dens invaginatus.

abrasion, this tubercle wears off fast causing early exposure of accessory pulp horn that extends into the tubercle. This may further result in periradicular pathology in otherwise caries free teeth even before completion of the apical root development. This condition is commonly seen in premolar teeth.

Variation in Shape of Pulp Cavity

Curved Canals

Curvature in canal can be gradual (root canal gradually curves from orifice to the apical foramen) **(Fig. 14.28)** or apical (root canal is generally straight but at apex it shows a curve, commonly seen in maxillary lateral incisors and mesiobuccal root of maxillary molars) **(Fig. 14.29)**.

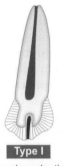 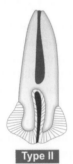 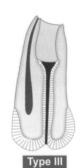

Type I	Type II	Type III
Minor invagination within crown not extending beyond CEJ	Invagination invades the root as a blind sac and may communicate with pulp	Invagination extends through root and opens in apical region without connection with pulp

Fig. 14.26 Types of dens invaginatus.

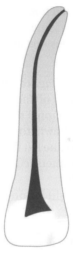

Fig. 14.28 Gradual curve in root canal.

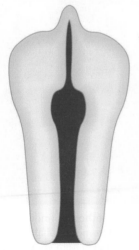

Fig. 14.27 Dens evaginatus.

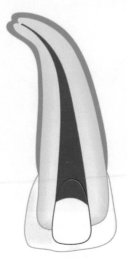

Fig. 14.29 Apical curve.

Classification of Curved Canals

According to anatomic location	Schneider's classification	According to shape of curvature
Apical third curvature	Straight (if angle <5)	Apical gradual curve
Middle third curvature	Moderately curve (if angle is 10–20)	Sickle-shaped curve
Coronal third curvature	Severely curved (if angle is >20)	Bayonet curve
		Dilacerated curve

Determination of Canal Curvature

Periapical radiographs
Though radiographs can be used to assess the root curvature, misinterpretation can occur because radiographs produce a two-dimensional image of a three-dimensional object. Curvatures present buccolingually may not be visible on radiographs.

Cone beam computed tomography (CBCT)
CBCT helps in assessing the true size, extent, nature and position of the lesions as compared to conventional radiography.

Schneider's method (Fig. 14.30)
In Schneider's method of finding root curvature, a straight line is drawn along coronal third of the canal and marked as A. Second line is drawn from apical foramen to intersect the point where first line left the long axis of the canal. The angle formed by the intersection of these lines is measured as Schneider's angle.

Schneider's classification on the basis of degree of curvature:
- Straight: 5° or less
- Moderate: 10–20°
- Severe: 25–70°

Weine's method (Fig. 14.31)
It is similar to Schneider's method but shows the differences in the angles according to curvature of the canal. In this method, a straight line is drawn from the canal orifices to the point of curvature and a second line is drawn from the apex for the apical curvature and the angle is measured at the point of intersection between the two lines.

C-shaped Canal (Fig. 14.32)
- These are called C-shaped due to their morphology as pulp chamber appears single ribbon-shaped with an arc of 180° or more. These are commonly seen in mandibular second molars and then in maxillary first molars and mandibular premolars, especially when the roots of these teeth appear very close or fused.
- Pulp chambers of teeth with C-shaped canals have greater apico-occlusal width with low bifurcation. This results in a deep pulp chamber floor
- Root canal system shows broad, fan-shaped communications from coronal to the apical third of the canal. Canal changes shape from coronal aspect of the root. For example, a continuous C-shaped canal would change to a semicolon configuration in the midroot and become continuous C-shape in the apical third of the root or vice versa

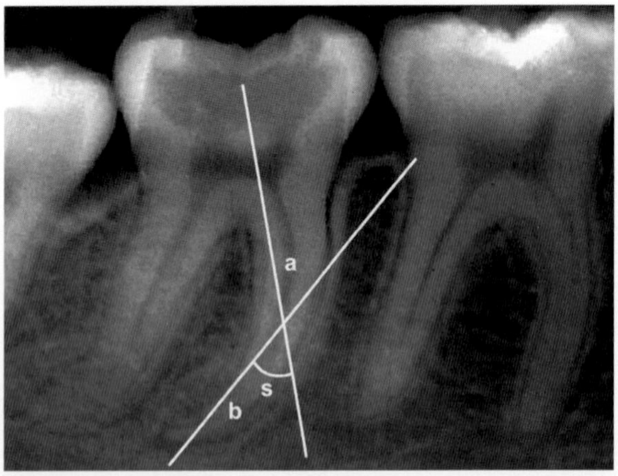

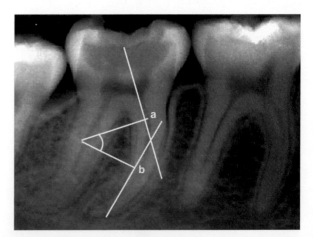

Fig. 14.30 Schneider's method of finding root curvature. Here, a straight line is drawn along coronal third of the canal: a, second line is drawn from apical foramen to intersect the point where first line left the long axis of the canal.

Fig. 14.31 Weine's method of finding canal curvature. Here, a straight line is drawn from the canal orifices to point of curvature and a second line is drawn from apex for apical curvature and the angle is measured at the point of intersection between the two lines.

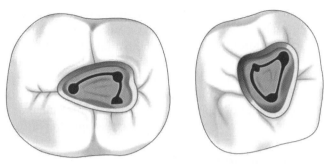

Fig. 14.32 Line diagram showing C shaped canals.

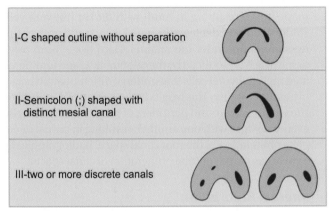

Fig. 14.33 Melton's classification of C shaped canals.

Classification

Melton's classification (Fig. 14.33)

It is based on cross-sectional shape.

- ❑ *Category I:* Continuous C-shaped canal running from the pulp chamber to the apex defines a C-shaped outline without any separation
- ❑ *Category II:* Semicolon shaped (;) in which dentin separates the main C-shaped canal from a mesial distinct canal
- ❑ *Category III:* Refers to two or more discrete and separate canals
  - • Subdivision I: C-shaped orifice in the coronal third that divides into two or more discrete and separate canals that join apically
  - • Subdivision II: C-shaped orifice in the coronal third that divides into two or more discrete and separate canals in the midroot to the apex
  - • Subdivision III: C-shaped orifice that divides into two or more discrete and separate canals in the coronal third to apex

Fan's classification (Anatomic classification) (Fig. 14.34)

Fan et al. in 2004 modified Melton's classification into the following categories:

- ❑ *Category I (C1):* The shape with an interrupted "C" with no separation or division
- ❑ *Category II (C2):* The canal shape resembles a semicolon resulting from a discontinuation of the "C" outline but either angle α or β should not be less than 60°
- ❑ *Category III (C3):* Two or three separate canals and both angles, α and β, were less than 60°
- ❑ *Category IV (C4):* Only one round or oval canal in that cross-section
- ❑ *Category V (C5):* No canal lumen can be observed (which is usually near the apex only)

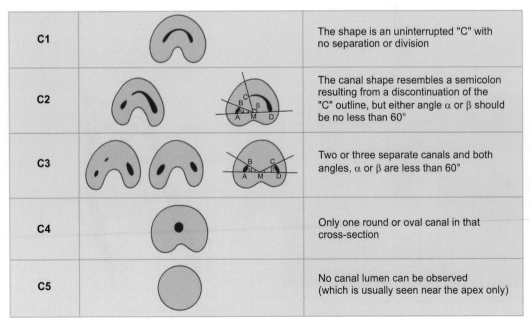

Fig. 14.34 Fan's classification.

Bayonet/S-shaped Canal

S-shaped or bayonet-shaped canals pose great problems while endodontic therapy, since they involve at least two curves, with the apical curves having maximum deviations in anatomy **(Figs. 14.35A and B)**. These double curved canals are usually identified radiographically if they cross in mesiodistal direction. If these traverse in a buccolingual direction, they are recognized using multiangled radiographs, or when the initial apical file is removed from the canal and simulates multiple curves. S-shaped canals are commonly found in maxillary lateral incisors, maxillary canines, maxillary premolars and mandibular molars.

Sickle-shaped Canals

In this, canal is sickle-shaped. It is commonly seen in mandibular molars. Cross-section of this canal is ribbon-shaped.

Variation in Pulp Cavity Due to Pathology

Pulp Stones and Calcifications

Pulp canal obliteration is pulpal response to trauma which is characterized by deposition of hard tissue within the root canal space **(Fig. 14.36)**.

It is characterized by an osteoid tissue that is produced by the odontoblasts at the periphery of pulp space or undifferentiated pulpal cells that undergo differentiation. This results in deposition of a dentin-like tissue along the periphery of the pulp space and within the pulp space, causing obliteration of pulp chamber and canal. Presence of pulp stones may alter the internal anatomy of the pulp cavity, making the access opening difficult.

Calcific Metamorphosis

Calcific metamorphosis is defined as a pulpal response to trauma that is characterized by deposition of hard tissue within the root canal space. Most common etiology is traumatic injury resulting in tooth with darker hue and yellow color because of decrease in translucency and greater thickness of dentin under the enamel. Hard tissue is an osteoid tissue which is produced by the odontoblasts and undifferentiated mesenchymal cells that undergo differentiation because of traumatic injury. This results in deposition of dentin-like tissue within and around periphery of pulp space. These tissues eventually fuse with one another, resulting in partial or complete obliteration of the root canal space. Radiographically, it appears as partial or total obliteration of canal space.

Internal Resorption

"Internal resorption is an unusual form of tooth resorption that begins centrally within the tooth, initiated in most cases by a peculiar inflammation of the pulp." It is characterized by an oval-shaped enlargement of root canal space **(Figs. 14.37 and 14.38)**. It is commonly seen in maxillary central incisors, but can affect any tooth in the arch.

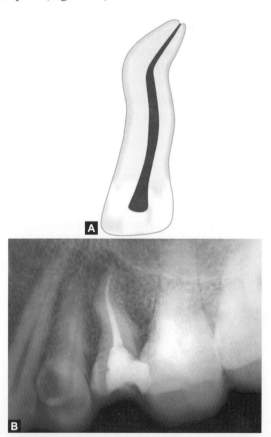

Figs. 14.35 A and B (A) Line diagram showing bayonet-shaped canal; (B) radiograph showing bayonet shaped maxillary second premolar.

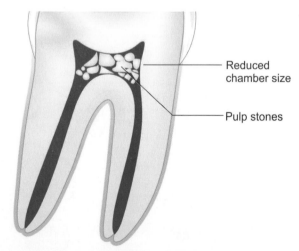

Reduced chamber size

Pulp stones

Fig. 14.36 Line diagram showing pulp stones in pulp chamber.

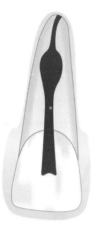

Fig. 14.37 Line diagram showing ballooning of pulp space in internal resorption.

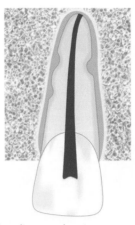

Fig. 14.39 Line diagram showing external resorption.

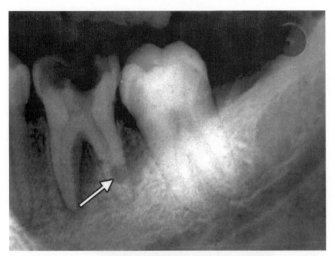

Fig. 14.38 Radiograph showing internal resorption in distal root of mandibular molar.

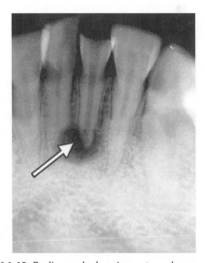

Fig. 14.40 Radiograph showing external resorption.

External Resorption

External root resorption is initiated in the periodontium and affects the external or lateral surface of the root **(Figs. 14.39 and 14.40)**.

Variation in Apical Third

Different Locations of Apical Foramen

Apical foramen may exit on mesial, distal, buccal or lingual surface of the root. It may also lie 2-3 mm away from the anatomic apex.

Accessory and Lateral Canals

These are lateral branches of the main canal that form a communication between the pulp and periodontium. They can be seen anywhere from furcation to apex but tend to be more common in apical third of posterior teeth.

Open Apex

It occurs when there is periapical pathology before completion of roof development or as a result of trauma or injury causing pulpal exposure. In this, canal is wider at apex than at cervical area. It is also referred to as blunderbuss canal **(Fig. 14.41)**. In vital teeth with open apex, treatment is apexogenesis, and in nonvital teeth, it is apexification.

Variation in Size of Root

Macrodontia

In this condition, pulp space and teeth are enlarged throughout the dentition. This condition is commonly seen in gigantism.

Microdontia

In this condition, pulp space and teeth appear smaller in size. It is commonly seen in cases of dwarfism.

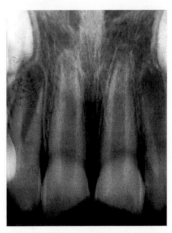

Fig. 14.41 Radiograph showing open apex of maxillary incisor tooth.

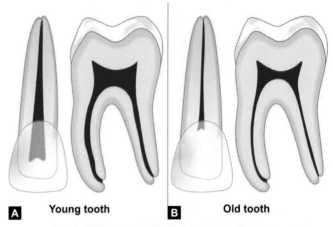

Figs. 14.42A and B (A) Root canal anatomy of young patient; (B) In older patient, pulp cavity decreases in size.

Factors Affecting Internal Anatomy

Though internal anatomy of teeth reflects the tooth form, yet various environmental factors whether physiological or pathological affect its shape and size because of pulpal and dentinal reaction to them. These factors can be enlisted as

Age

With advancing age, there is continued dentin formation causing regression in the shape and size of pulp cavity **(Figs. 14.42A and B)**. Clinically, it may pose problems in locating the pulp chamber and canals.

Irritants

Various irritants like caries, periodontal disease, attrition, abrasion, erosion, cavity preparation and other operative procedures may stimulate dentin formation at the base of tubules resulting in change in shape of pulp cavity.

Calcific Metamorphosis

It commonly occurs because of trauma to a recently erupted tooth **(Fig. 14.43)**.

Calcifications

Pulp stones or diffuse calcifications are usually present in chamber and the radicular pulp. These alter the internal anatomy of teeth and may make the process of canal location difficult.

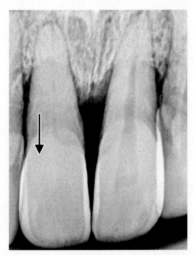

Fig. 14.43 Calcific metamorphosis of right maxillary central incisor showing radiopacity of pulp space.

Resorption

Chronic inflammation or internal resorption may result in change of shape of pulp cavity making the treatment of such teeth challenging.

Individual Tooth Anatomy

Maxillary Central Incisor (Fig. 14.44)

It has a single root with a single canal system. Canal form is usually Type 1.
- Average length: 22.5 mm
- Average crown length: 10.5 mm
- Average root length: 12 mm

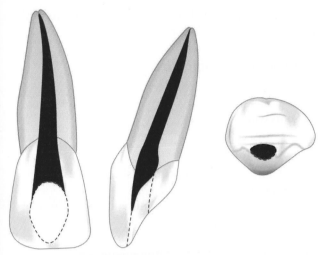

Fig. 14.44 Maxillary central incisor.

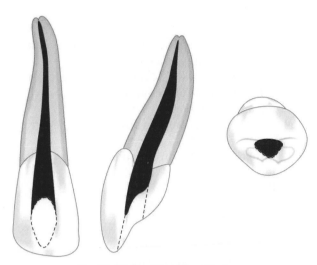

Fig. 14.45 Maxillary lateral incisor.

❑ Average pulp volume: 12.4 mm³

Pulp Chamber

❑ Located in the center of the crown and equidistant from the dentinal walls
❑ Mesiodistally broad with broadest part facing incisally
❑ In young patient, it shows three pulp horns correspond to enamel mamelons on the incisal edge

Root Canal

❑ Usually one root with one straight root canal
❑ Cross-section of canal
  • In cervical/coronal part: ovoid
  • Middle third: ovoid or round
  • Apical third: round

Commonly Found Anomalies

❑ Palatogingival groove
❑ Talon's cusp
❑ Fusion
❑ Gemination

Clinical Considerations

❑ Pulp horn can be exposed following a relatively small fracture of an incisal corner in the young patient
❑ Placing the access cavity too far palatally makes straight line access difficult
❑ Most canals are straight, but 15% -20% of roots show labial or palatal curve
❑ Labial perforation is most commonly seen during access cavity preparation

Maxillary Lateral Incisor (Fig. 14.45)

It has a single root with a single canal system. Canal form is usually Type 1.
❑ Average length: 21.5 mm
❑ Average crown length: 9 mm
❑ Average root length: 12.5 mm
❑ Average pulp volume: 11.4 mm³

Pulp Chamber

It is similar to central incisor except that
❑ Incisal outline is more rounded
❑ Two pulp horns are present

Root Canal

❑ Single root with smaller canal is seen when compared to central incisor
❑ Cross-section of canal
  • In cervical/coronal part: ovoid
  • Middle third: ovoid to round
  • Apical third: round
❑ Apical region of the canal is usually curved in a palatal direction

Commonly Found Anomalies

❑ Palatogingival groove
❑ Peg laterals
❑ Fusion
❑ Gemination
❑ Dens invaginatus

Clinical Considerations

❏ Cervical constriction is removed during coronal preparation to have a straight line access
❏ Palatal curvature of apical part can cause ledge formation, complicate surgical procedures like root end cavity preparation and root resection
❏ Lateral canals are more common than maxillary central incisors
❏ Labial perforation is common error during access cavity preparation

Maxillary Canine (Fig. 14.46)

It has a single root with a single canal system. Canal form is usually Type 1.
❏ Average length: 27 mm (*longest tooth*)
❏ Average crown length: 10 mm
❏ Average root length: 17 mm
❏ Average pulp volume: 14.7 mm³

Pulp Chamber

❏ Labiopalatally, pulp chamber is almost triangular in shape with apex pointed incisally
❏ Mesiodistallys it is narrow, resembling a flame
❏ One pulp horn corresponding to one cusp is seen

Root Canal

❏ A single root canal which is wider labiopalatally than mesiodistalky
❏ Cross-section of canal
  • In cervical/coronal part: ovoid
  • Middle third: ovoid
  • Apical third: round
❏ Cross-section at cervical and middle third show its oval shape, and at the apex it becomes circular

Commonly Found Anomalies

❏ Dens invaginatus
❏ Dilacerations
❏ Two roots with two canals

Clinical Considerations

❏ Cervical constriction needs to be shaped during uniformly tapered preparation
❏ Surgical access sometimes becomes difficult because of the long length of the tooth
❏ 32% canals may show distal apical curvature
❏ Abscess of maxillary canine perforates the labial cortical plate below insertion of levator muscles of the upper lip and drains into the buccal vestibule
❏ If perforation occurs above the insertion of levator muscles of lip, drainage of abscess occurs into the canine space, resulting in cellulitis

---

POINTS TO REMEMBER

• Because of the big size of canine root, there is bulge in the maxilla. It is called canine or alveolar eminence
• Root of canine is located between the nasal cavity and the maxillary sinus called canine pillar

---

Maxillary First Premolar (Fig. 14.47)

It has two roots with two canals. Canal form is usually Type 1.
❏ Average length: 21.5 mm
❏ Average crown length: 8.5 mm

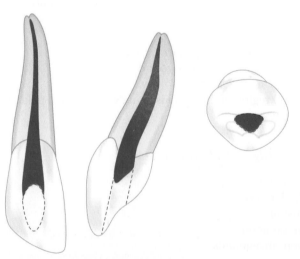

Fig. 14.46 Maxillary canine

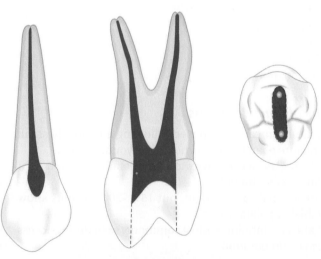

Fig. 14.47 Maxillary first premolar

- Average root length: 14 mm
- Average pulp volume: 18.2 mm³

Pulp Chamber

- It is wider buccopalatally with two pulp horns, corresponding to buccal and palatal cusps
- Palatal canal is usually larger than buccal canal
- Roof of pulp chamber is coronal to the cervical line
- Floor is convex with two canal orifices

Root Canal

- Two roots with two canals are seen commonly. In case of fused roots, a groove running in occlusoapical direction divides the roots into buccal and palatal portion each containing single canal
- Buccal canal is directly under the buccal cusp and palatal canal is directly under the palatal cusp
- Cross-section of canal:
  - In cervical/coronal part: ovoid
  - Middle third: round
  - Apical third: round

Commonly Found Anomalies

- Dens evaginatus
- Dilacerations

Clinical Considerations

- Good quality radiograph with different angulations is taken to avoid superimposition of canals
- Avoid overflaring of the coronal part of buccal root to avoid the perforation of mesial groove present on it
- Failure to observe distoaxial inclination of tooth may lead to perforation
- Palatal canal is usually larger than buccal canal

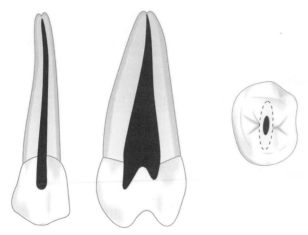

Fig. 14.48 Maxillary second premolar

Maxillary Second Premolar (Fig. 14.48)

It has a single root with single canal system. Canal form is usually of Type 1 and Type 2.
- Average length: 21.5 mm
- Average crown length: 8.5 mm
- Average root length: 13 mm
- Average pulp volume: 16.5 mm³

Pulp Chamber

- One root with a single canal is most commonly seen
- Pulp chamber is wider buccopalatally and narrower mesiodistally
- Cross-section shows a narrow and ovoid shape

Root Canal

- In more than 60% of cases, a single root with a single canal is found
- If two canals are present, they may be separated along the entire length of the root or merge to form a single canal as they approach apically
- Cross-section of canal:
  - In cervical/coronal part: ovoid
  - Middle third: round
  - Apical third: round

Commonly Found Anomalies

- Dens invaginatus
- Taurodontism
- Two roots with two or three canals

Clinical Considerations

- Narrow ribbon-like canal is difficult to clean and obturate
- If one canal is present, orifice is indistinct, but if two canals are present, two orifices are seen

Maxillary First Molar (Fig. 14.49)

It has three roots with three to four canals.
- Average length: 21.3 mm
- Average crown length: 7.5 mm
- Average root length: 14 mm
- Average pulp volume: 68.2 mm³

Pulp Chamber

- *Largest pulp chamber*
- Four pulp horns, namely, mesiobuccal, mesiopalatal, distobuccal and distopalatal
- Bulk of pulp chamber lies mesial to the oblique ridge

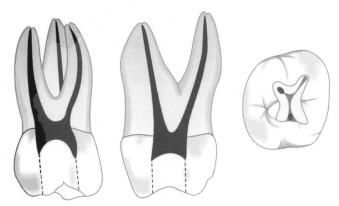

Fig. 14.49 Maxillary first molar

- Pulp horns are arranged to give rhomboidal shape in the cross-section
- Roof converges and lingual wall disappears, forming triangular form
- Orifices of root canals are located in the three angles of the floor; palatal orifice is the largest and easiest to locate and appears funnel-like in the floor of pulp chamber
- Distobuccal canal orifice is located more palatally than mesiobuccal canal orifice
- More than 80% of teeth show presence of two canals in mesiobuccal root. MB_2 is located 3 mm palatally and 2 mm mesially to the MB_1 orifice

Root Canal

- Three roots with three or four canals
- Two canals in mesiobuccal root are closely interconnected and sometimes merge into one canal
- Mesiobuccal canal is the narrowest of the three canals, flattened in mesiodistal direction at cervix but becomes round as it reaches apically. Distal curvature is seen in more than 78% of the canals
- Distobuccal canal is narrow, tapering canal, sometimes flattened in mesiodistal direction but generally it is round in cross-section
- Palatal root canal has the largest diameter which has a rounded triangular cross-section coronally and becomes round apically
- Palatal canal can curve buccally in the apical one third
- Lateral canals are found in 40% of the molars at apical third and at trifurcation area

Anomalies present
- Two palatal canals
- Two palatal roots
- Two distal canals
- Taurodontism

Clinical Considerations (Figs. 14.50A to D)

- Buccal curvature of palatal canal (56% of cases) may not be visible on radiographs, leading to procedural errors
- MB_2 should be approached from distopalatal angle since the initial canal curvature is mesial
- Sometimes isthmus is present between mesiobuccal canals, and should be cleaned properly for successful treatment
- Fundus of the alveolar socket of maxillary first molar may protrude into the maxillary sinus, producing a small, bony prominence in the floor of sinus
- Because of close proximity to sinus, pulpal inflammation can result in sinusitis.
- Since pulp chamber lies mesial to oblique ridge, pulp cavity is made mesial to oblique ridge
- Perforation of palatal root is commonly caused by assuming canal to be straight

Maxillary Second Molar (Fig. 14.51)

It has three roots with three to four canals almost similar to first molar.
- Average length: 17.5 mm
- Average crown length: 7 mm
- Average root length: 12.5 mm
- Average pulp volume: 44.3 mm^3

Pulp Chamber

- Similar to first molar except that it is narrower mesiodistally
- Roof is more rhomboidal in cross-section and floor is an obtuse triangle
- Mesiobuccal and distobuccal canal orifices lie very close to each other, sometimes all the three canal orifices lie in a straight line

Root Canal

Similar to first molar except that roots tend to be less divergent and may be fused.

Anomalies present
- Two palatal canals and two palatal roots
- Fusion of roots
- Taurodontism

Clinical Considerations

- Similar to maxillary first molar
- Maxillary second molar lies closer to the maxillary sinus than first molar

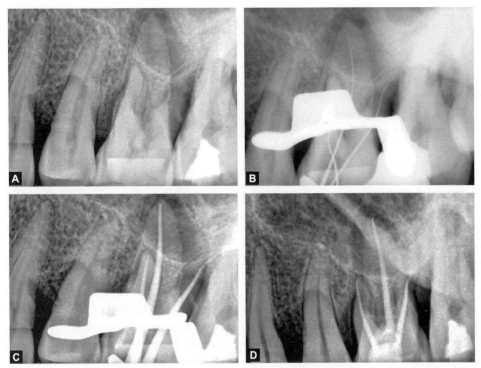

Figs. 14.50A to D Management of irreversible pulpitis in maxillary first molars: (A) Preoperative radiograph; (B). Working length radiograph; (C) Master cone radiograph; (D) Post- obturation radiograph.
Courtesy: Jaydev.

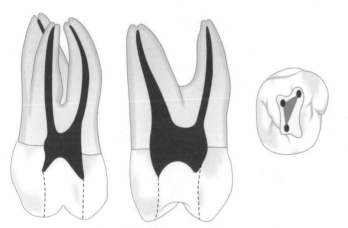

Fig. 14.51 Maxillary second molar.

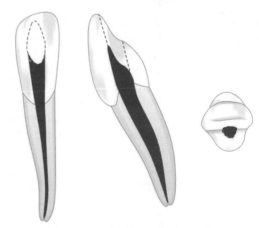

Fig. 14.52 Mandibular central incisor.

Maxillary Third Molar

- ❑ Average length: 16.5 mm
- ❑ Average crown length: 6.5 mm
- ❑ Average root length: 12 mm
- ❑ Average pulp volume: 40.3 mm³

Pulp Chamber and Root Canal

It is similar to second molar but displays great variations in shape, size and form of pulp chamber with presence of one, two, three or more canals at times.

Clinical Considerations

Maxillary third molar is closely related to maxillary sinus and maxillary tuberosity.

Mandibular Central Incisor (Fig. 14.52)

It is the smallest tooth in the arch. It has a single root with Type 1 canal configuration most prevalent, Type 2 and 3 less common.

- ❑ Average length: 21 mm
- ❑ Average crown length: 9 mm

- Average root length: 12 mm
- Average pulp volume: 6.1 mm^3

Pulp Chamber

- It is wider labiolingually than mesiodistally
- Cross-section shows an ovoid shape

Root Canal

There can be
- Single canal with one foramen in 65% cases
- Two canals with one foramen in 28% cases and two canals with separate foramen in 7% cases

Cross-Section of Canal

- In cervical/coronal part: ovoid
- Middle third: ovoid
- Apical third: round

Since canal is flat and narrow mesiodistally and wide buccopalatally, ribbon-shaped configuration is formed.

Commonly Found Anomalies

- Dens invaginatus
- Germination
- Fusion

Clinical Considerations

- Because of groove along the length of root and narrow canals, weakening of the tooth structure or chances of strip perforations are increased
- It is common to miss presence of two canals on preoperative radiograph if they are superimposed
- Second canal is usually found lingual to the main canal
- Since apex of mandibular central incisor is inclined lingually, the surgical access may become difficult to achieve

Mandibular Lateral Incisor (Fig. 14.53)

- Average length: 22.5 mm
- Average crown length: 9.5 mm
- Average root length: 13.0 mm
- Average pulp volume: 7.1 mm^3

Pulp Chamber

It is similar to central incisor except that it has larger dimensions.

Root Canal

- Similar to central incisor
- Root is straight or distally curved

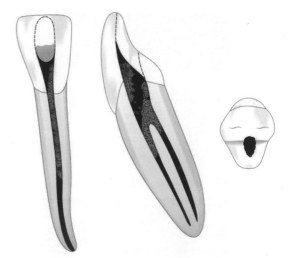

Fig. 14.53 Mandibular lateral incisor.

Cross-Section of Canal

- In cervical/coronal part: ovoid
- Middle third: ovoid
- Apical third: round

Clinical Considerations

These are similar to central incisor.

Mandibular Canine (Fig. 14.54)

It has single root with single canal system. Canal form is usually Type 1 and rarely has two roots but may display Type 4 configuration.
- Average length: 25.5 mm

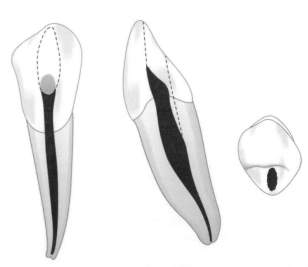

Fig. 14.54 Mandibular canine.

- Average crown length: 11 mm
- Average root length: 16 mm
- Average pulp volume: 14.2 mm^3

Pulp Chamber

- Ovoid in cross-section broader labiolingually and narrower mesiodistally
- One pulp horn present

Root Canal

- It has one root and one canal in 94% cases but two roots with separate foramen are present in 6% cases

Cross-Section of Canal

- In cervical/coronal part: ovoid
- Middle third: ovoid
- Apical third: round

Commonly Found Anomalies

- Dilaceration
- Dens invaginatus
- Two roots with two canals
- Two canals in single root

Mandibular First Premolar (Fig. 14.55)

It has single root with single canal but occasionally division of root is present in apical third.
- Average length: 21.5 mm
- Average crown length: 8.5 mm
- Average root length: 13.5 mm
- Average pulp volume: 14.9 mm^3

Pulp Chamber

- Buccolingually, wider and ovoid in cross-section
- Mesiodistally narrow
- Two pulp horns present, buccal horn being more prominent

Root Canal

- One root and one canal is commonly seen (70%), one canal and two foramina are seen in 24% cases
- Lateral canals are present in 44% cases

Cross-Section of Canal

- In cervical/coronal part: ovoid
- Middle third: round
- Apical third: round

Commonly Found Anomalies

- Dens evaginatus
- Dens invaginatus
- Two roots with two canals
- Single root splits into two, of which buccal is straight and lingual splits at right angle, giving letter "h" appearance **(Fig. 14.56)**.

Clinical Considerations

- Surgical access to the apex of the mandibular first premolar is often complicated due to proximity of the mental nerve
- Due to close proximity of root apex to mental foramen, one may mimic its radiographic appearance to periapical pathology

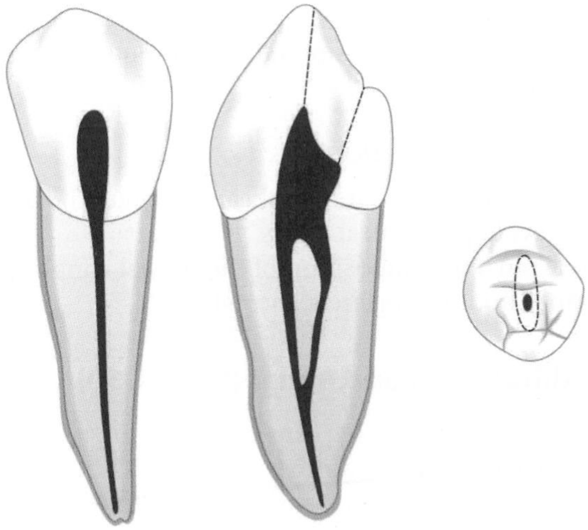

Fig. 14.55 Mandibular first premolar.

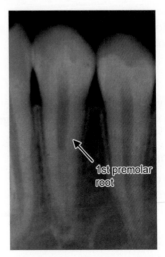

Fig. 14.56 In mandibular 1st premolar, single root splits into two, giving letter "h" appearance.

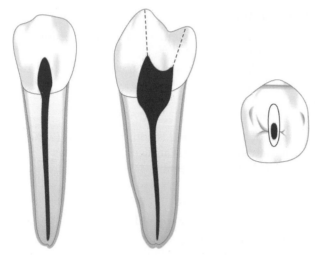

Fig. 14.57 Mandibular second premolar

- Lingual canal when present, is difficult to instrument. Access can usually be gained by running a fine instrument down the lingual wall of the main buccal canal until the orifice is located
- Perforation at distogingival margin is caused by failure to recognize the distal tilt of premolar

Mandibular Second Premolar (Fig. 14.57)

- Average length: 22.5 mm
- Average crown length: 8 mm
- Average root length: 14.5 mm
- Average pulp volume: 14.9 mm³

Pulp Chamber

- It is similar to first premolar except that lingual pulp horn is more prominent
- Cross-section shows an oval shape with greater dimensions buccolingually

Root Canal

- Usually only one root and one canal is seen, but in 11% of the cases, a second canal can be seen **(Figs. 14.58A to D)**

Cross-Section of Canal

- In cervical/coronal part: ovoid
- Middle third: less ovoid
- Apical third: round

Clinical Consideration

They are similar to mandibular first premolar.

Mandibular First Molar (Fig. 14.59)

It has two roots with three to four canals.
- Average length: 21.5 mm
- Average crown length: 7.5 mm
- Average root length: 14 mm
- Average pulp volume: 52.4 mm³

Pulp Chamber

- It is quadrilateral in cross-section at the level of the pulp floor being wider mesially than distally
- Roof is rectangular in shape with straight mesial and rounded distal wall. Walls converge to form rhomboidal floor
- Four or five pulp horns are present
- Mesiobuccal orifice is present under the mesiobuccal cusp
- Mesiolingual orifice is located in a depression formed by the mesial and lingual walls
- Distal orifice is the widest of all three canals. It is oval in shape with greater diameter in buccolingual direction

Root Canal

- Two roots with three canals are present, but three roots and four or five canals are also seen
- Mesial root has two canals, namely, mesiobuccal and mesiolingual which may exit in two foramina (>41% cases), single foramen (30%) and in different pattern
- Mesiobuccal canal is usually curved and often exit in pulp chamber in a mesial direction
- Distal root has one canal in >70% cases, but two canals are also seen in some cases
- Single distal canal is ribbon shaped and has larger diameter buccolingually. But when two canals are present in distal root, they tend to be round in the cross-section

Anomalies present
- Taurodontism
- Radix entomolaris—supernumerary roots
- C shaped canals

Clinical Considerations

- Over enlargement of mesial canals should be avoided to prevent procedural errors
- To avoid superimposition of the mesial canals, radiograph should be taken at an angle

Mandibular Second Molar (Fig. 14.60)

It has two roots with three canals.
- Average length: 21.5 mm
- Average crown length: 7 mm
- Average root length: 13.5 mm
- Average pulp volume: 32.9 mm³

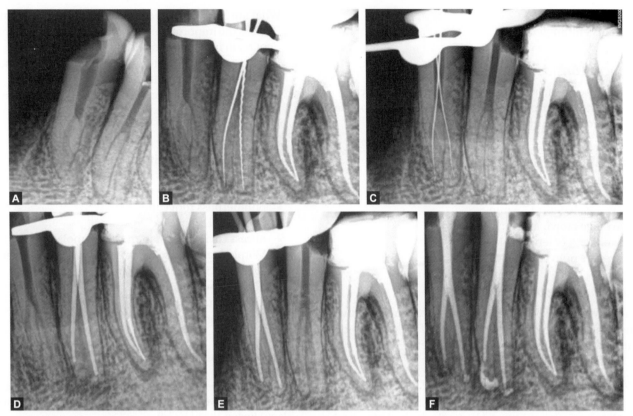

Figs. 14.58A to F Management of mandibular 1st and 2nd premolars with bifurcation of canals: (A) Preoperative radiograph; (B) working length radiograph of first premolar; (C) working length radiograph of second premolar; (D) Master cone radiograph of first premolar; (E) Master cone radiograph of second premolar; (F) Post obturation radiograph.

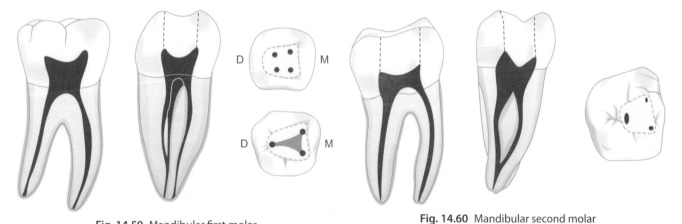

Fig. 14.59 Mandibular first molar   **Fig. 14.60** Mandibular second molar

Pulp Chamber

❑ It is similar to the first molar but smaller in size
❑ Root canal orifices are smaller and lie closer

Root Canal

❑ Two roots with two or three canals seen. If two canals are seen, both orifices are in mesiodistal midline

❑ If two orifices are not in mesiodistal midline, one should search for another canal on opposite side

Anomalies present

❑ C-shaped canals, that is, mesial and distal canals become fused into a fin
❑ Taurodontism
❑ Fused roots

❑ Single canal
❑ Radix entomolaris

Clinical Considerations

❑ C-shaped canals should be treated with proper care
❑ Perforation can occur at mesiocervical region if one fails to recognize the mesially tipped molar

Mandibular Third Molar

Average Tooth Length

❑ Average length: 17.5 mm
❑ Average crown length: 6 mm
❑ Average root length: 11.5 mm
❑ Average pulp volume: 44.4 mm^3

Pulp Chamber and Root Canals

Pulp cavity resembles the first and second molar but with enormous variations, that is, presence of one, two, or three canals and "C-shaped" root canal orifices

Clinical Considerations

❑ Root apex is closely related to the mandibular canal
❑ Alveolar socket may project onto the lingual plate of the mandible

▌Conclusion

For successful and predictable endodontics, apart from correct diagnosis and treatment planning, the clinician must have knowledge of internal anatomy of the tooth. The populations around the world have some peculiarities which must be taken care of. Anatomical variations can occur in any tooth. This necessitates the use of more precise technology to complete evaluation and treatment planning. The frequencies of root, root canals and apical foramina should be taken care of for individual teeth because outcomes of non-surgical and surgical endodontic procedures are influenced by highly variable anatomic structures. Therefore clinicians should be aware of complex root canal structures, dimensions and alterations of canal anatomy

▌Questions

1. Define root canal anatomy. Classify root canal configuration.
2. What are the different factors affecting root anatomy?
3. Discuss the importance of internal anatomy of permanent teeth in relation to endodontic treatment.
4. Discuss root canal anatomy and its corelation for success in endodontic treatment.
5. Discuss structure of root apex and its significance in endodontics.
6. Write short notes on:
   - Root canal anatomy of maxillary first molar
   - Principles of preparing access cavity
   - Root canal apex
   - Root canal anatomy of central incisor
   - Blunderbuss root canal
   - Root canal types
   - Access cavity design in maxillary molar teeth
   - Morphology and access cavity design in anterior teeth
   - Access cavity design in mandibular molar teeth
   - Accessory canals
   - Apical delta
   - Clinical significance of the apical third.

▌Bibliography

1. Bellizi R, Hartwell G. Radiographic evaluation of root canal anatomy of in vivo endodontically treated maxillary premolars. J Endod 1985;11:37–9.
2. Fan B, Yang J, Gutmann JL, Fan M, "Root canal systems in mandibular first premolars with C-shaped root configurations. Part I: microcomputed tomography mapping of the radicular groove and associated root canal cross-sections," Journal of Endodontics, 2008;34(11)1337–41.
3. Melton DC, Krall KV, Fuller MW. Anatomical and histological features of C-shaped canals in mandibular second molars. J Endod 1991; 17: 384–8.
4. Skidmore AE, Bjorndal AM. Root canal morphology of the human mandibular first molar. Oral Surg 1971;32:778–84.
5. Stropko JJ. Canal morphology of maxillary molars: clinical observations of canal configurations. J Endod 1999; 25: 446–50.
6. Tikku AP, Pandey PW, Shukla I. Intricate internal anatomy of teeth and its clinical significance in endodontics: A review. Endodontology 2012;24:160–9.
7. Vertucci FJ, Seeling A, Gillis R. Root canal morphology of the human maxillary second premolar. Oral Surg 1974;38: 456–64.
8. Vertucci FJ, "Root canal morphology and its relationship to endodontic procedures," Endodontic Topics, 2005;10:3–29.
9. Vertucci FJ. Root canal morphology of mandibular premolars. J Am Dent Assoc 1978; 97: 47–50.
10. Weine F. Endodontic therapy. 3rd edition St Louis: CV Mosby; 1982.pp.256–340.

Access Cavity Preparation

Introduction

Endodontic treatment starts with an ideal access cavity preparation and further steps of root canal treatment are based on accuracy and correctness of the access cavity preparation which decide straight line access to the apical foramen. This preliminary step permits the localization, cleaning, shaping, disinfection and three-dimensional obturation of the root canal system. Knowledge of pulp chamber morphology, examination of preoperative radiograph should be put together when going to prepare access cavity. An improperly prepared access cavity in terms of position, extent or depth affects the final outcome of endodontic treatment.

Definition

Access cavity preparation is defined as an endodontic coronal preparation which enables unobstructed access to the canal orifices, a straight line access to apical foramen, complete control over instrumentation and accommodates obturation technique.

An ideal coronal access forms the foundation of pyramid of endodontic treatment **(Fig. 15.1)**. It allows straight entry into canal orifices with line angles forming a funnel which drops smoothly into the canals **(Fig. 15.2)**. Removal of coronal interferences on instruments reduces the adverse unidirectional forces directed on

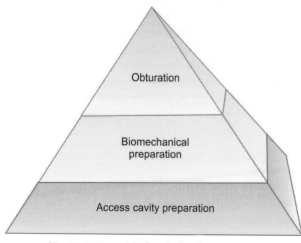

Fig. 15.1 Pyramid of endodontic treatment.

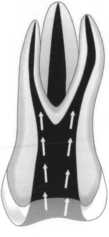

Fig. 15.2 Smooth, straight line access to root canal system.

the instruments which may result in instrumental errors like ledging and perforation **(Figs. 15.3A and B)**. An improperly prepared access cavity can impair the instrumentation, disinfection and obturation, therefore affecting prognosis of the endodontic treatment.

Before going for access cavity preparation, a study of preoperative periapical radiograph is necessary because it helps in knowing
- Morphology of the tooth **(Fig. 15.4)**
- Anatomy of root canal system
- Number of canals
- Curvature and branching of the canal system
- Length of the canal

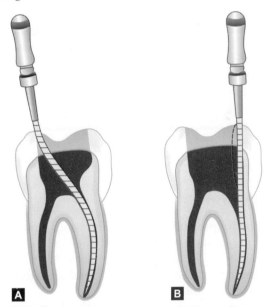

Figs. 15.3A and B (A) Not removing dentin from mesial wall causes bending of instrument while inserting in canal leading to instrumental errors; (B) Removal of dentin interference from access opening gives straight line access to the canal without any undue bending.

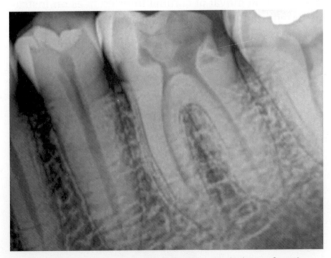

Fig. 15.4 Radiograph helps to know morphology of teeth.

- Position and size of the pulp chamber and its distance from occlusal surface
- Position of apical foramen
- Calcification, resorption present if any

Objectives of access cavity preparation
- *Direct straight line access to the apical foramen.* It helps in
  - Improved instrument control because of minimal instrument deflection and ease of instrumentation in the canal
  - Improved obturation
  - Decreased incidence of iatrogenic errors
- *Complete deroofing of pulp chamber.* It helps in
  - Complete debridement of pulp chamber
  - Improved visibility
  - Locating canal orifices
  - Permitting straight line access
  - Preventing discoloration of teeth because of remaining pulpal tissue
- *Conserve sound tooth structure as much as possible* so as to avoid weakening of the remaining tooth structure. Presence of walls allows
  - Proper application of rubber dam
  - Stable reference point
  - Flooding of chamber with irrigant
  - Support for temporary restoration
- *Provide a positive support for temporary filling* so as to avoid any contamination of the cavity. Walls of cavity should be flared in a shallow funnel shape with the occlusal surface wider than floor

---

Instruments for Access Cavity Preparation

To achieve access cavity preparation, every dentist should have following set of instruments.

Endodontic Explorer

DG 16: DG 16 was designed by Dr. David Green in 1951. It is designed because a straight explorer and cowhorn explorer did not help in locating canal orifices specially in case of posterior teeth. But, the design of DG 16 helps to identify canal orifices and to determine canal angulation **(Fig. 15.5)**.

CK (Clark-Khademi) 17: It is used to identify calcified canals because of being thinner and stiffer in nature.

Endodontic spoon excavator: It is double ended excavator with long shank so as to reach deep into the prepared cavities **(Fig. 15.6)**. It is used to excavate base of the pulp chamber.

Access Opening Burs

Diamond Round Burs

Nos. 2 and 4 round diamond burs are used to gain entry into tooth structure and restorative materials **(Figs. 15.7A and B)**.

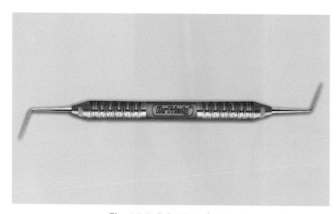

Fig. 15.5 DG 16 explorer.
Courtesy: HuFriedy.

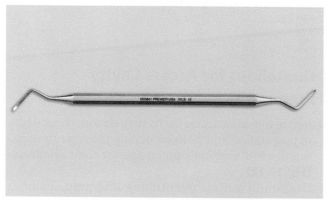

Fig. 15.6 Endodontic spoon excavator.

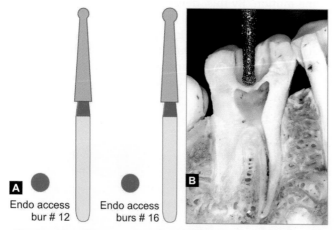

A — Endo access bur # 12
— Endo access burs # 16
B

Figs. 15.7A and B Round bur is used to gain entry into the tooth structure.

No. 2 size burs are used for anterior and premolars, whereas No. 4 is used for molars.

Carbide Round Burs

Nos. 2 and 4 surgical length round burs are used to reach pulp. These have longer shanks, so provide better visibility.

No. 2 size burs are used for anterior and premolars, whereas No. 4 is used for molars. These burs are used to gain entry through dentin, restorative materials, etc. **(Fig. 15.8)**.

Transmetal Bur

This is used for cutting any type of metal. It has saw tooth blade configuration which provides efficiency without vibrations **(Fig. 15.9)**. This bur is especially helpful for entering in hot tooth.

Endo Z Bur

It is safe-ended tapered carbide bur **(Figs. 15.10A and B)**. Lateral cutting edges of Endo Z bur are used to flare, flatten and refine the internal axial walls. Its noncutting tip can be safely placed on the pulpal floor without the risk of perforation.

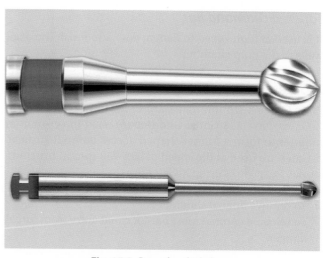

Fig. 15.8 Round carbide burs.

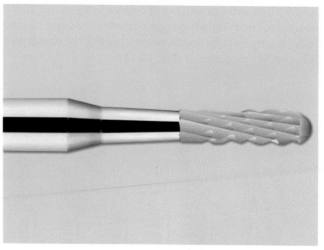

Fig. 15.9 Transmetal bur.

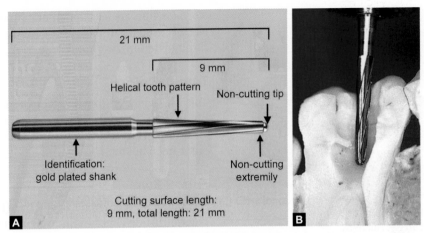

Figs. 15.10A and B (A) Endo Z bur is a long tapered, safe ended with noncutting tip tungsten carbide bur; (B) Working with Endo Z bur.

Tapered Diamond Bur

It is used at high speed to flatten, flare and finish the axial walls of the pulp chamber.

X-Gates

Four Gates-Glidden drills are combined to form one X-Gates. Nos. 1–4 Gates-Glidden are used in sequential manner to form a funnel-shaped access coronal surface. X-Gates are used at the speed of 500–750 rpm in brushing stroke. Purpose of using X-Gates is
- To flare and blend canal orifices
- To remove lingual shoulder
- To relocate coronal most part of canal away from furcal danger

Ultrasonic Instruments

Ultrasonic tips of various length, diameters and tapers are used with or without water port delivery. In general, these are used to create trough along the grooves to expose hidden orifices, remove pulp stones, negotiate calcified canals and finish access preparation **(Fig. 15.11)**.

Guidelines for Access Cavity Preparation

- Before initiating access cavity preparation, check depth of preparation and position of pulp chamber by aligning the bur and handpiece against the radiograph **(Fig. 15.12)**
- Use round bur for penetrating into pulp chamber **(Fig. 15.13)**. Once "drop in" into the pulp chamber is obtained, round bur is moved inside to outside in brushing motion. By this, dentinal overhangs are removed. **(Fig. 15.14)**
- After this, finishing and flaring of the preparation is done using nonend cutting bur. It creates smooth transition between access cavity and walls of pulp chamber and flaring of pulp chamber occlusally

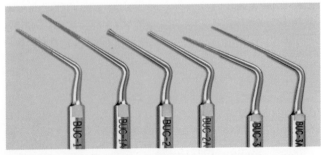

Fig. 15.11 Ultrasonic tips used in access cavity preparation.

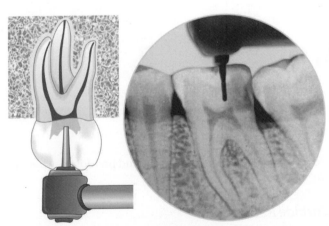

Fig. 15.12 Preoperative radiograph can help to note the position and depth of pulp chamber.

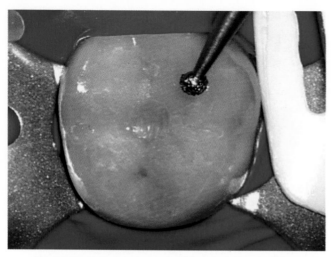

Fig. 15.13 Gain entry to pulp chamber with round bur.

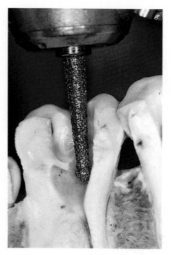

Fig. 15.15 Removal of chamber roof.

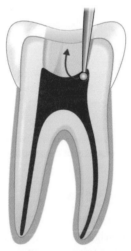

Fig. 15.14 Once "drop in" into pulp chamber is obtained, bur is moved inside to outside.

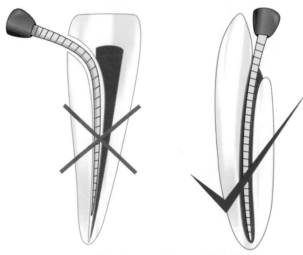

Fig. 15.16 An adequate access cavity preparation should permit straight line access to apical foramen.

- Diamond burs are preferred over tungsten carbide burs because they cut more smoothly, produce lesser vibrations and are well tolerated by patients. Complete removal of chamber roof facilitates the removal of pulp tissue, calcifications, caries or any residuals of previous restorations **(Fig. 15.15)**
- Walls of pulp chamber are flared and tapered to form a gentle funnel shape with larger diameter toward occlusal surface. Shape of access cavity differs from that used in restorative dentistry. For restorations, focus is on pits, fissures, sulci, fossae and one must avoid underlying pulp. For access cavity, one must uncover the pulp by removing the roof of pulp chamber
- Access cavity is prepared through the occlusal or lingual surface never through proximal or gingival surface. Improper access cavity results in inadequate canal instrumentation, iatrogenic errors and poor prognosis **(Fig. 15.16)**

Shape of access cavity is determined by
- *Size of pulp chamber:* In young patients, access preparation is wider than older ones
- *Shape of pulp chamber:* Final outline form should reflect the shape of pulp chamber. It is triangular in anteriors, ovoid buccolingually in premolars and trapezoidal or triangular in molars
- *Number, position and curvature of the canal:* It can lead to modified access preparation, like shamrock preparation in maxillary molar

Laws of Access Cavity Preparation for Locating Canal Orifices

- **Law of centrality:** Floor of pulp chamber is almost always located in the center of tooth at the level of cementoenamel junction **(Fig. 15.17)**
- **Law of cementoenamel junction(CEJ):** Distance from external surface of clinical crown to the wall of pulp

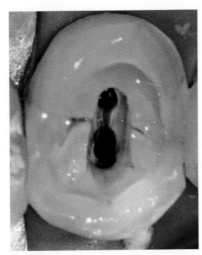

Fig. 15.17 *Law of centrality:* Floor of pulp chamber is located in center of tooth at level of cementoenamel junction.

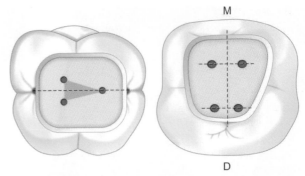

Fig. 15.19 *Law of symmetry:* Canal orifices are equidistant from a line drawn in mesiodistal direction through the floor of pulp chamber.

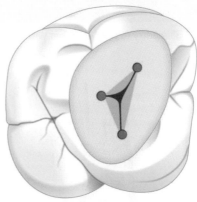

Fig. 15.20 Canal orifices are located at the junction of floor and walls and at terminus of root development fusion lines.

chamber is same throughout the tooth circumference at the level of CEJ **(Fig. 15.18)**

❑ **Law of concentricity:** Walls of pulp chamber are always concentric to external surface of the tooth at level of CEJ. This indicates anatomy of external tooth surface reflects the anatomy of pulp chamber

❑ **Law of color change:** Color of floor of pulp chamber is darker than the cavity walls

❑ **Law of symmetry:** Except for the maxillary molars, canal orifices are equidistant from a line drawn in mesiodistal direction through the floor of pulp chamber **(Fig. 15.19)**

❑ **Law of orifice location:** Canal orifices are located at the junction of floor and walls and at the terminus of root development fusion lines **(Fig. 15.20)**

Tests For Locating Canals

In case of vital pulp: Droplet of blood at orifice or a red line within a groove that originates from orifices **(Fig. 15.21)**.

If pulp is nonvital: A white line that can be seen as one trough along a groove.

Access Cavity of Anterior Teeth (Fig. 15.22)

i. Remove all the caries and any defective restorations so as to prevent contamination of pulp space and have a straight line access into the canals.

ii. Access opening is initiated at occlusal to the cingulum by using round bur almost perpendicular to palatal surface **(Figs. 15.22A and B)**. Due to its constant position, cingulum is choice of landmark because other areas like gingival margin can retract and incisal margin can abrade, causing loss of landmark.

iii. Once enamel is penetrated, bur is directed 45° to the long axis of the tooth, until "a drop in" is felt **(Fig. 15.22 C)**.

iv. Now chamber roof is removed by moving round bur from inside to outside. Locate the canal orifices using sharp endodontic explorer **(Fig. 15.22 D)**.

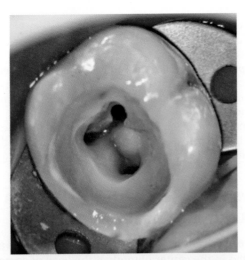

Fig. 15.18 Law of CEJ; Distance from external surface of clinical crown to the wall of pulp chamber is same throughout the tooth circumference at the level of CEJ.

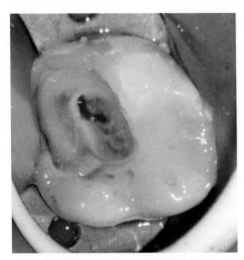

Fig. 15.21 In case of vital pulp, drop of blood at orifice indicates pulp.

v. Once the canal orifices are located, remove the lingual shoulder using Gates-Glidden drills or safe tipped diamond or carbide burs **(Fig. 15.22E)**. Lingual shoulder is a prominence of dentin formed by removal of lingual roof which extends from the cingulum to approximately 2 mm apical to the orifice. During removal of the lingual shoulder, orifice should also be flared so that it becomes confluent with all the walls of access cavity

preparation. By this a straight line access to the apical foramen is achieved **(Fig. 15.22 F)**. Since the outline form of access cavity reflects the internal anatomy of the pulp space, technique of the access opening of anterior teeth is the same, the shape may vary according to internal anatomy of each tooth.

Maxillary Central Incisor

❑ Outline form of access cavity of maxillary central incisor is a rounded triangular shape with base facing the incisal aspect **(Fig. 15.22 F)**
❑ Width of base depends upon the distance between mesial and distal pulp horns
❑ Shape may change from triangular to slightly oval in mature tooth because of less prominence of mesial and distal pulp horns

Maxillary Lateral Incisor

Shape of access cavity is almost similar to that of maxillary central incisor except that **(Fig. 15.22G)**
❑ It is smaller in size
❑ When pulp horns are present, shape of access cavity is rounded triangle
❑ If pulp horns are missing, shape is oval

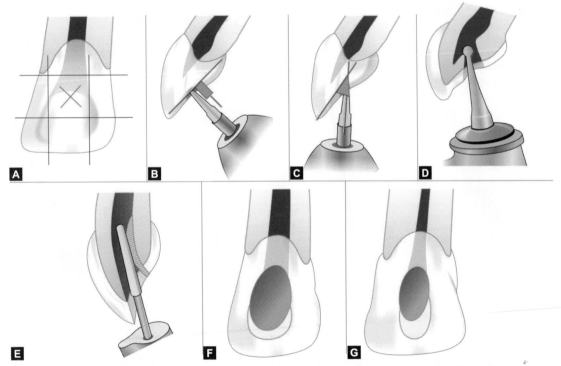

Figs. 15.22 A to G Schematic representation of access cavity preparation for maxillary anterior teeth: (A) Initial point for entry of bur is middle of middle third of palatal surface; (B) keep round bur perpendicular to the long axis of the tooth; (C) Bur is directed 45° to the long axis of the tooth to penetrate the pulp chamber; (D) removal of chamber roof; (F) final access cavity shape of maxillary central incisor; (G) Access cavity shape of maxillary lateral incisor.

□ Frequently, distal or palatal curvature of apical third of root is found. This explains the reason for often found lesion of endodontic origin on palatal surface of lateral incisor

Maxillary Canine

Shape of access cavity of canine is oval with greater dimensions labiopalatally.

Mandibular Incisors

Access cavity of mandibular central and lateral incisors is almost similar in steps and shape **(Figs. 15.23A to E)**. It is different from maxillary incisors in the following aspects:
□ Smaller in shape
□ Shape is long oval with greater dimensions directed incisogingivally

Mandibular Canine

Shape of access opening of mandibular canine is similar to maxillary canine except that
□ It is smaller in size
□ Root canal outline is narrower in mesiodistal dimension
□ Two canals are often present in mandibular canine
Commonly seen errors during access cavity preparation of anterior teeth are shown in **Figures 15.24A to D**:

Access Cavity Preparation for Premolars (Figs. 15.25A to F)

□ In premolars, pulp chamber is located in the center of occlusal surface between buccal and lingual cusp tips. Two pulp horns are located within the peaks of their cusps and orifices are located within the horns

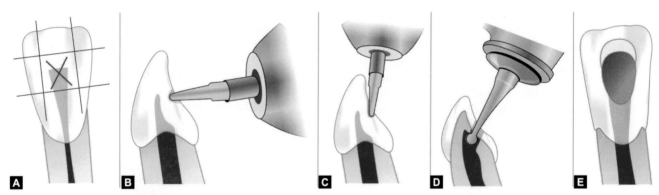

Fig. 15.23A to E Schematic representation of access cavity preparation for mandibular anterior teeth (A) Initial point of entry for bur; (B) bur is directed perpendicular to long axis of the tooth; (C) direct the bur at 45° to long axis of the tooth; (D) Deroofing of the pulp chamber; (E) oval-shaped access cavity of mandibular incisor.

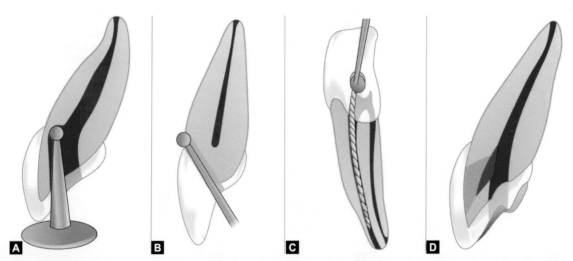

Figs. 15.24A to D Errors during access cavity preparation of anterior teeth: (A) Gouging due to not recognizing the 29° linguoaxial inclination of the tooth; (B) Perforation due to improper angulation of the bur; (C) Missed canal due to underextension of cavity; (D) Discoloration due to failure to remove pulp debris

(Fig. 15.25A). So, access cavity can be prepared without involving the cusps

❏ Penetrate the enamel with No. 4 round bur directed parallel to long axis of tooth. The bur is moved in buccolingual direction to widen the orifice **(Fig. 15.25 B)**

❏ Once the "drop in" is felt, locate the canal orifices with the help of sharp endodontic explorer **(Fig. 15.25 C)**

❏ Remove the roof of pulp chamber using a round, tapered fissure or nonend cutting bur alongside the walls of pulp chamber working from inside to outside **(Fig. 15.25 D)**

❏ Remove any remaining cervical bulges or obstructions using safety tip burs or Gates-Glidden drills and obtain a straight line access to canals

❏ Final preparation has larger dimensions buccolingually. Two canals are often joined by a shallow groove located at floor of pulp chamber **(Fig. 15.25E)**

Clinical Tips

- Extension of orifices to the axial walls results in "mouse hole effect" **(Figs. 15.26 A and B)**
- It is caused by under extension of access cavity
- Mouse hole effect results in hindrance to straight line access which may cause procedural errors

---

Maxillary First Premolar

Shape of access cavity is ovoid where boundaries should not exceed beyond half the lingual incline of buccal cusp and half the buccal incline of lingual cusp **(Fig. 15.27)**.

Maxillary Second Premolar

It is similar to that of maxillary first premolar. Weine stated that second premolar has single root with ovoid canal in

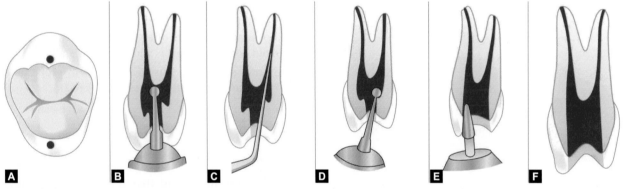

Figs. 15.25A to F Schematic representation of access cavity preparation for premolars: (A) Pulp chamber is located in center of occlusal surface and pulp horns are located within the peaks of their cusps. (B) Penetrate the enamel using round bur and move it in buccolingual direction; (C) locate the canal orifice using endodntic explorer; (D) Move the bur inside to outside for removing roof of the pulp chamber; (E) Removal of coronal bulges for straight line access; (F) Final preparation with coronal flare and larger dimensions buccolingually.

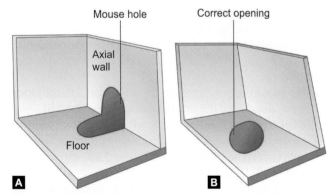

Figs. 15.26A and B Mouse hole effect: (A) Mouse hole effect—due to under extension of axial wall, orifice opening appears partly in axial wall and partly in floor; (B) Correct opening.

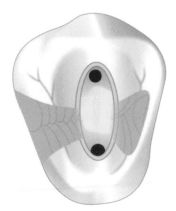

Fig. 15.27 Occlusal view of access cavity preparation of maxillary premolar.

60% of the cases. Finding of single, eccentric canal orifice indicates presence of another canal **(Fig. 15.28)**.

Mandibular First Premolar

Access cavity of mandibular first premolar differs from maxillary premolar in following aspects:

- There is *presence of 30° lingual inclination* of the crown to the root; hence the starting point of bur penetration should be halfway up the lingual incline of the buccal cusp on a line connecting the cusp tips **(Fig. 15.29)**
- Shape of access cavity is *oval which is wider mesiodistally,* when compared to its maxillary counterpart **(Fig. 15.30)**

Mandibular Second Premolar

The access cavity preparation is similar to mandibular first premolar except that in mandibular second premolar

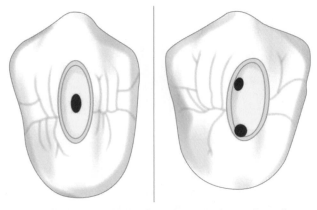

Fig. 15.28 Occlusal view of access cavity shape of maxillary second premolar with one and two canals.

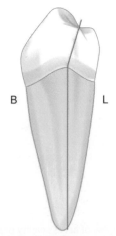

Fig. 15.29 Due to lingual inclination of mandibular premolar, initial entry point of bur should be halfway up the lingual incline of the buccal cusp on a line connecting the cusp tip.

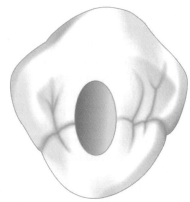

Fig. 15.30 Occlusal view of access cavity preparation of mandibular premolar.

- Enamel penetration is initiated in the central groove because its crown has smaller lingual tilt
- Because of better developed lingual half, the lingual boundary of access opening extends halfway up to the lingual cusp incline, making pulp chamber wider buccolingually
- Root canals are more often oval than round
- Ovoid access opening is wider mesiodistally

Commonly seen errors during access cavity preparation of premolars are shown in **Figures 15.31A to D.**

Access Cavity Preparation for Maxillary Molars (Figs. 15.32A to G)

- Determine shape and size of the access opening by measuring boundaries of pulp chamber mesially and distally
- Mesial boundary is a line joining the mesiobuccal and mesiolingual cusps and the distal boundary is the oblique ridge. The starting point of bur penetration is on the central groove midway between mesial and distal boundaries **(Fig. 15.32 A)**
- Penetrate the enamel with No. 4 round bur in the central groove directed palatally and prepare an external outline form
- Penetrate the bur deep into the dentin until the clinician feels "drop" into the pulp chamber **(Fig. 15.32 B)**
- Explore the canal orifices with sharp endodontic explorer. All the canal orifices should be positioned entirely on the pulp floor and should not extend to the axial walls **(Fig. 15.32 C)**
- Now remove the complete roof of pulp chamber using tapered fissure, round bur, safety tip diamond or the carbide bur working from inside to outside **(Fig. 15.32 D)** The shape and size of the internal anatomy of pulp chamber guides the cutting

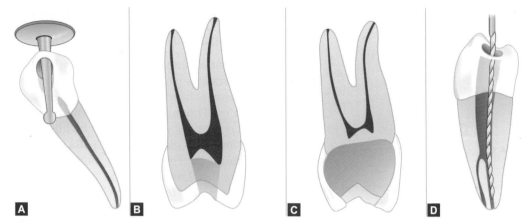

Fig. 15.31A to D Errors in cavity preparation of premolars: (A) Perforation caused by ignoring lingual tilt of premolar; (B) Under extended preparation; (C) Over extended preparation; (D) Failure to locate extra canal.

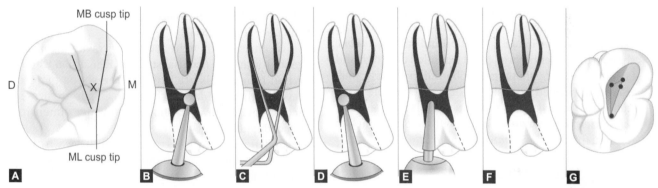

Figs. 15.32A to G Schematic representation of access cavity preparation for maxillary molars: (A) Mesial boundary is a line joining the mesial cusps and distal boundary is the oblique ridge. Initial point of bur penetration is on the central groove midway between mesial and distal boundaries; (B) Penetrate the enamel with No. 4 round bur in the central groove directed palatally until "drop" into the pulp chamber is felt; (C) Explore the canal orifices with sharp endodontic explorer; (D) De-roof the pulp chamber moving bur from inside to outside; (E) Remove any cervical bulges or obstructions if present; (F) Final access cavity shows confluent walls of pulp chamber and occlusal surface; (G) Occlusal view showing rhomboid shaped pulp chamber with acute mesiobuccal angle, obtuse distobuccal angle and palatal right angle.

❑ Now remove any cervical bulges, ledges or obstruction if present **(Fig. 15.32E)**
❑ Smoothen and finish the access cavity walls so as to make them confluent within the walls of pulp chamber and slightly divergent toward the occlusal surface **(Fig. 15.32 F)**

Maxillary First Molar

❑ Shape of pulp chamber is rhomboid with acute mesiobuccal angle, obtuse distobuccal angle and palatal right angles **(Fig. 15.32 G)**
❑ Palatal canal orifice is located palatally. Mesiobuccal canal orifice is located under the mesiobuccal cusp. Distobuccal canal orifice is located slightly distal and palatal to the mesiobuccal orifice **(Fig. 15.33)**
❑ A line drawn to connect all three orifices (i.e., MB, DB and palatal) forms a triangle, termed as **_molar triangle_** **(Figs. 15.34A to C)**

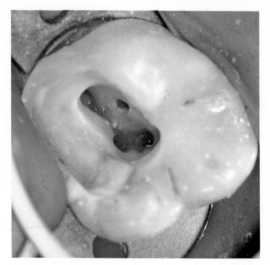

Fig. 15.33 Access cavity of maxillary first molar showing MB1, MB2, distal and palatal canals.

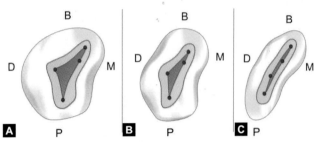

Figs. 15.34A to C Different patterns of molar triangle.

- Almost always a second mesiobuccal canal, that is, MB2 is present in first maxillary molars, which is located palatal and mesial to the MB1. Though its position can vary, sometimes it can lie a line between MB1 and palatal orifices
- Because of presence of MB2, the access cavity acquires a rhomboid shape with corners corresponding to all the canal orifices, that is, MB1, MB2, DB and palatal. *Luebke* showed that an entire wall is not extended to search and facilitate cleaning, shaping and obturation of extracanal. He recommended extension of only that portion of the wall where extracanal is present and this may result in "*cloverleaf appearance*" in the outline form. Luebke referred this to as a *shamrock preparation*

Maxillary Second Molar

Basic technique is similar to that of first molar but with the following differences:
- Three roots are found closer which may even fuse to form a single root
- MB2 is less likely to be present in second molar
- Three canals form a rounded triangle with base toward buccal side
- Mesiobuccal orifice is located more toward mesial and buccal than in first molar **(Fig. 15.35)**

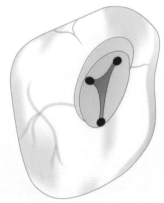

Fig. 15.35 Access cavity preparation of maxillary second molar here mesiobuccal orifice is located more mesial and buccal than first molar.

Access Cavity Preparation for Mandibular Molars (Figs. 15.36A to F)

- Remove caries and any restorative material if present
- Enamel is penetrated with No. 4 round bur on central fossa midway between the mesial and distal boundaries. Mesial boundary is a line joining the mesial cusp tips and the distal boundary is the line joining buccal and the lingual grooves **(Fig. 15.36A)**
- Bur is penetrated in the central fossa directed toward the distal root. Once the "drop" into pulp chamber is felt, remove roof of pulp chamber working from inside to outside with the help of round bur, tapered fissure, safety tip diamond or the carbide bur **(Fig. 15.36B)**
- Explore canal orifices with sharp endodontic explorer **(Fig. 15.36C)**
- Move the bur from inside to outside to deroof the chamber **(Fig. 15.36D)**
- Finish and smoothen the access cavity with slight divergence toward the occlusal surface **(Figs. 15.36 E and F)**
- When four canals are present, the shape of access cavity is rhomboid, but when two canals are present, access cavity is oval in shape with wider dimensions buccolingually
- Second molars with fused roots usually have two canals, buccal and lingual though the number, type, shape and form of canals may vary.

Mandibular First Molar

- Mesiobuccal orifice is under mesiobuccal cusp. Mesiolingual orifice is located in a depression formed by mesial and lingual walls. Distal orifice is oval in shape with largest diameter buccolingually located distal to the buccal groove **(Figs. 15.37 and 15.38)**
- Orifices of all the canals are usually located in the mesial two-thirds of the crown
- Cases have also been reported with an extramesial canal, that is, middle mesial canal (1%–15%) lying in the developmental groove between mesiobuccal and mesiolingual canals. Distal root has also shown to have more than one orifice, that is, distobuccal, distolingual and middle distal. These orifices are usually joined by the developmental grooves
- Shape of access cavity is usually trapezoidal or rhomboid irrespective of number of canals present
- The mesial wall is straight, the distal wall is round. The buccal and lingual walls converge to meet the mesial and distal walls.

Mandibular Second Molar

Access opening of mandibular second molar is similar to that of first molar except for following differences:

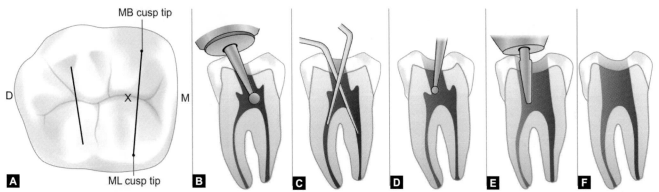

Figs. 15.36A to F Schematic representation of access cavity preparation for mandibular molars: (A) Initial point of entry of bur is central fossa midway between the mesial boundary (line joining the mesial cusp tips) and distal boundary (line joining buccal and the lingual grooves); (B) bur is penetrated in central fossa directed toward distal root; (C) explore canal orifices with sharp endodontic explorer; (D) Deroofing of pulp chamber; (E) Removal of coronal ledges or obstructions; (F) Final shape of access cavity with chamber walls flared occlusally.

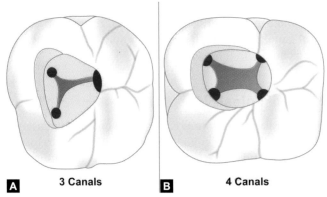

Figs. 15.37A and B Mandibular first molar showing: (A) Three canals; (B) Four canals.

- ☐ Pulp chamber is smaller in size
- ☐ One, two or more canals may be present
- ☐ Mesiobuccal and mesiolingual canal orifices are usually located closer
- ☐ When three canals are present, shape of access cavity is almost similar to mandibular first molar, but it is more triangular and less of rhomboid shape
- ☐ When two canal orifices are present, access cavity is rectangular, wider mesiodistally and narrower buccolingually
- ☐ Because of buccoaxial inclination, sometimes it is necessary to reduce a large portion of the mesiobuccal cusp to gain convenience form for mesiobuccal canal

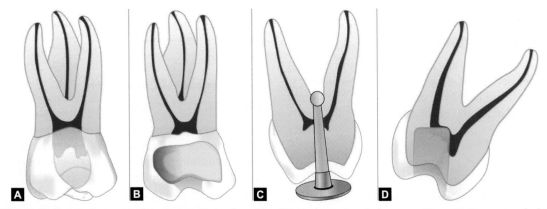

Figs. 15.38A to D Errors during cavity preparation of molars: (A) Under extended preparation; (B) Overextended preparation; (C) perforation due to over cutting of tooth structure; (D) Perforation resulting from not keeping the bur parallel to long axis of the tooth.

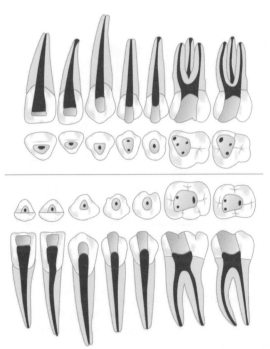

Fig. 15.39 Shapes of access opening of maxillary and mandibular teeth.

Commonly seen errors during access cavity preparation of molars are shown in **Figure 15.38.**

Figure 15.39 shows shape of access opening of maxillary and mandibular teeth.

Clinical Management of Difficult Cases for Access Opening

For optimal treatment of teeth with abnormal pulpal anatomy, the following are required:

Good Quality Radiographs

Good quality radiographs with angled views and contrast are required for better assessment of root canals anatomy. If canal disappears midway from orifice to apex, one should always suspect bifurcation **(Fig. 15.40)**. If radiograph shows presence of canal at unusual place, one should suspect abnormal anatomy of pulp space.

Magnification

Use of surgical operating microscope is recommended for endodontic treatment **(Fig. 15.41)**.

Knowledge of Clinical Anatomy

One should evaluate gingival contour for abnormal anatomy of tooth. For example, broad labiogingival wall in maxillary

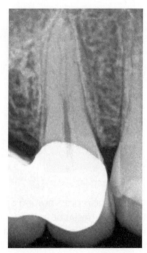

Fig. 15.40 If sharp break is seen in main canal in radiograph, one should suspect bifurcation or trifurcation of the canal.

premolar may suggest a broad buccal root and thus two root canals. Teeth with extra cusp may indicate aberrant pulp chamber.

Color of Pulpal Floor

In general, pulpal floor is dark gray in color, whereas axial dentin is lighter in color. This color difference helps the clinician to be very accurate in removing axial dentin so as to expose pulpal floor.

Extension of Access Cavity

Initial access shape is determined by shape of the pulpal floor but later it is extended to gain straight line access to the canals. Sometimes modified access cavity is prepared to locate MB2 in maxillary molars or second buccal canal in maxillary premolars.

Management of Cases with Extensive Restorations

If extensive restorations or full veneer crowns are marginally intact with no caries, then they can be retained with access cavity being cut through them. For cutting porcelain restorations, diamond burs are effective and for cutting through metal crowns, a fine cross-cut tungsten carbide bur is very effective. Restorative materials often alter the anatomic landmarks making the access cavity preparation difficult. If possible, complete removal of extensive restoration allows the most favorable access to the root canals. When access cavity is made through restoration, the following can occur:

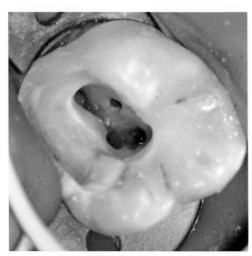

Fig. 15.41 Magnification helps in better visualization of canal anatomy.

❑ Coronal leakage because of loosening of fillings due to vibrations while access preparation
❑ Poor visibility and accessibility
❑ Blockage of canal if restoration pieces get stuck into canal system
❑ Misdirection of bur penetration (because in some cases restorations are placed to change the crown to root angulations so as to correct occlusal discrepancies)

Tilted and Angulated Crowns (Figs. 15.42A and B)

If tooth is severely tilted, access cavity should be prepared with great care to avoid perforations. Preoperative radiographs are of great help in evaluating the relationship of crown to the root. Sometimes it becomes necessary to open up the pulp chamber without applying the rubber dam so that bur can be placed at the correct angulation.

If not taken care, the access cavity preparation in tilted crowns can result in
❑ Failure to locate canals
❑ Gouging of the tooth structure
❑ Procedural accidents such as
  • Instrument separation
  • Perforation
  • Improper debridement of pulp space

Calcified Canals

Pulp canal obliteration in form of calcific metamorphosis or calcification is characterized by deposition of hard tissue within the root canal space. These can cause obliteration of pulp chamber and canal making management of the root canal difficult. Steps to manage teeth with calcified canals.

Access Preparation of Calcified Canals

❑ Success in negotiating small or calcified canals is predicted on a proper access opening and identification of the canal orifice
❑ To locate the calcified orifice, mentally visualize and plan the normal spatial relationship of the pulp space onto a radiograph of calcified tooth. Measure the distance from occlusal surface to the pulp chamber from preoperative radiograph
❑ Start with the access preparation using small No. 2 or 4 round bur. Avoid removing large amount of dentin in the hope of finding a canal orifice (**Fig. 15.43A**). By doing this all the pulp floor landmarks are lost, also the strength and dentinal thickness of tooth gets compromised. Small round burs should be used to create a path to the orifice. This will further ease the instruments into the proper lane to allow effortless introduction of files into the canals

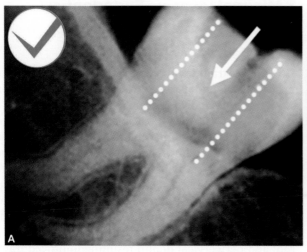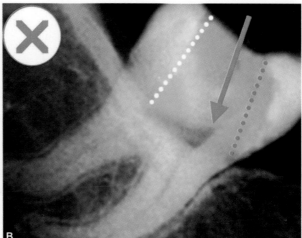

Figs. 15.42A and B To avoid perforations, the direction of access preparation should be according to the angle of tilted crown. (A) Proper angulation of bur according to tilted crown; (B) Perforation if bur is misdirected.

Location of the Canal Orifice

- If an orifice is present, use DG 16 explorer and apply firm pressure to force the instrument slightly into the orifice, **(Fig. 15.43B)** where it will "stick." At this suspected point, place No. 8 or 10 K-file or canal pathfinder into the orifice and try to negotiate the canal
- Probing with the explorer yields a characteristic "stick," but if explorer lies too close to the root surface, it actually penetrates a thin area of remaining dentin. The most common sign of accidental perforation is bleeding, but bleeding may also indicate that the pulp in the calcified canal is vital. If there is any doubt, place a small instrument in the opening and take a radiograph
- Sometimes, not anesthetizing the patient while performing access opening can be useful. Patient should be told to indicate when he/she feels a sharp sensation during access with a bur. At that point, a sharp DG 16 Endo Explorer is used to locate the canal. It is easy to tell the difference between PDL and pulp with a small file. Reaction to pain is sharper if file gets inserted into pulp than if it is in PDL
- Once the orifice has been located, a No. 8 K-file is penetrated into the canal to negotiate the calcified canal **(Fig. 15.43C)**. A No. 10 K-file is too large and a No. 6 K-file is too weak to apply any firm apical pressure. Use of nickel–titanium files is not recommended for this purpose because of lack of strength in the long axis of the file. Forceful probing of the canal with fine instruments and chelating agents results in formation of a false canal and continued instrumentation in a false canal results in perforation

For guidelines of negotiating calcified canals, refer to page number Page no 276.

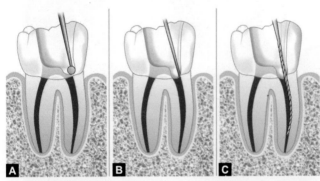

Figs. 15.43A to C Schematic representation of management of calcified canal: (A) Use a small No. 2 or 4 round bur to penetrate the enamel, taking care not to do over cutting; (B) Use DG 16 explorer and apply firm pressure check the presence of orifice; (C) If canal is suspected, place # 8 or #10 file in the canal to negotiate it.

Sclerosed Canals

Sclerosed canals make the endodontic treatment a challenge. Management:
- For visualization, magnification and illumination are the main requirements. Dyes can be used to locate the sclerotic canals
- While negotiation, précised amount of dentin should be removed with the help of ultrasonic tips to avoid over cutting
- Long shank low speed No. 2 round burs can also be used
- Use of chelating agents in these cases is not of much help because it softens the dentin indiscriminately, resulting in procedural errors such as perforations

Teeth with No or Minimal Crown

Though it seems to be quite simple to prepare access cavity in such teeth, the following precautions are needed while dealing such cases:
- Evaluate the preoperative radiograph to assess root angulation and depth of preparation
- Start the cavity preparation without applying rubber dam
- Apply rubber dam as soon as the canals are located
- If precautions are not taken in case of missing crown, there are chances of occurrence of iatrogenic errors like perforations due to misdirection of the bur
- In such cases, sometimes it becomes imperative to rebuild the tooth previous to endodontic treatment
- In teeth with weakened walls, it is necessary to reinforce the walls before initiating endodontic treatment so as to achieve the following goals:
  - Return the tooth to its normal form and function
  - Prevent coronal leakage during treatment
  - Allow use of rubber dam clamps
  - Prevent fracture of walls which can complicate the endodontic procedure

Minimal Invasive Endodontics/ Recent Trends in Endodontic Access Preparation

According to **traditional access preparation**, access is based on the radiographs that are 2D views of the 3D objects. Dentin is sacrificed liberally for expedient removal of debris and necrotic tissue with the straight line access to avoid iatrogenic errors. But, due to extensive loss of tooth structure, such preparations have shown fractures under functional loads. Extended access cavity preparations reduce the amount of sound dentin, increase deformability of the tooth, compromise the strength to fracture of endodontically treated teeth.

Conservative endodontic cavity (CEC) is prepared to minimize the loss of tooth structure, preserve chamber roof and pericervical dentin resulting improved fracture resistance of teeth.

Ninja is an extremely conservative approach which improves the fracture resistance of endodontically treated teeth **(Figs. 15.44 and 15.45)**.

Minimal removal of the tooth structure from inside to outside from the coronal to apical region is required to provide endo-endorestorative prosthodontic (EERP) continuum. A tooth may fail not because of poor endodontic treatment but due to irreparable microcracks/fractures due to removal of considerable amount of pericervical/pericingulum dentin (PCD). Hence, conservation of dentin and enamel is the best and only proven method to buttress the endodontically treated tooth.

Importance of Dental Hard Tissues

Importance	Posterior teeth	Anterior teeth
High	Pericervical dentin	Pericingulum dentin and enamel
	Soffit	Axial wall dentinoenamel junction
		Cervical enamel
Medium	Enamel	Enamel around incisal edge
Low	Unsupported enamel	Unsupported enamel
		Secondary/tertiary dentin
	Secondary/tertiary dentin	Exposed dentin in incisal area

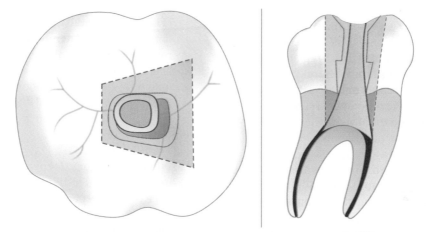

Fig. 15.44 Schematic representation of traditional, conservative and ninja access; green line depicts traditional cavity preparation, red line as conservative and blue line as ninja access cavity preparation.

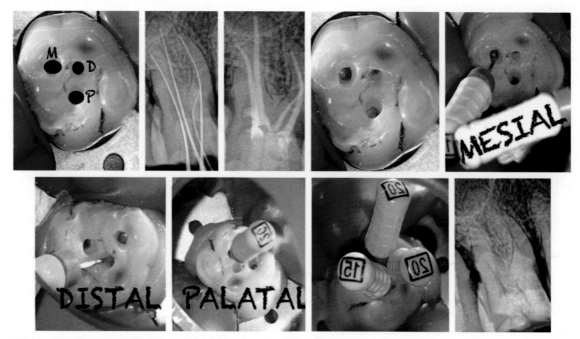

Fig. 15.45 Management of maxillary first molar by Ninja access. Note the ultraconservative access cavity preparation of first molar.
Courtesy: Jaydev.

Newer Guidelines for Access Preparation

Visualize the internal anatomy of tooth using
- Normal and angled periapical radiographs
- Position of CEJ
- Palpation along the attached gingiva to determine the root location direction
- Follow the caries

Important areas to consider:

i. **Pericervical/ pericingulum dentin (PCD)**

It is the area near the alveolar crest and is irreplaceable. This is the critical zone, roughly 4 mm above and 4 mm below the crestal bone and is important for giving ferrule and preventing fracture of the tooth at the cervical area **(Fig. 15.46)**. Also, CEJ is the most ideal area for transmitting the stress from crown to the apex. Apex of the tooth can be resected, coronal one third of the tooth can be replaced prosthetically, but PCD is irreplaceable

ii. **Avoid use of GG drills and round burs**

GG drills are not end cutting and are self-centring. But cervical self-centring can be dangerous. Also, due to thin shank, it is difficult to move it away from high-risk anatomy leading to strip perforations

- **Round burs**
  - Dropping round bur into a scant/non-existent chamber can lead to furcation perforation
  - Omnidirectional cutting blades can lead to severe loss of PCD
  - Flat walls in three dimensions cannot be cut with round bur because it only point cut but does not do planing

iii. **Preserve tooth structure for three-dimensional ferrule**

- 3D ferrule is mandatory for long-term survival of the tooth **(Fig. 15.47)**. Sufficient amount of tooth structure should be present to have minimum 1.5–2.5 mm of vertical height, 1 mm of thickness and almost parallel walls for success of postendodontic restoration

- **Cavosurface design**
  - *Cala lilly preparation*: If abundant highly bondable structure such as etchable porcelain or enamel is available and a highly filled composite is to be placed, the cavosurface should be cala-lillied (generously beveled on those areas). Enamel is cut back at 45° with cala lilly shape. Preparation is in middle and apical portion of coronal tooth **(Figs. 15.48A and B)**

- **Posterior teeth**
  - **Banking/Soffit/Stepped access**

    Soffit is a small piece of chamber roof near a point where it curves 900 and becomes the wall left behind. This tiny lip of 0.5 to 3.0 mm thickness gives strength to the tooth **(Figs. 15.49A and B)**. Its removal can lead to collateral damage to PCD. Attempting to remove pulp chamber roof doesn't accomplish any real endodontic objective. Rather, it gouges the walls that are responsible for long-term survival of the tooth. This 360° soffit can also be compared with a metal ring that stabilizes a wooden barrel. Pulp beneath it can be removed with an explorer

- **Anterior teeth**
  - **Traditional**

    When access goes deeper in the tooth, inverse funneling is created resulting in decreased fracture resistance of tooth especially with all ceramic preparation which require deep axial reduction and finish lines. Also, removal of lingual shoulder to explore lingual canal results in greater loss of tooth structure

  - **New model by Clark Khademi (CK)**

    Loading of maxillary anterior teeth results in severe tensile forces at cingulum. Pericingulum dentin

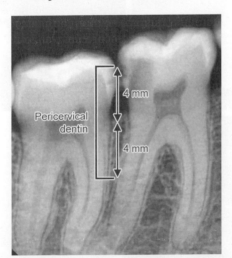

Fig. 15.46 Markings on radiograph showing pericervial dentin 4 mm above and below the crestal bone.

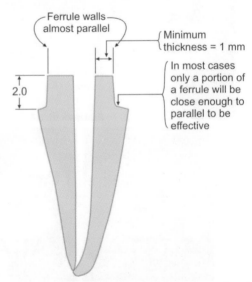

Fig. 15.47 Minimum required dimensions for ferrule.

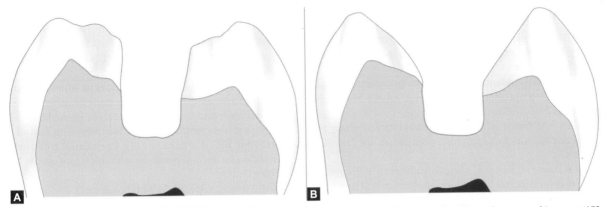

Figs. 15.48A and B (A) Showing traditional parallel-sided access; (B) cala Lilly enamel preparation. Here, the enamel is cut at 45° with the cala lilly shape, engaging almost the entire occlusal surface.

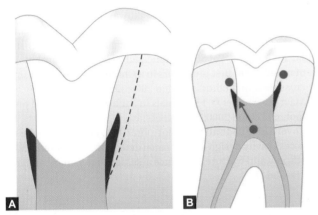

Figs. 15.49A and B (A) Dotted lines show where dentin is removed to have straight-line access; (B) Area between two lines should be maintained, called soffit.

should be preserved. So, CK suggested access preparation closer to incisal edge. In worn teeth/calcified teeth access may be made through the incisal edge. Incisal placement preserves pericingulum dentin. Beveled margin is created and access is started. Smaller internal shape is compensated by funnel shape externally. Shape forms a true funnel wherein narrow portion of funnel is in PCD zone and cavosurface with 45° angle becomes mouth/top of the funnel. In same anterior teeth, labial access may be better suited

Labial access can be made in the following cases:
- ❑ Presence of two canals (incidence as high as 41.4%)
- ❑ Patients with limited mouth opening (post-trauma maxillomandibular fixation)
- ❑ Crowded teeth
- ❑ Patients with Class II, division 2 dentition

Advantages
- ❑ Preservation of dentin in cingulum area which is essential for adequate resistance and retention of crown

- ❑ Visibility and accessibility which prevents gouging of labial wall

Conclusion

To have optimal straight line endodontic access cannot be overemphasized. A compromised access cavity design could lead to inadequate cleaning, shaping and obturation compromising the successful outcome. Successful access cavity preparation relies on a sound knowledge of the internal and external anatomy of teeth. The use of magnification, ultrasonic endodontic tips and diagnostic aids improves the ability of an operator to identify the root canal orifices more precisely. According to contemporary techniques, minimal removal of tooth structure should be done to provide EERP continuum for their long-term survival because iatrogenic removal of tooth structure may lead to retrograde vertical/oblique/horizontal fracture of the tooth. Therefore, precise balance between providing adequate access and preservation of tooth structure should be aim of access cavity preparation, enhancing both successful outcome and long-term survival of the tooth

Questions

1. Define access cavity preparation. What are objectives of access cavity preparation?
2. How will you do access preparation for mandibular molar?
3. What is minimally invasive endodontics?
4. Write short notes on:
   - Mouse-hole effect
   - Shamrock preparation
   - Soffit
   - Management of calcified canals
   - Guidelines for access cavity preparation.

Bibliography

1. Abbott PV. Assessing restored teeth with pulp and periapical for the presence of cracks, caries and marginal breakdown. Aust Dent J 2004;49:33.

2. Agwan AS, Sheikh Z. Identification and endodontic treatment of threecanalled maxillary first premolar. J Ayub Med Coll Abbottabad 2016;28:627–9.

3. Al-Qudah AA, Awawdeh LA. Root canal morphology of mandibular incisors in a Jordanian population. Int Endod J 2006;39:873.

4. Allwani V, Pawar M, Pawar A, Abrar S, Ambhore S. Permanent maxillary central incisor with dilacerated crown and root and C-shaped root canal. J Clin Diagn Res 2017.

5. Arora V, Yadav MP, Singh SP. Per-cervical dentin (PCD): a new paradigm for endodontic success. GJRA 2015;4:490–3.

6. Awawdeh LA, Al-Qudah AA. Root form and canal morphology of mandibular premolars in a Jordanian population. Int Endod J 2008;41:240.

7. Awawheh L, Abdullah H, Al-Qudah A. Root forms and canal morphology of Jordanian maxillary first premolars. J Endod 2008;34:956.

8. Bahcall JK, Barss JT. Fiberoptic endoscope usage for intracanal visualization. J Endod 2001;27:128.

9. Calberson FL, DeMoor RJ, Deroose CA. The radix entomolaris and paramolaris: a clinical approach in endodontics. J Endod 2007;33:58.

10. Clark D, Khademi J. Modern endodontic access and dentin conservation, Part 2. Dent Today 2009.pp.2–5.

11. Clark D, Khademi J. Modern molar endodontic access and directed dentin conservation. Dent Clin North Am 2010;54:249–73.

12. Coelho de Carvalho MC, Zuolo ML. Orifice locating with a microscope. J Endod 2000;26:532.

13. Connert T, Zehnder MS, Amato M, et al. Microguided endodontics: a method to achieve minimally invasive access cavity preparation and root canal location in mandibular incisors using a novel computer-guided technique. Int Endod J 2017.

14. DeMoor RJG, Calberson FLG. Root canal treatment in a mandibular second premolar with three root canals. J Endod 2005;31:310.

15. Gopikrishna V, Reuben J, Kandaswamy D. Endodontic management of a maxillary first molar with two palatal roots and a fused buccal root diagnosed with spiral computed tomography: a case report. Oral Surg Oral Med Oral Pathol Oral Radiol Endod 2008;105:e74.

16. Hargreaves K, Cohen S. Cohen's pathways of the pulp. 10th ed.

17. Krishna VG. Access cavity preparation—an anatomical and clinical perspective. Famdent Pract Dent Handb 2010;10:1–10.

18. Lu TY, Yang SF, Pai SF. Complicated root canal morphology of mandibular first premolars in a Chinese population using cross section method. J Endod 2006;32:932.

19. Macri E, Zmener O. Five canals in a mandibular second premolar. J Endod 2000;26:304.

20. Rover G, Belladonna FG, Bortoluzzi EA, et al. Influence of access cavity design on root canal detection, instrumentation efficacy and fracture resistance assessed in maxillary molars. J Endod 2017.

Irrigation and Intracanal Medicaments

Successful endodontic treatment depends on combinaton of proper instrumentation, irrigation and three dimensional obturation of root canal system. Among these, irrigation plays an indispensable role in endodontic treatment. It is truly said, "Instruments shape, irrigants clean." Irrigation is the only way to clean those areas of root canal wall that are not touched by mechanical instrumentation. These areas are fins, isthmuses, anastomosis and large lateral canals **(Fig. 16.1)**.

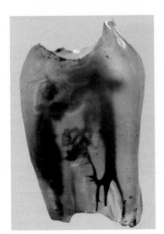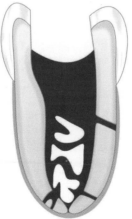

Fig. 16.1: Root canal system is complicated with fins, webs and anastomosis. It can be cleaned by effective use of an irrigating solution.

Objective of using an irrigant is chemical dissolution/disruption, mechanical detachment, removal of pulp tissue, dentin debris and smear layer, microorganisms and their products out of the root canal system.

Ideal Requirements for an Irrigant

It should
- Have broad-spectrum antimicrobial properties
- Aid in the debridement of the canal system
- Have the ability to dissolve necrotic tissue or debris
- Have low toxicity level
- Be a good lubricant
- Have low surface tension so that it can easily flow into inaccessible areas
- Be able to effectively sterilize the root canal (or at least disinfect them)
- Be able to prevent formation of smear layer during instrumentation or dissolve the latter once it is formed
- Inactivate endotoxin

Other desirable properties of an ideal irrigant are that it should
- Be able to penetrate root canal periphery
- Be able to dissolve pulp tissue, smear layer and biofilm
- Be bactericidal even for microorganisms in biofilm
- Be fungicidal

- Not weaken the tooth structure
- Be easily available
- Be cost-effective
- Be easy to use
- Have adequate shelf life
- In addition to these properties, if endodontic irrigants come in contact with vital tissue, these should be systemically nontoxic, noncaustic to the periodontal tissue and have little potential to cause an anaphylactic reaction

Functions of Irrigants

- Irrigants perform physical and biologic functions. They remove dentin shavings from canals and thus prevent blockage of canal apex (Fig. 16.2)
- Efficiency of instruments increases in wet canals and they are less likely to break in lubricated canals

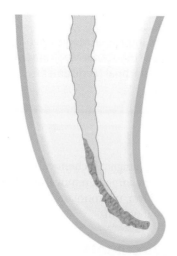

Fig. 16.2 Irrigants remove dentin shavings from the canal preventing it's blockage.

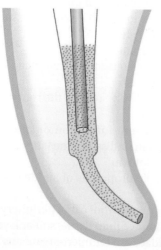

Fig. 16.3 Irrigation helps in loosening of debris.

- Irrigants act as a solvent of necrotic tissue, so they loosen debris, pulp tissue and microorganisms from irregular dentinal walls (Fig. 16.3)
- Irrigants help in removing the debris from fins, anastomosis, accessory and lateral canals where instruments cannot reach
- Most irrigants are germicidal and have antibacterial action
- Bleaching action of irrigants lighten the teeth discolored due to trauma or extensive silver restorations

Factors that Modify Activity of Irrigating Solutions

Efficacy of irrigating solutions depends on the following factors (Fig. 16.4):

Concentration

Studies have shown that though tissue dissolving ability of sodium hypochlorite increases linearly with concentration, it is preferred to use lower concentration due to it's cytotoxic effects.

Contact

To be effective, the irrigant must contact the substrate (organic tissue or microbes). When canals are sufficiently enlarged, irrigant can be deposited directly in the apical area with a fine irrigating needle to increase its effect.

Presence of Organic Tissue

Presence of organic tissues decreases the effectiveness of intracanal medicaments. The protein content of organic tissues form a coagulate when reacts with medicament. This coagulant serves as a barrier to prevent further penetration of medicament, thus limiting its effectiveness.

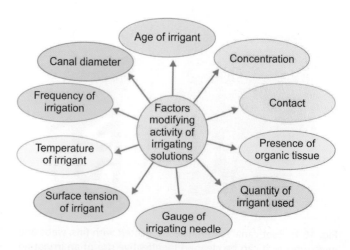

Fig. 16.4 Factors that modify activity of irrigating solutions.

Quantity of Irrigant Used

Quantity of irrigant used is directly related to its ability to remove the debris from the canal.

Gauge of Irrigating Needle

27- or 28-gauge needle is preferred as it can go deeper in canal for better delivery and debridement action.

Surface Tension of Irrigant

Lower surface tension of an irrigant increases its wettability, hence better penetration in narrow areas for effective debridement.

Temperature of Irrigant

As the temperature of irrigant is increased, its efficacy increases.

Frequency of Irrigation

Copious irrigation has the following advantages:
- ❑ More irrigation causes better debridement of tissues
- ❑ Each time a fresh potent irrigants plays an action

Canal Diameter

Wider the canal, better is the debridement action of irrigant.

Age of Irrigant

Freshly prepared solutions are more efficient, than older ones.

▌ Commonly used Irrigating Solutions

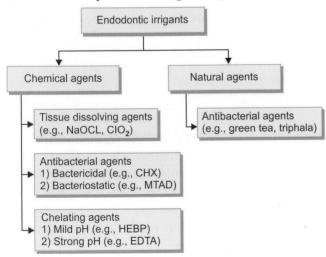

▌ Normal Saline (Fig. 16.5)

Normal saline as 0.9% w/v is commonly used in endodontics for gross debridement and lubrication of root canals

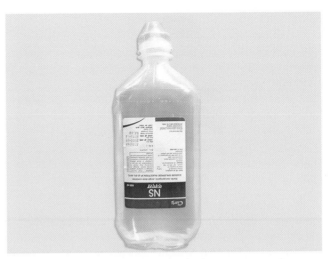

Fig. 16.5 Normal saline.

because it acts by flushing action. Since it is very mild in action, it can be used as an adjunct to chemical irrigant. It can also be used as final rinse for root canals to remove any chemical irrigant left after root canal preparation.

Advantages

It is biocompatible in nature. No adverse reaction even if extruded periapically because osmotic pressure of normal saline is same as that of the blood.

Disadvantages
- Does not possess dissolution and disinfecting properties
- Too mild to thoroughly clean the canals
- Cannot clear microbial flora from inaccessible areas like accessory canal
- Does not possess antimicrobial activity
- Does not remove smear layer

▌ Sodium Hypochlorite

Sodium hypochlorite is a clear, pale, green yellow liquid with strong odor of chlorine (**Fig. 16.6**). It was introduced during the World War I by chemist Henry Drysdale Dakin for treating infected wounds. It is known as Dakin's solution. Original concentration suggested by Dakin was 0.5%. Beside being wide spectrum, it is sporicidal, has tissue dissolving properties. Due to these properties, Coolidge suggested use of hypochlorite as an endodontic irrigant in 1919.

Availability

- ❑ Unbuffered at pH 11 at conc. 0.5% to 5%
- ❑ Buffered with bicarbonate at pH 9.0 as 0.5% or 1% solution

Mechanism of Action of Sodium Hypochlorite

At body temperature, reactive chlorine in aqueous solution exists in two forms—hypochlorous acid (HOCl) and hypochlorite (OCl) depending on pH of solution. On coming in contact with organic tissues:

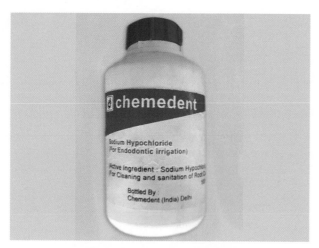

Fig. 16.6 Sodium hypochlorite.

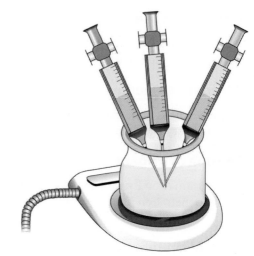

Fig. 16.7 To warm NaOCl, syringes filled with NaOCl are placed in 60–70°C (140°F) water bath.

❑ It forms glycerol and fatty acid salts (saponification reaction), resulting in surface tension of the solution.

❑ It causes amino acid neutralization reaction resulting in formation of salt and water. pH decreases due to release of hydroxyl ions.

❑ When hypochlorous acid comes in contact with organic tissue, it releases chlorine which combines with amino acids forming chloramines. This chloramination reaction between chlorine and amino acids causes interference in cell metabolism.

Together these three reactions that occur in presence of organic tissues lead to tissue dissolution and antibacterial effect.

Methods to Increase the Efficacy of Sodium Hypochlorite (Flowchart 16.1)

Time

Antimicrobial effectiveness of sodium hypochlorite is directly related to its contact time with the canal.

Flowchart 16.1 Factors affecting the efficacy of sodium hypochlorite.

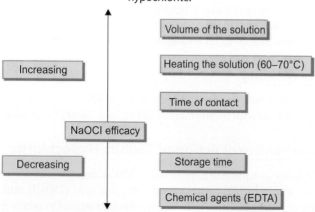

Heat

Increase in temperature by 25°C enhances efficacy by factor of 100 **(Fig. 16.7)**. But one should be careful not to overheat the solution because this can cause breakdown of sodium hypochlorite constituents and thus may damage the solution.

pH

If NaOCl is diluted, its tissue dissolving property decreases. In aqueous solution, hypochlorous acid dissociates into hypochlorite:

$$HOCl \leftrightarrow H^+ + OCl^-$$

HOCl is stronger oxidant than hypochlorite ion, i.e. HOCl is responsible for strong chlorination, oxidizing action and tissue dissolution. This dissociation of HOCl to OCl depends on pH. At pH 10, OCl form exists and at pH of 4.5, HOCl form dominates. So, antibacterial properties of hypochlorite are more in acidic pH.

Ultrasonic Activation of Sodium Hypochlorite

Ultrasonic activation of sodium hypochlorite has shown to accelerate chemical reaction, create cavitational effect and thus achieve a superior cleansing action **(Fig. 16.8)**.

Precautions to be Taken while Using Sodium Hypochlorite Solution

It is important to remember that though sodium hypochlorite is nontoxic during intracanal use but 5.25% NaOCl can cause serious damage to tissue if injected periapically **(Fig. 16.9)**.

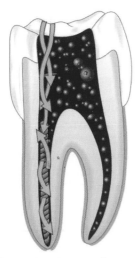

Fig. 16.8 Ultrasonic activation of irrigating solution.

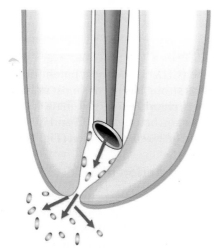

Fig. 16.9 Forceful irrigation can cause periapical extrusion of sodium hypochlorite solution.

If sodium hypochlorite gets extruded into periapical tissues, it causes excruciating pain, periapical bleeding and swelling. As potential for spread of infection is related to tissue destruction, medication like antibiotics, analgesics, antihistamine should be prescribed accordingly. In addition to these, reassurance to the patient is the prime consideration.

Therefore, to avoid accidental extrusion of hypochlorite, care should be taken to do passive irrigation especially in cases with large apical openings.

Advantages
- Causes tissue dissolution
- Remove organic portion of dentin for deeper penetration of medicament
- Removes biofilm
- Causes dissolution of pulp and necrotic tissue
- Shows antibacterial and bleaching action
- Causes lubrication of canals
- Economical
- Easily available

Disadvantages
- Because of high surface tension, its ability to wet dentin is less
- Irritant to tissues, if extruded periapically, it can cause tissue damage
- If comes in contact, it cause inflammation of gingiva because of its caustic nature
- It can bleach the clothes, if spillage occurs
- It has bad odor and taste
- Vapors of sodium hypochlorite can irritate the eyes
- It can be corrosive to instruments
- It is unable to remove inorganic components of smear layer
- Long time of contact with dentin has determined effect on flexural strength of dentin
- Exudate and microbial biomass inactivates NaOCl. So, continuous irrigation and time are important when irrigation is done with NaOCl

Hydrogen Peroxide

It is a clear, odorless liquid and mainly 3% solution of hydrogen peroxide is used as an irrigating agent (**Fig. 16.10**).

Mechanism of Action

- It is highly unstable and easily decomposed by heat and light. It rapidly dissociates into $H_2O + [O]$ (water and nascent oxygen). On coming in contact with tissue enzymes catalase and peroxidase, the liberated [O] produces bactericidal effect but this effect is transient and diminishes in presence of organic debris
- It causes oxidation of bacterial sulfhydryl group of enzymes and thus interferes with bacterial metabolism
- Rapid release of [O] on contact with organic tissue results in effervescence or bubbling action which is thought to aid in mechanical debridement by dislodging particles of necrotic tissue and dentinal debris and floating them to the surface

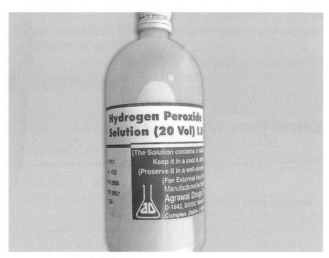

Fig. 16.10 Hydrogen peroxide.

Uses

It is used as an irrigating solution either alone or alternatively with sodium hypochlorite. The advantage of using alternating solutions of 3% H_2O_2 and 5.2% NaOCl are

- ❏ Effervescent reaction by hydrogen peroxide bubbles pushes debris mechanically out of root canal
- ❏ Solvent action of sodium hypochlorite on organic debris
- ❏ Disinfecting and bleaching action by both solutions

> **Clinical Tips**
>
> While using combination of sodium hypochlorite and hydrogen peroxide, always use sodium hypochlorite in the last because hydrogen peroxide can react with pulp debris and blood to produce gas (nascent oxygen) which builds up pressure on closing the tooth, this can result in severe pain.

▌ Urea

It is a white, odorless, crystalline powder. It was used in the World War I as a therapeutic agent for infected wounds. Urea solution (40% by weight) is mild solvent of necrotic tissue and pus and is mild antiseptic too. In 1951, Blechman and Cohen suggested that 30% urea solution can be used as root canal irrigant in patients with vital pulp as well as those with necrotic pulp.

Mechanism of Action

- ❏ *Denaturation of protein:* Urea denatures the protein by destroying bonds of the secondary structure resulting in loss of functional activity of protein. This mode of action is responsible for its antiseptic property
- ❏ It has the property of chemically debriding the wound by softening the underlying substrate of fibrin

Uses

- ❏ It is excellent vehicle for antimicrobials such as sulfonamides
- ❏ It has low toxicity
- ❏ It can be used in teeth with open apices or areas with resorptive defects

▌ Urea Peroxide

It is white crystalline powder with slight odor. It is soluble in water, alcohol and glycerine.

Mechanism of Action

- ❏ It decomposes rapidly when exposed to heat, light, or moisture. It dissociates into urea and hydrogen peroxide

$$Urea\ peroxide \rightarrow Urea + H_2O_2$$

Its mechanism of action combines the effects of urea and hydrogen peroxide.
- ❏ Anhydrous glycerol increases the stability of urea peroxide

Uses

- ❏ 10% solution of urea peroxide in anhydrous glycerol base is available as glyoxide. Advantages of adding glycerol are
  - • It increases stability of solution, thus increases shelf life
  - • It acts as a good lubricant, so facilitates negotiation and instrumentation of thin, tortuous root canals
  - • Glyoxide can be used along with EDTA-Ethylenediaminetetraacetic acid to clean the walls of the canal

Disadvantages

It dissociates more slowly than hydrogen peroxide (H_2O_2). So, its effervescence is prolonged but not pronounced. This can be overcome by alternating irrigation with sodium hypochlorite.

▌ Chlorhexidine

Chlorhexidine (CHX) is the most potent of tested bisbiguanides. It has strong base and is most stable in the form of its salts, that is, chlorhexidine gluconate. It shows optimal antimicrobial action between pH 5.5 and 7.0. For canal irrigation, it is used in 2% concentration **(Fig. 16.11)**.

Mechanisms of Action (Fig. 16.12)

- ❏ Chlorhexidine is broad-spectrum antimicrobial agent which is due to its cationic bisbiguanide molecular structure
- ❏ Cationic molecule is absorbed to negatively charged phosphate groups of microbial cell wall. This alters the cell's osmotic equilibrium and causes leakage of intracellular components

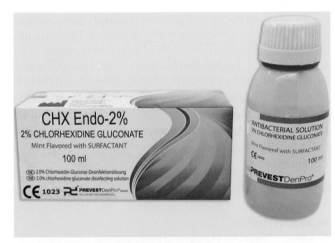

Fig. 16.11 2% Chlorhexidine used as root canal irrigant.
Courtesy: PrevestDenPro.

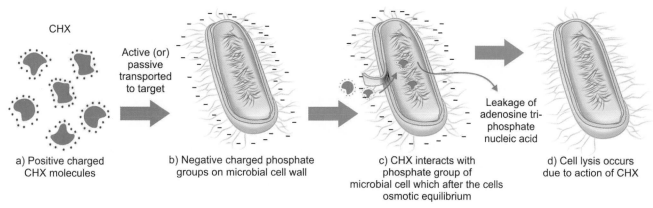

CHX

a) Positive charged CHX molecules

Active (or) passive transported to target

b) Negative charged phosphate groups on microbial cell wall

c) CHX interacts with phosphate group of microbial cell which after the cells osmotic equilibrium

Leakage of adenosine tri-phosphate nucleic acid

d) Cell lysis occurs due to action of CHX

Fig. 16.12 Mechanism of action of chlorhexidine.

- At low concentration, it acts as a bacteriostatic, whereas at higher concentrations, it causes coagulation and precipitation of cytoplasm and therefore acts as bactericidal **(see Fig. 16.11)**
- Chlorhexidine has the property of substantivity (residual effect). It can show residual antimicrobial activity for 72 h or even up to 7 days if used as an endodontic irrigant

Disadvantages
- It is unable to dissolve necrotic tissue remnants
- It is less effective on Gram-negative than on Gram-positive bacteria
- Does not show effect on biofilms

Combination of NaOCl and CHX is preferred to enhance their antimicrobial properties. However, presence of NaOCl in the canals during irrigation with CHX produces an orange–brown precipitate known as parachloroaniline (PCA) **(Fig. 16.13)**. This precipitate occludes the dentinal tubules and may compromise the seal of the obturated root canal. Moreover, leaching of PCA from the insoluble precipitate has shown to be cytotoxic in rats and carcinogenic in humans. Formation of precipitate can be prevented by minimizing the chance for two irrigants to come in contact with each other. Basrani et al. advocated flushing of remaining NaOCl with alcohol or EDTA, before using CHX.

▌Chelating Agents

Chelating agent is defined as a chemical which combines with a metal to form chelate. Chelating agents were introduced in dentistry in 1957 for aid in preparation of narrow and tortuous canals to soften the canal dentin, increase dentin permeability and remove smear layer.

EDTA

Ethylenediaminetetraacetic acid (EDTA) is the most commonly used chelating agent. It was introduced in dentistry by Nygaard-Ostby for cleaning and shaping of the canals. It contains four acetic acid groups attached to ethylenediamine **(Flowchart 16.2)**. EDTA is relatively nontoxic and slightly irritating in weak solutions. Effect of EDTA on dentin depends on its concentration and duration of contact with dentin.

Clinical Tips

- EDTA and citric acid are used for 2–3 min at the end of instrumentation to remove the smear layer so as to improve the antibacterial effect of locally used disinfecting agents in deeper layer of dentin
- EDTA or citric acid should never be mixed with sodium hypochlorite because EDTA and citric acid strongly interact with sodium hypochlorite. This immediately reduces the available chlorine in solution and thus making it ineffective against bacteria

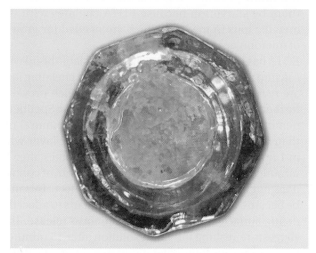

Fig. 16.13 contact of sodium hypochlorite and chlorhexidine produces an orange–brown precipitate known as parachloroaniline (PCA).

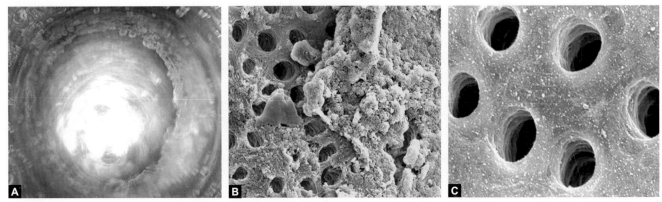

Figs. 16.14A to C (A) Dentin tubules blocked with smear layer; (B) Application of chelating agent causes removal of smear layer; (C) Opening of dentinal tubules.
Courtesy: Dentsply, India.

Flowchart 16.2 Structural formula of EDTA

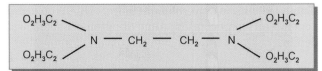

Functions of EDTA
- Lubrication
- Emulsification
- Holding debris in suspension
- Smear layer removal **(Figs. 16.14A to C)**

Mechanism of Action

☐ It inhibits growth of bacteria and ultimately destroys them by starvation because EDTA chelates with the metallic ions in medium which are needed for growth of microorganisms

☐ EDTA has self-limiting action. It forms a stable bond with calcium and dissolves dentin, but when all chelating ions are reacted, an equilibrium is reached which prevents further dissolution. According to Goldberg & Speilberg, demineralization effect of EDTA is more at neutral pH than at alkaline pH. EDTA removes smear layer with in 1 minute of exposure and this effect doubles after 15 minutes of exposure. Further increase in time of contact does not increase the demineralization effect. This may be because of chelating material which starts to affect the dentin surface causing slower phosphorus release. This suggests refreshing the EDTA solution after 15 minutes.

☐ Calt and Serper found that increasing the contact time along with concentration from 10% to 17% and pH 7.5 to 9.0 has shown to increase the dentin demineralization.

Uses of EDTA
☐ It has dentin dissolving properties
☐ It helps in enlarging narrow canals
☐ Makes easier manipulation of instruments
☐ Reduces time needed for debridement

Different Preparations of EDTA (Fig. 16.15)

Liquid type:
1. **REDTA:** In this, 17% EDTA is combined with cetrimide, that is, cetyltrimethylammonium bromide to reduce the surface tension.
2. **EDTAT:** EDTA is combined with sodium lauryl ether sulphate (Tergentol) which reduces the surface tension.
3. **EDTAC:** It is commercially available as 15% solution and pH of 7.3 under the name EDTAC because it contains cetavlon, a quaternary ammonium compound

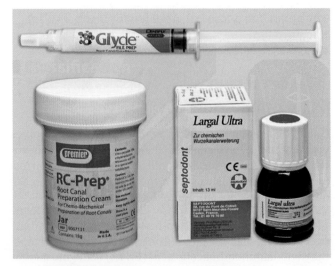

Fig. 16.15 Chelating agents in form of gel and liquid.

which is added due to its disinfecting properties. It reduces the contact angle of EDTA when placed on dentin surface and thus enhances its cleaning efficacy.

4. **Largal Ultra:** It contains 15% EDTA solution as disodium salt, cetrimide and sodium hydroxide to adjust pH value to 7.4.

Paste type:

1. **Calcinase slide:** It contains 15% sodium EDTA and 58%–64% water but no peroxides or preservatives. It has stable pH of 8–9. This gel is thixotropic in nature, so it is firm at room temperature and forms creamy consistency when agitated. So it sticks to the instrument very well and spreads well in the root canal.
2. **RC prep:** It consists of 10% urea peroxide, 15% EDTA and glycol in an ointment base. Presence of glycol makes it a lubricant and coats the instrument which facilitates its movement in the canal.
3. **Glyde file:** It consists of 10% urea peroxide, 15% EDTA in aqueous solution. On reaction with NaOCl, oxygen is released from urea peroxide which causes effervescence. This facilitates the removal of the pulpal remnants and debris.
4. **File-Eze:** It contains 19% EDTA in aqueous water soluble solution.

> **Clinical Tips**
>
> Collagen is major constituent of vital pulp which can be packed into glue-like mass which contributes to iatrogenic blocks. Without the use of a chelator, vital tissue tends to collapse and readheres to itself, but use of chelator does not allow this phenomenon to occur and accelerate emulsification of tissue

Citric Acid

- ❑ Use of 10% citric acid has shown to remove the smear layer. It reacts with metals to form non-ionic chelate. It shows antimicrobial activity against facultative and obligative anaerobes
- ❑ Citric acid should not be used with sodium hypochlorite as it interacts with NaOCl and reduces the available chlorine making it ineffective against microorganisms

Polyacrylic Acid

It is commercially available as Durelon and Fuji II liquid (**Fig. 16.16**). Polyacrylic acid and 7% malic acid may be used to remove smear layer.

Hydroxyethylidene Bisphosphonate

- ❑ It is also known as etidronate or etidronic acid
- ❑ Hydroxyethylidene bisphosphonate (HEBP) is nontoxic chelating agent and shows only short-term interference with sodium hypochlorite.

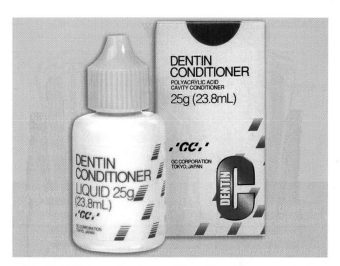

Fig. 16.16 Polyacrylic acid conditioner to remove smear layer.

Maleic Acid

It is a mild organic acid used as conditioner in adhesive dentistry.

Salvizol

- ❑ It belongs to surface acting materials like quaternary ammonium group. It shows antibacterial property even in presence of organic materials
- ❑ It is most effective against Gram-positive and Gram-negative microorganisms and fungi

Tetraclean

It is a mixture of doxycycline hyclate [lower concentration than mixture of a tetracycline isomer, an acid and a detergent (MTAD)], an acid and a detergent. It has shown to remove microorganisms and smear layer from dentinal tubules with a final 5-min rinse.

Chlorine Dioxide

Chlorine dioxide is similar to hypochlorite and studies have shown that ClO_2 is equally efficient to NaOCl for dissolving organic tissue. Since, ClO_2 produces little or no trihalomethanes (carcinogen), it might prove as better dental irrigant than NaOCl.

■ Ultrasonic Irrigation

Ultrasonic irrigation has shown to clean the root canals or eliminates bacteria from the walls better than conventional methods. Use of ultrasonics causes continuous flow of an irrigant in the canal, thus prevents accumulation of debris in the canal (**Fig. 16.17**).

Summary of irrigants used during endodontic therapy

Irrigant	Normal saline	Sodium hypochlorite	Hydrogen peroxide	EDTA	Chlorhexidine
Concentration	0.9%	0.5%, 1%, 2.5%, 5.25%	3%	15%, 17%	2%
pH	7.3	10.8–12	6	7.3–8	5.5–7
Mechanism of action	Physical flushing	Bactericidal	Bactericidal • Dissociates in H_2O and [O][O] has bactericidal activity • Causes oxidation of sulfhydryl groups of enzymes • Effervescent reaction of H_2O_2 bubbles causes mechanical debridement	• Lubrication, emulsification and holding debris in suspension • Forms chelates with calcium ions of dentin making it more friable and easier to manipulate	• At low concentration bacteriostatic • Bactericidal by causing coagulation and precipitation of cytoplasm
Advantages	No side effects, if extruded periapically	Has dissolution, disinfectant and antimicrobial properties.	Has disinfectant and antimicrobial property	• Dentin dissolving property • Makes easier manipulation of canals	• Property of substantivity • More effective against Gram-positive bacteria • Less effective on Gram-positive bacteria
Disadvantages	Too mild to be disinfectant	Can cause tissue injury if extruded periapically			• Unable to dissolve necrotic tissue remnants • Less effective on Gram-positive bacteria

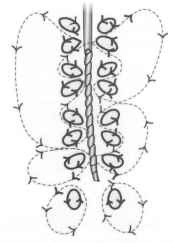

Fig. 16.17 Ultrasonic irrigation showing continuous flow of irrigation in the canal.

Mechanism of Action

When a small file is placed in canal and ultrasonic activation is given, ultrasonic energy passes through irrigating solution and exerts its "acoustic streaming or scrubbing" effect on the canal wall. This mechanical energy warms the irrigant (sodium hypochlorite) and dislodges debris from canal. Combination of activation and heating of irrigating solution is adjunct in cleaning the root canal.

Advantages
• It cleans the root canal walls better than conventional ones
• It removes the smear layer efficiently
• It dislodges the debris from the canal better due to acoustic effect

Disadvantages
• Ultrasonic preparation of the canal is found to be unpredictable
• It can lead to excessive cutting of canal walls and may damage the finished preparation

Newer Irrigating Solutions

Electrochemically Activated Solution (Flowchart 16.3)

- It is produced from the tap water and low concentrated salt solutions
- Principle of electrochemically activated (ECA) is transferring liquid into metastable state via electrochemical unipolar action using a reactor
- Electrochemical treatment in anode and cathode chambers results in synthesis of two type of solutions, that is, anolyte (produced in anode chamber) and catholyte (produced in cathode chamber)
- Anolyte solution has also been termed as super oxidized water or oxidative potential water. The pH of anolyte can be acidic (anolyte), neutral (anolyte neutral), or alkaline (anolyte neutral cathodic). Earlier, acidic anolyte was used but now neutral and alkaline solutions are preferred

Advantages of electrochemically activated solution:
- Nontoxic to biological tissues
- Less or no allergic reaction
- Effective with wide range of microbial spectra
- Combined use of NaOCl and ECA solution has shown to remove the smear layer

Ozonated Water Irrigation

- Ozone is an unstable gas which can oxidize any biological unit. Ozonated water is shown to be powerful antimicrobial agent against bacteria, fungi, protozoa and viruses

Advantages of ozonated water:
- Its potency
- Ease of handling
- Lack of mutagenicity
- Rapid microbial effects

Ruddle's Solution

It is of 17% EDTA, 5% NaOCl and hypaque.

Mechanism of Action

- Hypaque is an aqueous radiopaque solution of iodide salts, namely, ditrizoate and sodium iodine
- Use of EDTA lowers the surface tension and allows better penetration of sodium hypochlorite
- Solvent action of sodium hypochlorite clears the contents of root canal system and thus enables hypaque component to flow into every nook and corner of the canal system such as fracture, perforation, missed canals and defective restoration

Uses:
- Useful for visualization of root canal anatomy, missed canal, perforation, etc.
- Helps in diagnosis of internal resorption, its size and site
- Helps in visualization of blockage, perforation, ledge and canal transportation
- Helps in management of iatrogenic errors

Photoactivated Disinfection (Fig. 16.18)

Photoactivated disinfection (PAD) is based on the concept that nontoxic photosensitizers can be localized in certain tissues and activated by light of the suitable wavelength to produce oxygen and free radicals which are cytotoxic to cells of the target tissue. Methylene blue, toluidine blue and chlorine p6 are commonly used photosensitizers which release oxygen when exposed to low power laser.

Advantages of PAD:
- Most effective antimicrobial agent
- Effectively kills Gram-negative, Gram-positive, aerobic and anaerobic bacteria

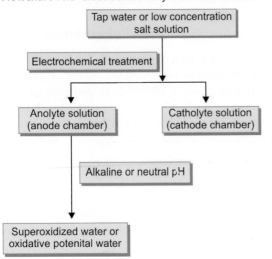

Flowchart 16.3 Electrochemically activated solution.

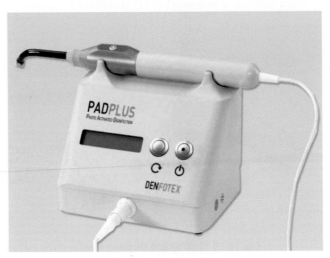

Fig. 16.18 PAD system.

- Overcomes the problems of antibiotic resistance
- Kills bacteria present in complex biofilm such as sub-gingival plaque which is typically resistant to action of antimicrobial agents
- Does not pose any thermal risk due to low power of PAD laser
- Does not cause any sensitization
- Nontoxic

A Mixture of a Tetracycline Isomer, an Acid and a Detergent (MTAD) (Fig. 16.19)

MTAD was introduced in 2000 as a final rinse for disinfection of root canal system. Torabinejad et al. have shown that MTAD is able to safely remove the smear layer and is effective against *Enterococcus faecalis.*

Composition

- *Tetracycline:*
  - It is bacteriostatic broad-spectrum antibiotic
  - It has low pH and acts as calcium chelator
  - It removes smear layer
  - It has property of substantivity
  - It promotes healing
- *Citric acid:* It is bactericidal in nature and removes smear layer
- *Detergent (Tween 80):* It decreases surface tension

Advantages of MTAD

- It is an effective solution for removal of smear layer
- It kills *E. faecalis* which has been shown to be resistant to many intracanal medicaments and irrigants
- It is biocompatible
- MTAD has similar solubilizing effects on pulp and dentin to those of EDTA
- High binding affinity of doxycycline present in MTAD for dentin allows prolonged antibacterial effect (it is the main difference between MTAD and EDTA)

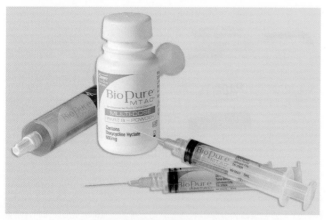

Fig. 16.19 Photograph showing MTAD.
Courtesy: Dentsply Sirona.

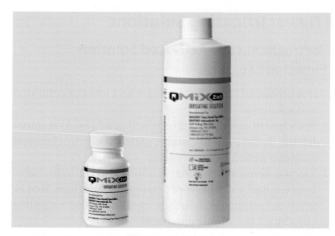

Fig. 16.20 Q-Mix.

Q-MIX (Fig. 16.20)

Q-Mix 2 in 1 is a colorless and odorless solution which consists of 17% EDTA and 2% chlorhexidine which can kill 99.99% of the bacteria.

To be used as a final rinse, continuous irrigation of root canal is done for 60–90 s.

Functions

- Kills 99.99% planktonic bacteria
- Penetrates biofilm

Advantages of Q-MIX

- Less demineralization of dentin as compared to EDTA
- It does not cause erosion of dentin like NaOCl, when NaOCl is used as a final rinse after EDTA

▌ Herbal Irrigants

Herbal irrigants are becoming popular now due to their biocompatibility, antimicrobial activity, antioxidative and anti-inflammatory nature.

Following are commonly used herbal irrigants:

Triphala and Green Tea Polyphenols

Triphala's fruit is rich in citric acid. It has chelating property which helps in removing the smear layer. Green tea polyphenols possess antioxidant, anticariogenic, anti-inflammatory and antimicrobial properties. J. Prabhakar et al. showed that Triphala and Green tea polyphenols have significant antimicrobial activity against *E. faecalis* biofilm.

Turmeric

It possesses anti-inflammatory, antioxidant, antimicrobial and anticancer activity. Studies have shown its antibacterial activity against *E. faecalis* and thus can be used as for root canal irrigation.

German Chamomile and Tea Tree Oil

The active component of tea tree oil is terpinen-4-ol which possesses anti-inflammatory, analgesic and antimicrobial properties. It helps in removing smear layer and has activity against *E. faecalis*.

Allium sativum (Garlic)

Its active component is allicin which destroys the bacterial cell wall and thus can be used as root canal irrigant.

Azadirachta indica (Neem)

Neem possesses antifungal, antibacterial, antioxidant and anticarcinogenic activity. Naiyak Arathi et al. in their study showed that ethanolic extract of neem has significant activity against *E. faecalis*.

Propolis

Propolis is a resinous substance which honey bees collect from poplars and conifers. It shows antioxidant, anti-inflammatory and antibacterial activities against *Streptococcus sobrinus* and *Streptococcus mutans*. Studies have shown its antimicrobial activity comparable to that of sodium hypochlorite.

Myristica fragrans (Nutmeg)

Its main constituent myristic acid has antibacterial property.

Spilanthes calva DC

Moulshree Dube et al. showed that antibacterial efficacy of methanolic extract of *Spilathes calva* DC is comparable to sodium hypochlorite.

Acacia nilotica (Babool)

Acacia nilotica have antimicrobial, antioxidant and antibiotic properties. Researches have shown that 50% concentration acacia shows the highest activity against *E. faecalis*.

Aloe vera

Aloe vera has antibacterial and antifungal activity. It has been found to be effective against *E. faecalis* and resistant microorganisms of root canal.

▌Method of Irrigation

- ❑ Solution should be introduced slowly and passively into the canal
- ❑ Needle should never be wedged into the canal and should allow an adequate backflow **(Fig. 16.21)**

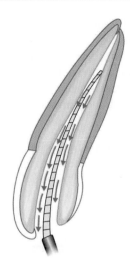

Fig. 16.21 Loose fitting needle providing space for optimal flow of irrigant.

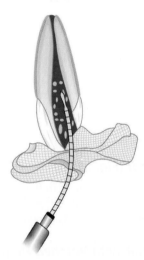

Fig. 16.22 A sterile gauge piece is placed near access opening to absorb excess irrigating solution and to check the debris from root canal.

- ❑ Blunted needle of 26 gauge or 27 gauge are preferred
- ❑ In case of small canals, deposit the solution in pulp chamber. Then file carries the solution into the canal. Capillary action of narrow canal will stain the solution. To remove the excess fluid, either the aspirating syringe or 2 × 2 inches folded gauge pad is placed near the chamber **(Fig. 16.22)**. To further dry the canal, remove the residual solution with paper point
- ❑ Regardless of delivery system, irrigants must never be forcibly inserted into apical tissues
- ❑ For effective cleaning, the needle delivering the solution should be in close proximity to the debris to be removed
- ❑ In case of large canals, tip of needle should be introduced until resistance is felt, then withdraw the needle 2–3 mm away from that point and irrigate the canal passively.

For removal of the solution, sterile gauge pack or paper points should be used

❑ In order to clean effectively in both anterior and posterior teeth canals, a blunt bend of 30° in the center of needle can be given to reach the optimum length to the canal

❑ Volume of irrigant is more important than concentration or type of irrigant

Various delivery systems for irrigation
- Stropko irrigator
- 27-gauge needle with notched tip
- Needle with bevel
- Monojet endodontic needle
  – 23-gauge
  – 27-gauge
- ProRinse—25-, 28-, 30-gauge probes
- Ultrasonic handpiece

Ideal properties of irrigating needle
An irrigating needle should
- Blunt
- Allow backflow
- Flexible
- Longer in length
- Easily available
- Cost-effective

Different Needle Designs

Stropko Irrigator (Fig. 16.23)

In this system, combination of delivery and recovery of irrigant is present in one probe. It is specially used when surgical operating microscope is used for procedures.

27-Gauge Needle with Notched Tip (Fig. 16.24)

This needle is preferred as its notched tip allows backflow of the solution and does not create pressure in the periapical area. So, it ensures optimum cleaning without damage to periapical area (**Figs. 16.25A and B**).

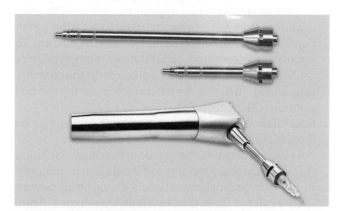

Fig. 16.23: Stropko irrigator

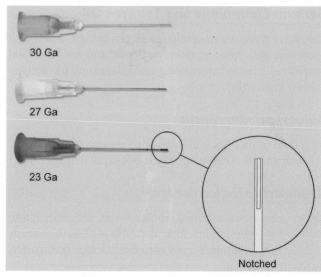

Fig. 16.24: Needle with notched tip.

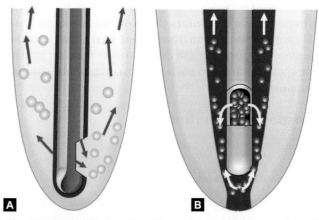

Figs. 16.25A and B: Needle with notched tip allows back flow of solution and does not create pressure in periapical area.

Needle with Bevel

Needle with bevel, if gets lodged into the canal, there is risk of forcing irrigant past the apex (**Fig. 16.26**).

Monojet Endodontic Needle

This is an efficient irrigant long blunt needle which can be inserted to the full length of the canal to ensure optimum cleaning (**Fig. 16.27**).

ProRinse probe

❑ Design of this needle produces upward flushing motion for complete canal irrigation. Its side port dispersal prevents solution and debris from being expressed through the apex and closed, rounded end reduces the risk of apical damage

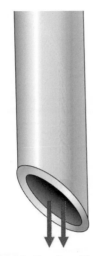

Fig. 16.26: Needle with bevel.

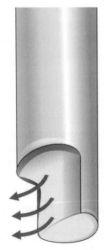

Fig. 16.27: Monojet endodontic needle.

Microbrushes and Ultrasonic

In this, bristles are attached to braided wires or flexible plastic cores. An optimal sized microbrush can be attached to rotary or ultrasonic handpiece. These microbrushes have tapers like nonstandardized gutta-percha cones. These are used in conjunction with sodium hypochlorite and EDTA to produce clean canals.

Endovac (Apical Negative Pressure Irrigation System) (Figs. 16.28A to D)

The EndoVac apical negative pressure irrigation system draws fluid apically by way of evacuation. Instead of applying positive pressure, it uses suction to pull the

irrigant down the canal. This system is comprised of the following parts:
1. **Master delivery tip**, which allows constant flow of irrigant without overflow
2. **Macrocannula**, which removes coarse debris left in the canal from instrumentation
3. **Microcannula**, which removes microscopic debris at the apical 1 mm via 28 gauze needle with 12 laser-drilled microscopic evacuation holes

Precautions

❑ Confirm the integrity of rubber dam seal
❑ Protect patient's eyes and clothing from sodium hypochlorite spill
❑ Never place the MDTs delivery tip closer than 5 mm from the coronal opening of canal
❑ For optimal use of EndoVac system, canal should be instrumented to minimum of 35 No. at a 4% taper or 45 No, if 2% taper
❑ Make sure no air bubbles are trapped in the prefilled syringes, as this will cause uncontrolled irrigant extrusion after releasing the plunger pressure

Positive Pressure versus Apical Negative Pressure (Figs. 16.29A and B)

Irrigation involves placement of an irrigating solution into the canal system and its evacuation from the tooth. It is done by placing an end-port or side-port needle into the canal and expressing solution out of the needle to be suctioned coronally. This creates a positive pressure system with force created at the end of the needle, which may lead to solution being forced into the periapical tissues. In an apical negative pressure irrigation system, the irrigation solution is expressed coronally and suction at the tip of the irrigation needle at the apex creates a current flow down the canal toward the apex and is drawn up the needle. But true apical negative pressure only occurs when the needle is used to aspirate irrigants from the apical termination of the root canal. The apical suction pulls irrigating solution down the canal walls toward the apex, creating a rapid, turbulent current force toward the terminus of the needle.

▌Intracanal Medicaments

Originally, endodontics was mainly a therapeutic procedure in which drugs were used to destroy microorganisms, fix or mummify vital tissue and affect the sealing of the root canal space.

The drugs commonly used were caustics such as phenol and its derivatives which were shown to produce adverse effects on the periapical tissues. Gradually, the reliance on drugs has been replaced by emphasis on thorough canal

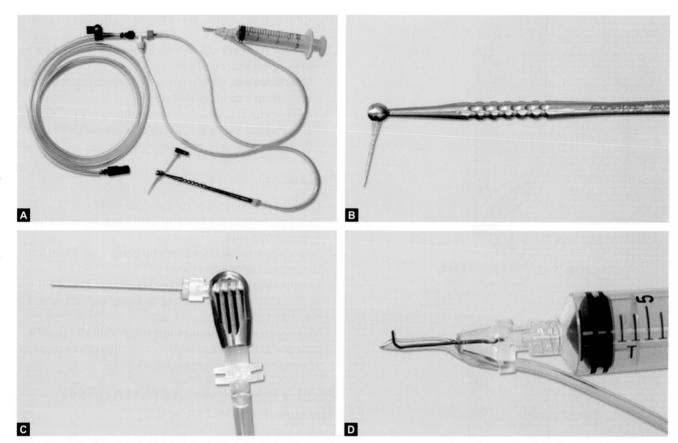

Figs. 16.28A to D: (A) The complete EndoVac system; (B) The macrocannula attached to its handle used for initial flushing of the coronal portion of the canal; (C) The microcannula attached to its handle used for irrigation at the apical portion of the canal; (D) The evacuation tip attached to a syringe. Irrigant is delivered by the metal needle, and excess is suctioned off through the plastic tubing surrounding the metal that is attached to the suction tubing.

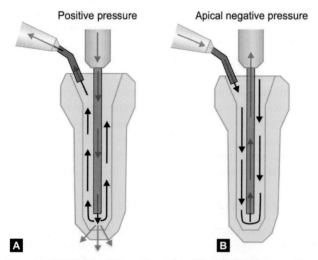

Figs. 16.29A and B: Comparison of positive and apical negative pressure in relation to endodontic irrigation.

debridement. But drugs are still being used as intratreatment dressings, although an ever increasing number of endodontists use them only for symptomatic cases.

Functions of Intracanal Medicaments

- ❑ Destroy the remaining bacteria and limit the growth of new arrivals
- ❑ In cases of apical periodontitis, for example, in cases of inflammation caused due to overinstrumentation

Indications of Using Intracanal Medicaments

- ❑ Remove the remaining microorganisms from the pulp space
- ❑ Dry the weeping canals
- ❑ Act as barrier against leakage from an interappointment dressing
- ❑ Neutralize the tissue debris

Desirable Properties of an Intracanal Medicaments

It should
- ❑ Be effective germicide and fungicide
- ❑ Be nonirritating to pulpal tissue

- ❏ Remain stable in the solution
- ❏ Have prolonged antimicrobial action
- ❏ Remain active in presence of blood, pus, etc.
- ❏ Have low surface tension
- ❏ Not interfere with repair of periapical tissue
- ❏ Non-staining to tooth
- ❏ Be capable of inactivation in the culture media
- ❏ Not induce immune response

Classification of Intracanal Medicaments

Classification

- • Essential oils: Eugenol
- • Phenolic compounds
  - • Phenol
  - • Paramonochlor
  - • Camphorated phenol
  - • Cresatin
  - • Aldehydes
    - – Formocresol
    - – Paraformaldehyde
    - – Glutaraldehyde
- • Calcium hydroxide
- • Halogens
  - • Chlorine–sodium Hypochlorite
  - • Iodine
    - – 2% I_2 in 5% KI solution, that is, Iodophors
    - – 5% I_2 in tincture of alcohol
- • Chlorhexidine gluconate
- • Antibiotics
- • Corticosteroid–antibiotic combination

Characteristics of Intracanal Medicaments

Essential Oils

Eugenol(Fig.16.30)

It has been used in endodontics for many years. It is a constituent of most root canal sealers and is used as a part of many temporary sealing agents. This substance is the chemical essence of oil of clove and is related to phenol. Effects of eugenol are dependent on tissue concentrations of the eugenol and can be divided into low dose (beneficial effects) and high dose (toxic effects).

Eugenol

Low dose (beneficial effects)	High dose (toxic effects)
• Inhibits prostaglandins synthesis	• Induces cell death
• Inhibits nerve activity	• Inhibits cell respiration
• Inhibits white cell chemotaxis	

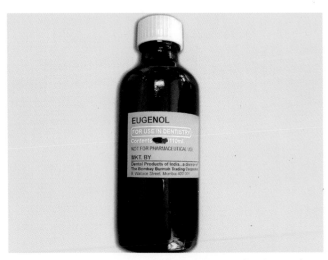

Fig. 16.30: Eugenol is used as constituent of sealers and temporary restorative materials.

Uses of eugenol
- ❏ Used as an intracanal medicament
- ❏ Used as root canal sealers
- ❏ Part of temporary sealing agents

Phenolic Compounds

Phenol

It was used for many years for its disinfectant and caustic action. However, it has strong inflammatory potential, so, at present, it is rarely used as an intracanal medicament.

Liquefied phenol (carbolic acid) consists of nine parts of phenol and one part of water.

Uses
- ❏ It is used for disinfection before periapical surgery
- ❏ It is also used for cauterizing tissue tags that resist removal with broaches or files

Parachlorophenol

Parachlorophenol (PCP) has been a very popular component of dressing as phenol is no longer used in endodontics because of its high toxicity-to-efficacy ratio.

Composition
- ❏ It is substitution product of phenol in which chlorine replaces one of the hydrogen atoms (C_6H_4OHCl)
- ❏ On trituration with gum camphor, these products combine to form an oily liquid

Concentration: 1% aqueous solution is preferred.

Uses: Used as a dressing of choice for infected tooth

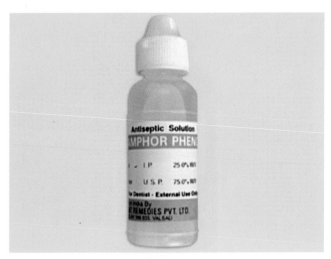

Fig. 16.31: Camphorphenol.

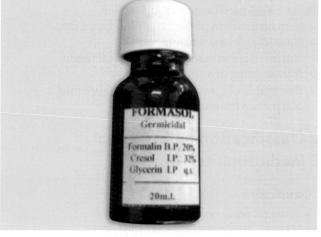

Fig. 16.32: Formocresol.

Camphorated Monoparachlorophenol (CMCP)

It is probably the most commonly used medicament in endodontics, presently, even though its use has decreased considerably in the past few years **(Fig. 16.31)**.

Composition

Two parts of PCP
+
Three parts gum camphor
↓
Camphorated monochlorophenol (CMCP)

Camphor is added to PCP because it

- Has diluent action
- Prolongs the antimicrobial effect
- Reduces the irritating effect of PCP
- Serves as a vehicle for the solution

Uses: Used as a dressing of choice for infected teeth.

Cresatin

Schilder and Amsterdam showed that Cresatin possesses same desirable qualities and actions as that of CMCP, but less irritating to periapical tissues

Composition: It is a clear, stable, oily liquid of low volatile nature known as metacresyl acetate.

Aldehydes

- Formaldehyde, paraformaldehyde and glutaraldehyde are commonly used intracanal medicaments in root canal therapy
- These are water-soluble protein denaturing agents and are considered among the most potent disinfectants
- They are mainly applied as disinfectants for surfaces and medical equipment which cannot be sterilized, but

they are quite toxic and allergic and some even may be carcinogenic

Formocresol

Formocresol contains formaldehyde as its main ingredient and is still widely used medicament for pulpotomy procedures in primary teeth but its toxic and mutagenic properties are of concern **(Fig. 16.32)**.

Composition of formocresol

- Formaldehyde—19%
- Cresol—35%
- Water and glycerine—46%

Uses: Used as dressing for pulpotomy to fix the retained pulpal tissue.

Paraformaldehyde

- It is polymeric form of formaldehyde and is commonly found as component of some root canal obturating material like endomethasone
- It slowly decomposes to give out formocresol, its monomer
- Its properties are similar to formaldehyde that is toxic, allergenic and genotoxic in nature

---

Clinical Tips

All phenolic and similar compounds are highly volatile with low surface tension. If they are placed on a cotton pellet in the pulp chamber, vapors will penetrate the entire canal preparation. Therefore, paper point is not needed for their application. Only small quantity of medication is needed for effectiveness, otherwise, chances of periapical irritation are increased.

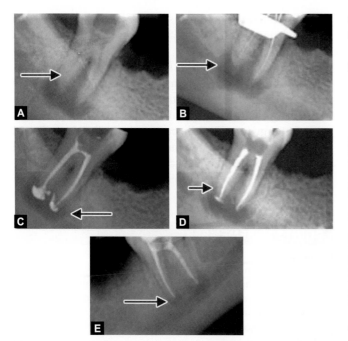

Figs. 16.33A to E Management of mandibular molar with periapical infection using Calcium hydroxide as intracanal medicament (A) Preoperative radiograph showing mandibular molar with periapical radiolucency; (B) Root canal treatment initiated and working length radiograph taken; (C) Ca(OH)2 placement for 2 months; (D) Obturation done; (E) Follow-up after 6 months shows healing of periapical area
Courtesy: Anil Dhingra.

Calcium Hydroxide (Figs. 16.33A to E)

Use of calcium hydroxide in endodontics was introduced by Hermann in 1920. It acts as a strong base in contact with aqueous solution and dissociate into calcium and hydroxyl ions.

Effects of Calcium Hydroxide

Physical
❑ Acts as a physical barrier for ingress of bacteria
❑ Destroys the remaining bacteria by limiting space for multiplication and holding substrate for growth

Chemical
❑ It shows antiseptic action because of its high pH and leaching action on necrotic pulp tissues. It also increases the pH of circumpulpal dentin when placed into the root canal
❑ Suppresses enzymatic activity and disrupts cell membrane
❑ Inhibits DNA replication by splitting it
❑ It hydrolyses the lipid part of bacterial lipopolysaccharide (LPS) and thus inactivates the activity of LPS. This is a desirable effect because dead cell wall material remains after the killing of bacteria which may cause infection

Calcium hydroxide is available in
❑ *Paste form:* Single paste or in combination with iodoform
❑ *Powder form:* Powder form is mixed with saline and anesthetic solution. For placement in root canals, it is coated with the help of paper points, spreaders, or lentulo spirals.

Indications of calcium hydroxide
• In weeping canals
• In treatment of phoenix abscess
• In resorption cases
• For apexification
• During pulpotomy
• For nonsurgical treatment of periapical lesion
• In cases of direct and indirect pulp capping
• As sealer for obturation
• To decrease postoperative pain after overinstrumentation, it is used in combination with Ledermix (1:1)

Advantages of Ca(OH)$_2$
❑ Inhibits root resorption
❑ Stimulates periapical healing
❑ Encourage mineralization

Disadvantages of Ca(OH)$_2$ as intracanal medicament
❑ Difficult to remove from canals
❑ Decreases setting time of zinc oxide eugenol based cements
❑ It has a little or no effect on severity of postobturation pain

Use of Calcium Hydroxide in Weeping Canal Cases

Sometimes, a tooth undergoing root canal treatment shows constant clear or reddish exudation associated with periapical radiolucency. Tooth can be asymptomatic or tender on percussion. When opened in next appointment, exudates stops but it again reappears in next appointment. This is known as "weeping canal."

In these cases, tooth with exudates is not ready for filling, since culture reports normally show negative bacterial growth, so antibiotics are of no help in such cases. For such teeth, dry the canals with sterile absorbent paper points and place calcium hydroxide in the canal. By next appointment, one finds a dry canal, ready for obturation. It happens because pH of periapical tissues is acidic in weeping stage which gets converted into basic pH by calcium hydroxide. Some say that caustic effect of calcium hydroxide burns the residual chronic inflamed tissue and also calcium hydroxide builds up the bone in the lesion due to its calcifying action.

Halogens

Halogens include chlorine and iodine which are used in various formulations in endodontics. They are potent oxidizing agents with rapid bactericidal effects.

Chlorine

Sodium hypochlorite: Disinfectant action of halogens is inversely proportional to their atomic weights. So, when compared to iodine, chlorine shows better disinfectant action. But chlorine disinfectants are not stable compounds because they interact rapidly with organic matter. Mentz found sodium hypochlorite as effective intracanal medicament as well as irrigant. As the activity of sodium hypochlorite is intense but of short duration, the compound should be changed in root canal every other day.

Iodides

Iodine is highly reactive in nature. It combines with proteins in a loosely bound manner so that its penetration is not impeded. It destroys microorganisms by forming salts that are *unfavorable* to the life of the organism. Iodine is used as iodine potassium iodide and in iodophors, which are organic iodine containing compounds that release iodine over time. It is also a very potent antibacterial agent of low toxicity but may stain clothing if spilled. It is used as an irrigating solution and short-term dressing in a 2% solution of iodine in 4% aqueous potassium iodide and as a constituent of gutta-percha points for filling.

2% Chlorhexidine Gluconate

Antibacterial activity of chlorhexidine gluconate is comparable to sodium hypochlorite. Substantivity, broad-spectrum activity and low toxicity of CHX make it suitable for irrigation. Attempts are being made to utilize its disinfecting properties in gutta-percha points.

PBSC Paste

As mentioned by Grossman, PBSC has enjoyed wide use among dentists. The constituents of PBSC paste are as follows:

Penicillin—effective against Gram-positive microorganisms
Bacitracin—effective against penicillin-resistant microorganisms
Streptomycin—effective against the Gram-negative microorganisms
Caprylate (sodium salt)—effective against fungi

Nystatin replaces sodium caprylate as the antifungal agent and is available in form of PBSN. Both are available in a paste form that may be injected into root canals or impregnated on paper points. Because there is no volatility, the drug must be placed in the canal to have effect in that area.

PBSC may interfere with subsequent culturing procedures; therefore, penicillinase may be added to culture media to inactivate penicillin. Reports of allergic reaction to the drug have been presented, if the patient reports history of allergy to any of the constituents, the drug should not be used. With the decline in popularity of intracanal drugs in general and because of the potential for sensitivity due to topical use of antibiotics, PBSN largely has fallen into disuse.

POINTS TO REMEMBER

PBSC paste
- By Grossman
- **P**enicillin—against Gram-positive microorganisms
- **B**acitracin—against penicillin-resistant microorganisms
- **S**treptomycin—against the Gram-negative microorganism
- **C**aprylate (sodium salt)—against fungi

PBSN
- **N**ystatin—replaces sodium caprylate as antifungal agent
- PBSC interferes culturing procedures—penicillinase is added to culture media to inactivate penicillin

Sulfonamides

Sulfanilamide and sulfathiazole are used as medicaments by mixing with sterile distilled water or by placing a moistened paper point into a fluffed jar containing the powder. Yellowish tooth discoloration has been reported after use. Sulfonamides are usually recommended while giving closed dressing in a tooth which had been left open after an acute periapical abscess.

N$_2$ by Sargenti

It is a compound consisting of paraformaldehyde as the main ingredient. It contains eugenol, phenyl mercuric borate and perfumes. Antibacterial effect of N$_2$ is short lived and dissipated in 7–10 days.

Grossman Paste

Composition
- Potassium penicillin G	1,000,000 units
- Bacitracin	100,00
- Streptomycin sulfate	1.0 g
- Sodium caprylate	1.0 g
- Silicon fluid	3 mL
- Nystatin	10,000 units

Chloramines-T

It is a chlorine compound with good antimicrobial. It is used in the concentration of 5%. It remains stable for long period of time and is used to disinfect gutta-percha points. It can be used in patients allergic to iodine.

Quaternary Ammonium Compounds

These are positively charged compounds which attract negatively charged microorganisms; they have low surface tension, for example, aminoacridine.

Aminoacridine is a mild antiseptic which is more effective than creation but less effective than CMCP. It is used more as an irritant than intracranial medicament.

Corticosteroid–Antibiotic Combinations

- ❑ Medications that combine antibiotic and corticosteroid elements are highly effective in cases of overinstrumentation
- ❑ They must be placed into the inflamed periapical tissue by a paper point or reamer
- ❑ Tetra-Cortril, Cortisporin, Mycolog and other combinations are available for their use in endodontics
- ❑ Ledermix is one of best known antibiotic-corticosteroid combination.
- ❑ Schroeder and Triadan developed Ledermix in 1960. It contains an antibiotic demeclocycline—HCl (3.2%) and a corticosteroid, triamcinolone acetonide (1%), in a polyethylene glycol base.
- ❑ Corticosteroid constituent reduces the periapical inflammation and gives almost instant relief of pain to the patient who complains of extreme tenderness to percussion after canal instrumentation
- ❑ Antibiotic constituents present in the corticosteroid–antibiotic combination prevent the overgrowth of microorganisms when the inflammation subsides

Root canal disinfectants

Halogens

Chlorine
Irrigating solution: Sodium hypochlorite 0.5–5.25% in aqueous solution.

Iodine
Irrigating solution: 2% I_2 in 5% KI aqueous solution; iodophors.
Surface disinfection: 5% I_2 in tincture of alcohol.

Chlorhexidine
Chlorhexidine gluconate Irrigating solution: 2.0% aqueous solution.

Calcium hydroxide
Dressing: Aqueous or viscous formulation with varying amounts of salts added. Antibacterials like iodine, chlorophenols, chlorhexidine may also be added.

Aldehydes
Formocresol
Dressing: 19% formaldehyde, 35% cresol, 46% water and glycerine.

Phenols
Camphorated phenol
Paramonochlorphenol (PMCP)
Irrigating solution; 2% aqueous solution.
Dressing: CMCP; 65% camphor, 35% PMCP.

Eugenol
Formation of electrochemically activated solution.

Placement of Intracanal Medicament

- ❑ Copiously irrigate the canal to remove debris present if any **(Fig. 16.34A)**
- ❑ Place the master apical file in the canal **(Fig. 16.34B)**
- ❑ Dry the canal using absorbent paper points **(Fig. 16.34C)**
- ❑ Place the intracanal medicament on a sterile cotton pellet and place it in the pulp chamber **(Fig. 16.34D)**
- ❑ Over this, another sterile cotton pellet is placed, which is finally sealed with a temporary restorative material **(Fig. 16.34E)**

Limitations of Intracanal Medicaments

- ❑ For an intracanal, medicament to be effective, it should remain active during the time of interappointment, which does not happen not in every case
- ❑ Clinical effectiveness of sustained release delivery systems is unknown
- ❑ Therapeutic action of medicament depends upon its direct contact with tissues, but it can be prevented due to presence of organic tissue/matter

Conclusion

The success of endodontic treatment depends on the eradication of microbes from the root-canal system and prevention of reinfection. Instrumentation and irrigation are the most important parts for successful endodontic treatment. Irrigant performs many functions, the most important of which are to dissolve tissue and to have an antimicrobial effect. Commonly used during cleaning and shaping include sodium hypochlorite, chlorhexidine, EDTA, MTAD etc. None of these irrigants has all of the characteristics of an ideal irrigant. Many chemicals used for irrigation have been chemically modified and several mechanical devices have been developed to improve the penetration and effectiveness of irrigation. Intracanal medicaments have been used to disinfect root canals between appointments and reduce interappointment pain. The major intracanal medications

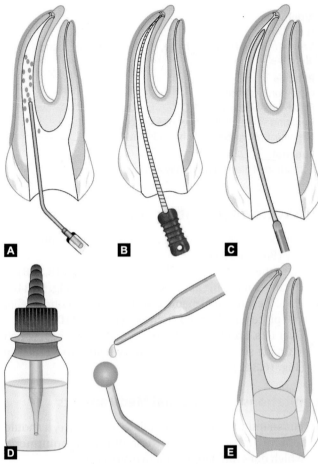

Figs. 16.34A to E: (A) Copiously irrigate the canal; (B) Place the master apical file in the canal; (C) Dry the canal using absorbent paper points; (D) Intracanal medicament; (E) Intracanal medicament on a cotton pellet is applied and placed in pulp chamber. Over it, a sterile dry cotton pellet is placed which is finally sealed with a temporary filling material.

currently used in endodontics include calcium hydroxide, though search for an ideal material and/or technique to completely clean infected root canals continues.

Questions

1. What are properties of ideal irrigating solutions?
2. What are functions of irrigating solution? Enumerate various irrigants used in endodontics.
3. Define chelating agents. Write in detail about EDTA.
4. Classify intracanal medicaments. What are ideal requirements for intracanal medicament?
5. Explain role of calcium hydroxide in endodontics.
6. Write short notes on
   - Sodium hypochlorite
   - Hydrogen peroxide

- MTAD
- Ozonated water
- Grossman paste
- Ultrasonic irrigation
- Enumerate newer irrigating solutions
- Electrochemically activated solution
- Ruddle's solution
- Photoactivated disinfection
- Q-mix
- Discuss different needle designs
- EndoVac
- Formocresol
- PBSC paste

Bibliography

1. Abbott PV. Medicaments: aids to success in endodontics. Part I. A review of literature. Aust Dent J 1990;35:438–48.
2. Bryce G, Donnell DO, Ready D. Contemporary root canal irrigants are able to disrupt and eradicate single- and dual-species biofilms. J Endod 2009;35:1243–8.
3. Chong BS, Pitt Ford TR. The role of intracanal medication in root canal treatment. Int Endod J 1996;25:97–106.
4. Estrela C, Estrela CR, Barbin EL, et al. Mechanism of action of sodium hypochlorite. Braz Dent J 2002;13113–7.
5. Foreman PC, Barnes IE. Review of calcium hydroxide. Int Endod J 1990;23:283–97.
6. Grossman LI. Polyantibiotic treatment of pulpless teeth. J Am Dent Assoc 1951;43:265–78.
7. Haenni S, Schmidlin PR, Mueller B, et al. Chemical and anti-microbial properties of calcium hydroxide mixed irrigating solutions. Int Endod J 2003;36:100–5.
8. Kandaswamy D, Venkateshbabu N. Root canal irrigants. J Conserv Dent 2010;13(4):256–64.
9. Krithkmadatta J, Indira R, Dorothykalyani AL. Disinfection of dentinal tubules with 2 percent chlorhexidine, 2 percent metronidazole, bioactive glass when compared with calcium hydroxide as intracanal medicaments. J Endod 2007;33:1473–6.
10. Kuruvilla JR, Kamath MP. Antimicrobial activity of 2.5% sodium hypochlorite and 0.2% chlorhexidine gluconate separately and combined, as endodontic irrigants. J Endod 1998;24:472–76.
11. Mello I, Kammerer BA, Yoshimoto D. Influence of final rinse technique on ability of ethylenediaminetetraacetic acid of removing smear layer. J Endod 2010;36:512–4.
12. Pallotta RC, Ribeiro MS, de Lima Machado ME. Determination of the minimum inhibitory concentration of four medicaments used as intracanal medication. Aust Endod J 2007;33:107–11.
13. Retamozo B, Shabahang S, Johnson N. Minimum contact time and concentration of sodium hypochlorite required to eliminate *Enterococcus faecalis*. J Endod 2010;36:520–3.

Working Length Determination

Introduction

Determination of accurate working length and its maintenance during cleaning and shaping procedures are key factors for successful endodontic treatment. The cleaning, shaping, and obturation cannot be accomplished accurately unless the working length is determined correctly. Thus, predictable endodontic success demands an accurate working length determination of the root canal. The procedure for establishment of working length should be performed with skill, using techniques which have shown to give valuable and accurate results and are practical and successful.

Definitions

According to endodontic glossary, *working length* is defined as "the distance from a coronal reference point to a point at which canal preparation and obturation should terminate" **(Figs. 17.1A and B)**.

Reference point: Reference point is the site on occlusal or the incisal surface from which measurements are made.
❑ It should be stable and easily visualized during preparation
❑ Usually, it is the highest point on the incisal edge of anterior teeth and buccal cusp of posterior teeth **(Fig. 17.2)**
❑ It should not change between the appointments. Therefore to have stable reference point, undermined cusps and restorations should be reduced before access preparation
   Anatomic apex is "tip or end of root determined morphologically."
   Radiographic apex is "tip or end of root determined radiographically."

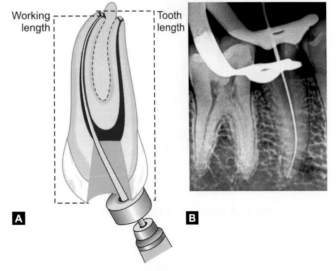

Figs. 17.1A and B Working length is distance from coronal reference point to a point where instrumentation and obturation should end: (A) Line diagram; (B) Radiograph showing working length determination.

Apical foramen is the main apical opening of the root canal which may be located away from anatomic or radiographic apex.

Apical constriction (minor apical diameter) is the apical portion of root canal having narrowest diameter. It is usually 0.5–1 mm short of apical foramen **(Fig. 17.3)**. The minor diameter widens apically to major diameter (apical foramen) **(Fig. 17.4)**. Dummer classified apical constriction as four types which need to be analyzed to prevent over and under-instrumentation **(Fig. 17.5)**.

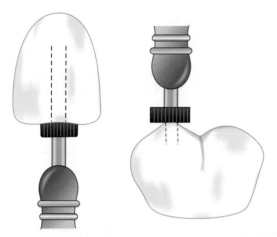

Fig. 17.2 Usually, the reference point is the highest point on incisal edge of anterior teeth and buccal cusp tip of posterior teeth.

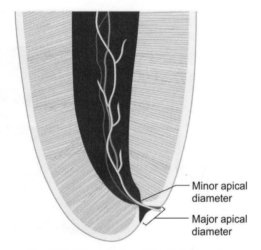

Minor apical diameter

Major apical diameter

Fig. 17.3 Minor and major apical diameter.

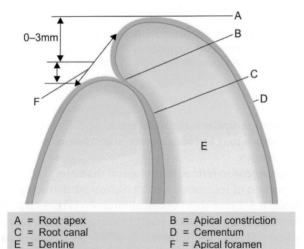

A = Root apex	B = Apical constriction
C = Root canal	D = Cementum
E = Dentine	F = Apical foramen

Fig. 17.4 Anatomy of root apex.

Cementodentinal junction (CDJ) is the region where the cementum and dentin are united, the point at which cemental surface terminates at or near the apex of tooth.

❑ It is not always necessary that CDJ always coincide with apical constriction (**Fig. 17.6**).

❑ Location of CDJ ranges from 0.5 mm to 3 mm short of anatomic apex.

Historical Perspectives

At the end of 19th century		Working length was usually calculated when file was placed in the canal and patient experienced pain
1899	Kells	Introduced X-rays in dentistry
1918	Hatton	Microscopically studied the diseased periodontal tissues
1929	Coolidge	Studied the anatomy of root apex in relation to treatment problem
1955	Kuttler	Microscopically investigated the root apices
1962	Sunada	Found electrical resistance between periodontium and oral mucous membrane
1969	Inove	Significant contribution in evolution of electronic apex locator

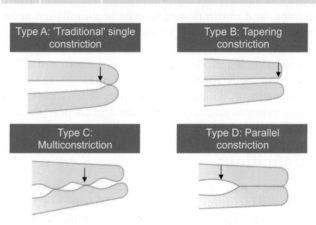

Figs. 17.5 Dummer classification of *apical constriction*.

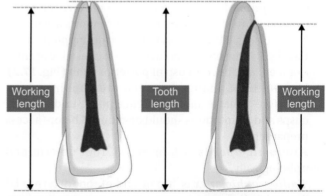

Figs. 17.6 CDJ need not to terminate at apical constriction. It can be 0.5–3 mm short of the apex.

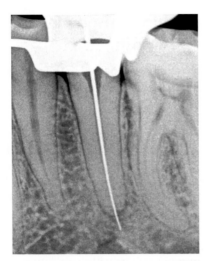

Fig. 17.7 Radiograph showing working length beyond the apex.

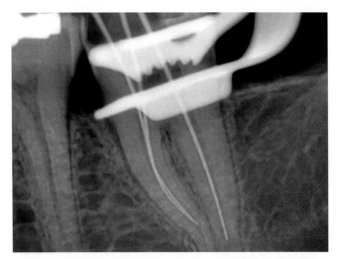

Fig. 17.8 Radiograph showing working length short of apex.

▌Significance of Working Length

❑ Working length determines how far into canal instruments can be placed and worked.
❑ If placed within correct limits, it plays an important role in determining the success of the treatment
❑ It affects the degree of pain and discomfort the patient will experience during or after the treatment.
❑ If proper care is not taken, over or underinstrumentation can occur.

Consequences of overinstrumentation

Overinstrumentation means extension of instruments into periapical tissue beyond apical constriction **(Fig. 17.7)**. It may cause
❑ Pain as a result of acute inflammatory response from mechanical damage to the periapical tissue
❑ In infected teeth, overinstrumentation leads to the extrusion of microbes and infected debris which aggravate the inflammatory responses in the periapical tissue
❑ Overfilling that causes mechanical and chemical irritation of the periapical tissue along with foreign body reaction
❑ Prolonged healing time and lower success rate because of incomplete regeneration of cementum, periodontal ligament, and alveolar bone

Consequences of underinstrumentation

❑ Underinstrumentation is working to a level shorter than actual length, leaving the apical part of the canal without proper instrumentation **(Fig. 17.8)**. It may cause:
❑ Accumulation of infected debris apically which impairs or prevents healing
❑ Incomplete apical seal which supports existence of viable bacteria resulting in poor prognosis of the treatment

▌Working Width

Working width is defined as "initial and postinstrumentation horizontal dimensions of the root canal system at working length and other levels." Minimum initial working width corresponds to initial apical file size which binds at working length. Maximum final working width corresponds to the master apical file size.

> **Definitions:**
> MinIWW(N): Minimal initial horizontal dimension *N* mm short of working length
> MinIWW0: Minimal initial horizontal dimension at working length
> MaxIWW(N): Maximal initial horizontal dimension *N* mm short of working length
> MaxIWW0: Maximal initial horizontal dimension at working length

Traditional Concept

For many years, two guidelines were considered for instrumentation:
1. Enlarge the root canal at least three sizes beyond the first instrument that binds the canal
2. Enlarge the canal until it is clean. It is indicated by white dentinal shavings on the instrument flutes

However, these guidelines are not considered sole criteria in all the cases. The color of dentinal shavings is not indication of presence of infected dentin. An ideal enlargement should provide debris removal throughout the canal and facilitate irrigation to the level of minor constriction. Final apical filing should not cause any apical transportation.

Current Concept

Ideally, master apical file, that is, the final file of prepared canal cannot be standardized and it varies according to different cases. Nowadays, use of NiTi rotary files with greater taper allows irrigants to reach apical third more effectively, so it is always recommended to prevent overenlargement of minor constriction. It can result in increased chances of preparation errors like extrusion of irrigants, obturating material, etc.

Final enlargement of the canal depends on the following factors:

- Gauging of canal: Initial canal width guides to a large extent the master apical file. If gauging file is 10 N, apex cannot be prepared to No. 60 MAF
- Presence or absence of periradicular pathology
- Vitality of the pulp
- Canal configuration like degree of curvature, C-shaped canal, etc.

Directional Stop Attachments

- Most commonly used stoppers for endodontic instruments are silicon rubber stops, though stop attachments can be made up of metal, plastic, or silicon rubber
- Stop attachments are available in tear drop or round shapes
- Irrespective of shape, the stop should be placed perpendicular to the instrument not at any other direction (oblique) so as to avoid variation in working length
- Advantage of using tear-shaped stopper is that in curved canal, it can be used to indicate the canal curvature by placing its apex toward the direction of curve

Different Methods of Working Length Determination

Methods of determining working length	
Radiographic methods	*Nonradiographic methods*
• Best's method	• Digital tactile sense
• Bregman's method	• Apical periodontal sensitivity
• Bramante's method	• Paper point method
• Grossman formula	• Electronic apex locators
• Ingle's method	
• Weine's method	
• Kuttler's method	
• Radiographic grid	
• Endometric probe	
• Direct digital radiography	
• Xeroradiography	
• Subtraction radiography	

Radiographic Method of Working Length Determination

Radiographic apex has been used as the termination point in working length determination since many years and it has showed promising results. However, there are two schools of thoughts regarding this:

Those who follow this concept say cementodentinal junction is impossible to locate clinically and the radiographic apex is the only reproducible site available for length determination. According to it, a patent root tip and larger files kept within the tooth may result in excellent prognosis.

Those who do not follow this concept say that the position of radiographic apex is not reproducible. Its position depends on number of factors like angulation of tooth, position of film, film holder, length of X-ray cone, and presence of adjacent anatomic structures, etc.

When radiographs are used in determining working length, the quality of the image is important for accurate interpretations. Among the two commonly used techniques, paralleling technique has been shown to be superior compared to bisecting angle technique in determination and reproduction of apical anatomy. As the angle increases away from parallel, the quality of image decreases. This occurs because as the angle increases, the tissue that X-rays must pass through includes a greater percentage of bone mass, therefore, the root anatomy becomes less apparent.

Clinical Tips

- When two superimposed canals are present (e.g., buccal and palatal canals of maxillary premolar, mesial canals of mandibular molar), one should take the following steps:
  - Take two individual radiographs with instrument placed in each canal
  - Take radiograph at different angulations, usually 20–40° at horizontal angulation
  - Insert two different instruments, e.g., K file in one canal, H file/reamer in other canal, and take radiograph at different angulations
  - Apply SLOB rule; expose tooth from mesial or distal horizontal angle; canal which moves to same direction is lingual, whereas canal that moves to opposite direction is buccal
- In curved canals, canal length is reconfirmed because final working length may shorten up to 1 mm as canal is straightened out by instrumentation

Advantages

- Anatomy of the tooth and curvature of root canal can be seen on radiograph
- Radiograph helps in analyzing the relationship with adjacent teeth and anatomic structures.

Disadvantages
- Varies with different observers
- Superimposition of anatomical structures
- Two-dimensional view of three-dimensional object
- Cannot interpret if apical foramen has buccal or lingual exit
- Risk of radiation exposure
- Time consuming
- Limited accuracy

Clinical Tips

Orthopantograph (OPG) radiographs are not advocated for calculating tentative working length because gross magnification of 13–28% employed in OPG may lead to errors in calculation of accurate readings.

Best's Method

It was introduced in 1960 by Best. In this, a steel 10 mm pin is fixed to the labial surfaces of root with utility wax, keeping it parallel to the long axis of the tooth
- Radiograph is taken and measurements were made using a gauge

Bregman's Method

- In this, 25-mm length flat probes are prepared which have a steel blade fixed with acrylic resin as a stop, leaving a free end of 10 mm for placing in root canal
- After this, radiograph is taken and working length is measured using the following formula:
$$RLT = RLI \times ALT/ALI$$
    RLT : Real length of tooth
    RLI : Real length of instrument
    ALT : Apparent length of tooth
    ALI : Apparent length of instrument

Bramante's Method

- It was introduced in 1974. Here, stainless steel probes are used, which are bent at a right angle at one end that is inserted into acrylic resin
- Probe is placed in the canal such that resin touches the cusp tip and bent part of probe is parallel to the mesiodistal diameter of the crown so that it can be seen on radiograph
- On the radiograph, the following reference points are made:
    A: Internal angle of intersection of incisal and radicular probe segment
    B: Apical part of probe
    C: Apex of tooth

Now working length is calculated in two ways:
1. From radiograph, AB (radiographic length of probe) and AC (radiographic length of tooth) and actual length of probe are measured and working length of tooth is calculated using the following equation (**Fig. 17.9**):
$$CRD = CRS \times CAD/CAS$$
    CRD: Real tooth length
    CRS: Real probe length
    CAD: Radiographic tooth length
    CAS: Radiographic probe length
2. Measure the distance between apical end of probe and radiographic apex and add or subtract accordingly that can be correct working length

Grossman Method/Mathematical Method of Working Length Determination

It is based on simple mathematical formulations to calculate the working length. In this, an instrument is inserted into the canal, stopper is fixed to the reference point and radiograph is taken. The formula to calculate actual length of the tooth is as follows:

$$\frac{\text{Actual length of the tooth}}{\text{Actual length of the instrument}} = \frac{\text{Apparent length of tooth in radiograph}}{\text{Apparent length of instrument in radiograph}}$$

$$\text{Actual length of the tooth} = \frac{\text{Actual length of the instrument} \times \text{Apparent length of tooth in radiograph}}{\text{Apparent length of instrument in radiograph}}$$

In the formula, three variables are known and by applying the formula, fourth variable, that is, the actual length of tooth can be calculated.

Ingle's Method of Length Determination

- Before access opening, fractured cusps, cusps weakened by caries, or restorations are reduced to avoid the fracture of weakened enamel during the treatment. This will avoid the loss of initial reference point and thus working length (**Figs. 17.9A and B**)
- Measure the estimated working length from preoperative periapical radiograph
- Adjust stopper of instrument to this estimated working length and place it in the canal up to the adjusted stopper (**Figs. 17.10A to D**)

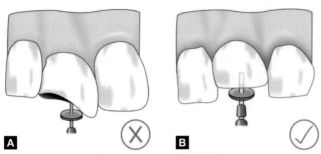

Figs. 17.9A and B Reference point should not be made of fractured tooth surface or carious tooth structure. These should be first removed for avoiding loss in working length.

- Take the radiograph
- On the radiograph, measure the difference between the tip of the instrument and root apex. Add or subtract this length to the estimated working length to get the new working length
- Correct working length is finally calculated by subtracting 1 mm from this new length

Weine's Modification

Weine modified calculation of working length according to presence or abscence of resorption as given below **(Fig. 17.11)**

- No resorption – subtract 1 mm
- Periapical bone resorption - subtract 1.5 mm
- Periapical bone + root apex resorption – subtract 2 mm

Kuttler's Method

In 1955, Kuttler described apical area both under anatomic and histological point of view. He discussed and

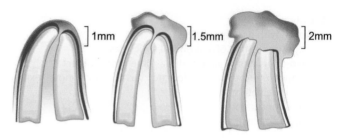

Fig. 17.11 Weine's modification in working length by subtraction in the case of root resorption.

explained dentinocemental junction (DCJ), anatomic apex, and apical foramen.

DCJ is explained histologically but not clinically. *Anatomic apex* is the apex of tooth and is just a geometric reference. *Apical Constriction (Minor Diameter)* is the narrowest part of root canal short of apical foramina or radiographic apex.

Apical foramen (Major diameter) is the main apical opening of root canal through which blood vessels enter the canal. It's diameter is almost double the apical constriction giving it a funnel shape appearance, which has been described as **morning glory or hyperbolic (Fig. 17.12)**. Apical foramen may not always be located at the centre of the apex. It may exit mesial, distal, buccal, or lingual.

According to Kuttler, canal preparation should terminate at apical constriction (minor diameter).

POINTS TO REMEMBER

In young patients, average distance between minor and major diameter is 0.524 mm, whereas in older patients it is 0.66 mm.

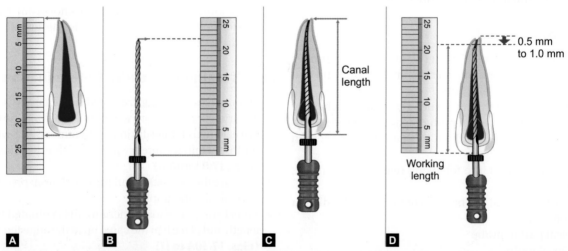

Figs. 17.10A to D Working length measurement by Ingle's method: (A) Measure estimated working length from preoperative radiograph; (B) adjust stopper of instrument to this length; (C) place it in canal up to the adjusted stopper; (D) take the radiograph and measure the difference between tip of the instrument and root apex. Add or subtract this length to estimated working length to get the new length.

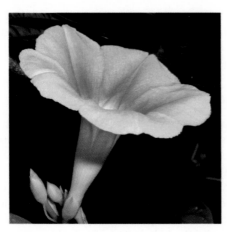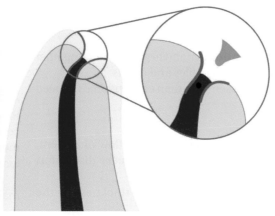

Fig. 17.12 Minor diameter widens apically towards major diameter giving rise to funnel shape appearance, described as Morning glory or hyperbolic.

Technique

- ❏ Locate minor and major diameter on preoperative radiograph
- ❏ Estimate length of roots from preoperative radiograph
- ❏ Estimate canal width on radiograph. If the canal is narrow, use 10 or 15 size instrument. If it is of average width, use 20 or 25 size instruments. If the canal is wide, use 30 or 35 size instrument
- ❏ Insert the selected file in the canal up to the estimated canal length and take a radiograph
- ❏ If the file is too long or short by >1 mm from minor diameter, readjust the file and take second radiograph
- ❏ If the file reaches major diameter, subtract 0.5 mm from it for younger patients and 0.67 for older patients

Advantages
- ❏ Minimal errors
- ❏ Has shown many successful cases

Disadvantages
- ❏ Time consuming and complicated
- ❏ Requires excellent quality radiographs

Radiographic Grid

- ❏ It was designed by Everett and Fixott in 1963. It is a simple method in which a millimeter grid is superimposed on the radiograph **(Fig. 17.13)**
- ❏ This overcomes the need for calculation
- ❏ But it is not a good method if the radiograph is bent during exposure

Endometric Probe

- ❏ In this method, one uses the graduations on diagnostic file which are visible on radiograph
- ❏ But its main disadvantage is that the smallest file size to be used is number 25

Direct Digital Radiography

Here, digital image is formed which is represented by spatially distributed set of discrete sensors and pixels.

Two types of digital radiography:
1. Radiovisiography
2. Phosphor imaging system

Xeroradiography

- ❏ It is a new method for recording images without film in which image is recorded on an aluminum plate coated with selenium particles
- ❏ Plate is removed from the cassette and subjected to relaxation which removes old images, then these are electrostatically charged and inserted into the cassette
- ❏ Radiations are projected on film which cause selective discharge of the particles
- ❏ This forms the latent image and is converted to a positive image by a process called "development" in the processor unit

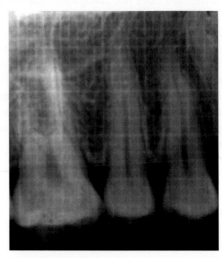

Fig. 17.13 Radiographic grid superimposed on a radiograph.

Advantages

❑ This technique offers "edge enhancement" and good detail
❑ Ability to have both positive and negative prints together
❑ Improves visualization of files and canals
❑ It is two times more sensitive than conventional D-speed films

Disadvantages

❑ Since saliva may act as a medium for flow of current, the electric charge over the film may cause discomfort to the patient
❑ Exposure time varies according to thickness of the plate
❑ The process of development cannot be delayed beyond 15 min

Nonradiographic Methods of Working Length Determination

Digital Tactile Sense

In this, clinician may see an increase in resistance as file reaches the apical 2–3 mm.

Advantages
❑ Time saving
❑ No radiation exposure

Disadvantages
❑ Does not always provide the accurate readings
❑ In the case of narrow canals, one may feel increased resistance as file approaches apical 2–3 mm
❑ In the case of teeth with immature apex, instrument can go periapically

Apical Periodontal Sensitivity Test

❑ This method is based on patient's response to pain
❑ But this method does not always provide the accurate readings
❑ For example, in the case of narrow canals, instrument may feel increased resistance as file approaches apical 2–3 mm and in the case of teeth with immature apex, instrument can go beyond the apex
❑ In the cases of canal with necrotic pulp, instrument can pass beyond apical constriction and in the case of vital or inflamed pulp, pain may occur several mm before periapex is crossed by the instrument

Paper Point Measurement Method

❑ In this method, paper point is gently passed in the root canal to estimate the working length
❑ It is most reliable in cases of open apex where apical constriction is lost because of perforation or resorption

❑ Moisture of blood present on the apical part of paper point indicates that paper point has passed beyond estimated working length
❑ It is used as supplementary method

Electronic Apex Locators

Electronic apex locator (EAL) is used to locate the apical constriction or cementodentinal junction, or apical foramen, but not the radiographic apex. Hence, the term apex locator is a misnomer one.

Ability to distinguish between minor diameter and major diameter of apical terminus is the most important for creation of apical control zone. *Apical control zone* is mechanical alteration of apical terminus of root canal space which provides resistance and retention form to the obturating material against the condensation pressure of obturation.

Components of EALs
❑ Lip clip
❑ File clip
❑ Electronic device
❑ Cord which connects above three parts

Historical review of EALs

1918	Custer	Use of electric current for working length
1942	Suzuki	Studied flow of current through teeth of dogs
1960's	Gordon	Use of clinical device for measurement of length
1962	Sunada	Found electrical resistance between periodontium and oral mucous membranes
1969	Inove	Significant contribution in evolution of EAL
1996	Pratten and McDonald	Compared the efficacy of three parallel radiographs and Endex apex locators in cadaver

Advantages of apex locators
• Provide objective information with high degree of accuracy
• Accurate in reading (90–98% accuracy)
• Some apex locators are also available in combination with pulp tester and can be used to test pulp vitality

Disadvantages of apex locators
• Can provide inaccurate readings in the following cases:
  – Presence of pulp tissue in canal
  – Too wet or too dry canal
  – Use of narrow file
  – Blockage of canal
  – Incomplete circuit
  – Low battery
• Chances of overestimation
• May pose problem in teeth with immature apex
• Incorrect readings in teeth with periapical radiolucencies and necrotic pulp associated with root resorption, etc. because of lack of viable periodontal ligament

Uses of apex locators
❑ Provide objective information with high degree of accuracy
❑ Useful in conditions where apical portion of canal system is obstructed by
  • Impacted teeth
  • Zygomatic arch
  • Tori
  • Excessive bone density
  • Overlapping roots
  • Shallow palatal vault
❑ Useful in patients who cannot tolerate X-ray film placement because of gag reflex
❑ Useful in pregnant patients, to reduce the radiation exposure
❑ Useful in children who may not tolerate taking radiographs, disabled patients and patients who are heavily sedated
❑ Valuable tool for
  • Detecting site of root perforations
  • Diagnosis of external and internal resorption which have penetrated root surface
  • Detection of horizontal and vertical root fracture
  • Determination of perforations caused during postpreparation
  • Testing pulp vitality

Contraindications to the use of apex locator
Older apex locators were contraindicated in the patients who have cardiac pacemaker functions. Electrical stimulation to such patients could interfere with pacemaker function. But this problem has been overcome in newer generation of apex locators.

Classification of EALs

McDonald[1] classified apex locators on the basis of type of current flow as following:

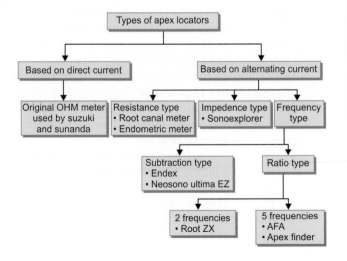

Classification According to Generations of EALs (Evolution of EALs)

1. **First-generation apex locator (resistance apex locator)**
   • It is also known as resistance apex locator which measures opposition to flow of direct current, that is, resistance
   • It is based on the *principle* that resistance offered by periodontal ligament, and oral mucous membrane is the same, that is, 6.5 kΩ
   • Examples of 1st generation apex locators are root canal meter, endometric meter (Onuki Medical Co., Japan), Dentometer, Endo Radar.

Technique for Using Resistance-Based EAL
❑ Turn on the device and attach the lip clip near the arch being treated. Hold a 15 number file and insert it approximately 0.5 mm into sulcus of tooth (like periodontal (PD) probe). Adjust the control knob until the reference needle is centered on the meter scale and produces audible beeps. Note this reading **(Figs. 17.14A to D)**
❑ Using preoperative radiograph, estimate the working canal width. Clean the canal if bleeding form vital pulp is excessive, dry it with paper points
❑ Insert the file into canal unless the reference needle moves from extreme left to center of scale and alarm beeps sound. Reset the stop at reference point and record the lengths
❑ Take the radiograph with file in place at the length indicated by apex locator. If length is longer/shorter, it is possible that preoperative film can be elongated or apex locator is inaccurate

---

Advantages
• Easily operated
• Digital read out
• Audible indication
• Detect perforation
• Can be used with K-file
• May incorporate pulp tester

Disadvantages
• Requires a dry field
• Patient sensitivity
• Requires calibration
• Requires good contact with lip clip
• Cannot estimate beyond 2 mm
• File should fit snugly in the canal
• File should not contact metal restorations

---

2. **Second-generation apex locator (impedance-based apex locator)/low-frequency apex locator**
   • Inoue introduced the concept of *impedance-based apex locator* which measure opposition to flow of alternating current or impedance
   • This apex locator indicates the apex when two impedance values approach each other. Examples of second-generation apex locators are:

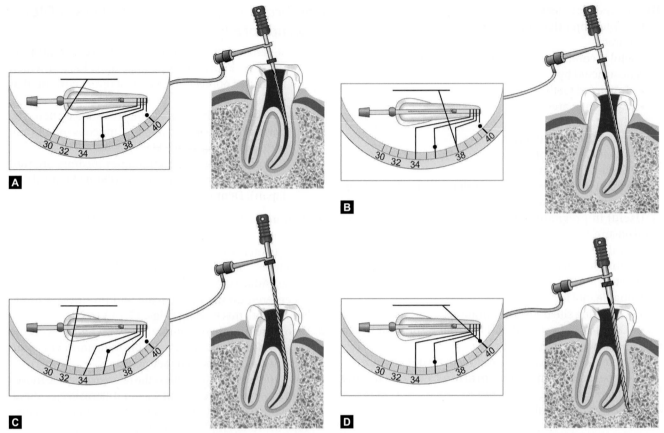

Figs. 17.14A to D (A) File being introduced in the canal; (B) Steady increase in the reading as file approaches apex; (C) Reading showing that file has reached at apex; (D) Sudden increase in reading indicates perforation.

- Sonoexplorer
- Apex finder
- Exact-A-Pex
- Endoanalyzer (combination of apex locator and pulp tester)
- Digipex (has digital LED indicator but requires calibration)

Advantages
- Does not require lip clip
- No patient sensitivity
- Analog meter
- Detects perforations

Disadvantages
- No digital read out
- Difficult to operate
- Canal should be free of electroconductive irrigants and tissue fluids
- Requires coated probes
- Cannot use files

3. **Third-generation apex locator/high-frequency apex locator**

- It is based on the fact that different sites in canal give difference in impedance between high (8 kHz) and low (400 Hz) frequencies
- The difference in impedance is least in the coronal part of canal
- As the probe goes deeper into canal, difference increases
- It is the greatest at the cementodentical junction
- Since impedance of a given circuit may be substantially influenced by the frequency of current flow, these are also known as frequency dependent
- More appropriately, they should be termed as **"*comparative* impedance"** because they measure relative magnitudes of impedance which are converted into length information. Various third-generation apex locators are:
  - Endex (Original third-generation apex locator)
  - Neosomo ultimo EZ apex locator
  - Mark V plus
  - Root ZX **(Fig. 17.15)**
  - Root ZX II **(Fig. 17.16)**
  - Root ZX mini

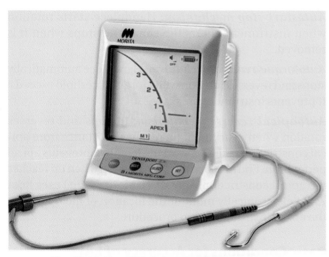

Fig. 17.15 Root ZX -3rd generation apex locator
Courtesy: J Morita.

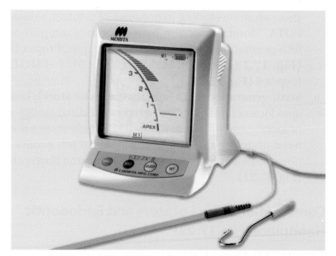

Fig. 17.16 Root ZX II -3rd generation apex locator.
Courtesy: J Morita.

- Endo analyser 8005
- Apex pointer
- Apex Finder

Advantages
- Easy to operate
- Uses K-type file
- Audible indication
- Can operate in presence of fluids
- Analog read out

Disadvantages
- Requires lip clip
- Chances of short circuit
- Needs fully charged battery
- Must calibrate each canal
- Sensitive to canal fluid level

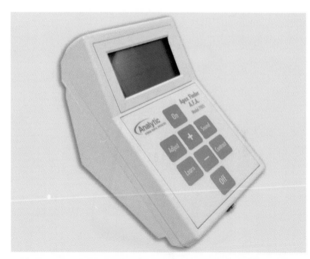

Fig. 17.17 AFA Apex Finder – 4th generation apex locator.
Courtesy: Sybron Endo.

Combination of apex locator and endodontic handpiece

Tri Auto ZX	Cordless electrical handpiece with three safety mechanism
Endy 7000	Reverses the rotation when tip reaches apical constriction
Sofy ZX	Monitor the location of file during instrumentation

4. **Fourth-generation apex locator**
   - Fourth-generation EAL measures resistance and capacitance separately rather than the resultant impedance value
   - There can be different combination of values of capacitance and resistance that provides the same impedance and the same foraminal reading
   - However, by using fourth-generation apex locator, this can be broken down into primary components

and measures separately for better accuracy and thus less chances of occurrence of errors
   - Examples of fourth-generation apex locators are AFA apex finder **(Fig. 17.17)**, i-Pex, Rayapex 4, Propex, Elements Diagnostic Unit

The main problem with fourth-generation EALs is that they can perform well in relatively dry canals, so difficult to use in cases of heavy exudates or weeping canals.

5. **Fifth-generation EALs (dual-frequency ratio type):** To overcome the disadvantages of previous generations of apex locators, fifth-generation EALs have been developed which are based on comparison of data taken from the electrical characteristic of the canal and additional mathematical processing. These

show accurate reading in presence of dry, wet, saline, EDTA, blood, or sodium hypochlorite. Examples of fifth generation apex locators are Rayapex, Propex II **(Fig. 17.18)**, Propex Pixi **(Fig. 17.19)**, I -ROOT, Joypex 5 **(Fig. 17.20)**

6. **Sixth-generation EALs (adaptive apex locators):** This apex locator is intended to overcome the disadvantages of fourth- and fifth-generation EALs. It eliminates the need of drying the canals. Examples of 6th generation apex locator are Adaptive apex locator, Raypex 6 **(Fig. 17.21)**

Combination Apex Locators and Endodontic Handpiece (Fig. 17.22)

Tri Auto ZX (J. Morita Calif) is cordless electric endodontic handpiece with built-in root ZX apex locator. It has three safety mechanisms:

Autostart-stop mechanism: Handpiece starts rotation when instrument enters the canal and stops when it is removed.

Autotorque-reverse mechanism: Handpiece automatically stops and reverses rotation when torque threshold exceeds. It prevents instrument breakage.

Autoapical-reverse mechanism: It stops and reverses rotation when instrument tip reaches a distance from apical constriction taken for working length. It prevents apical perforation. Endy 7000 reverse the rotation when tip reaches the apical constriction. Sofy ZX (J. Morita Calif) uses Root ZX to electronically monitor the location of file tip during the entire instrumentation procedure.

Basic Conditions for Accuracy of EALs

Whatever is the generation of apex locator, there are some basic conditions, which ensure accuracy of their usage.
- Canal should be free from most of the tissue and debris

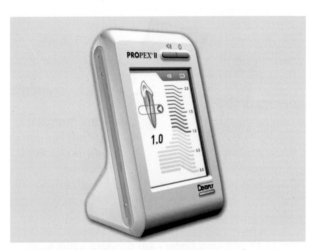

Fig. 17.18 Propex II – 5th generation apex locator. *Courtesy:* Dentsply, India.

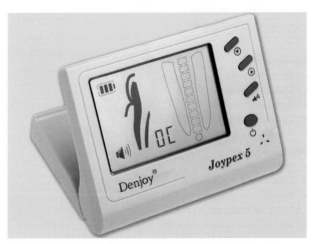

Fig. 17.20 Joypex 5 – 5th generation apex locator. *Courtesy:* Denjoy.

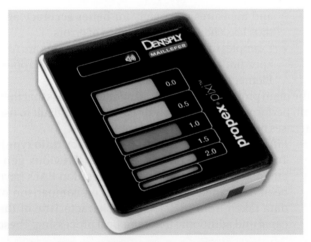

Fig. 17.19 Propex Pixi – 5th generation apex locator. *Courtesy:* Dentsply Maillefer.

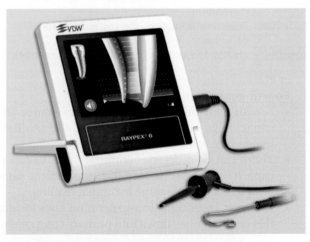

Fig. 17.21 Raypex 6–6th generation apex locator. *Courtesy:* VDW Dental.

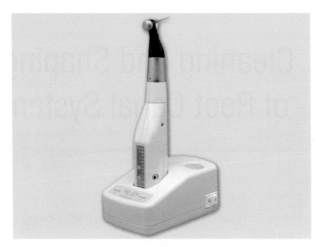

Fig. 17.22 Tri-Auto ZX – combination of Apex locator and endodontic handpiece.
Courtesy: J Morita.

- Apex locator works best in a relatively dry environment. But extremely dry canals may result in low readings, that is, long working length
- Cervical leakage must be eliminated and excess fluid must be removed from the chamber as this may cause inaccurate readings
- If residual fluid is present in the canal, it should be of low conductivity value, so that it does not interfere the functioning of apex locator
- Descending order of conductivity of various irrigating solutions is
  - 5.25% NaOCl > 17% EDTA > saline
- Since EALs work on the basis of contact with canal walls and periapex. Better the adaptation of file to the canal walls, more accurate is the reading
- Canals should be free from any type of blockage, calcifications, etc.
- Battery of apex locator and other connections should be proper

Conclusion

To establish a precise working length is mandatory for success of the endodontic treatment. Cementodentinal junction (CDJ) is the anatomic point where instrumentation and obturation should end. Many techniques are available for determination of accurate working length. The CDJ, termination point for the preparation, and obturation of the root canal and this cannot be determined radiographically. Modern electronic apex locators can determine this position with accuracies of greater than 90% but still have some limitations. Knowledge of apical anatomy, careful use of radiographs, and the correct use of an electronic apex locator will assist clinicians to achieve predictable results.

Questions

1. Define working length. What is significance of working length?
2. Enumerate different methods of working length determination. Write in detail Ingle's method of working length determination.
3. Classify apex locators. What are third-generation apex locators.
4. Write short notes on:
   - Paper point sensitivity test
   - Advantages of apex locators

Bibliography

1. Bramante CM, Berbert A. Critical evaluation of methods of determining working length. Oral Surg 1974;37:463.
2. Cluster LE. Exact methods of locating the apical foramen. J Nat Dent Assoc 1918;5:815.
3. Cohen S, Burns RC. Pathways of the pulp. 4th edition St Louis: CV Mosby, 1987:164-9.
4. Ingle JI, Bakland LK. Endodontic cavity preparation. In: Textbook of endodontics. 5th edition Philadelphia, PA: BC Decker; 2002.
5. Kim E, Lee SJ. Electronic apex locator. Dent Clin North Am 2004;48:35–54. (Review).
6. Kuttler Y. A precision and biologic root canal filling technique. J Am Dent Assoc 1958; 58:38-50.
7. Kuttler Y. Microscopic investigation of root apexes. J Am Dent Assoc 1955;50:544–52.
8. McDonald NJ. 'The electronic determination of working length.' Dent Clin North Am. 1992;36:293.
9. Mello I. Use of electronic apex locators may improve determination of working length. Evid Based Dent 2014.
10. Sunada I. New method for measuring the length of root canals. J Dent Res 1962;41:375–87.
11. Weine FS. Endodontic therapy. 2nd edition St Louis: CV Mosby, 1976.pp.206-14.

Cleaning and Shaping of Root Canal System

Introduction

Endodontic treatment mainly consists of three steps:
1. Cleaning and shaping of the root canal system
2. Disinfection
3. Obturation

Cleaning and shaping is one of the most important steps in the root canal therapy for obtaining success in the root canal treatment **(Fig.18.1)**.

Cleaning and Shaping of the Root Canal System

Cleaning and shaping of the canals means:
❑ To remove all the contents from root canal which may cause growth of microorganisms or breakdown of toxic products into the periradicular tissues.

❑ To prepare the root canal not only for disinfection but also to develop a shape that permits a three-dimensional sealing of the canal.
❑ To remove all the irregularities, obstructions and old fillings from the canals, if present.

Cleaning of canals can be assessed by presence of clean dentinal shavings, color of the irrigant whereas a properly shaped canal should feel smooth in all dimensions when tip of file is pushed against the canal walls **(Fig. 18.1)**.

For success of endodontic treatment, one must remove all the contents of the root canal completely because any communication from root canal system to periodontal space acts as portal of exit which can lead to formation of lesions of endodontic origin **(Fig. 18.2)**.

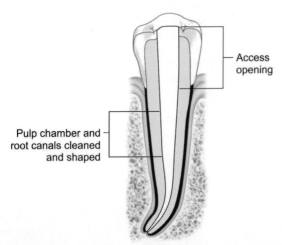

Fig. 18.1 Diagrammatic representation of cleaned and shaped root canal system.

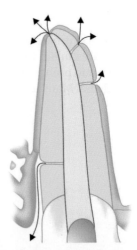

Fig. 18.2 Portals of communication of root canal system and periodontium.

Biomechanical preparation of the root canal system was a hit and trial method, before **Dr Schilder** gave the concept of cleaning and shaping.

With changing concepts of root canal treatment, the preparation is described as instrumentation, chemomechanical instrumentation, biomechanical preparation, etc. which describes the mode of root canal therapy, but the ultimate goal is of cleaning and shaping of the root canal system.

Objectives of Biomechanical Preparation

Mechanical Objectives of Root Canal Preparation

The mechanics of cleaning and shaping may be viewed as an extension of the principles of coronal cavity preparation to the full length of the root canal system. *Schilder* gave the following five mechanical objectives:

1. ***Root canal preparation should develop a continuously tapering cone (Fig. 18.3):*** This shape mimics the natural canal shape. Here, funnel-shaped preparation of canal merges with the access cavity so that instruments will slide into the canal, thus forming a continuous channel.
2. ***Making the preparation in multiple planes which introduces the concept of "flow":*** This objective preserves the natural curve of the canal.
3. ***Making the canal narrower apically and widest coronally:*** To create continuous taper up to apical third which creates the resistance form to hold gutta-percha in the canal **(Figs. 18.4A and B).**
4. ***Avoid transportation of the foramen:*** There should be gentle and minute enlargement of the foramen while maintaining its position.

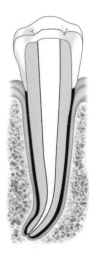

Fig. 18.3 Prepared root canal shape should be continuously tapered.

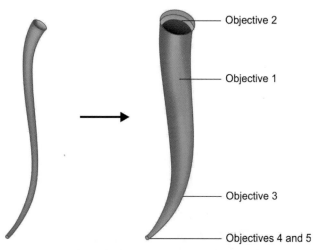

Figs. 18.4A and B Diagrammatic representation of objectives of canal preparation.

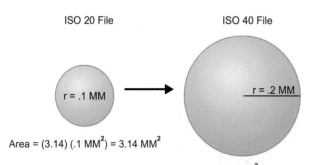

Fig. 18.5 Doubling the file size apically increases the surface area of foramen four times.

5. ***Keep the apical opening as small as possible:*** The foramen size should be kept as small as possible as overlapping of foramen contributes to number of iatrogenic problems. Doubling the file size apically increases the surface area of foramen four folds (πr^2) **(Fig. 18.5).** Thus overenlarging of apical foramen should be avoided.

Biologic Objectives of Root Canal Preparation

❏ Procedure should be confined to the root canal space
❏ All infected pulp tissue, bacteria and their by-products should be removed from the root canal
❏ Necrotic debris should not be forced periapically
❏ Sufficient space for intracanal medicaments and irrigants should be created

Clinical Objectives of Biomechanical Preparation

❏ The clinician should evaluate the tooth to be treated to ensure that the particular tooth has favorable prognosis

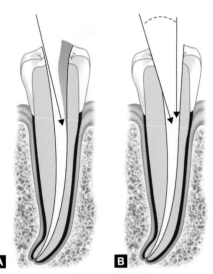

Figs. 18.6A and B Removal of overlying dentin causes smooth internal walls and provides straight-line access to root canals.

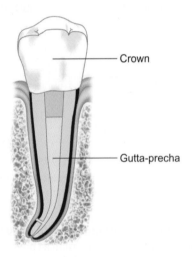

Fig. 18.7 Obturation of root canals followed by crown placement.

- Before performing cleaning and shaping, the straight-line access to canal orifice should be obtained
- All the overlying dentin should be removed and there should be flared and smooth internal walls to provide straight-line access to root canals **(Figs. 18.6A and B)**
- Since shaping facilitates cleaning, in properly shaped canals, instruments and irrigants can go deeper into the canals to remove all the debris and contents of root canal
- This creates a smooth tapered opening to the apical terminus for obtaining three-dimensional obturation of the root canal system **(Fig. 18.7)**
- After obturation, there should be complete sealing of the pulp chamber and the access cavity so as to prevent microleakage into the canal system
- Tooth should be restored with permanent restoration to maintain its form, function and esthetics

- Patient should be recalled on regular basis to evaluate the success of the treatment

Different Movements of Instruments

Reaming

- To ream means use of sharp-edged tool for enlarging holes
- It involves clockwise rotation of an instrument (reamer is most commonly used) **(Fig. 18.8)**

Filing

- Term filing indicates push–pull motion of an instrument **(Fig. 18.9)**
- This active pushing of file with apically directed pressure may result in iatrogenic errors like ledge formation.

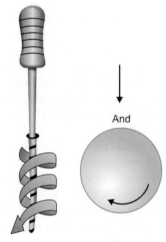

Fig. 18.8 Reaming motion involving clockwise rotation of instrument.

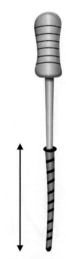

Fig. 18.9 Filing motion showing push and pull action of instrument.

Combination of Reaming and Filing (Fig. 18.10)

- In this technique, file is inserted with a quarter turn clockwise and apically directed pressure (i.e., reaming) and then is subsequently withdrawn (i.e., filing)
- File edges get engaged into dentin while insertion and breaks the loose dentin during its withdrawal
- By performing this combination of reaming and filing repeatedly, canal enlargement takes place
- This technique has also shown to cause frequent ledge formation, perforation and other procedural errors
- To overcome these shortcomings, this technique was modified by Schilder. He suggested giving a clockwise rotation of half revolution followed by directing the instrument apically. In this method, every time when a file is withdrawn, it is followed by next in the series. Though this method is effective in producing clean canals, it is very laborious and time consuming

Balanced Force Technique

- This technique involves oscillation of instrument right and left with different arcs in either direction
- Instrument is first inserted into the canal by moving it clockwise with one quarter turn
- Then to cut dentin, file is rotated counterclockwise simultaneously pushing apically to prevent it from backing out of the canal
- Finally, the file is removed by rotating file clockwise simultaneously pulling the instrument out of the canal **(Figs. 18.11A and B)**
- This technique offers most efficient dentin cutting but care should be taken not to apply excessive force with this technique because it may lock the instrument into the canal

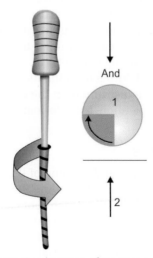

Fig. 18.10 Combination of reaming and filing.

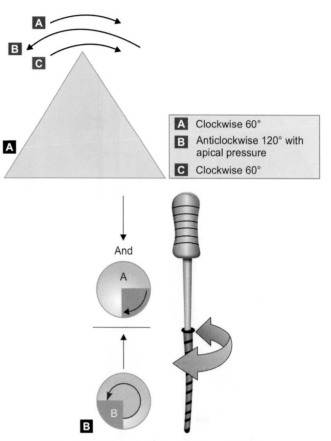

A	Clockwise 60°
B	Anticlockwise 120° with apical pressure
C	Clockwise 60°

Figs. 18.11A and B A balanced force technique.

- Since H-files and broaches do not possess left-hand cutting efficiency, they are not used with this technique
- Simultaneous apical pressure and anticlockwise rotation of the file maintains the balance between tooth structure and the elastic memory of the instrument, this balance locates the instrument near the canal axis and thus avoids transportation of the canal

Watch-Winding

- It is back and forth oscillation of the endodontic instrument right and left as it is advanced into the canal
- Angle of rotation is usually 30–60° **(Figs. 18.12A and B)**
- This technique is efficient with K-type instruments
- Watch-winding motion is less aggressive than quarter turn and pull motion because in this motion, instrument tip is not forced into the apical area with each motion, thereby reducing the frequency of instrumental errors

Watch-Winding and Pull Motion

- In this, first instrument is moved apically by rotating it right and left through an arc
- When the instrument feels any resistance, it is taken out of the canal by pull motion **(Fig. 18.13)**

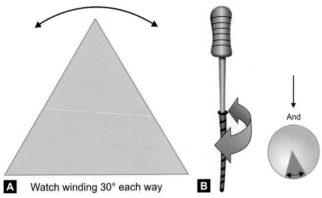

A Watch winding 30° each way   **B**

Figs. 18.12A and B (A) Watch-winding motion; (B) Rotation of file in watch-winding motion.

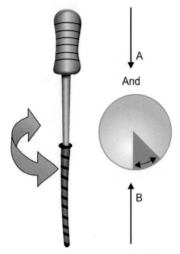

Fig. 18.13 Watch-winding and pull motion.

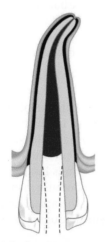

Fig. 18.14 Straight-line access to root canal system.

□ This technique is primarily used with Hedstorm files. When used with H-files, watch-winding motion cannot cut dentin because these can cut only during pull motion

Motions of instruments for cleaning and shaping

1. Follow: It is performed using files during initial cleaning and shaping. In this, file is precurved so as to follow canal curvatures
2. Follow withdraw: It is performed with files when apical foramen is reached. In this, simple in and out motion is given to the instrument. It is done to create a path for foramen and no attempt is made to shape the canal
3. Cart: Cart means transporting. In this, precurved reamer is passed through the canal with gentle force and random touch with dentinal wall up to the apical foramen. It is done to transport pulp remnants and dentinal debris
4. Carve: Carve is performed with reamers to do shaping of the canals. In this a precurved reamer as touched with dentinal wall and canal is shaped on withdrawal
5. Smooth: It is performed with files. In this, circumferential motion is given to smoothen the canal walls
6. Patency: It is performed with files or reamers. Patency means that apical foramen has been cleared of any debris in its path

Basic Principles of Canal Instrumentation

□ There should be a straight-line access to the canal orifices **(Fig. 18.14)**
□ Establish the apical patency by passing a #10 file across the apex (0.5 mm) so as to make minor constriction patent. Patency keeps the clear passage to apical foramen by removing debris from apical area
□ Files always work within the canal along with copious irrigation
□ Preparation of canal should be completed while retaining its original form and the shape
□ Canal enlargement should be done in the sequential order without skipping file sizes
□ All the working instruments should be kept in confines of the root canal to avoid any procedural accidents
□ After each insertion and removal of the file, its flutes should be cleaned and inspected
□ Fine instruments should be used extravagantly
□ Recapitulation is regularly done to loosen debris by returning to working length (WL). Canal walls should not be enlarged during recapitulation
□ Never force the instrument in the canal, it may cause instrument separation, ledge formation, etc.

Apical Gauging

For optimal cleaning and shaping of the root canal, it is imperative to accurately determine the endodontic WL and working width (WW) of each root canal. Inadequate determination of the width of the canal and subsequently the WW amplifies the possibilities of its insufficient cleaning and shaping. Therefore, the final instrument size must be large enough to touch all walls. Because most canals are oval in their cross-sectional shape, so goal should be to make the final apical instrument size correspond to the largest diameter of the oval, whenever possible. This is done by apical gauging.

Apical gauging is a mechanical term which clinically indicates the measuring of the apical diameter prior to obturation of the root canal system. It is important as it gives us a fairly good approximation of canal diameter in the critical apical 3–5 mm.

Tuning verifies if there is a uniform taper in the apical one third of the shaped canal.

Apical gauging helps in
1. Choosing the best master cone that closely matches canal length and taper
2. Achieving true tug back—as opposed to false tug back!
3. Minimizing gutta-percha (GP) extrusions during obturation, especially with warm vertical compaction

How to measure apical gauging?
1. Establish the position of apical constriction and keep working length (WL) 0.5 mm – 1 mm short of this
2. After cleaning and shaping, passively insert 02 taper hand files, starting from #15. If the file goes past the apical constriction, then choose the next largest file and repeat

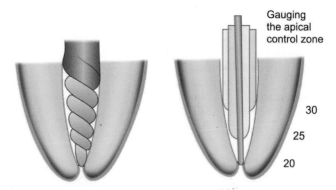

Fig. 18.15 Apical gauging of root canal. Diagrammatic representation of apical gauging. Here, #20 passively goes beyond the constriction and #25 binds short of the constriction, indicating that apical constriction has a diameter of >20 but <25.

3. When a file passively binds short of the apical constriction, that will be the upper limit of the apical constriction diameter. The smaller file before that would be the lower limit **(Fig. 18.15)**

Techniques of Root Canal Preparation

There are *three approaches* used for cleaning and shaping **(Figs. 18.16A to C)**.

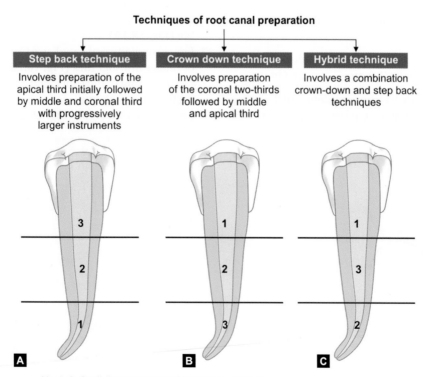

Techniques of root canal preparation

Step back technique	Crown down technique	Hybrid technique
Involves preparation of the apical third initially followed by middle and coronal third with progressively larger instruments	Involves preparation of the coronal two-thirds followed by middle and apical third	Involves a combination crown-down and step back techniques

No.1, 2, 3 tell the sequence of canal preparation

Figs. 18.16A to C Line diagram showing sequence of canal preparation in step back, crown down and hybrid technique.

Step-back	Crown-down	Hybrid
• Conventional step back • Modified step back • Passive step back	• Crown-down pressureless • Double flare • Modified double flare • Balanced force • Reverse balanced force	Hybrid technique

Step-Back Technique/Telescopic Canal Preparation/Serial Root Canal Preparation

Step-back technique emphasizes keeping the apical preparation small, in its original position and producing a gradual taper coronally.

Clem was first to describe a stepped preparation of the curved canal in which the apical portion was prepared using small, relatively flexible instruments. Coronal portion was shaped with larger instruments to obtain an adequate flare without undue enlargement at apical portion. Weine, Martin, Walton and Mullaney were early advocates of step-back preparation.

Mullaney (in 1960) divided the step-back preparation into two phases:

Phase I: It is the apical preparation starting at the apical constriction **(Fig. 18.17)**.

Phase II: It is the preparation of the remainder of the root canal, gradually stepping back while increasing in size.

Refining Phase IIA and IIB: It is the completion of the preparation to produce the continuing taper from apex to cervical.

Phase I

❑ Cleaning and shaping begins after gaining straight-line access and determination of WL
❑ A #10 file is inserted into the canal with watch-winding motion. In watch-winding motion, a gentle clockwise and anticlockwise rotation of file with minimal apical pressure is given **(Fig. 18.17)**. Don't use the instrument in filing motion as it can result in ledge formation
❑ Remove the instrument and irrigate the canal
❑ Do not forget to lubricate the instrument for use in apical area because lubricant emulsifies fibrous pulp tissue allowing the instrument to remove it, whereas irrigants may not reach the apical area to dissolve the tissues
❑ Place the next larger size files to the WL in similar manner and again irrigate the canal
❑ Repeat the procedure until at least size 25 K-file reaches the WL **(Fig. 18.18)**
❑ Always recapitulate the canal with previous smaller number instrument to break the collected debris which are then washed away with the irrigant

Phase II

❑ Place next file in the series 1 mm short of WL. Insert the instrument into the canal with watch-winding motion, remove it after circumferential filing, irrigate and recapitulate. Repeat the same procedure with successively larger files at 1 mm increments from previously used file **(Fig. 18.19)**
❑ For coronal third of canal, use Gates-glidden (GG) drills or bigger number files **(Fig. 18.20)**
❑ Final refining of the root canal is done using master apical file with push–pull strokes to achieve a smooth taper form of the root canal **(Fig. 18.21)**

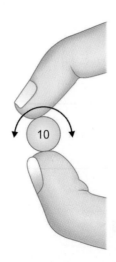

Fig. 18.17 Watch-winding motion with gentle clockwise and anticlockwise motion of the file.

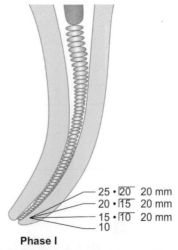

25 • 20 20 mm
20 • 15 20 mm
15 • 10 20 mm
10

Phase I

Fig. 18.18 Place #10 file in watch-winding motion, place the next larger size files to working length and irrigate the canal. Repeat the procedure till size 25 K-file reaches the working length.

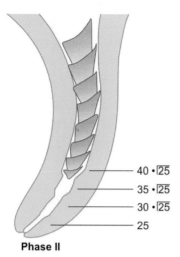

40 • 25
35 • 25
30 • 25
25

Phase II

Fig. 18.19 Use next file 1 mm short of working length, remove it after circumferential filing, irrigate, recapitulate and repeat the same procedure with successively larger files at 1 mm increments from previously used file.

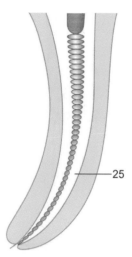

25

Fig. 18.21 Final refining of the root canal is done by using master apical file in push and pull strokes.

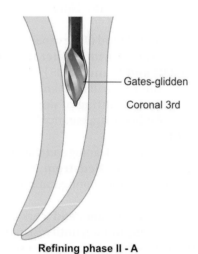

Gates-glidden

Coronal 3rd

Refining phase II - A

Fig. 18.20 Coronal part of the canal is flared using Gates-glidden drills.

Advantages of Step-Back Techniques

❑ This technique creates small apical preparation with larger instruments used at successively decreasing lengths to create a taper
❑ Taper of canal preparation can be altered by changing the interval between consecutive instruments, for example, taper of prepared canal can be increased by reducing the intervals between each successive file from 1 mm to 0.5 mm

Disadvantages of Step-Back Technique

❑ Difficult to irrigate apical region
❑ More chances of pushing debris periapically

❑ Time consuming
❑ It has a tendency to straighten the curved canal
❑ Increased chances of iatrogenic errors; ledge formation, instrument separation, zipping of the apical area, apical blockage, etc. **(Figs. 18.22A to D)**
❑ Since, curvature of the canal is reduced during mid-root flaring, there will be a loss in the WL
❑ Difficult to insert instruments in canal

Modified Step-Back Technique

❑ In this technique, preparation is completed in apical third of the canal
❑ After this, step-back procedure is started 2–3 mm short of minor diameter/apical constriction so as to give an almost parallel retention form at apical area

Advantage
❑ Less chances of apical transportation

Disadvantage
❑ Less space for irrigants, leads to accumulation of debris in the canals

Passive Step-Back Technique

Torabinejad developed this technique; it involves combination of hand and rotary instruments to obtain an adequate coronal flare and preparation of apical part. It provides gradual enlargement of the root in an apical to coronal direction without applying force, thereby reducing the occurrence of procedural errors like transportation of the canal, ledge, or zip formation.

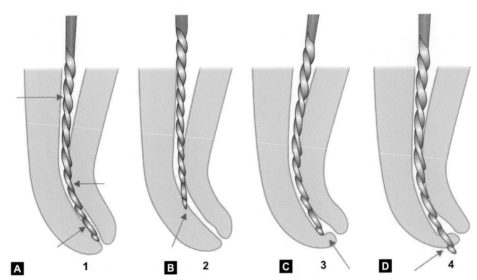

Figs. 18.22A to D Procedural errors. (A) Stiffness in curved canals; (B) Ledge formation causing loss of working length; (C) Apical transportation; (D) Apical perforation.

Technique

- ❏ Establish the apical patency using #10 file
- ❏ Use #20, 25, 30, 35 and 40 into the canal passively. This step removes the debris and creates a mildly flared preparation for insertion of Gates-glidden (GG) drills
- ❏ Now use #2 GG drill into mildly flared canal to a point, where it binds slightly. Here, it is pulled back 1–1.5 mm and then activated. In similar fashion, use #3 and 4 GG drill coronally **(Fig. 18.23)**
- ❏ Place #20 file up to WL and prepare the canal. Narrow canal should not be enlarged beyond size 25 or 30.

▌Crown-Down/Step-Down Technique

It was first suggested by Goerig et al. In crown-down technique, coronal one-third is instrumented before apical shaping

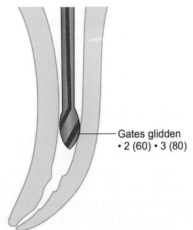

Fig. 18.23 Gates-glidden drill is used to prepare the coronal one-third of the canal.

- ❏ A #10 file is placed in the canal to *establish patency* **(Fig. 18.24 A)**
- ❏ Prepare the coronal third of the canal with progressively smaller GG drills or with greater taper instruments **(Figs. 18.24B and C and 18.25)**. One should avoid carrying all the GG drills to same level which may result in excessive cutting of dentin, weakening of roots and "coke-bottle appearance" in the radiographs **(Fig. 18.26)**
- ❏ Begin with step-down cleaning and shaping using **K-flex**, **Triple-flex**, or **Safety Hedstrom** instruments in the 0.02, 0.04, or 0.06 taper configurations depending on the canal size
- ❏ Start with a #50 instrument and work down the canal in a watch-winding motion until resistance is encountered. Then use sequentially smaller size instruments for step-down preparation. Irrigation and recapitulation after every instrumentation is done to prevent canal from being blocked with dentinal debris **(Figs. 18.24D and E)**
- ❏ Now enlarge the apical third to recommended master apical file size **(Fig. 18.24F)**

Modifications of Crown-Down Technique

Crown-Down Pressureless Technique

Marshall and **Pappin** advocated a "Crown-Down Pressureless Preparation" which involves early coronal flaring with GG drills, followed by preparation in apical direction, hence the term "**crown-down.**" K-files are used from large to small sequence without apical pressure, thus term is "**pressureless.**"

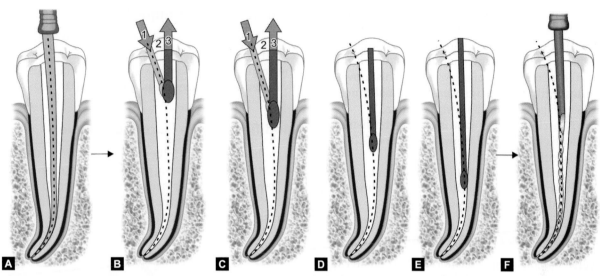

Figs. 18.24A to F Schematic representation of crown down technique: (A) Place a No. 10 to establish patency; (B and C) Prepare coronal third of canal with progressively smaller GG drills; (D and E) Perform crown down cleaning and shaping using progressively smaller files. (F) Enlarge apical third to recommended master apical file size.

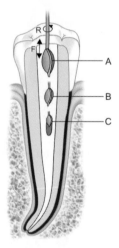

Fig. 18.25 Use of Gates-glidden for preflaring.

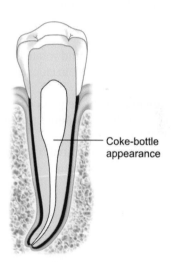

Fig. 18.26 "Coke-bottle appearance" caused by over use of Gates-glidden drills.

Balanced Force Technique

It was developed by *Roane and Sabala in 1985*. It involves the use of instrument with noncutting tip. Since K-type files have pyramidal tips with cutting angles which can be quite aggressive with clockwise rotation, for this technique triangular cross-sectioned instruments should be used. The decreased mass of instrument and deeper cutting flutes improves the flexibility of instrument and decrease restoring force of the instrument when placed in curved canals.

Flex-R file is recommended for this technique because this file has "safe tip design" with a guiding land area behind

the tip which allows the file to follow the canal curvature without binding in the outside wall of the curved canal **(Fig. 18.27)**.

Technique

☐ Coronal and middle thirds of canal are flared with GG drills

☐ After mechanical shaping with GG drills, balanced force hand instrumentation begins with triad of movements: placing, cutting and removing instruments using only rotary motions **(Fig. 18.28)**

- First file which binds short of WL is placed into the canal and rotated clockwise a quarter of a turn. This movement causes flutes to engage a small amount of dentin
- Now file is rotated counterclockwise with apical pressure at least one-third of a revolution, this movement provides cutting action by shearing off small amount of dentin engaged during clockwise rotation
- Then a final clockwise rotation is given to the instrument which loads the flutes of file with loosened debris and the file is withdrawn
- This movement is repeated (clockwise insertion and counterclockwise cutting) while advancing the instrument apically in shallow steps

Reverse Balanced Force Preparation

For reverse balanced force technique, NiTi greater taper hand files are used because flutes of these files are machined in a reverse direction unlike other files. Also handle of these files is increased in size to make the manipulation of files easier for reverse balanced technique.

Technique

- Insert GT file in the canal and rotate it 60° in anticlockwise direction and then 120° in clockwise direction with apical pressure
- These files are used in the sequence from largest to the smallest in crown-down sequence progressively toward the apex till WL is achieved
- Prepare apical portion of canal using 2% tapered ISO files in balance force technique

Double Flare Technique

It was introduced by *Fava*. In this, canal is prepared in crown-down manner using K-files in decreasing sizes and then to prepare apical part step-back technique is followed by increasing file sizes (**Figs. 18.29A to D**).

Modified Double Flared Technique

- In this, a #40 Flex-R file is instrumented in the straight part of the canal, using balanced force technique
- Sequentially, larger sizes of files are used to instrument the straight part of canal and coronal 4–5 mm of canal is instrumented with GG drills

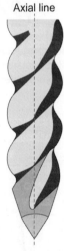

Axial line

Fig. 18.27 Flex-R file with safe tip design and guiding land.

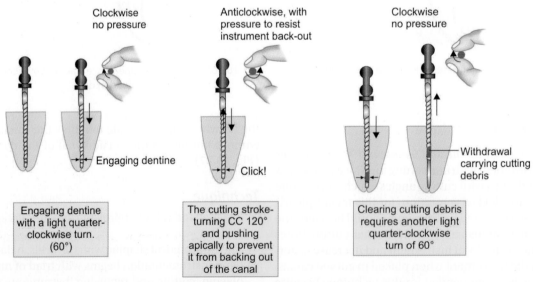

Clockwise no pressure

Anticlockwise, with pressure to resist instrument back-out

Clockwise no pressure

Engaging dentine

Click!

Withdrawal carrying cutting debris

Engaging dentine with a light quarter-clockwise turn. (60°)

The cutting stroke-turning CC 120° and pushing apically to prevent it from backing out of the canal

Clearing cutting debris requires another light quarter-clockwise turn of 60°

Fig. 18.28 Balanced force technique.

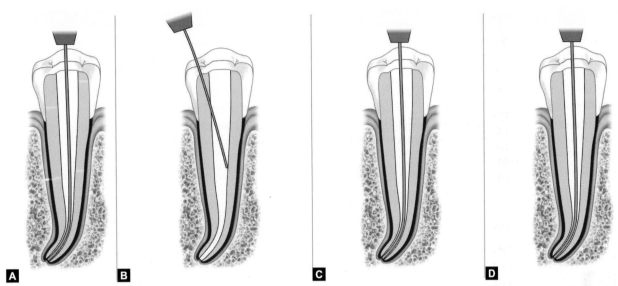

Figs. 18.29A to D Double flare technique: (A) Estimate the working length; (B) prepare coronal and middle third of the canal in crown-down method using K files in decreasing size; (C) Establish the working length; (D) Prepare apical part in step back manner.

- A #20 Flex-R file is taken to the working length and the canal is prepared using the balanced force technique by sequential use of files
- Preparation till the WL is continued until clean dentin is removed, the master apical varying between #40 and 45
- Step-back technique using balanced forces is then used to prepare the remaining curved portion of the canal

Advantages of crown-down technique
- Permits straighter access to the apical region
- Eliminates coronal interferences which allows better determination of apical canal sizes
- Removes bulk of the tissue and microorganisms before apical shaping
- Allows deeper penetration of irrigants
- Less likely to alter working length
- Eliminates the amount of necrotic debris that could be extruded through the apical foramen during instrumentation
- Freedom from constraints of the apical enlarging instruments
- Increased access allows greater control and less chance of zipping near the apical constriction
- It provides a coronal escapeway that reduces the "piston in a cylinder effect" responsible for debris extrusion from the apex

Biological benefits
- Removal of tissue debris coronally, thus minimizing the extrusion of debris periapically
- Reduction of postoperative sensitivity which could result from periapical extrusion of debris

- Greater volumes of irrigants can reach in canal irregularities in early stages of canal preparation because of coronal flaring
- Better dissolution of tissue with increased penetration of the irrigants
- Rapid removal of contaminated and infected tissues from the root canal system

Disadvantages
- More time consuming than step-back technique
- Excessively flared preparation in the coronal and middle thirds may weaken the root
- Use of end cutting rotary instruments in small or partially calcified canals may cause perforation as instrument moves apically
- In severely curved canals, rotary instrumentation is difficult because these can't be precurved
- If less flexible rotary instruments are used too rapidly and forcefully in canal, a ledge may form

Hybrid Technique of Canal Preparation (Step Down/Step Back)

In this, combination of crown-down preparation followed by step-back technique is used.

Technique
- Check the patency of canal using #10 or 15 K files
- Prepare the coronal third of canal using GG drills (in sequence of #3 followed by nos. 2 and 1) till the point of curvature without applying excessive pressure
- Establish the WL using #15

Differences between Step-back and crown-down technique	
Step-back/serial/telescopic technique	*Crown-down/step-down technique*
• Given by Clem and Weine	• Introduced by Riitano in 1976 and later by Goerig et al. and Marshall and Pappin
• Advocated with use of hand instruments, 2% standardized hand files	• Advocated with the use of both hand and rotary instruments, greater taper rotary NiTi files
• Apico-coronal technique, i.e. apical preparation is followed by preparation of middle and coronal one-third with ascending instrument sizes	• Corono-apical technique, i.e coronal preparation is followed by preparation of middle and apical one-third with descending instrument sizes
• Produces apical stop before preparing middle and coronal part	• Produces apical stop after preparing coronal and middle part
• Coronally placed interferences affect optimal instrumentation	• Early removal of coronal interferences allows ease of instrumentation, decreases torsional loads on instruments, increase tactile feedback, less deviation of instruments in canal
• More chances of instrument fracture because of torsional loads	• Less chance of instrument fracture
• Chances of alteration of WL	• Since coronal curvature is eliminated, there are less chances of change in WL
• More apical blockages due to debris	• Less apical blockage as rapid removal of debris and microorganism with coronal preparation first
• Less irrigant preparation in apical area	• Better dissolution of tissue with increased irrigant preparation especially in apical area
• More apical extrusion of debris	• Less apical extrusion of debris
• More postoperative pain	• Less postoperative pain
• Time consuming	• Takes less time

- ❑ Prepare apical portion of canal from size #15 till the recommended Master Apical File (MAF) size using step-back technique
- ❑ Recapitulate and irrigate the canal at every step so as to maintain patency of the canal
- ❑ Perform the step-back procedure till middle third of the canal so as to have continuous funnel shaped preparation

Advantages
- ❑ It has advantages of both crown-down and step-back procedure
- ❑ This technique maintains the integrity of dentin by avoiding excessive removal of radicular dentin

Canal Preparation Using Ultrasonic Instruments

Concept of using ultrasound in endodontic therapy was suggested in 1957 by **Richman**. But, it was the late 1970s, when ultrasonic scaling units became common for use in endodontics resulting in **endosonics (Fig. 18.30)**. The machines used for this purpose are designed to transmit low frequency ultrasonic vibration by conversion of electromagnetic energy to the mechanical energy to produce oscillation of file. File oscillates at the frequency of 20,000–25,000 vibrations/s. For

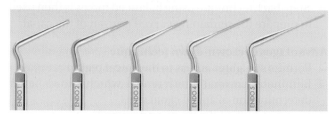
Fig. 18.30 Endosonic tips.

free movement of file in the canal, it should not have any binding specially at the apical end **(Figs. 18.31A and B)**. During the oscillation of file, there is continuous flow of irrigants solutions from the handpiece along the file. This causes formation of cavitation.

Technique

- ❑ Before starting with ultrasonic instrumentation, apical third of the canal should be prepared to at least size 15 file
- ❑ After activation, ultrasonic file is moved in the *circumferential* manner with push–pull stroke along the walls of canal
- ❑ File is activated for 1 minute. This procedure is repeated till the apex is prepared

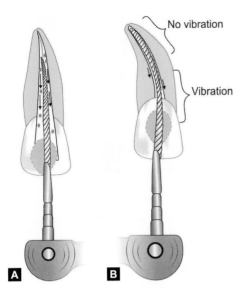

Figs. 18.31A and B (A) Ultrasonic instrument and irrigation work actively in straight canal; (B) Curvature in canal may impede vibration.

Advantages
- Less time consuming
- Produces cleaner canals because of synergetic relationship between the ultrasound and the sodium hypochlorite
- Heat produced by ultrasonic vibration increases the chemical effectiveness of the sodium hypochlorite

Disadvantages
- Increased frequency of canal transportations
- Increased chances of overinstrumentation

Canal Preparation Using Sonic Instruments

Design of sonic instruments is similar to that of ultrasonics. They consist of a driver on to which an endosonic file is attached. The oscillatory pattern of driver determines the nature of movement of attached file. In sonic instruments, on activation, there is longitudinal pattern of vibration.

Sonic system uses three types of file system for root canal preparation, viz; Heliosonic, Rispisonic and the canal shaper instruments. These files have spiral blades protruding along their length and noncutting tips.

Technique

- After gaining the straight-line access to the canal orifices, penetrate small number file in the canal. Enlarge the canal #20 or 25 up to 3 mm of apex to make some space for sonic file
- Now place sonic file 0.5–1 mm short of #20 file and do circumferential filling with up and down motion for 30–40 seconds
- After this, use the larger number sonic file and do the coronal flaring
- Now determine the WL and prepare the apical third of the canal using hand files
- Finally, blend the apical preparation with coronal flaring using smaller number sonic file

Laser-Assisted Root Canal Therapy

Weichman and Johnson in 1971 were the first to suggest the use of lasers in endodontics. Neodymium-doped yttrium aluminum garnet (Nd: YAG), Ar, Excimer, Holmium, Erbium (Er) laser beam are delivered through the optical fiber with the diameter of 200–400 mm equivalent to size #20–40 file. Studies have shown different results with lasers.

Bahcall et al. in 1992 found that though the use of Nd:YAG laser can produce cleaner canals, but heat produced by it may damage the surrounding supporting tissues, that is, bone and periodontal ligament (PDL). Hibst et al. showed that use of Er:YAG laser may pose less thermal damage to the tissues because it causes localized heating thereby minimizing the absorption depth.

Er, Cr:YSGG (erbium, chromium:Yttrium scandium gallium garnet) is used to reduce anxiety and discomfort to the patient. Waterlase—hydrokinetic hard and soft tissue laser uses specialized fibers of various diameters and lengths to effectively clean the root canal walls and prepare the canal for obturation. By using hydrokinetic process in which water is energized by YSGG laser photons to cause molecular excitation and localized microexpansion, hard tissues are removed precisely with no thermal side effects.

With this technique, there is minimal patient discomfort and postoperative complications. Intracanal irradiation with laser reduces microbial flora, inflammation and other postoperative complications, simultaneously providing the comfort to patient. However, performance of the equipment safety measures, temperature rise and level of microbial reduction should be well documented before it becomes a current method of choice for treatment.

Evaluation Criteria of Canal Preparation

- Spreader should be able to reach within 1 mm of the WL **(Fig. 18.32)**

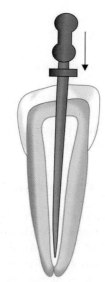

Fig. 18.32 Spreader should reach 1 mm short of apex in a well prepared canal.

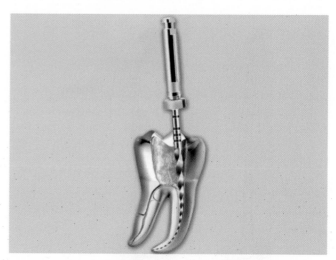

Fig. 18.33 Master apical file should feel smooth in a well prepared canal.

☐ After canal preparation, when master apical file is pressed firmly against each wall, it should feel smooth (**Fig. 18.33**)

☐ A microcomputed tomography scanner is used to record the precise canal anatomy before and after the instrumentation. A three-dimensional analysis of root canal geometry by high-resolution CT is then performed

Management of Difficult Cases

☐ Management of curved canals
☐ Management of calcified canals
☐ Management of C-shaped canals
☐ Management of S-shaped canals

Management of Curved Canals

For anatomy of curved canals, please refer to page number 185. Challenges encountered during the treatment of curved canals are

☐ Negotiating the canal curvature
☐ Enlarging the canal space and maintaining the original anatomy
☐ Creating a taper-shaped canal

Steps

In curved canals, frequently seen problem is occurrence of uneven cutting. File can cut dentine evenly only if it engages dentine around its entire circumference. Once it becomes loose in a curved canal, it will tend to straighten

up and will contact only at certain points along its length. These *areas are usually outer portion of curve, apical to the curve, on inner part of curve at the height of curve and outer or inner curve coronal to the curve.* All this can lead to occurrence of procedural errors like formation of ledge, transportation of foramen, perforation, or formation of elbow and zip in a curved canal. To avoid occurrence of such errors, there should be even contact of file to the canal dentine.

Factor affecting success of negotiation of a curved canal:
• Degree of curvature
• Flexibility of instrument
• Length of root canal
• Width of root canal
• Skill of operator

This can be done by
1. Decreasing the force which makes the straight file bend against the curved dentine surface
2. Decreasing the length of file which aggressively cuts at a given span

1. *Decrease in the filing force:* It can be done in following ways:
   • *Precurving the file:* A precurved file has shown to traverse the curve better than a straight file. Precurving can be done by (**Fig. 18.34**)
     – Placing gradual curve for entire length of the file
     – Placing a sharp curve of nearly 45° at apical end of the instrument. It is then used when a sharp curve or an obstruction is present in the canal.

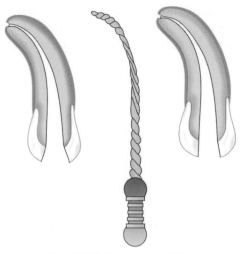
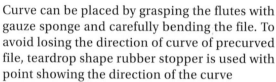

Fig. 18.34 Precurving of file.

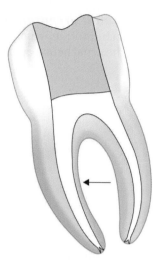

Fig. 18.35 Arrow showing area where chances of strip perforation are more.

Curve can be placed by grasping the flutes with gauze sponge and carefully bending the file. To avoid losing the direction of curve of precured file, teardrop shape rubber stopper is used with point showing the direction of the curve

- **Extravagant use of smaller number files:** Small-sized instruments can follow the canal curvature because of their flexibility; they should be used extravagantly till the larger files are able to negotiate the canal without force

- **Use of intermediate sizes of files:** Increment of 0.05 mm between two consecutive instruments is too large to reach the correct working length in curved canals. To solve this problem, cut off a portion of file tip to create a size intermediate to two consecutive instruments. There is increase of 0.02 mm of diameter per millimeter of the length, cutting 1 mm of tip creates a new instrument size. For example, cutting 1 mm of #15 file makes it #17 file. In severely curved canals, cut 0.5 mm of the file to increase the instrument diameter by 0.01 mm to allow smoother transition of the instrument sizes for even cutting

- **Use of flexible files:** Flexible files help in maintaining the shape of the curve and avoid occurrence of procedural errors like formation of ledge, elbow, or zipping of the canal

2. **Decrease in Length of Actively Cutting File:** *It can be achieved by following means.*
   - **Anticurvature filing** (given by Lim and Stock)
     - Anticurvature filing prevents excessive dentin removal from thinner part of curved canals. If care is not taken while cleaning and shaping, strip formation can occur in danger zone area. Danger zone has less dentin thickness than safety zone, for

example, on mesial side of mesial root of mandibular molar **(Figs. 18.35 and 18.36)**
   - Anticurvature filing involves lesser filing of the canal wall which is facing the curvature. For example, in case of mesial root of mandibular molar, more filing is done on mesial side than on distal side **(Figs. 18.37 and 18.38)**

- **Modifying cutting edges of the instrument:** Cutting edges of curved instrument can be modified by dulling the flute of outer portion of apical third and inner portion of middle third with the help of diamond file **(Figs. 18.39)**

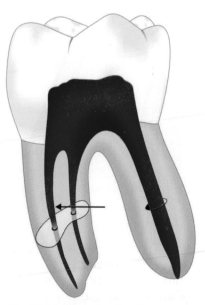

Fig. 18.36 Arrow showing danger zone.

- *Changing the canal preparation techniques:* Crown-down technique in which preparation of coronal part of the canal before apical part removes the coronal interferences and allows the files to reach up to the apex more effectively **(Fig. 18.40)**. **Figures 18.41 to 18.43** are showing management of curved root canals.

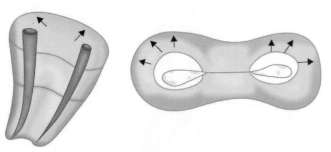

Fig. 18.37 Removal of dentin should be done more in shaded area to avoid perforation.

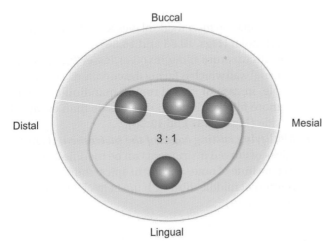

Fig. 18.38 In mesiobuccal canal of mandibular molars, more filing is done on mesial and buccal wall than on lingual and distal wall.

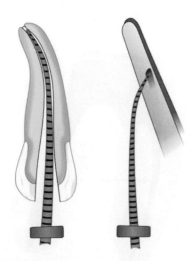

Fig. 18.39 Modifying the cutting edges of instrument

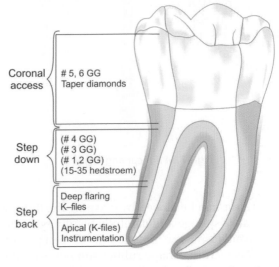

Fig. 18.40 Crown-down technique for curved canals.

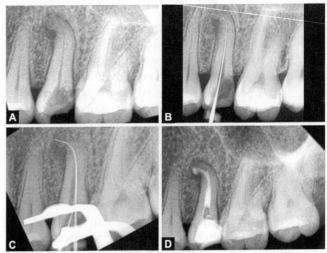

Figs. 18.41A to D Management of dilacerated roots of maxillary second premolar: (A) Radiograph showing carious pulp exposure with widening of periodontal ligament space of maxillary second premolar; (B) 10# K-file was precurved in accordance with curvature of the canal and glide path was established till WL; (C) Both canals negotiated till working length and coronal flaring was done with rotary files. Shaping of canals was done using S_1 and S_2 till working length. Canals were finished with F_1; (D) Final obturation with calamus dual for downpack and backfill.
Courtesy: Punit Jindal

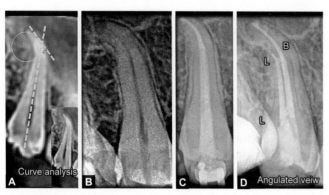
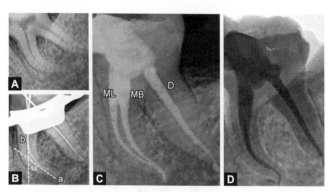

Figs. 18.42A to D Endodontic treatment of maxillary premolar with curved canals. (A) Estimation of root canal curvature; (B) Preoperative radiograph; (C) Postobturation radiograph; (D) Postobturation radiograph at different angle.
Courtesy: Jaydev

Figs. 18.43A to D Management of mandibular molar with curved canals. (A) Preoperative radiograph; (B) Estimation of root canal curvature; (C) Postobturation radiograph; (D) Postobturation radiograph at different angle.
Courtesy: Jaydev

Management of Calcified Canals

For anatomy of calcified canals, please refer to page no. 188.

For access opening of calcified canals, please refer to page no. 215.

- Take a proper radiograph of calcified tooth to visualize the location of pulp chamber floor. Measure the distance from occlusal surface to the pulp chamber from preoperative radiograph
- Start with the access preparation using long shank #2 or #4 round bur **(Fig. 18.44)**
- Use DG–16 explorer and apply firm pressure to force the instrument slightly into the orifice, where it will "stick." At this suspected point, place #8 or 10 K-file or canal pathfinder into the orifice and try to negotiate the canal **(Figs. 18.45 and 18.46)**
- Always advance instruments slowly in calcified canals and clean the instrument on withdrawal and inspect before reinserting it into the canal
- When a fine instrument reaches the approximate canal length, do not remove it; rather obtain a radiograph to ascertain the position of the file
- Use chelating agents to assist canal penetration
- Do copious irrigation with NaOCl which enhances dissolution of organic debris, lubricates the canal and keeps dentin chips and pieces of calcified material in solution

Figures 18.47A to D shows case management of nonvital maxillary central incisor with calcified canal.

Management of C-Shaped Canals

For anatomy of C-shaped canal, please refer to page no. 186

Diagnosis: Following radiographic characteristics can predict the presence of C-shaped canals: radicular fusion,

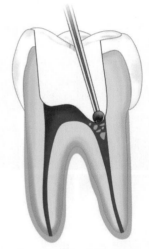

Fig. 18.44 Direct the small round bur to assumed pulp space.

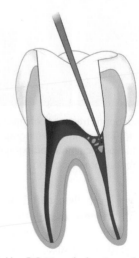

Fig. 18.45 Use DG 16 endodontic explorer in orifice.

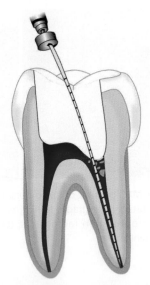

Fig. 18.46 Use #8 or 10 file to negotiate calcified canal.

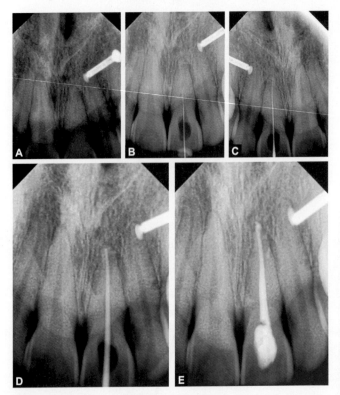

Figs. 18.47A to D Endodontic treatment of maxillary central incisor with calcified canal: (A) Preoperative radiograph; (B) Explore the canal using #10 file; (C) Working length radiograph; (D) Master cone radiograph; (E) Postobturation radiograph

radicular proximity, a large distal canal, or a blurred image of a third canal in between. In a continuous C-shaped canal, it is possible to pass an instrument from the mesial to the distal aspect without hindrance. In semicolon type,

when an instrument is inserted into any side of the canal, it always ends in the distal foramen of the tooth and a file introduced in this canal could probe the whole extension of the C.

Negotiation of canals: When the orifice is continuous C-shaped or arced, number of canals can vary from one to three, when the orifice is oval, number of canals can be one or two and when orifice is round, one canal is suspected. Explore the canals with small size endodontic files (nos. 8, 10, 15 K-file) so as not to miss irregularities.

Cleaning and shaping: To gain access to irregularities in the C-shaped canal system, coronal third is prepared using GG drills. Care should be taken to avoid perforation in C1 (continuous C type) and C2 (semicolon type) type canals. In narrow, interconnecting isthmus areas, GG drills should not be used and cleaning should be using a #25 instrument. Anticurvature filing is recommended to avoid danger zones. Caution should be taken to prevent strip perforation during cleaning and shaping of mandibular premolars, which has thin dentinal walls in the radicular groove area.

Cleaning of C-shaped canal with rotary instruments should be assisted by ultrasonic irrigation.

Obturation: Cleaning and shaping of C-shaped canals leave a very less remaining dentin thickness of 0.2–0.3 mm, forces of compaction during obturation can cause root fracture. So, thermoplasticized gutta-percha technique is preferred.

Figures 18.48 and 18.49 show management of C-shaped canals.

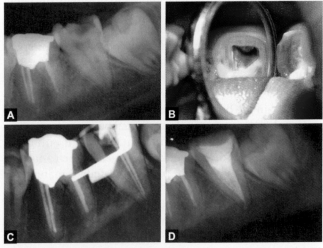

Figs. 18.48A to D Root canal treatment of mandibular second molar with C-shaped canal. (A) Preoperative radiograph; (B) after access preparation; (C) working length radiograph; (D) postobturation radiograph.
Courtesy: JaidevDhillon

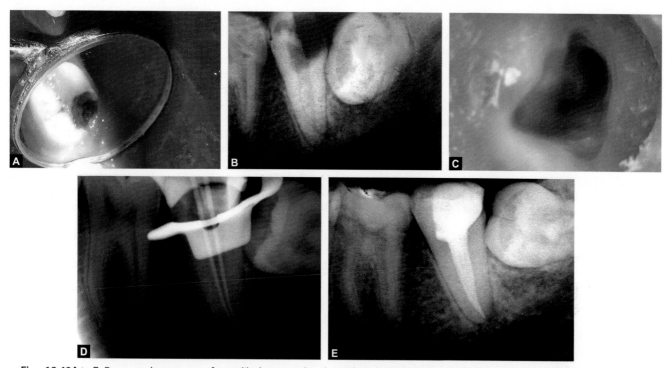

Figs. 18.49A to E Root canal treatment of mandibular second molar with C-shaped canals. (A) Preoperative photograph; (B) preoperative radiograph; (C) After access preparation; (D) Working length radiograph; (E) Postobturation radiograph.
Courtesy: Jaidev Dhillon.

Management of S-Shaped/ Bayonet-Shaped Canals

For anatomy of S-shaped canal, please refer to page no. 185

For optimal cleaning and shaping of S-shaped canals, the three-dimensional nature of these canals must be visualized with special consideration and evaluation to the multiple concavities along the external surfaces of the root. Failure to know these may result in stripping of the canal along the inner surface of each curve. During initial canal penetration, it is essential that there be an unrestricted approach to the first curve. For this, the access preparation is flared to allow a more direct entry. Once the canal is negotiated, passive shaping of coronal curve is done first to facilitate the cleaning and shaping of the apical curve. Constant recapitulation with small files and copious irrigation is necessary to prevent blockage and ledging. Over curving the apical 3 mm of the file aids in maintaining the curvature in the apical portion of the canal as the coronal curve becomes almost straight during the later stages of cleaning and shaping. Gradual use of small files with short amplitude strokes is essential to manage these canals effectively. To prevent stripping in the coronal curve, anticurvature or reverse filing is recommended, with primary pressure being placed away from curve of coronal curvature.

▌Questions

1. What are Schilder's concept of root canal preparation?
2. What are biologic and clinical objectives of root canal preparation?
3. What are different movements of instruments?
4. Write in detail about step-back technique of canal preparation with its advantages and disadvantages.
5. What is crown-down technique? What are its advantages over step-back technique?
6. How will you manage a case of nonvital maxillary first molar with curved canals?
7. Describe in detail crown-down technique of root canal preparation.
8. Discuss your line of treatment for an infected nonvital tooth with calcified root canal.
9. Write short notes on:
   - Balanced force technique
   - Management of calcified canals
   - Step-back technique
   - Crown-down technique

- Anticurvature filing technique
- Difference between step-back, crown-down, and hybrid technique of canal preparation.

Bibliography

1. Abou-Rass M, Jastrab RJ. The use of rotary instruments as auxiliary aids to root canal preparation of molars. J Endod 1982;8:78–82.
2. Balani P, Niazi F, Rashid H. A brief review of the methods used to determine the curvature of root canals. J Restor Dent 2015;3:57–63.
3. Charles TJ, Charles JE. The 'balanced force' concept for instrumentation of curved canals revisited. Int Endod J 1998;31:166–72.
4. Fava LR. The double-flared technique: an alternative for biomechanical preparation. J Endod 1983;9:76–80.
5. Gambarini G. Shaping and cleaning the root canal system: a scanning electron microscopic evaluation of a new instrumentation and irrigation technique. J Endod 1999;25:800.
6. Jafarzadeh H, Abbott PV. Dilaceration: review of an endodontic challenge. J Endod 2007;33:1025–30.
7. Miserendino LJ, Miserendino CA, Moser JB, Heuer MA, Osetek EM. Cutting efficiency of endodontic instruments. Part III: Comparison of sonic and ultrasonic instrument systems. J Endod 1988;14:24–30.
8. Miserendino LJ, Moser JB, Heuer MA, Osetek EM. Cutting efficiency of endodontic instruments. Part II: Analysis of tip design. J Endod 1986;12:8–12.
9. Piattelli A. Generalized "complete" calcific degeneration or pulp obliteration. Endod Dent Traumatol 1992;8:259–63.
10. Schilder H. Cleaning and shaping of the root canals. Dent Clin North Am 1974;18:269–96.
11. Stock CR, Gulabiwala WK. Endodontics. 3rd edition St Louis, MI: Mosby; 2004.
12. Wiene FS. Endodontic therapy. 6th edition St Louis, MI: Mosby; 2004.

Obturation of Root Canal System

Success of endodontic treatment is based on proper diagnosis, treatment planning, biomechanical preparation followed by obturation. Obturate means to fill the shaped and disinfected canal with a temporary or permanent filling material. It can be achieved by using cements, pastes, plastics, or solids. Gutta-percha, in its various forms, has remained material of choice for obturation.

Why to Obturate?

Microorganisms and their byproducts are the major cause of pulpal and periapical diseases. However, it is difficult to consistently and totally disinfect root canal systems. Therefore, the goal of three-dimensional (3-D) obturation is to provide an impermeable fluid tight seal within the entire root canal system, to prevent oral and apical microleakage.

Objectives of obturation are:
- Elimination of coronal leakage of microorganisms or potential nutrients to support their growth in dead space of root canal system
- To confine any residual microorganisms that have survived the chemomechanical cleaning and shaping, to prevent their proliferation and pathogenicity
- To prevent percolation of periapical fluids into the root canal system and feeding microorganism

History
1757—Carious teeth were extracted, filled with gold/lead and replanted again.
1847—Hill's stopping was developed.
1867—CA Bowman claimed to be the first to use gutta-percha for root canal filling.
1883—Perry claimed that he had been using a pointed gold wire wrapped with some gutta-percha (roots of present day core carrier technique).
1887— SS White Company began to manufacture GP points.

Timing of Obturation

Patient Symptoms

Sensitivity on percussion—indicates inflammation of periodontal ligament space, hence canal should not be obturated before the inflammation has subsided.

Pulp and Periradicular Status

Vital Pulp Tissue

In case of vital pulp, obturation can be done in single visit after complete cleaning and shaping

Necrotic Pulp Tissue

❑ Single-visit endodontics can be done if tooth is asymptomatic
❑ If patient presents with sensitivity on percussion, it indicates inflammation of periodontal ligament space, hence canal should be obturated after the inflammation has subsided.

Purulent Exudates

If obturation is done in tooth with purulent exudate, pressure and subsequent tissue destruction may occur rapidly. In such cases, calcium hydroxide should be placed as an intracanal medicament.

Negative Culture

Dependence on negative culture has decreased now because studies have shown that false negative results can give inaccurate assessment of microbial flora; also the positive results do not indicate the potential pathogenicity of bacteria.

Extent of Root Canal Filling

❑ Anatomic limit of pulp space is cementodentinal junction (CDJ) apically and pulp chamber coronally. Kuttler (1995) described CDJ as minor apical diameter which ends 0.5 mm short of apical foramen in young patients and 0.67 mm short in older patients. According to Cohen, apical point of termination should be 1 mm from the radiographic apex. Radiographically, the root canal filling should have appearance of a dense, 3-D

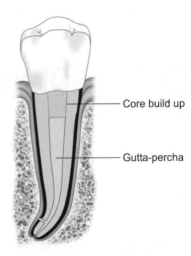

Fig. 19.2 Diagrammatic representation of an obturated tooth.

Core build up
Gutta-percha

filling up to cementodentinal junction (**Figs. 19.1 and 19.2**)

So an ideal obturation should
❑ Fill the entire root canal three dimensionally as close to CDJ as possible
❑ Reflect a continuously tapered funnel same as external root morphology
❑ Radiographically appear as 3-D filling that extends close to CDJ

Overextended obturation is vertical dimension of root filling beyond the apex (**Fig. 19.3**).

Overfilling is total obturation of root canal system with excess material extruding beyond apical foramen (**Figs. 19.4A and B**).

Underfilling is filling of root canal system >2 mm short of radiographic apex (**Fig. 19.5**).

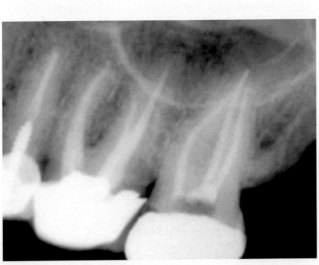

Fig. 19.1 Radiograph showing obturation in maxillary premolar and molars.

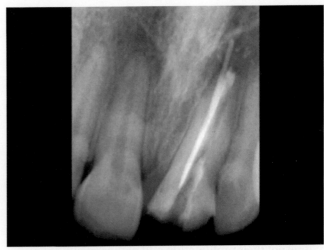

Fig. 19.3 Radiograph showing overextended obturation in maxillary central incisor beyond the apex.

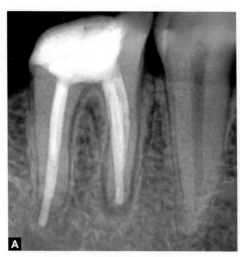
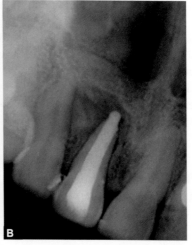

Figs. 19.4A and B Radiograph showing overfilled: (A) Distal canal of mandibular molar; (B) Maxillary central incisor.

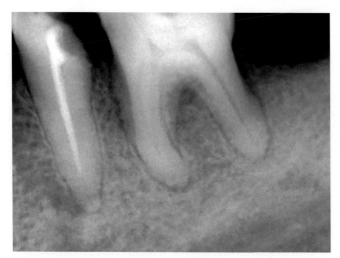

Fig. 19.5 Radiograph showing underfilled canal of mandibular second premolar.

Evaluation of obturation

Radiographically, an obturated tooth should show
- Three-dimensionally filled root canal
- Dense radiopaque filling of root canal system
- Filling close to apical terminus without overextending periapically

But there can be difficulty in radiographic interpretation due to radiopacity of sealer, overlying bony anatomy and 2-D view.

▌Materials Used for Obturation

An ideal root canal filling should be capable of completely preventing communication between the oral cavity and periapical tissue. Root canal sealers should be biocompatible or well tolerated by the tissues in their set state and are used in conjunction with the core filling material to establish an adequate seal.

Grossman (1982) grouped acceptable filling materials into plastics, solids, cements, and pastes. He gave the following 10 requirements for an ideal root canal filling material:

1. Easily introduced into root canal
2. Seal the canal laterally as well as apically
3. Not shrink after being inserted
4. Impervious to moisture
5. Bacteriostatic or at least do not encourage bacterial growth
6. Radiopaque
7. Nonstaining the tooth structure
8. Nonirritating
9. Sterile/easily sterilized immediately before obturation
10. Easily removed from the root canal if necessary

Materials used for root canal obturation are:
- Silver cones
- Gutta-percha
- Custom cones
- Resilon
- Root canal sealers

Silver Cones

- Jasper (1941) introduced silver cones with same success rate as gutta-percha and easier to use
- Rigidity provided by the silver cones made them easy to place and permitted length control
- Due to stiffness of silver cones, these were mainly used for teeth with fine, tortuous, and curved canals like canals

of maxillary first premolars, mesial canal of mandibular molars

- Since silver cones lack plasticity, these are not used in oval canals like single canal premolars and teeth with oval canals in young persons
- But nowadays their use has been declined, due to corrosion caused by them. Presence of traces of copper, nickel, etc. in silver points add up the corrosion

Gutta-Percha

Gutta-percha is derived from two words:
"GETAH"—meaning gum
"PERTJA"—name of the tree in Malay language

Gutta-percha was initially used as a restorative material and later developed into an indispensable endodontic filling material. Being biologically inert, resilient, and electric insulator, it was used for various purposes such as coating the transatlantic telegraph cable, cores of golf balls, handles of knives, splints for holding fractured joints, to control hemorrhage in extracted sockets, in various skin diseases such as psoriasis and eczema.

Historical background
1843—Sir Jose d'Almeida first introduced gutta-percha to Royal Society of England.
In Dentistry—Edwin Truman introduced gutta-percha as temporary filling material.
1847—Hill introduced Hill's stopping (a mixture of bleached gutta-percha and carbonate of lime and quartz).
1867—Bowman first used gutta-percha as root canal filling material.
1883—Perry packed gold wire wrapped with gutta-percha in root canals.
1887—SS White Company started the commercial manufacture of gutta-percha points.
1893—Rollins used gutta-percha with pure oxide of mercury in root canals.
1914—Callahan softened the gutta-percha by using rosins and then used it for obturation of the root canals.
1959—Ingle and Levine proposed standardization of root canal instruments and filling materials.
1976—A group evolved into present day ISO for approval of specification of root canal instruments and filling materials.
ADA specification for gutta-percha points is no. 78

Sources

Gutta-percha is a rigid natural latex produced from sap of trees of genus *Palaquium*. These trees are found in Southeast Asia, especially in Malaysia and Indonesia. In India, these are found in Assam and Western Ghats.

Chemistry

It is an isomer of natural rubber and the natural chemical form of gutta-percha is *trans*-1,4-polyisoprene. The *cis*-form belongs to latex elastomer.

Composition of commercially available gutta-percha (given by Friedman et al.)

• Matrix (organic)	Gutta-percha	20%
• Filler (inorganic)	Zinc oxide	66%
• Radiopacifiers (inorganic) sulfates	Heavy metal	11%
• Plasticizers (organic)	Waxes or resins	3%

In other words
- Organic content – Gutta-percha + waxes = 23%
- Inorganic content – ZnO + metal sulfates = 77%

Phases of gutta-percha

Chemically pure gutta-percha exists in two different crystalline forms, that is, α and β, which differ in molecular repeat distance and single bond form. Natural gutta-percha coming directly from the tree is in α-form while the most commercial available product is in β-form. These phases are interconvertible.

α-Form	β-Form
• Brittle at room temperature	• Stable and flexible at room temperature
• Becomes tacky and flowable when heated (low viscosity)	• Becomes less adhesive and flowable when heated (high viscosity)
• Thermoplasticized gutta-percha for warm compaction technique is in α-form	• Gutta-percha points used with cold compaction are in β-form

Properties of Gutta-percha

- **Biocompatibility:** It is inert, highly biocompatible
- **Ductility:** Depending on phase existence, it is a ductile material
- **Melting point:** It is 60°C
- **Dimensional stability:** Expansion and shrinkage occurs due to heating and cooling, otherwise it is dimensionally stable material
- **Ease of handling:** It can be used both in α- and β-form for obturation depending upon handling features

Clinical Considerations

- On heating, gutta-percha expands that accounts for its increased volume which can be compacted into the root canal
- Gutta-percha shrinks as it returns to normal temperature. So, vertical pressure should be applied in all warm gutta-percha technique to compensate for volume change when cooling occurs (Schilder et al.)

- Aging of gutta-percha causes brittleness because of the oxidation process **(Fig. 19.6)**. Storage under artificial light also speeds up their deterioration. Brittle gutta-percha can be rejuvenated by a technique described by Sorien and Oliet. In this, gutta-percha is immersed in hot water (55°C) for 1 or 2 s and then immediately immersed in cold water for few seconds
- Gutta-percha cannot be heat sterilized. For disinfection of gutta-percha points, they should be immersed in 5.25% NaOCl for 1 min **(Fig. 19.7)**
- After this, gutta-percha should be rinsed in hydrogen peroxide or ethyl alcohol to remove crystallized NaOCl before obturation, as these crystallized particles impair the obturation

- Gutta-percha should always be used with sealer and cement to seal root canal space as gutta-percha lacks adhering qualities
- Gutta-percha is soluble in certain solvents like chloroform, eucalyptus oil, etc. This property can be used to plasticize gutta-percha by treating it with the solvent for better filling in the canal. But it has shown that gutta-percha shrinks (1–2%) when solidified
- Gutta-percha also shows some tissue irritation which is due to high content of zinc oxide

Current Available Forms of Gutta-percha

- *Gutta-percha points*: Standard cones are of same size and shape as that of ISO endodontic instruments **(Fig. 19.8)**
- *Auxiliary points:* Non-standardized cones; perceive form of root canal
- *Greater taper gutta-percha points:* Available in 4%, 6%, 8%, and 10% taper **(Fig. 19.9)**

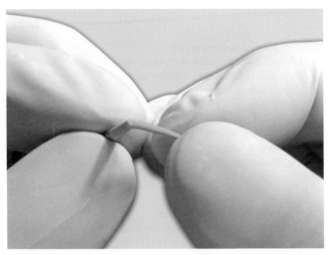

Fig. 19.6 Aging causes gutta-percha to become brittle which breaks upon bending.

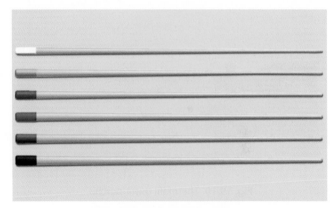

Fig. 19.8 Gutta-percha points.

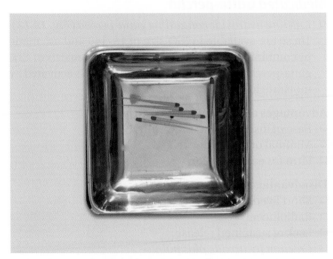

Fig. 19.7 Sterilization of gutta-percha by immersing in 5.25% sodium hypochlorite for 1 min.

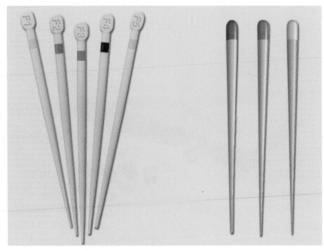

Fig. 19.9 Greater taper gutta-percha points.

- **Gutta-percha pellets/bars:** They are used in thermoplasticized gutta-percha obturation, for example, obtura system
- **Precoated core carrier gutta-percha:** In these stainless steel, titanium or plastic carriers are precoated with α-phase gutta-percha for use in canal, for example, thermafil **(Fig. 19.10)**
- **Syringe systems:** These use low viscosity gutta-percha, for example, α-seal
- **Gutta flow:** In this gutta-percha powder is incorporated into resin-based sealer **(Fig. 19.11)**
- **Gutta-percha sealers like chloropercha and eucopercha:** In these, gutta-percha is dissolved in chloroform/eucalyptol to be used in the canal
- **Medicated gutta-percha:** Calcium hydroxide, iodoform, or chlorhexidine diacetate containing gutta-percha points

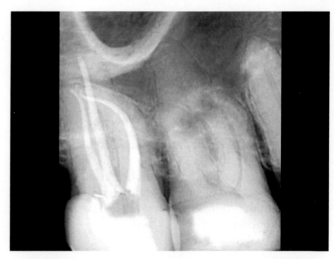

Fig. 19.12 Radiograph showing radiopaque gutta-percha.

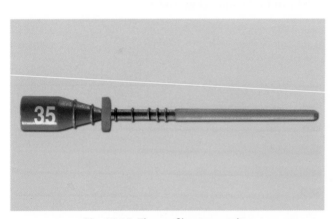

Fig. 19.10 Thermafil gutta-percha.

Advantages of gutta-percha
- *Compatibility:* Adaptation to canal walls
- *Inertness:* Makes it non reactive material
- *Dimensionally stable*
- *Tissue tolerance*
- *Radiopacity:* Easily recognizable on radiograph **(Fig. 19.12)**
- *Plasticity:* Becomes plastic when heated
- Dissolve in some solvents like chloroform, eucalyptus oil, etc. This property makes it more versatile as canal filling material

Disadvantages of gutta-percha
- *Lack of rigidity:* Bending of gutta-percha is seen when lateral pressure is applied. So, difficult to use in smaller canals
- Easily displaced by pressure
- Lacks adhesive quality

Medicated Gutta-percha

- *Calcium hydroxide containing gutta-percha (**Fig. 19.13**):* These are available in ISO size of 15–140 and are made by combining 58% of calcium hydroxide in matrix of 42% gutta-percha. Action of calcium hydroxide is activated by moisture in canal

Advantages of calcium hydroxide points
- Ease of insertion and removal
- Minimal or no residue left
- Firm for easy insertion

Disadvantages
- Short lived action
- Radiolucent
- Lack of sustained release
- *Calcium hydroxide plus points*
  - Along with calcium hydroxide and gutta-percha, they contain tenside which reduces the surface tension

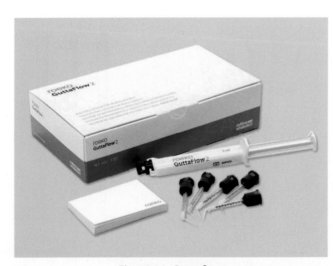

Fig. 19.11 Gutta flow.

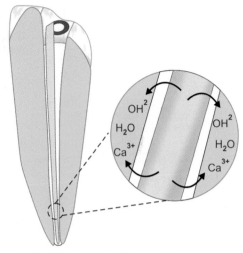

Fig. 19.13 Calcium hydroxide containing gutta-percha.

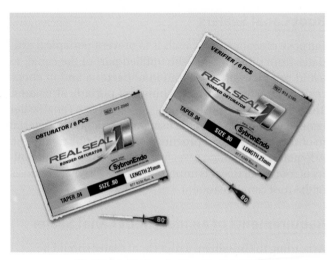

Fig. 19.14 Real seal obturation system.

- Due to presence of water soluble components, such as tenside and sodium chloride, they are three times more reactive than calcium hydroxide points
- They have superior pH and increases wettability of canal surface with increased antibacterial property
- They have sustained alkaline pH for one week

❑ *Iodoform containing gutta-percha*
- Iodoform containing gutta-percha remains inert till it comes in to contact with the tissue fluids
- On coming in to contact with tissue fluids, free iodine is released, which is antibacterial in nature

❑ Chlorhexidine diacetate containing gutta-percha
- In this, gutta-percha matrix is embedded in 5% chlorhexidine diacetate
- This material is used as an intracanal medicament

Resilon (Fig. 19.14)

❑ A resin-based obturation system was introduced as an alternative to gutta-percha. It consists of a resin core material (Resilon) composed of polyester, difunctional methacrylate, bioactive glass and radiopaque fillers, and a resin sealer. Core material is available in conventional and standardized cones and pellets
❑ Resilon core bonds to resin sealer, which attaches to the etched root surface forming a "monoblock." This results in a gutta-percha–sealer interface and a tooth–sealer interface. This bonding provides a better coronal seal and may strengthen the root
Resilon is discussed in detail on page no. 290.

Custom Cones (Fig. 19.15)

❑ When apical foramen is open or canal is large, a custom cone is made which allows adaptation of the cone to canal walls and improves the seal

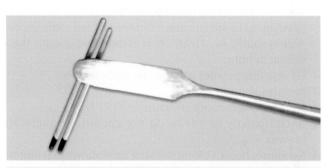

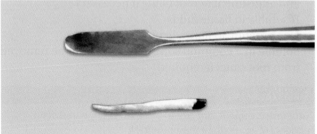

Fig. 19.15 Custom cone made according to shape of canal.

❑ Technique involves customization of gutta-percha cones according to the canal shape by:
- Softening it in chloroform, eucalyptol, or halothane for 1–2 seconds
- Heating several large gutta-percha cones and rolling the mass between two glass slabs until an appropriate size is obtained
❑ Softened cone is then placed into the canal and gently packed to the length. This process is repeated until an adequate impression of the canal is obtained at the prepared length

Root Canal Sealers

Purpose of sealing root canals is to prevent periapical exudates from diffusing into the unfilled part of the canal, to avoid re-entry and colonization of bacteria and to check residual bacteria from reaching the periapical tissues. Therefore to accomplish a fluid tight seal, a root canal sealer is needed. Though sealer is used only as adjunct material in obturation, it affects prognosis of endodontic treatment. Adequate combination of sealing ability and biocompatibility of root canal sealer is important for a favorable prognosis of the root canal treatment.

Requirements of an Ideal Root Canal Sealer

According to Grossman, a root canal sealer should be
- Tacky when mixed so as to provide good adhesion between it and canal wall
- Able to create hermetic seal
- Radiopaque so as to be visible on radiograph. According to ANSI/ADA specification number 57, all endodontic sealers should be at least 2 mm Al more radiopaque than dentin or bone
- Of very fine powder particles for optimal mix
- Not shrink upon setting
- Nonstaining to tooth structure
- Bacteriostatic or atleast do not encourage bacterial growth
- Set slowly because long working time allows placement and adjustment of root filling if necessary
- Insoluble in tissue fluids
- Nonirritating to periradicular tissue
- Soluble in a common solvent so that it can be removed from root canal if required

Stains caused by different sealers	
Grossman's cement, zinc oxide–eugenol (ZOE), endomethasone and N$_2$	Orange–red stain
Diaket and Tubli-Seal	Mild pink discoloration
AH-26	Gray color
Riebler's paste	Dark red stain

The following were added to Grossman's basic requirements:
- It should not provoke an immune response in periradicular tissue
- It should be neither mutagenic nor carcinogenic

Functions of Root Canal Sealers

- ***Antimicrobial agent:*** Sealers show antibacterial effect which is excreted immediately after its placement
- ***Fill in the discrepancies*** between the obturating material and dentin walls **(Fig. 19.16)**

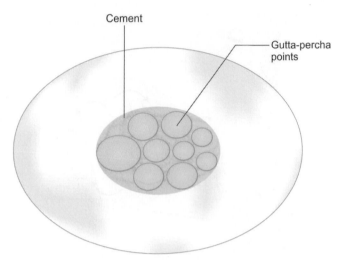

Fig. 19.16 Sealer fills the space between gutta-percha points.

- ***Binding agent:*** Act as binding agent between obturating material and dentin walls
- ***As lubricant:*** When used with semisolid materials, sealer acts as a lubricant
- ***Radiopacity:*** Due to radiopacity, sealer can be seen on radiograph and thus can show presence of auxiliary canals, resorptive areas, root fractures, and shape of apical foramen
- ***Certain techniques dictate use of particular sealer:*** For example, chloropercha technique uses material as sealer as well as a solvent for the master cone. It allows the shape of normal gutta-percha cone to be altered according to the shape of the prepared canal

Classification

Classification of Sealers According to their Composition

- Eugenol
  - Silver containing cements:
    - Kerr sealer (Rickert, 1931)
    - Procosol radiopaque silver cement (Grossman, 1936)
  - Silver free cements:
    - Procosol nonstaining cement (Grossman, 1958)
    - Grossman's sealer (Grossman, 1974)
    - Tubliseal (Kerr, 1961)
    - Wach's paste (Wach)
- Noneugenol
  - Diaket
  - AH-26
  - Chloropercha and eucapercha
  - Nogenol

- Hydron
- Endofil
- Glass ionomer
- Polycarboxylate
- Calcium phosphate cement
- ❏ Medicated: These sealers have therapeutic properties and normally used without core materials
  - Diaket-A
  - N_2
  - Endomethasone
  - SPAD
  - Iodoform paste
  - Riebler's paste
  - Mynol cement
  - $Ca(OH)_2$ paste

Classification According to Grossman

- ❏ Zinc oxide resin cement
- ❏ Calcium hydroxide cements
- ❏ Paraformaldehyde cements
- ❏ Pastes

According to Cohen

ADA specification no. 57 classifies endodontic filling materials as follows:
- ❏ Type I: Material intended to be used with core material
  Subtypes:
  - Class 1: Includes materials in the form of powder and liquid that sets through a nonpolymerizing process
  - Class 2: Includes material in the form of two pastes that sets through a nonpolymerizing process
  - Class 3: Includes polymers and resin systems that set through polymerization
- ❏ Type II: Material intended to be used with or without core material or sealer
  - Class 1: Powder and liquid nonpolymerizing
  - Class 2: Paste and paste nonpolymerizing
  - Class 3: Metal amalgams
  - Class 4: Polymer and resin systems—polymerization

According to Ingle

- ❏ Cements
- ❏ Pastes
- ❏ Plastics

According to Harty FJ

1. ZOE-based
2. *Resin-based:* Consists of an epoxy resin base which sets upon mixing with an activator. For example, AH-26, Diaket, hydron
3. Gutta percha-based cements consist of solutions of gutta-percha in organic solvents, for example, chloropercha, eupercha
4. Dentin adhesive materials, like cyanoacrylate cements, glass ionomer cements, polycarboxylate cements, calcium phosphate, composite materials
5. Materials to which medicaments have been added; these are divided into two groups:
   i. Those in which strong disinfectants are added to decrease possible postoperative pain, like paraformaldehyde and corticosteroid preparation
   ii. Those in which calcium hydroxide is to induce cementogenesis and dentinogenesis at foramen, thus creating a permanent biological seal. For example, calcibiotic root canal sealer (CRCS), sealapex and biocalex

Zinc Oxide Eugenol (ZOE) Sealers

Chisolm in 1873 introduced zinc oxide and oil of clove cement in dentistry.

Setting reaction: It sets because of a combination of physical and chemical reaction, yielding a hardened mass of zinc oxide embedded in matrix of long sheath-like crystals of zinc eugenolate. Hardening of the mixture is due to formation of zinc eugenolate. Presence of free eugenol tends to weaken the set and shows cytotoxicity. Practically, all ZOE sealer cements are cytotoxic and invoke an inflammatory response in connective tissue.

Sealer	Composition		Features	Problems
Kerr root canal sealer or Rickert's formula (developed by Rickert)	*Powder* Zinc oxide Precipitated silver Oleo resins Thymol iodide *Liquid* Oil of clove Canada balsam	34–41.2% 25–30.0% 30–16% 11–12% 78–80% 20–22%	• Excellent lubricating properties • Greater bulk than any other sealer and thus makes it ideal for warm vertical compaction to fill voids, auxiliary canals and irregularities present lateral to gutta-percha cones	It stains the tooth due to presence of silver

Contd...

Contd...

Sealer	Composition		Features	Problems
Procosol radiopaque-silver cement (Grossman, 1936)	*Powder* • Zinc oxide • Precipitated silver • Hydrogenated resins • Magnesium oxide *Liquid* • Eugenol • Canada balsam	45% 17% 36% 2% 90% 10%		Precipatated silver leads to staining of tooth
Procosol nonstaining cement (Grossman, 1958)	*Powder* • Zinc oxide (reagent) • Staybelite resin • Bismuth subcarbonate • Barium sulfate *Liquid* • Eugenol • Sweet oil of almond	40% 27% 15% 15% 80% 20%	• Cement hardens in approximately 2 h at room temperature • Setting time in canal is less • Begins to set in root canal within 10 to 30 min because of the moisture present in dentin	
Grossman's sealer	*Powder* • Zinc oxide (reagent) • Staybelite resin • Bismuth subcarbonate • Barium sulfate • Sodium borate *Liquid* • Eugenol	42 parts 27 parts 15 parts 15 parts 1 part	It has plasticity and slow setting time (2 h at 37°C) due to presence of sodium borate anhydrate	• Due to coarse particle size of resin, vigorous spatulation is done during mixing • Zinc eugenolate is decomposed by water through continuous loss of eugenol, which makes it a weak unstable compound
Wach's sealer	*Powder* • Zinc oxide • Tricalcium phosphate • Bismuth subnitrate • Bismuth subiodide • Heavy magnesium oxide *Liquid* • Canada balsam • Oil of clove	10 g 2 g 3.5 g 0.3 g 0.5 g 20 mL 6 mL	• Increase in thickness of sealer reduces its lubricating effect. So, it is indicated when there is a possibility of overextension beyond the confines of root canal	• Odor of liquid • Sticky due to presence of Canada balsam
Tubliseal (1961)	*Base* • Zinc oxide • Oleo resins • Bismuth trioxide • Thymol iodide • Oil and waxes *Catalysts* • Eugenol • Polymerized resin • Annidalin	57–59% 18.5–21.25% 7.5% 3.75–5% 10%	• Because of good lubricating property, it is used in cases where it is difficult for a master cone to reach apical third of root canal • Does not stain the tooth structure	• Irritant to periapical tissue • Very low viscosity makes extrusion through apical foramen • Short working time
Endoflas	*Powder* • Zinc oxide • Iodoform • Calcium hydroxide • Barium sulfate *Liquid* • Eugenol • Parachlorophenol		• It includes the advantages of zinc oxide, iodoform and calcium hydroxide • Resorption is only limited to excess material pushed periapically	

Root Canal Sealers without Eugenol

Kloroperka N-Ø Sealers (given by Nyborg and Tullin, 1965)	*Power* • Canada balsam 19.6% • Rosin 11.8% • Gutta-percha 19.6% • Zinc oxide 49% *Liquid* • Chloroform
Chloropercha mixture of gutta-percha (9%) and chloroform 91% *Modified chloropercha methods* *Johnston-Callahan method*	Canal is flooded with Callahan resin chloroform solution for 2–3 min and gutta-percha cone is placed and compressed laterally and apically with a plugger until it gets dissolved completely in the chloroform solution in the root canal. Additional points are added and dissolved in the same way
Nygaard-Ostby	Consists of Canada balsam; colophonium and zinc oxide powder mixed with chloroform. Here, canal walls are coated with Kloroperka, cone is dipped in sealer and placed apically
Hydron (Wichterle and Lim, 1960)	Rapid setting hydrophilic, plastic material used as sealer without using a core. It is available as an injectable root canal filling material
Nogenol	Developed to overcome the irritating quality of eugenol. Base is ZnO with barium sulfate as radiopacifier along with vegetable oil. Set is accelerated by hydrogenated rosin, chlorothymol, and salicylic acid
Appetite root canal sealer	*Type I* • Tricalcium phosphate 80% • Hydroxyapatite 20% | • Polyacrylic acid 25% • Water 75% *Type II* • Tricalcium phosphate 52% • Hydroxyapatite 14% • Iodoform 30% | • Polyacrylic acid 25% • Water 75% *Type III* • Tricalcium phosphate 80% • Hydroxyapatite 14% • Iodoform 5% • Bismuth subcarbonate 1% | • Polyacrylic acid 25% • Water 75%

Resin-Based Sealers

Sealer	Composition	Features	Problems
Diaket **(Schmidt in 1951)**	*Powder:* • Zinc oxide • Bismuth phosphate *Liquid* • Dihydroxy di-chlorodiphenylmethane • B-diketone • Triethanolamine • Caproic acid • Copolymers of vinyl chloride, vinyl acetate, and vinyl isobutyl ether	• Good adhesion • Fast setting • Stable in nature • Superior tensile strength	• Toxic in nature • Tacky material; so difficult to manipulate • If extruded, can lead to fibrous encapsulation • Setting is adversely affected by presence of camphor or phenol
AH-26 **(Schroeder, 1957)**	*Powder* • Bismuth oxide 60% • Hexamethylenetetramine 25% • Silver powder 10% • Titanium oxide 5% *Liquid* • Bisphenol diglycidyl ether	• Good adhesive property • Good flow • Low toxicity and well tolerated by periapical tissue • Setting time is 36–48 h at body temperature and 5–7 days at room temperature	• Allergic/mutagenic potential • Silver present in powder causes discoloration of tooth

Contd...

Contd...

Sealer	Composition	Features	Problems
AH Plus	*Paste A contains* • Epoxy resins • Calcium tungstate • Zirconium oxide • Silica • Iron oxide pigments *AH Plus paste B contains* • Aminoadamantane • Dibenzyldiamine • Calcium tungstate • Zirconium oxide • Silica • Silicone oil	• Because of color and shade stability, material of choice where esthetic is required • Adapts closely to canal walls • Minimum shrinkage on setting	
Fiberfill (composition resembles to dentin bonding agents)	• Mixture of UDMA, PEGDMA, HDDMA, Bis-GMA resins • Treated barium borosilicate glasses • Barium sulfate and silica • Calcium hydroxide and phosphates • Initiators, stabilizers, pigments • Benzoyl peroxide *Fiberfill primer A* • Mixture of acetone and active monomer, NTG-GMA magnesium *Fiberfill primer B* • Mixture of acetone and PMGDMA, HEMA initiator • Mix equal number of drops of fiberfill primer A and B and apply to root canal		

Calcium Hydroxide Sealers

Sealer	Composition	Features	Problems
Sealapex	*Base* • Calcium hydroxide, zinc oxide, calcium oxide, butyl benzene, fumed silica *Catalyst* • Barium sulfate, titanium dioxide, zinc stearate, isobutyl salicylate, disalicylate, trisalicylate, bismuth trioxide	• Good therapeutic effect and biocompatible • Extruded material resorbs in 4–5 months	• In 100% humidity, it takes 3 weeks to final set. It never sets in a dry atmosphere • Absorbs water and expands on setting
CRCS	*Powder* • Zinc oxide • Hydrogenated resin • Barium sulfate • Calcium hydroxide • Bismuth subcarbonate *Liquid* • Eugenol • Eucalyptol	• Biocompatible • Takes 3 days to set • Stable in nature • Little water resorption	• Extruded sealer is resistant to resorption by tissue fluids • It shows minimal antibacterial activity

Contd...

Contd...

Apexit Plus	*Base* • Calcium hydroxide/calcium oxide, hydrated collophonium, and fillers *Activator* • Disalicylate, bismuth hydroxide/carbonate, bismuth oxide, and fillers	• Excellent tissue tolerance • Durable sealing of the root canal due to the slight setting expansion • Its easy flowing composition allows the material to adapt well even to morphologically complicated canals • Convenient application (automix syringe and intra canal tip enable easy direct application) • Long working time (mixed Apexit Plus can be used over 3 h at room temperature)	
Medicated sealers N_2 (Sargenti and Ritcher, 1961) N_2 refers to second nerve *(Pulp is referred to as first nerve).*	*Powder* • Zinc oxide 68.51 g • Lead tetraoxide 12.00 g • Paraformaldehyde 4.70 g • Bismuth subcarbonate 2.60 g • Bismuth subnitrate 3.70 g • Titanium dioxide 8.40 g • Phenylmercuric borate 0.09 g *Liquid* • Eugenol • Oleum Rosae • Oleum Lavandulae	• Corticosteroids are added to cement separately as hydrocortisone powder or Terra-Cortril • Continued release of formaldehyde gas causes prolonged fixation and antiseptic action	• Degree of irritation is severe with overfilling when N_2 gets pushed into maxillary sinus or mandibular canal, it can result in persisting paresthesia
Endomethasone (composition is almost similar to N_2)	*Powder* • Zinc oxide 100.00 g • Bismuth subnitrate 100.00 g • Dexamethasone 0.019 g • Hydrocortisone 1.60 g • Thymol iodide 25.0 g • Paraformaldehyde 2.20 g *Liquid* Eugenol	• Radiopaque • Neither resorbable after setting nor retractable to allow stable root canal obturation. • Antiseptic and anti-inflammatory	
Silicone-based sealers **Endo-fill**	• Silicone monomer, silicone-based catalyst, bismuth subnitrate filler • Active ingredients are hydroxyl terminated dimethyl polysiloxane, benzyl alcohol, and hydrophobic amorphous silica • Catalysts are tetraethyl orthosilicate and polydimethylsiloxane	• Ease of penetration • Adjustable working time • Low working viscosity • Rubbery consistency • Nonresorbable	• Cannot be used in presence of hydrogen peroxide • Canal must be absolutely dry • Shrinks upon setting but has affinity for flowing into open dentinal tubules • Difficult to remove from the canals
Roeko seal	• Main constituent is polydimethylsiloxane	• Low film thickness, good flow, biocompatibility, and low solubility	• Shows 0.2% expansion on setting
Glass ionomer sealer (Ketac-Endo)	*Powder* • Calcium aluminum lanthanum flurosilicate glass • Calcium volframate • Silicic acid • Pigments *Liquid* • Polyethylene polycarbonic acid/maleic acid • Copolymer • Tartaric acid • Water	• Shows bonding to dentin • Optimal flow property	• It cannot be removed from root canal if retreatment is required

Abbreviation: CRCS: calcibiotic root canal sealer.

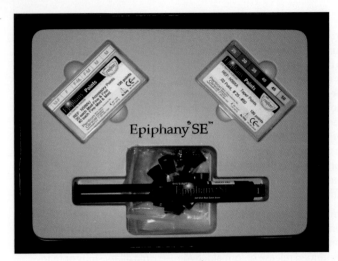

Fig. 19.17 Resilon.

Resilon (Fig. 19.17)

Resilon (Epiphany, Pentron Clinical Technologies; Wallingford, CT; RealSeal, SybronEndo; Orange, CA) is developed to overcome the problems associated with gutta-percha, viz

- Shrinkage of gutta-percha on cooling
- Gutta-percha does not bind physically to the sealer, it results in gap formation between the sealer and the gutta-percha

Resilon core shrinks only 0.5% and bonds to sealer by polymerization, so no gaps are seen. It is biocompatible, noncytotoxic, and nonmutagenic. The excellent sealing ability of resilon system is attributed to the "monoblock" which is formed by adhesion of the resilon cone to epiphany sealer, which adheres and penetrates into the dentin walls of root canal system.

Components of Resilon System

- **Primer:** It is a self-etch primer, which contains a sulfonic acid terminated functional monomer, HEMA, water, and a polymerization initiator
- **Resilon sealer:** It is a dual-cure, resin-based sealer. Resin matrix contains Bis-GMA, ethoxylated Bis-GMA, UDMA, and hydrophilic difunctional methacrylates. It contains fillers of calcium hydroxide, barium sulfate, barium glass, bismuth oxychloride, and silica. Total filler content is 70% by weight
- **Resilon core material:** It is a thermoplastic synthetic polymer-based (polyester) core material which contains bioactive glass, bismuth oxychloride, and barium sulfate. Filler content is 65% by weight

Method of Use

- **Smear layer removal:** Sodium hypochlorite should not be the last irrigant to be used due to compatibility issues with resins. Use 17% EDTA or 2% chlorhexidine as a final rinse
- **Placement of primer:** After drying the canal using paper points, primer is applied up to apex. Use dry paper points to wick out the excess primer from canal. Primer is very important because it creates a collagen matrix that increases the surface area for bonding. Low viscosity primer also draws the sealer into the dentinal tubules
- **Placement of sealer:** Sealer can be placed into canal using a lentulo spiral or by coating the master cone
- **Obturation:** Obturate the canals by lateral or warm vertical compaction
- **Curing:** Resilon is cured with a halogen curing light for 40 s
- **Coronal restoration:** A coronal restoration is done to seal the access cavity

Advantages of epiphany

- Biocompatible
- Good coronal seal; so less microleakage
- Nontoxic
- Nonmutagenic
- Forms monoblock
- Increases resistance to fracture in endodontically treated teeth

Disadvantage of epiphany

- Does not retain its softness after heating

Monoblock Concept

Literal meaning of monoblock is a single unit.

Monoblock concept means the creation of a solid, bonded, continuous material from one dentin wall of the canal to the other. Monoblock phenomenon strengthens the root by approximately 20%.

Classification of monoblock concept based on number of interfaces present between core filling material and bonding substrate:

Primary: In this, obturation is completely done with core material, for example, use of Hydron, MTA, BioGutta as en masse materials **(Fig. 19.18A)**.

Secondary: These have two circumferential interfaces, one between sealer and the primed dentin and other between the sealer and core material **(Fig. 19.18B)**. For example, resilon-based system.

Tertiary: In this, conventional gutta-percha surface is coated with resin which bonds with the sealer, which further bonds to canal walls. So, there are three circumferential interfaces **(Fig. 19.18C)**:

1. Between the sealer and primed dentin
2. Between the sealer and coating which has been applied over gutta-percha to make them bondable to the root surface
3. Between the coating and the core material
   For example, EndoRez and Activ GP system.

Two prerequisites for a monoblock to function as mechanically homogenous unit:

1. Material should be able to bond strongly and mutually to each other and substrate used for monoblock
2. Monoblock material should have same modulus of elasticity as that of substrate (dentin/restoration)

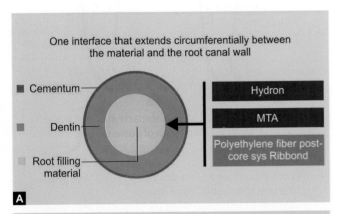

One interface that extends circumferentially between the material and the root canal wall

- Cementum
- Dentin
- Root filling material

Hydron

MTA

Polyethylene fiber post-core sys Ribbond

A

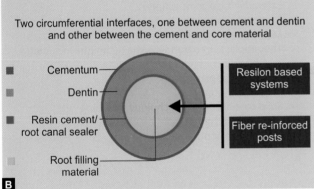

Two circumferential interfaces, one between cement and dentin and other between the cement and core material

- Cementum
- Dentin
- Resin cement/ root canal sealer
- Root filling material

Resilon based systems

Fiber re-inforced posts

B

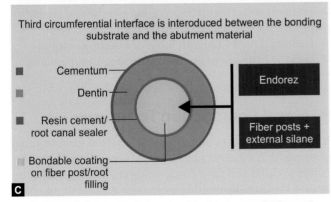

Third circumferential interface is introduced between the bonding substrate and the abutment material

- Cementum
- Dentin
- Resin cement/ root canal sealer
- Bondable coating on fiber post/root filling

Endorez

Fiber posts + external silane

C

Figs. 19.18A to C (A) Primary monoblock concept; (B) Secondary monoblock concept; (C) Tertiary monoblock concept.

Methods of Sealer Placement

- Coating the master cone and placing the sealer in canal with a pumping action. (**Fig. 19.19**)
- Placing the sealer in canal with a lentulo spiral (**Fig. 19.20**)
- Placing the sealer on master apical file and turning the file counterclockwise (**Fig. 19.21**)
- Injecting the sealer with special syringes (**Fig. 19.22**)
- Sealer placement techniques vary with the status of apical foramen
- If apex is open, only apical one-third of master cone is coated with sealer to prevent its extrusion into periapical tissues
- If apex is closed, any of above techniques can be used

Obturation Techniques

Material of choice for obturation is gutta-percha in conjunction with sealer. Obturation methods vary by direction of compaction (lateral/vertical) and/or temperature of gutta-percha used either cold or warm (plasticized) (**Figs. 19.23A and B**).

There are two basic procedures:
1. Lateral compaction of cold gutta-percha
2. Vertical compaction of warm gutta-percha

Other methods are the variations of warmed gutta-percha technique.

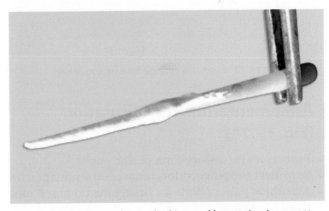

Fig. 19.19 Sealer can be applied in canal by coating it on gutta-purcha cone.

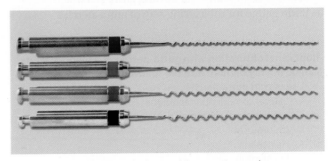

Fig. 19.20 Lentulo spiral for carrying sealer.

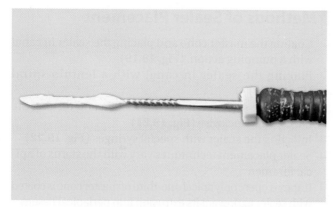

Fig. 19.21 Sealer can be placed in canal by applying it on master apical file and turning counter clockwise.

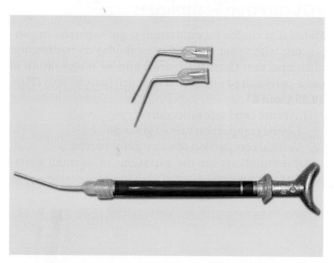

Fig. 19.22 Injectable syringe for carrying sealer.

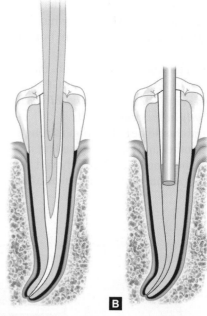

Figs. 19.23A and B (A) Lateral compaction of gutta-percha; (B) Vertical compaction of gutta-percha.

- Use of heat softened gutta-percha
  - Vertical compaction technique
  - System B continuous wave condensation technique
  - Lateral/vertical compaction
  - Sectional compaction technique
  - McSpadden compaction of gutta-percha
  - Thermoplasticized gutta-percha technique including
    - Obtura II
    - Ultrasonic plasticizing
    - Ultrafil system
  - Solid core obturation technique including
    - Thermafil system
    - Silver point obturation

Armamentarium for Obturation (Fig. 19.24)

- ❑ Primary and accessory gutta-percha points
- ❑ Spreaders and pluggers for compaction of guttapercha
- ❑ Absorbent paper points for drying the prepared root canal before applying sealer
- ❑ Lentulo spirals for placing sealer
- ❑ Scissors or GP cutter for cutting gutta-percha
- ❑ Endo gauge for measuring size of gutta-percha

- ❑ Endo block for measuring gutta-percha points
- ❑ Endo organizer for arranging gutta-percha and accessory points of various sizes
- ❑ Heating device like spirit lamp or butane gas torch
- ❑ Heating instrument like ball burnisher, spoon excavator, etc.

Root canal obturation with gutta-percha as a filling material can be mainly divided into the following groups:
- Use of cold gutta-percha
  - Lateral compaction technique
- Use of chemically softened gutta-percha
  - Chloroform
  - Halothane
  - Eucalyptol

Lateral Compaction Technique

It is one of the most common methods used for root canal obturation. It involves placement of tapered gutta-percha cones in canal and then compacting them under pressure against the canal walls using a spreader. A canal should have continuous tapered shape with a definite apical stop, before it is ready to be filled by this method.

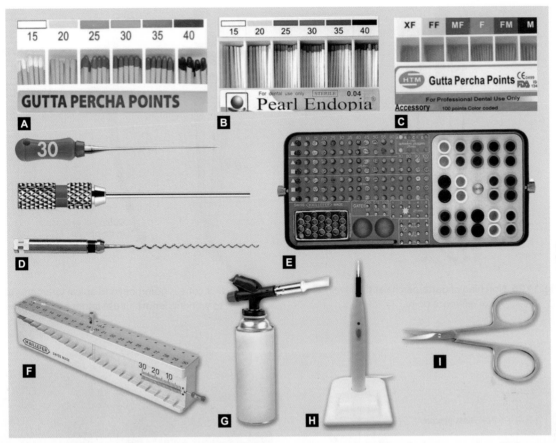

Figs. 19.24A to I Armamentarium for obturation: (A) Primary gutta-percha points; (B) Absorbent paper points; (C) Accessory gutta-percha points; (D) Spreader, plugger and Lentulo spiral; (E) Endo organizer for keeping files and gutta-percha; (F) Endo gauge for measuring size of gutta-percha; (G) Butane gas torch; (H) Gutta-percha cutter; (I) Scissor.

Technique

❑ Following the canal preparation, select the master gutta-percha cone whose diameter is same as that of master apical file. One should feel the tugback with master gutta-percha point **(Fig. 19.25)**. Master gutta-percha point is notched at the working distance analogous to the level of incisal or occlusal edge reference point **(Fig. 19.26)**

❑ Check the fit of cone radiographically. If found satisfactory, remove the cone from the canal and place it in sodium hypochlorite:
  • If cone fits short of the working length, check for dentin chip debris, any ledge, or curve in the canal and treat them accordingly **(Figs. 19.27A and B)**
  • If cone selected is going beyond the foramen, either select the larger number cone or cut that cone to the working length **(Fig. 19.28)**
  • If cone shows "s" shaped appearance in the radiograph, it means cone is too small for the canal. In that case, a larger cone should be selected to fit in the canal **(Fig. 19.29)**

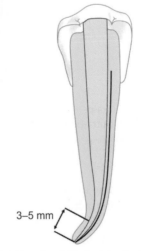

3–5 mm

Fig. 19.25 One should feel tugback with master gutta-percha cone.

❑ Select the size of spreader to be used for lateral compaction of that tooth. It should reach 1–2 mm of true working

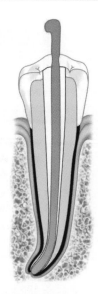

Fig. 19.26 Notching of gutta-percha at the level of reference point.

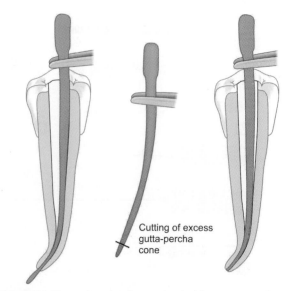

Cutting of excess gutta-percha cone

Fig. 19.28 If cone is going beyond apical foramen, cut the cone to working length or use larger number cone.

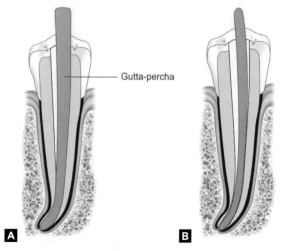

Gutta-percha

A   **B**

Figs. 19.27A and B (A) Gutta-percha showing tight fit in middle and space in apical third; (B) Gutta-percha cone showing tight fit only on apical part of the canal.

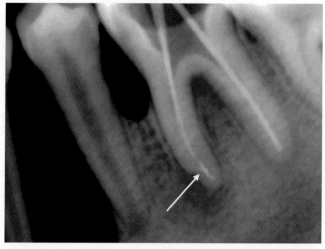

Fig. 19.29 S-shaped appearance of cone in mesial canal shows that cone is too small for the canal, replace it with bigger cone.

length without binding in the canal should occur, there is a chance for tooth fracture with excessive pressures **(Fig. 19.30A)**.

❑ Dry the canal with paper points and apply sealer in canal. Place master gutta-percha cone in the canal **(Fig. 19.30B)**

❑ Coat the premeasured cone with sealer and place into the canal. After master cone placement, place spreader into the canal alongside the cone **(Fig. 19.30C)**. Spreader helps in compaction of gutta-percha. It acts as a wedge to squeeze the gutta-percha laterally under vertical pressure

not by pushing it sideways. It should reach 1–2 mm of the prepared root length

❑ Remove spreader by rotating it back and forth. This compacts the gutta-percha and creates a space for accessory cones lateral to the master cone **(Figs. 19.30D and E)**

❑ Place accessory cone in this space and repeat the above procedure until spreader no longer penetrates beyond the cervical line **(Fig. 19.30F)**

❑ Now sever the protruding gutta-percha points at canal orifice with hot instrument

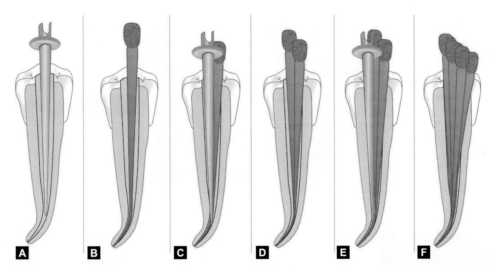

Figs. 19.30A to F (A) Check the fit of the spreader; (B) place the master gutta-percha cone in sealer coated canal; (C) place the spreader alongside the master cone to compact the cone; (D and E) Add accessory cones in the prepared space and repeat the step C to create space for more accessory cones; (F) Place accessory cone in this space and repeat the above procedure until spreader no longer penetrates beyond the cervical line.

Advantages
- Can be used in most clinical situations
- Positive dimensional stability of root filling
- During compaction of gutta-percha, it provides length control, thus decreases the chances of overfilling

Disadvantages
- Presence of voids
- Increased sealer: GP ratio
- Does not produce homogenous mass
- Space may exist between accessory and master cones **(Fig. 19.31)**
- Time-consuming
- Less able to seal lateral canals and intracanal defects

Variation in Lateral Compaction Technique

Use of Vibration, Heat, and Ultrasonics

An alternative to cold lateral compaction is ultrasonics, combination of vibration and heat. Lateral compaction done with alternating heat after placing accessory gutta-percha cone can result in better compaction.

Gutta-percha is soluble in number of solvents, namely, chloroform, eucalyptol, xylol. This property of gutta-percha is used to adapt it in various canal shapes which are amenable to be filled by lateral compaction of gutta-percha technique.

Indications

- In teeth with blunderbuss canals and open apices.
- Root ends with resorptive defects **(Figs. 19.32A to J)**
- In teeth with internal resorption

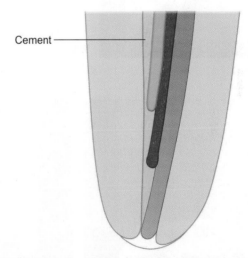

Fig. 19.31 In lateral compaction of gutta-percha, cones never fit as homogeneous mass, sealer occupies the space in between the cones.

Technique (Figs. 19.33A to H)

- Root canal is cleaned and shaped properly
- Cone is held with a locking tweezer which has been adjusted to the working length
- Apical 2–3 mm of cone is dipped into solvent for 3–5 s
- Softened cone is inserted in the canal with slight apical pressure until the beaks of locking tweezer touches the reference point
- Here care is taken to keep the canal moistened by irrigation, otherwise some of softened gutta-percha may stick to the desired canal walls, though this detached segment can be easily removed by using H-file

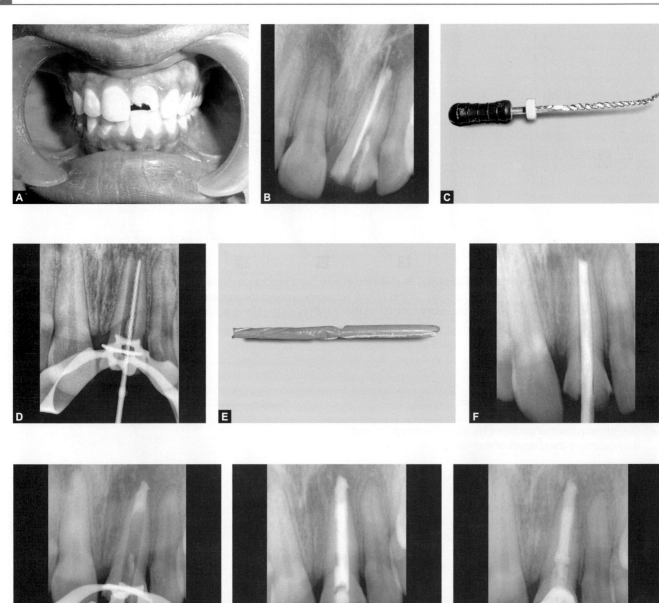

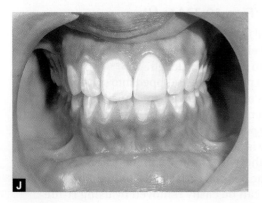

Figs. 19.32A to J Esthetic rehabilitation of maxillary central incisor by endodontic retreatment and crown placement. (A) Preoperative photograph; (B) Preoperative radiograph; (C) Old gutta-percha removed; (D) working length radiograph; (E) custom-made gutta-percha cone; (F) Radiograph taken with master cone; (G) MTA plug given for apical stop; (H) Obturation done using gutta-percha and MTA; (I) Postobturation radiograph; (J) Postobturation photograph.

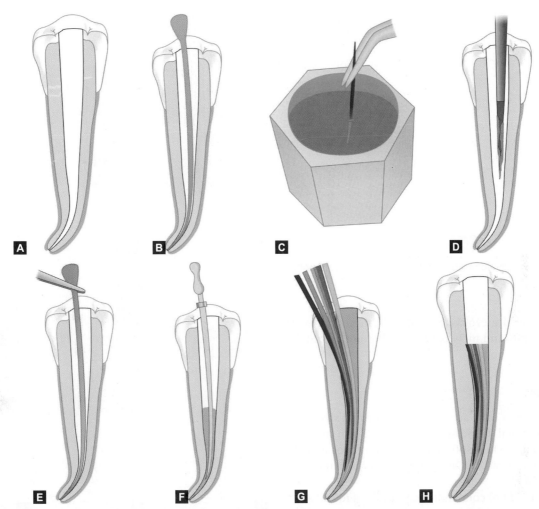

Figs. 19.33A to H (A) Thoroughly clean and shape the canal; (B) adjust the cone to working length; (C) dip apical 2 to 3 mm of cone into solvent for 3 to 5 s; (D) Coat the canal with sealer; (E) Place the softened cone in the canal; (F and G) Compact the cone using spreader and place the accessory gutta-percha cones; (H) Sever the protruding gutta-percha cones using hot burnisher.

- Radiograph is taken to verify the fit and correct working length of the cone. When found satisfactory, cone is removed from the canal and canal is irrigated with sterile water or 99% isopropyl alcohol to remove the residual solvent
- After this canal is coated with sealer. Cone is dipped again for 2–3 s in the solvent and thereafter inserted into the canal with continuous apical pressure until the plier touches the reference point
- A finger spreader is then placed in the canal to compact the gutta-percha laterally
- Accessory gutta-percha cones are then placed in the space created by spreader
- Protruding gutta-percha points are cut at canal orifice with hot instrument

Though this method is considered good for adapting gutta-percha to the canal walls, chloroform dip fillings have shown to produce volume shrinkage which may lead to poor apical seal.

Warm Vertical Compaction Technique

Vertical compaction of warm gutta-percha method of filling the root canal was introduced by Schilder with an objective of filling all the portals of exit with maximum amount of gutta-percha and minimum amount of sealer. This is also known as **Schilder's technique of obturation**. In this technique using heated pluggers, pressure is applied in vertical direction to heat softened gutta-percha which causes it to flow and fill the canal space.

Basic requirements of a prepared canal to be filled by vertical compaction technique are
- Continuous tapering funnel shape from orifice to apex **(Fig. 19.34)**
- Apical opening to be as small as possible so as to prevent extrusion of obturating material

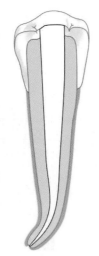

Fig. 19.34 Canal should be continuous funnel shape from orifice to apex.

❑ Decreasing the cross-sectional diameter at every point apically and increasing at each point as canal is approached coronally

Technique

❑ Select a master cone according to shape and size of the prepared canal. Cone should fit in 1–2 mm of apical stop because when softened material moves apically into prepared canal, it adapts better to the canal walls **(Fig. 19.35A)**
❑ Confirm the fit of cone radiographically, if found satisfactory, remove it from the canal and place in sodium hypochlorite
❑ Irrigate the canal and then dry by rinsing it with alcohol and latter using the paper points
❑ Select the heat transferring instrument and pluggers according to canal shape and size **(Figs. 19.35B to D)**
❑ Pluggers are prefitted at 5 mm intervals so as to capture maximum cross-section area of the softened gutta-percha
❑ Lightly coat the canal with sealer
❑ Cut the coronal end of selected gutta-percha at incisal or occlusal reference point
❑ Now use heated plugger to force the gutta-percha into the canal. Blunt end of plugger creates a deep depression in the center of master cone **(Fig. 19.35E)**. The outer walls of softened gutta-percha are then folded inward to fill the central void; at the same time, mass of softened gutta-percha is moved apically and laterally. This procedure also removes 2–3 mm of coronal part of gutta-percha
❑ Once apical filling is done, complete obturation by doing backfilling. Obturate the remaining canal by heating small segments of gutta-percha, carrying them into the canal and then compacting them using heated pluggers as described above **(Figs. 19.35F to H)**

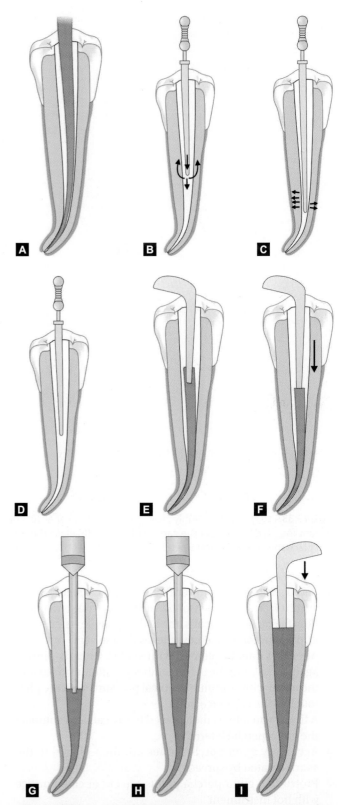

Figs. 19.35A to H (A) Select the master gutta-percha cone; (B) select the plugger according to canal shape and size; (C) Larger sized plugger may bind the canal and may split the root; (D) Small plugger is ineffective for compaction; (E) Heated plugger used to compact gutta-percha; (F to H) Back filling of the canal.

- Take care not to overheat the gutta-percha because it will become too soft to handle
- Do not apply sealer on the softened segments of gutta-percha because sealer will prevent their adherence to the body of gutta-percha present in the canal
- After completion of obturation, clean the pulp chamber with alcohol to remove remnants of sealer or gutta-percha

Advantages
- Excellent sealing of canal apically, laterally and obturation of lateral as well as accessory canals
- Oval canals get better filled than with lateral compaction technique

Disadvantages
- Increased risk of vertical root fracture
- Overfilling of canals with gutta-percha or sealer from apex
- Time-consuming
- Difficult to use in curved canals where rigid pluggers are unable to penetrate to required depth

Temperature Control

System B, Downpak cordless obturation device, and Touch and heat are the devices which permit temperature control.

System B: Continuous Wave Condensation Technique

System B is newly developed device by *Buchanan* for warming gutta-percha in the canal. It monitors temperature at the tip of heat carrier pluggers, thereby delivering a precised amount of heat (**Fig. 19.36**).

To have satisfactory 3-D obturation by using System B technique, following precautions should be taken:

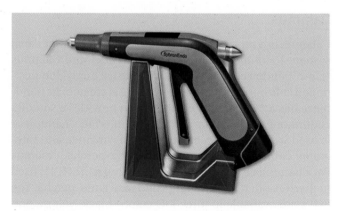

Fig. 19.36 System B cordless endodontic obturation system.
Courtesy: Kerr Sybron Endo.

- Canal shape should be continuous perfectly tapered
- Do not set the System B at high temperature because this may burn gutta-percha
- While down packing, apply a constant firm pressure

Technique (Figs. 19.37A to G)

- Select the Buchanan plugger which matches with the selected gutta-percha cone. Place rubber stop on the plugger and adjust it to its binding point in the canal 5–7 mm short of working length
- Confirm the fit of the gutta-percha cone
- Dry the canal, cut the gutta-percha 0.5 mm short of working length, and apply sealer in the canal
- With the System B turned on to "use," place it in touch mode, set the temperature at 200°C, and dial the power setting to 10. Sever the cone at the orifice with preheated plugger. Afterwards plugger is used to compact the softened gutta-percha at the orifice. Push the plugger smoothly through gutta-percha to 3–4 mm of binding point
- Release the switch. Hold the plugger here for 10 s with a sustained pressure to take up any shrinkage which might occur upon cooling of gutta-percha
- Maintaining the apical pressure, activate the heat switch for 1 sec followed by 1 sec pause and then remove the plugger
- After removal of plugger, introduce a small flexible end of another plugger with pressure to confirm that apical mass of gutta-percha has cooled, set and not dislodged. Following radiographic confirmation, canal is ready for the backfill by any means

Advantages
- It creates single wave of heating and compacting thereby. Compaction of filling material can be done at the same time when it has been heat softened
- Excellent apical control
- Less technique sensitive
- Fast, easy, predictable
- Thorough condensation of the main canal and lateral canals
- Compaction of obturating materials occurs at all levels simultaneously throughout the momentum of heating and compacting instrument apically

Lateral/Vertical Compaction of Warm Gutta-Percha

Vertical compaction causes dense obturation of the root canal, while lateral compaction provides length control and satisfactory ease and speed.

Advantages of both of these techniques are provided by a newer device, Endotec II, which helps the operator to

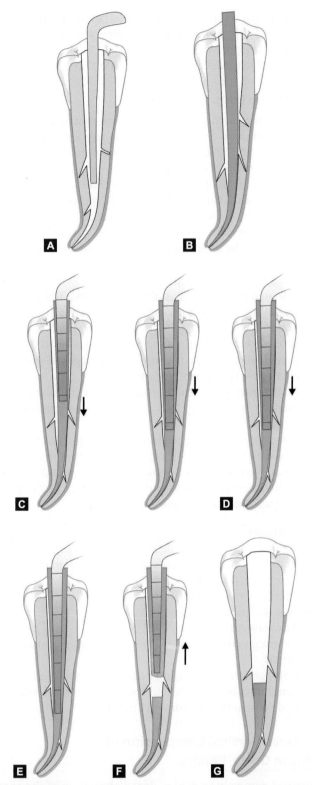

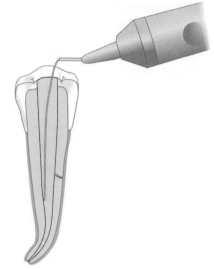

Fig. 19.38 Obturation using Endotec II device.

employ length control with warm gutta-percha technique. It comes with battery which provides energy to heat the attached plugger and spreader **(Fig. 19.38)**.

Technique

❑ Adapt master gutta-percha cone in canal, select endotec plugger, and activate the device
❑ Insert the heated plugger in canal beside master cone to be within 3–4 mm of the apex using light apical pressure
❑ Afterwards, unheated spreader can be placed in the canal to create more space for accessory cones. This process is continued until canal is filled

Advantages

❑ Three-dimensional obturation of canal
❑ Better sealing of accessory and lateral canals
❑ *Endotec* can also be used to soften and remove the gutta-percha

Calamus

Calamus is a recent technique of obturation of root canal system. It combines both Calamus "Pack" and Calamus "Flow" handpiece **(Fig. 19.39)**. With the Pack and Flow positioned side by side, a dense apical plug is created. Its handpiece has a 360° activation cuff, which provides a smooth, continuous flow of gutta-percha. Calamus Flow handpiece is used with a one-piece gutta-percha cartridge and integrated cannula to dispense warm gutta-percha. Calamus Pack handpiece with an electric heat plugger (EHP) is used to thermosoften, remove and condense gutta-percha. The EHPs are available in three ISO color—black, yellow, and blue—which correspond to working end diameters and tapers of 40/03, 50/05, and 60/06, respectively.

Figs. 19.37A to G (A) Selection of plugger according to shape and size of the canal; (B) Confirm fit of the cone; (C) Filling the canal by turning on System B; (D) compaction of gutta-percha by keeping the plugger for 10 s with sustained pressure; (E and F) Removal of plugger; (G) Apical filling of root canal completed.

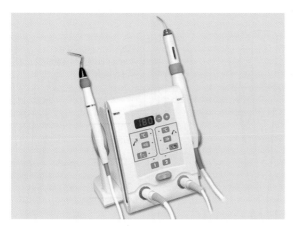

Fig. 19.39 Calamus dual obturation system.

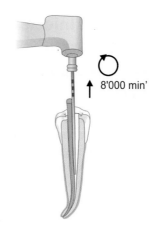

8'000 min'

Fig. 19.40 Thermomechanical compaction of gutta-percha, McSpadden compaction.

Sectional Method of Obturation/ *Chicago Technique*

In this technique, small pieces of gutta-percha cones are used to fill the sections of the canal. It is also known as *Chicago technique* because it was widely promoted by *Coolidge, Lundquist, Blayney*, all from *Chicago*.

Technique

- A gutta-percha cone of same size of the prepared root canal is selected and cut into sections of 3–4 mm long
- Select a plugger which loosely fits within 3 mm of working length
- Apply sealer in the canal
- One end of gutta-percha is mounted to heated plugger and is then carried into the canal and apical pressure is given. After this, disengage the plugger from gutta-percha by rotating it
- Radiograph is taken to confirm its fit. If found satisfactory, fill the remainder of the canal in the same manner

Advantages
- It seals the canals apically and laterally
- In case of post and core cases, only apical section of canal is filled

Disadvantages
- Time-consuming
- If canal gets overfilled, difficult to remove sections of gutta-percha

McSpadden Compaction/ Thermomechanical Compaction of the Gutta-Percha

McSpadden introduced a technique in which heat was used to decrease the viscosity of gutta-percha and thereby increasing its plasticity (**Fig. 19.40**). This technique involves the use of a compacting instrument *(McSpadden compacter)* which resembles inverted Hedstroem file. This is fitted into latch-type handpiece and rotated at 8,000–10,000 rpm alongside gutta-percha cones inside the canal walls **(see Fig. 19.39)**. At this speed, heat produced by friction softens the gutta-percha and designs of blade forces the material apically.

Because of its design, the blades of compaction break easily if it binds, so it should be used only in straight canals. But nowadays, its newer modification in the form of microseal condenser has come, which is made up of nickel–titanium. Because of its flexibility, it can be used in curved canals.

Advantages
- Requires less chair-side time
- Ease of selection and insertion of gutta-percha
- Dense, 3-D obturation

Disadvantages
- Liability to use in narrow and curved canals (canal has to be enlarged to a size no. 45)
- Frequent breakage of compactor blades
- Overfilling of canals
- Shrinkage of gutta-percha on cooling

Thermoplasticized Injectable Gutta-Percha Obturation

Obtura II Heated Gutta-Percha System/ High-Heat System

This technique was *introduced in 1977 at Harvard institute*. It consists of an electric control unit with pistol grip syringe and specially designed gutta-percha pellets which are heated to approximately 365–390°F (185–200°C) for obturation (**Fig. 19.41**). In this, regular β-phase of gutta-percha is used.

Prerequisites for Canal to be filled by Obtura II

❑ Continuous tapering funnel shape for unrestricted flow of softened gutta-percha (**Fig. 19.42A**)
❑ A definite apical stop to prevent overfilling

Indications for using Obtura II

❑ Roots with straight or slightly curved canals
❑ For backfilling of canals
❑ For obturation of roots with internal resorption, perforations, etc.

Technique

❑ Before starting the obturation, applicator needle and pluggers are selected. Needle tip should reach ideally 3–5 mm of the apical terminus passively (**Fig. 19.42B**)
❑ Apply sealer along the dentinal walls to fill the interface between gutta-percha and dentinal walls
❑ Place obtura needle loosely 3–5 mm short of apex, as warm gutta-percha flows and fills the canal, back pressure pushes the needle out of the canal (**Fig. 19.42C**)

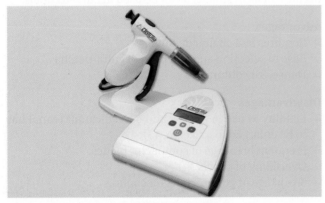

Fig. 19.41 Obtura II
Courtesy: Obtura Spartan, Fenton.

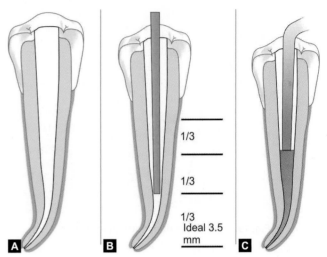

Figs. 19.42A to C (A) Tapering funnel shape of prepared canal is well suited for obturation using obtura II; (B) Needle tip of obtura II should reach 3–5 mm of apical end; (C) Compaction of gutta-percha using plugger

❑ Now use pluggers to compact the gutta-percha; pluggers are dipped in isopropyl alcohol or sealer to prevent sticking of the gutta-percha

Continuous compaction force should be applied throughout the obturation of whole canal to compensate shrinkage and to close any voids if formed.

Variations in Thermoplasticizing Technique of Gutta-Percha

Ultrasonic Plasticizing of Gutta-Percha

❑ It has been seen that ultrasonics can be used to fill the canals by plasticizing the gutta-percha
❑ Earlier, cavitron US scaler was used for this purpose but its design limited its use only in anterior teeth
❑ Recently, ENAC ultrasonic unit comes with an attached spreader which has shown to produce homogenous compaction of gutta-percha

Ultrafil System

❑ This system uses low temperature, (90°C) plasticized α-phase gutta-percha
❑ Here gutta-percha is available in three different viscosities for use in different situations
❑ Regular set and the firm set with highest flow properties primarily used for injection and need not be compacted manually. Endoset is more of viscous and can be condensed immediately after injection

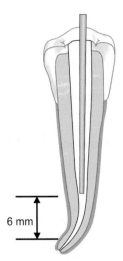

Fig. 19.43 Needle should reach 6–7 mm from the apical end.

6 mm

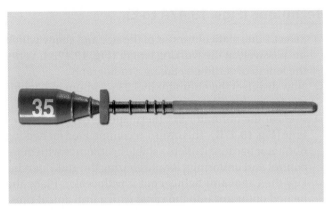

Fig. 19.44 Thermafil cones.

Technique

❑ Cannula needle is checked in canal for fitting. It should be 6–7 mm from apex **(Fig. 19.43)**. After confirming the fit, it is placed in heater which has a preset temperature of 90°C.

❑ Apply sealer in the canal and passively insert the needle into the canal. As the warm gutta-percha fills the canal, its backpressure pushes the needle out of the canal

❑ Once needle is removed, prefitted plugger dipped in alcohol is used for manual compaction of gutta-percha

Difference between Obtura II and Ultrafil II	
Obtura II	*Ultrafil II*
• Uses high temperature	• Uses low temperature
• Uses gun with heating element	• There is no heating element
• Uses needles of 18, 20, 22, and 25 gauze	• Uses needles of 22 gauze
• Digital display of temperature	• No digital read out
• Working time is 3–10 min	• Working time is <1 min

Solid Core Carrier Technique

Thermafil Endodontic Obturators

Thermafil endodontic obturators are specially designed of flexible steel, titanium, or plastic carriers coated with α-phase gutta-percha. Thermafil obturation was devised by **W. Ben Johnson in 1978**.

In this, carriers are made up of stainless steel, titanium, or plastic. They have ISO standard dimension with matching color coding in the sizes of 20–140 **(Fig. 19.44)**. Plastic carrier is made up of special synthetic resin which can be liquid

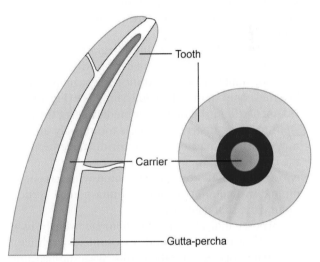

Tooth

Carrier

Gutta-percha

Fig. 19.45 The carrier is not primary cone for obturation. It acts as a carrier for carrying thermoplasticized gutta-percha.

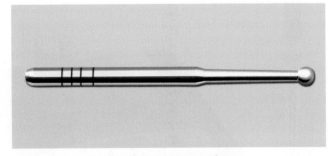

Fig. 19.46 Therma cut bur.

plastic crystal or polysulfone polymer. The carrier is not the primary cone for obturation. It acts as carrier and condenser for thermally plasticized gutta-percha **(Fig. 19.45)**. Plastic cores allow postspace to be made easily and they can be cut off by heated instrument, stainless steel bur, diamond stone, or therma cut bur **(Fig. 19.46)**.

Technique (Figs. 19.47A to E)

❑ Select a thermafil obturator of the size and shape which fits passively at the working length (**Fig. 19.47A**). Verify the length of verifier by taking a radiograph

❑ Now disinfect the obturator in 5.25% sodium hypochlorite for 1 min and then rinse it in 70% alcohol

❑ Preheat the obturator in "Thermaprep" oven for sometime (**Fig. 19.47B**). This oven is recommended for heating obturator because it offers a stable heat source with more control and uniformity for plasticizing the gutta-percha

❑ Dry the canal and lightly coat it with sealer. Place the heated obturator into the canal with a firm apical pressure (**Fig. 19.47C**) to the marked working length

❑ Working time is 8–10 s after removal of obturator from oven. If more obturators are required, insert them immediately

❑ Verify the fit of obturation in radiograph. When found accurate, while stabilizing the carrier with index finger, sever the shaft level with the orifice using a prepi bur or an inverted cone bur in high-speed handpiece (**Fig. 19.47D**)

❑ Do not use flame heated instrument to sever the plastic shaft because instrument cools too rapidly and thus may cause inadvertent obturator displacement from the canal

❑ Now use a small condenser coated with vaseline or dipped in alcohol, to condense gutta-percha vertically around the shaft (**Fig. 19.47E**)

❑ When post is indicated, sever the obturator with the fissure bur at the selected length and give counterclockwise rotation of shaft following insertion to disengage the instrument

Advantages

❑ Requires less chair-side time

❑ Provides dense 3-D obturation as gutta-percha flows into canal irregularities such as fins, anastomoses, and lateral canals

❑ No need to precure obturators because of flexible carriers

❑ Since this technique requires minimum compaction, so less strain while obturation with this technique

Ultrafil 3-D

Ultrafil 3-D is injectable gutta-percha system which provides three viscosities to accommodate different techniques. Success-Fil (Coltene/Whaledent, Inc.) utilizes high viscosity gutta-percha which comes in a syringe. Sealer is lightly coated on the canal walls and the carrier with gutta-percha is placed in the canal to the prepared length. Gutta-percha is then compacted around the carrier with various pluggers depending on the canal morphology. Then carrier is severed at the orifice with a bur.

Cold Gutta-Percha Compaction Technique

Gutta Flow

Gutta flow is eugenol-free radiopaque form which can be injected into root canals using an injectable system (**Fig. 19.48**). It is self-polymerizing filling system in which gutta-percha in powder form is combined with a resin sealer in one capsule.

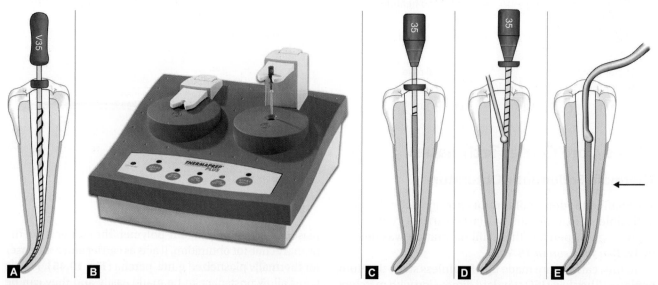

Figs. 19.47A to E (A) Select a thermafil obturator which fits into the canal passively at the working length; (B) Preheat the thermaprep oven; (C) Place the heated obturator into the canal with firm apical pressure; (D) Cut the thermafil using therma cut bur; (E) Condense gutta-percha vertically around the shaft.

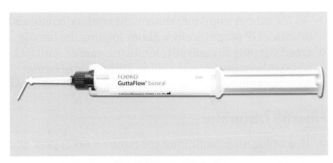

Fig. 19.48 Gutta Flow.

Composition: Gutta flow consists of polydimethylsiloxane matrix filled with powdered gutta-percha, silicon oil, paraffin oil, platinum, zirconium dioxide, and nano silver.

Advantages
- Easy to use
- Time saving
- Does not require compaction
- Does not require heating
- Biocompatible
- Can be easily removed for retreatment

▌Obturation with Silver Cone

Use of silver cones is not the preferred method of obturation, mainly because of corrosion. Their use is restricted to teeth with fine, tortuous, curved canals which make use of gutta-percha with difficulty **(Fig. 19.49)**.

Indications for use of silver cones
- In round and straight canals, like canals of maxillary premolars, mesial canals of mandibular molars, and buccal canals of maxillary molars
- In mature teeth with small calcified canals

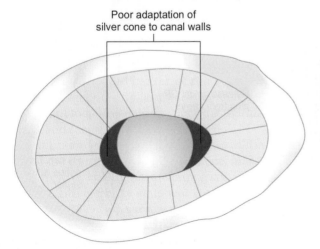

Fig. 19.49 Cross-section of canal obturated with silver cone showing poor adaptation of the cone in irregularly shaped canal.

Contraindications
- Teeth with open apex
- Large ovoid-shaped canals, like maxillary incisors, premolars with oval single canals, etc.

Steps

- Select a silver cone conforming the final shape and size of the prepared canal. Check if it fits radiographically. If found satisfactory, remove it from the canal and sterilize it over an alcohol flame
- Dry the canal and coat the canal walls with sealer
- Insert the cone into the canal with sterile cotton plier or Stieglitz forceps
- Take a radiograph to see the fit of cone. If satisfactory, fill the remaining canal with accessory gutta-percha cones
- Remove excess of sealer with cotton pellet and place restoration in the pulp chamber

Advantages
- Easy handling and placement
- Negotiates extremely curved canals
- Radiopaque in nature
- Mild antibacterial property

Disadvantages
- Prone to corrosion resulting in loss of apical seal
- Difficult to retrieve if it is snugly fitting
- Nonadaptable, so does not seal accessory canals

Stainless Steel

They are more rigid than silver points and are used for fine and tortuous canals. They cannot seal the root canals completely without use of sealer.

▌Apical Third Filling

Sometimes apical barriers are needed to provide apical stop in cases of teeth with incomplete root development, overinstrumentation, and apical root resorption. Various materials can be used for this purpose. They are designed to allow the obturation without apical extrusion of the material in such cases.

Apical third filling
- Carrier-based system
  - Simplifill obturator
  - Fiberfill obturator
- Paste system
  - Dentin chip filling
  - Calcium hydroxide filling
  - MTA filling

Simplifill Obturator

It was originally developed at light speed technology so as to complement the canal shape formed by using light speed instruments. In this, the apical gutta-percha size is the same ISO size as the light speed master apical rotary. Here a stainless steel carrier is used to place gutta-percha in apical portion of the canal **(Fig. 19.50)**.

Steps (Figs. 19.51A to D)

❑ Try the size of apical GP plug so as to ensure an optimal apical fitting. This apical GP plug is of same size as the light speed master apical rotary

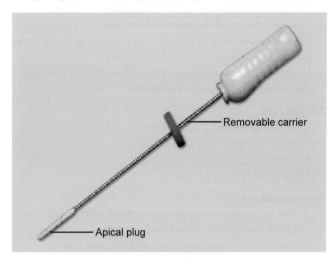

Removable carrier

Apical plug

Fig. 19.50 Simplifill stainless steel carrier with apical gutta-percha plug.

❑ Set the rubber stop 4 mm short of the working length and advance GP plug apically without rotating the handle
❑ Once GP plug fits apically, rotate the carrier anticlockwise without pushing or pulling the handle of carrier
❑ Now backfilling of canal is done using syringe system

Fiberfill Obturator

❑ This obturation technique combines a resin post and obturator forming a single until and apical 5–7 mm of gutta-percha
❑ This apical gutta-percha is attached with a thin flexible filament to be used in moderately curved canals
❑ Advantage of this technique is that due to presence of dual cure resin sealer, chances of coronal microleakage are less
❑ But it poses difficulty in retreatment cases

Dentin Chip Filling

Dentin chip filling forms a ***Biologic seal***. In this technique, after thorough cleaning and shaping of canal, H-file is used to produce dentin powder in central portion of the canal, which is then packed apically with butt end of paper point.

Technique (Figs. 19.52A to D)

❑ Clean and shape the canal
❑ Produce dentin powder using hedstroem file or Gates-Glidden drill

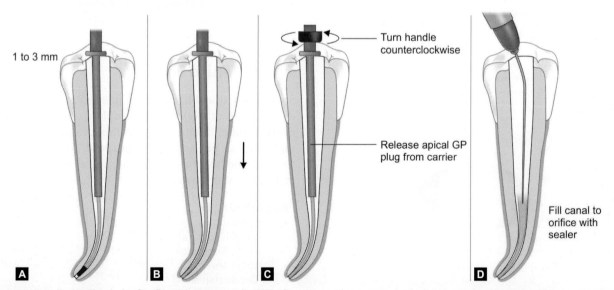

1 to 3 mm

Turn handle counterclockwise

Release apical GP plug from carrier

Fill canal to orifice with sealer

Figs. 19.51A to D (A) Check the fit of apical gutta-percha (GP) plug; (B) condense apical GP plug to working length; (C) Once GP plug fits apically, rotate the carrier anticlockwise without pushing or pulling the handle of carrier; (D) Backfilling of canal is done using syringe system.

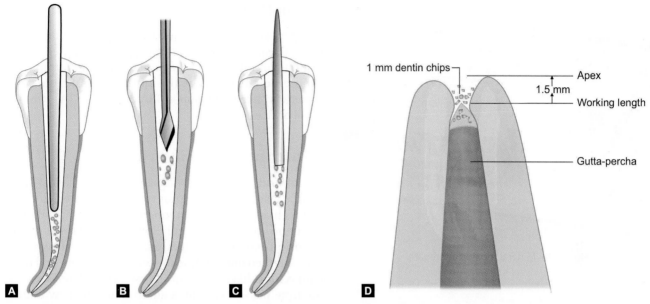

Figs. 19.52A to D (A) Compaction of dentin chips apically; (B) dentin chips produced by use of Gates-Glidden drills; (C) chips being compacted with blunt end of instrument/paper point; (D) compaction of dentin chips in apical 2 mm from working length to stimulate hard tissue formation.

❑ Using butt end of a paper point, push and compact dentin chips apically

❑ 1–2 mm of chips should block the apical foramen. The density of pack is checked by resistance to perforation by #15 or 20 file

❑ Backpacking is done using gutta-percha compacted against the plug

Advantages
❑ Biocompatible
❑ Promotes healing and decreases inflammation
❑ Prevents extrusion of filling material from the canal space

Disadvantage
Care must be taken in this technique, because infected pulp tissue can be present in the dentinal mass.

Calcium Hydroxide

It has also been used frequently as apical barrier. Calcium hydroxide has shown to stimulate cementogenesis. It can be used both in dry or moist state.

Moist calcium hydroxide is placed with the help of plugger and amalgam carrier, injectable syringes, or by lentulo spirals.

Dry form of $Ca(OH)_2$ is carried into canal by amalgam carrier which is then packed with pluggers **(Fig. 19.53)**. Calcium hydroxide has shown to be a biocompatible material with potential to induce an apical barrier in apexification procedures.

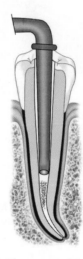

Fig. 19.53 Placement of $Ca(OH)_2$ in the canal.

Mineral Trioxide Aggregate

Mineral trioxide aggregate was developed by Dr Torabinejad in 1993 **(Fig. 19.54)**. It contains tricalcium silicate, dicalcium silicate, tricalcium aluminate, bismuth oxide, calcium sulfate, and tetracalcium aluminoferrite.

pH of MTA is 12.5, thus having its biological and histological properties similar to calcium hydroxide. Setting time is 2 h and 45 min. In contrast to $Ca(OH)_2$, it produces hard setting nonresorbable surface.

Because of being hydrophilic in nature, it sets in a moist environment. It has low solubility and shows resistance to

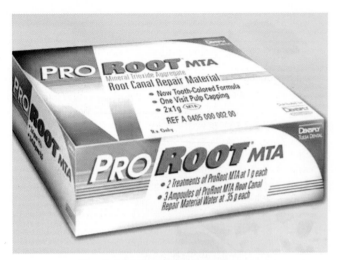

Fig. 19.54 Mineral trioxide aggregate.

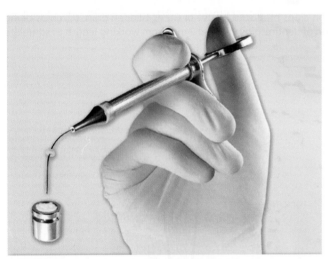

Fig. 19.55 Due to loose, granular nature of MTA, a special carrier like messing gun or amalgam carrier is used for carrying it.

marginal leakage. It also exhibits excellent biocompatibility in relation with vital tissues.

To use MTA, mix a small amount of liquid and powder to putty consistency. Since MTA mix is a loose granular aggregate, it cannot be carried out in cavity with normal cement carrier and thus has to be carried in the canal with messing gun, amalgam carrier, or specially designed carrier **(Fig. 19.55)**. After its placement, it is compacted with micropluggers.

Advantages of MTA include its excellent biocompatibility, least toxicity of all the filling materials, radiopaque nature, bacteriostatic nature, and resistance to marginal leakage. However, it is difficult to manipulate with long setting time (3–4 h).

Coronal Seal

Irrespective of the technique used to obturate the canal, coronal leakage can occur through well-obturated canals, resulting in infection of the periapical area. Coronal seal should be enhanced by the application of restorative materials (like Cavit, super EBA cement, MTA) over the canal orifice.

Postobturation Instructions

Postoburation pain can be seen in some cases. Since pain is a subjective symptom which is related to many factors like presence of preoperative pain, periradicular infection, retreatment, etc. Sometimes, pain is due to extrusion of root canal filling or a tiny bubble of air, which can be forced out periapically causing pressure and pain. Pain is most likely to occur in first 24 h and decreases as the time passes. Patient is advised not to chew unduly on the treated tooth until it is protected by permanent restoration.

Patient Recall

Patient should be recalled regularly to evaluate tissue repair and healing progresses.

In case of periapical radiolucency, radiographs should be taken at 3, 6, and 9 months interval period to see continued new bone formation. Radiograph of a successful endodontic treatment shows uniformly thickened periodontal ligament and continuous lamina dura along the root.

Repair Following Endodontic Treatment

Repair of tooth being treated begins as soon as infection is controlled.

Repair occurs in the following steps:
- Organization of blood clot
- Formation of granulation tissue
- Development of scar tissue by laying down of collagen fibers

❏ In periapical area, bone is there. Here healing process is more complicated because soft tissue must be converted to hard tissue
❏ Bone contains protein matrix filled with calcium compounds like calcium phosphate and calcium carbonate. This protein matrix is formed by osteoblasts
❏ Osteoblasts produce enzyme called alkaline phosphatase, which separates in organic phosphorus from organically bound phosphorus

- ❑ This increase of phosphate ions forms saturated solution of calcium phosphate, which precipitates into matrix. The precipitated areas of calcium phosphate join to form spongy trabeculae
- ❑ Resorption and deposition of bone may occur simultaneously depending upon degree of periapical damage; repair usually takes 6–12 months after endodontic treatment
- ❑ Since repair proceeds from periphery to center, the granulation tissue formation, fibrous connective tissue maturation, and finally matrix for bone formation occur in steps
- ❑ In some cases, connective tissue matures into dense fibrous tissue instead of bone. These areas represent as areas of rarefactions in radiographs, though histologically healing has taken place

Questions

1. What are the different materials used for obturation?
2. Write in detail about gutta-percha with its advantages and disadvantages?
3. What are the functions of root canal sealers? Classify different root canal sealers?
4. How would you know that root canal is ready for obturation?
5. Classify different obturation techniques. Explain in detail about lateral compaction technique?
6. What are the advantages and disadvantages of vertical compaction technique?
7. Describe biological considerations for selecting a filling material.
8. What are different endodontic obturation techniques? Describe in detail lateral compaction technique.
9. Why is it necessary to hermetically seal the root canal? Describe root canal sealers and obturating materials.
10. Describe prerequisite of root canal obturation and its various techniques.
11. Enumerate different methods of root canal obturation and describe in detail about vertical condensation technique highlighting merits and demerits?
12. What are the ideal requirements of root canal filling materials? Name various obturation techniques and describe vertical condensation techniques.
13. Write short notes on:
    - System B obturation system
    - Sectional method of obturation
    - Obtura II
    - Thermafil endodontic obturation
    - Timing of obturation
    - Gutta-percha.

Bibliography

1. Bailey GC, NgYL, Cunnington SA, et al. Part II: an in vitro investigation if the quality of obturation. Int Endod J 2004;37:694–8.
2. Bowman CJ, Baumgartner JC. Gutta-percha obturation of lateral grooves and depression. J Endod 2002;28:220–3.
3. Buchanan LS. Filling root canal system with centered condensation: concepts, instruments and techniques. Endod Prac 2005;8:9–15.
4. Cobankara FK, Orucoglu H, Sengun A, Belli S. The quantitative evaluation of apical sealing of four endodontic sealers J Endod. 2006;32(1):66–8.
5. Eldeniz AU, Mustafa K, Orstavik D, Dahl JE. Cytotoxicity of new resin-, calcium hydroxide– and silicone-based root canal sealers on fibroblasts derived from human gingiva and L929 cell lies. Int Endod J 2007;40:329–37.
6. Friedman CE, Sandrik JL, Heuer MA, Rapp GW. Composition and physical properties of gutta-percha endodontic filling materials. J Endod 1977;3:304–8.
7. Grossman L. Endodontics. 11th ed. Philadelphia, PA: Lea & Febiger; 1988
8. Grossman LI. Endodontic practice. Philadelphia, PA: Lea and Febiger, 1978.
9. Gutmann J, Witherspoon D. Chapter 9: obturation of the cleaned and shaped root canal system. Pathways of the pulp. 7th edition St Louis, MO: Cohen and Burns; 2002.pp. 293–364.
10. Gutmann JL, Rakusin H. Perspectives on root canal obturation with thermoplasticized injectable gutta-percha. Int Endod J 1987;20:261–70.
11. Juhasz A, Verdes E, Tokes L, Kobor A, Dobo-Nagy C. The influence of root canal shape on the sealing ability of two root canal sealers. Int Endod J 2006;39:282–6.
12. Kytridou V, Gutmann JL, Nunn MH. Adaptation and sealability of two contemporary obturation techniques in the absence of the dentinal smear layer. Int Endod J 1999;32:464–74.
13. Lacey S, Pitt Ford TR, Yuan XF, Sherrif M, Watson T. The effect if temperature on viscosity of root canal sealers. Int Endod J 2006;39:860–33.
14. ldeniz AU, Ørstavik D. Physical properties of newly developed root canal sealers. Int Endod J 2005;38:935.
15. Lohbauer U, Gambarini G, Ebert J, Dasch W, Petschelt A. Calcium release and pH-characteristics of calcium hydroxide plus points. Int Endod J 2005;38:683–9.
16. Mayer B, Roggendorf MJ, Ebert J, Petschelt A, Frankenberger R. Influence of sealer placement on apical extrusion of two root canal sealers. Int Endod J 2005;38:928.
17. Patel DV, Sherriff M, Ford TR, Watson TF, Mannocci F. The penetration of RealSeal primer and tubliseal into root canal dentinal tubules: a confocal microscopic study. Int Endod J 2007;40:67–71.
18. Santos MD, Walker III WA, Carnes Jr. DL. Evaluation of apical seal in straight canals after obturation using the Lightspeed sectional method. J Endod 1999;25:609–12.
19. Schilder H, Goodman A, Aldrich W. The thermomechanical properties of gutta-percha. V. Volume changes in bulk gutta-percha as a function of temperature and its relationship to

molecular phase transformation. Oral Surg Oral Med Oral Pathol 1985;59:285–96.

20. Schilder H. Filling root canals in three dimensions. Dent Clin North Am 1967;11:723–44.

21. Silver GK, Love RM, Purton DG. Comparison of two vertical condensation obturation techniques: touch 'n' heat modified and system B. Int Endod J 1999;32:287–95.

22. Tunga U, Bodrumlu E. Assessment of the sealing ability of a new root canal obturation material. J Endod 2006;32:876–8. associated with thermoplastic gutta percha. J Endod 2001;27:512–15.

23. Wollard RR, Brough SO, Maggio J, Seltzer S. Scanning electron microscopic examination of root canal filling materials. J Endod 1976;2:98–110.

Single Visit Endodontics

Single-visit endodontics (SVE) is defined as the conservative, nonsurgical treatment of an endodontically involved tooth consisting of cleaning, shaping and obturation of the root canal system in one visit.

The most common factors which appear to be responsible for not performing SVE are as follows:
- Doubt of postoperative pain
- Fear of failure of the endodontic therapy
- Discomfort to patient because he/she has to keep the mouth open for a long period of time
- Lack of time
- Lack of experience and equipment

Advantages of Single-Visit Endodontics

- **Convenience:** Patient does not have to endure the discomfort of repetitive local anesthesia, treatment procedure and postoperative recovery
- **Efficiency:** Clinician does not have to refamiliarize to patient's particular anatomy or landmarks
- **Patient comfort:** Because of the reduced number of visits and injections, it is more comfortable for patient
- **Reduced intra-appointment pain:** Due to reduced chances of leakage of temporary cements, there are less chances of intra-appointment pain
- **Economics:** Extra cost of multiple visits, use of fewer materials make single visit endodontics cost-effective for both operator and patient
- **Minimizes the fear and anxiety:** Especially beneficial for patients who have psychological trauma and fear of dentist

- **Reduces incomplete treatment:** Some patients do not return to complete the root canal therapy; SVE reduces this risk
- **Lesser errors in working length:** In multiple visits, chances of losing reference point due to fracture or grinding in case of flare-up are more, resulting in loss of actual working length
- **Restorative consideration:** In SVE, immediate placement of coronal restoration ensures effective coronal seal and esthetics

Disadvantages of Single-Visit Endodontics

- It is tiring for patient to keep mouth open for long duration
- If flare-up occurs, it is easier to establish drainage in a tooth which is not obturated
- Clinician may lack proficiency to do SVE
- Some case cannot be treated by single visit, for example, cases with very fine, curved, calcified, multiple canals and teeth with weeping canals

Criteria of Case Selection

- **Competence of the clinician:** Clinician should be able to perform all steps of root canal in single visit without compromising quality of the treatment
- **Positive patient acceptance:** Patient should be cooperative for SVE. Uncooperative patients and patients with TMJ problems, limited mouth opening should be avoided for SVE

- **Absence of anatomical interferences:** Anatomical problems like presence of fine, curved or calcified canals require more than usual time for the treatment and thus should be treated in multiple visits rather than a single visit
- **Accessibility:** Teeth for single visit should have an optimal accessibility and visibility
- **Availability of sufficient time to complete the case:** Both clinicians as well as patients should have sufficient time for SVE
- **Pulp status:** Vital teeth are better candidate for SVE than nonvital teeth because of less chances of flare-ups
- **Clinical symptoms:** Teeth with acute alveolar abscess should not be treated by single visit. But teeth with sinus tract are good candidate for SVE because the presence of sinus acts as safety valve and prevents buildup of pressure, so these teeth seldom show flare-ups

Criteria of case selection as given by Oliet includes
- Positive patient acceptance
- Absence of acute symptoms
- Absence of continuous hemorrhage or exudation
- Absence of anatomical interferences like presence of fine, curved or calcified canals
- Availability of sufficient time to complete the case
- Absence of procedural difficulties like canal blockage, ledge formation or perforations

Indications of Single-Visit Endodontics

- Vital teeth
- Fractured anteriors where esthetics is the concern **(Fig. 20.1)**
- Uncomplicated vital teeth

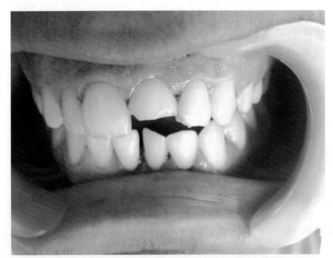

Fig. 20.1 In anterior teeth, single-visit endodontic therapy is indicated because of esthetic reasons.

- Patients who require sedation every time
- Nonvital teeth with sinus tract
- Nonsurgical retreatment cases
- Teeth with accidental pulp exposure
- Medically compromised patients who require antibiotics prophylaxis
- Physically compromised patients who cannot come to dental clinics frequently

Contraindications of Single-Visit Endodontics

- Teeth with anatomic anomalies such as calcified and curved canals **(Figs. 20.2 and 20.3)**
- Asymptomatic nonvital teeth with periapical pathology and no sinus tract **(Fig. 20.4)**
- Acute alveolar abscess cases with frank pus discharge

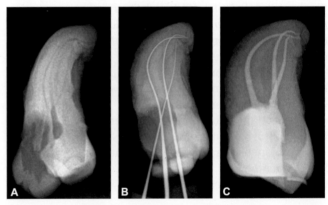

Figs. 20.2A to C Root canal treatment of maxillary molar with curved canals is a poor candidate for single visit endodontics: (A) Preoperative radiograph; (B) Working length; (C) Post obturation radiograph.

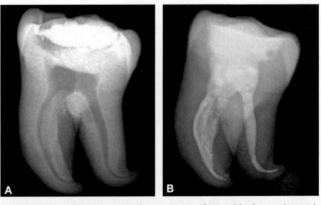

Figs. 20.3A and B Root canal treatment of Mandibular molar with curved canals is not a good choice for single visit endodontics: (A) Preoperative radiograph; (B) Post operative radiograph.

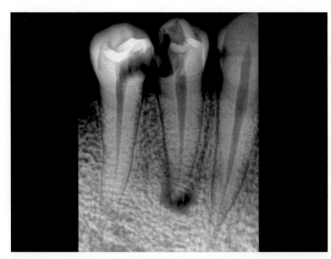

Fig. 20.4 Nonvital mandibular first premolar with periapical pathology is not indicated for single-visit endodontics, whereas uncomplicated mandibular second premolar with carious exposure can be completed in single-visit endodontics.

❑ Patients with acute apical periodontitis
❑ Symptomatic nonvital teeth and no sinus tract
❑ Patients with allergies or previous flare-ups
❑ Teeth with limited access
❑ Patients who are unable to keep mouth open for long durations such as patients with TMJ disorders

Questions

1. What are indications and contraindications of single-visit endodontics? Mention its advantages and disadvantages.
2. What is single-visit root canal treatment? What are its advantages, disadvantages, indications and contraindications?
3. Compare single-visit vis-à-vis multiple-visit root canal treatment. Add a note on "Oliet's criteria."

Bibliography

1. Ng YL, Mann V, Rahbaran S, Lewsey J, Gulabivala K. Outcome of primary root canal treatment: systematic review of the literature—Part 1. Effects of study characteristics on probability of success. Int Endod J 2007;40(12):921–39.
2. Ng YL, Mann V, Rahbaran S, Lewsey J, Gulabivala K. Outcome of primary root canal treatment: systematic review of the literature—Part 2. Influence of clinical factors. Int Endod J 2008;41(1):6–31.
3. Peters LB, Wesselink PR. Periapical healing of endodontically treated teeth in one and two visits obturated in the presence or absence of detectable microorganisms. Int Endod J 2002;35(8):660–7.
4. Sathorn C, Parashos P, Messer H. Effectiveness of single- versus multiple-visit endodontic treatment of teeth with apical periodontitis: A systematic review and meta-analysis. Int Endod J 2005;38(6):347–55. (Review).

Mid-treatment Flare-ups in Endodontics

Flare-up is described as the occurrence of pain, swelling, or the combination of these during the course of root canal therapy, which results in unscheduled visits by the patient.

American Association of Endodontics defines a flare-up "as an acute exacerbation of periradicular pathosis after initiation or in continuation of root canal treatment".

Etiology

Causative Factors

There can be *mechanical, chemical, and/or microbial injury* to the pulp or periapical tissues resulting in release of myriad of inflammatory mediators. Pain occurs due to the direct stimulation of the nerve fibers by these mediators or edema resulting in an increase in the hydrostatic pressure with consequent compression of nerve endings.

Mechanical Injury

Mechanical injury occurs due to
❏ Overinstrumentation (most common cause of mid-treatment flare-ups) **(Fig. 21.1)**
❏ Inadequate debridement or incomplete removal of pulp tissue **(Fig. 21.2)**
❏ Periapical extrusion of debris **(Fig. 21.3)**

Chemical Injury

Chemical injury to periapical tissue is caused by
❏ Irrigants
❏ Intracanal medicaments **(Fig. 21.4)**
❏ Overextended filling materials

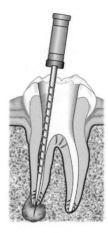

Fig. 21.1 Overinstrumentation is most common cause of mid-treatment flare-ups.

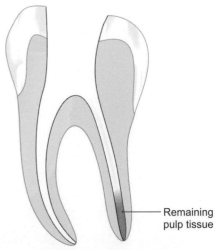

Remaining pulp tissue

Fig. 21.2 Inadequate debridement of pulp tissue.

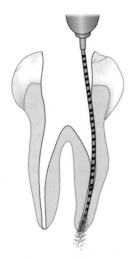

Fig. 21.3 Periapical extrusion of debris.

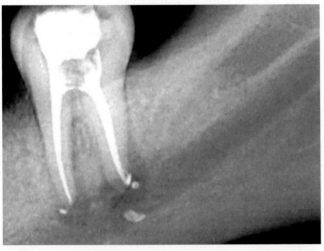

Fig. 21.4 Calcium hydroxide placed as intracanal medicament in mandibular second molar may act as an chemical irritant to the periapical tissues.

Microbial Induced Injury

Microbial factors in combination with iatrogenic errors cause interappointment pain.

Contributing Factors for Flare-ups

Age of the Patient

Patients aged 40–59 years experience more flare-ups than younger ones.

Gender

Females show more pain incidences than males.

Systemic Conditions

Patients with allergies to various substances (sulfa medication, pollen, dust, and food stuffs) have a higher frequency of interappointment pain.

Tooth Type

Mandibular teeth show more interappointment emergencies than maxillary teeth.

Anxiety

Anxious patients are likely to have more pain during the course of treatment.

Presence of Preoperative Pain and/or Swelling

Patients taking analgesics and anti-inflammatory drugs to prevent preoperative pain have shown higher incidence of flare-ups.

Pulpal/Periapical Status

Teeth with vital pulps show lower incidence of flare-ups as compared to teeth with necrotic pulp (**Fig. 21.5**).

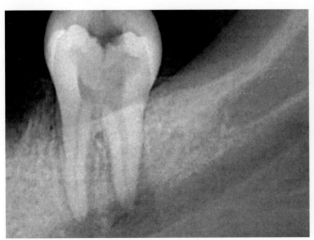
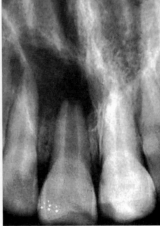

Fig. 21.5 Teeth with necrotic pulp and periapical radiolucency shows more incidence of flare-ups.

Periradicular status of the tooth can also predict the flare-up rates, with incidence of 3.4% in chronic apical periodontitis, 4.8% in acute apical periodontitis, and 13.1% in case of acute apical abscess. Presence of a sinus tract is not associated with the development of flare-up.

Number of Visits

If proper case selection is not done, more flare-ups occur after multivisit approach compared to single visit endodontics.

Retreatment Cases

Chances of flare-ups are 10-fold higher in retreatment cases because of extrusion of infected debris or solvents into periapical tissues.

Mechanisms for Flare-ups

Microbiological and Immunological Factors

The following microbiological and immunological factors are responsible for flare-ups (Seltzer et al., 2004):
- Alteration of local adaptation syndrome
- Changes in periapical tissue pressure
- Microbial factors
- Chemical mediators
- Changes in cyclic nucleotides
- Immunological responses
- Psychological factors

Alteration of Local Adaptation Syndrome

Selye showed that when a new irritant is introduced in a chronically inflamed tissue, a violent reaction may occur because of disturbance in local tissue adaptation to applied irritants. For example, in case of chronic pulpal diseases, the inflammatory lesion is adapted to irritants but during root canal therapy, a new irritant in form of medicament get introduced in the lesion leading to flare-up.

Changes in Periapical Tissue Pressure

In teeth with increased periapical pressure, exudate creates pain by causing pressure on nerve endings. In these cases pain is relieved when tooth is kept open to drain the exudate but in teeth with less periapical pressure, if kept open, microorganisms and other irritants gets aspirated into periapical area resulting in pain.

Microbial Factors

Gram-negative anaerobes like *Prevotella* and *Porphyromonas* species release endotoxins which are neurotoxic. These organisms also activate the Hageman factor to release bradykinin, a potent pain mediator. Teichoic acid, present in the cell wall and plasma membranes of Gram-positive bacteria produce humoral antibodies IgM, IgG, IgA, and releases various chemical mediators that cause pain.

Microbial Mechanisms in the Induction of Flare-ups

- *Apical extrusion of infected debris:* Extrusion of microorganisms and their products during the endodontic procedures may disrupt the balance between microbial aggression and host defense leading to acute periapical inflammation (**Figs. 21.6A and B**)
- *Changes in the endodontic microflora and/or in environmental conditions (Fig. 21.7):* Incomplete chemomechanical preparation disrupts the balance between different microbial communities within the root canal system resulting in flare-up

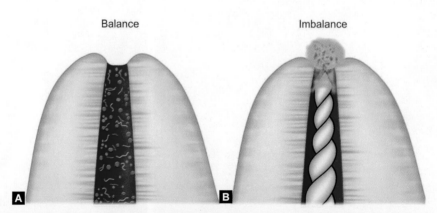

Balance Imbalance

Figs. 21.6A and B (A) Balance between host defense and microbes; (B) Imbalance between microbial aggression and host defense leads to acute periapical inflammation.

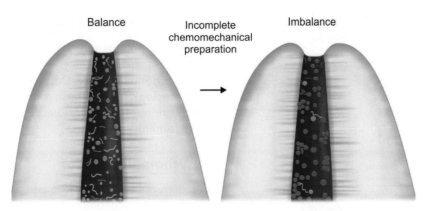

Fig. 21.7 Incomplete debridement of canal disrupts the balance between various microbial communities with in root canal system.

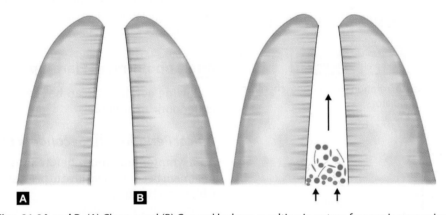

Figs. 21.8A and B (A) Clean canal (B) Coronal leakage resulting in entry of new microorganisms.

❑ *Secondary intraradicular infection (Figs. 21.8A and B):* Penetration of new microbial species, microbial cells, and substrate from saliva into the root canal system during treatment may lead to a secondary infection and can be a cause of flare-up

❑ *Increase of oxidation–reduction potential (Fig. 21.9):* Alteration of oxidation–reduction potential during endodontic treatment may favor overgrowth of facultative bacteria that resist chemomechanical procedures resulting in flare-ups.

Effect of Chemical Mediators

Chemical mediators are in form of cell mediators, plasma mediators and neutrophils products **(Fig. 21.10)**. Cell mediators include histamine, serotonin, prostaglandins, platelet activating factor, etc. which cause pain. Plasma mediators are present in circulation in inactive precursor form and get activated on coming in contact with irritants.

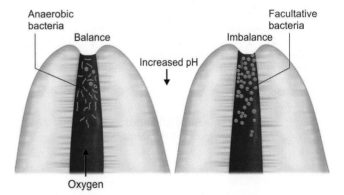

Fig. 21.9 Change in oxidation-reduction potential in root canal favors the overgrowth of facultative bacteria.

For example, Hageman factor when gets activated after coming in contact with irritants produce multiple effects like production of bradykinin and activation of clotting cascade, which may cause vascular leakage.

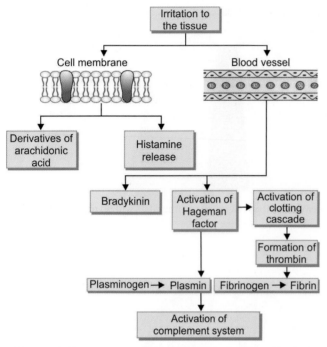

Fig. 21.10 Tissue response to irritation by releasing chemical mediators.

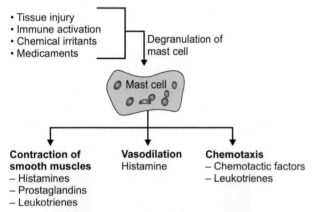

Fig. 21.11 Release of inflammatory mediators from mast cell degranulation.

Changes in Cyclic Nucleotides

Bourne et al. showed that the character and intensity of inflammatory and immune response is regulated by hormones and the mediators. In flare-up cases, there is increase in cGMP which stimulates mast cell degranulation and decrease in cAMP which inhibits mast cell degranulation (**Fig. 21.11**).

Immunological Response

In chronic pulpitis and periapical disease, presence of macrophages, and lymphocytes indicates both cell mediated and humoral response. Despite their protective effect, the immunologic response also contributes to destructive phase of reaction, which causes perpetuation and aggravation of inflammatory process.

Psychological Factor

Anxiety, apprehension, fear, and previous history of dental experience plays a contributory role in mid-treatment flare-ups.

▌ Clinical Conditions Related to Flare-up

Flare-ups in endodontics may be grouped as
- Interappointment flare-ups
- Postobturation flare-ups

Interappointment Flare-ups

Following conditions can be seen during the course of endodontic treatment.

Apical Periodontitis Secondary to Treatment

An asymptomatic tooth before initiation of endodontic treatment becomes sensitive to percussion during treatment which can be due to
❑ Overinstrumentation
❑ Overmedication
❑ Forcing debris into periapical tissues

Confirmatory test: Apply the rubber clamp and use a sterile paper point. Access and mark the working length. Then, place the paper point in the canal. In case of overinstrumentation, paper point will go beyond working length without obstruction. On withdrawal, the tip of paper point shows a reddish or brownish color indicating inflamed tissue in the periapical region and absence of stop in apical preparation (**Fig. 21.12**).

Management: An intracanal corticosteroid–antibiotic medication is given to the patient for symptomatic relief. Medication is carried on paper point and applied with a pumping action so as to reach the inflamed periapical

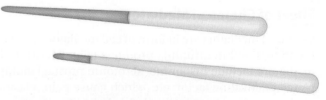

Fig. 21.12 Absorbent paper point showing reddish color indicating inflamed periapex.

tissues. Routine endodontic therapy may be continued after 2–5 days after readjusting the working length.

Incomplete Removal of the Pulp Tissue

Incomplete removal of inflamed pulp tissue can cause pain.

Confirmatory test: Apply rubber dam and place a sterile paper point; on removal, it shows brownish discoloration indicative of inflamed seeping tissue.

Management: Re-establish the working length and remove the remaining pulp tissue.

Recrudescence of Chronic Apical Periodontitis (Phoenix Abscess)

This condition occurs in teeth with necrotic pulps and asymptomatic apical lesions. Reason for pain in these cases is the alteration of internal environment of root canal space during instrumentation which activates the bacterial flora.

Management: Apply the rubber dam and allow it to drain. Drainage is allowed until exudation ceases or a slight clear serum drains. Irrigate the canal using sodium hypochlorite, dry with paper points, place an appropriate intracanal medicament, and seal it with a dry cotton pellet and temporary restoration.

Recurrent Periapical Abscess

It is a condition where a tooth with an acute periapical abscess is relieved by emergency treatment after which the acute symptoms return. In some cases, the abscess may recur more than once due to microorganism of high virulence or it results in resistance.

Management: Management is same as discussed above for phoenix abscess.

Flare-ups Related to Necrotic Pulp

Teeth with necrotic pulp often develop as acute apical abscess after the initial appointment. As the lesion is confined to bone, there occurs severe pain.

Management: The drainage is established, canal copiously irrigated and the tooth sealed after placing an intracanal medicament of calcium hydroxide. Increasing the appointment time allows more exposure of the bacteria to irrigants like hydrogen peroxide and sodium hypochlorite, thus reducing the chances of flare-ups.

Postobturation Flare-ups

Postobturation flare-ups are relatively infrequent as compared to interappointment flare-ups. Only one-third of the endodontic patients experience some pain after obturation. A mild pain is usually present which may resolve spontaneously. Patients experiencing preoperative pain are more likely to suffer from postobturation flare-ups. Another cause of postobturation flare-ups may be overextended root canal fillings.

Management: Mild-to-moderate pain may be controlled with analgesics. For severe pain, retreatment is indicated. When nonsurgical retreatment is not possible, surgical intervention is required.

▌Management of Flare-ups

As the etiology of flare-ups is multifactorial, many treatment options have been advocated for the prevention and alleviation of symptoms during the root canal therapy.

Management of flare-ups can be categorized as
- Preventive management
- Definitive management.

Preventive Management

Accurate Diagnosis

An accurate diagnosis of the condition should be made to prevent incorrect treatment that may cause pain/swelling to the patient.

Long-Acting Local Anesthetics

Long acting anesthetics, for example, bupivacaine, provide increased period of analgesia for up to 8 h during the immediate postoperative period.

Determination of Proper Working Length

Inaccurate measurement of working length may cause under or overinstrumentation and extrusion of debris, irrigants, medicaments, or obturating materials beyond apex.

Complete Debridement

Thorough cleaning and shaping of root canal system by crown-down preparation and maintaining apical patency reduce the incidence of flare-ups (**Fig. 21.13**).

Occlusal Reduction

Pain relief provided by occlusal reduction is due to the reduction of mechanical stimulation of sensitized nociceptors.

Placement of Intracanal Medicament in Multivisit Root Canal Treatment (Figs. 21.14A to C)

Calcium hydroxide is used as an intracanal medicament for the prevention or the treatment of flare-up. It serves the following purposes:

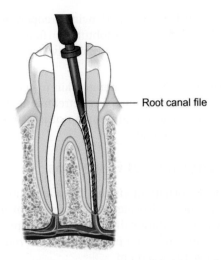

Fig. 21.13 Complete chemomechanical cleaning and shaping prevents incidence of flare ups.

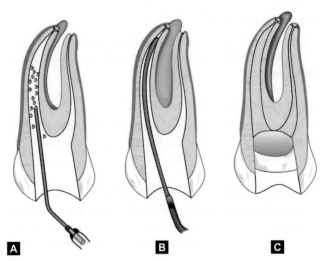

Figs. 21.14A to C (A) Irrigation of canal for final cleaning of the canal; (B) Drying of the canal using absorbent paper point; (C) Placement of intracanal medicament.

□ *Antimicrobial action:* Calcium hydroxide hydroxylates the lipid moiety of bacterial lipopolysaccharide, rendering it incapable of producing biologic effects and complement activation. It absorbs carbon dioxide thus nutritionally depriving the capnophilic bacteria in the root canal system. Antimicrobial effect of calcium hydroxide remains in the canal for one week

□ It obliterates the root canal space which minimizes the ingress of tissue exudates, a potential source of nourishment of remaining bacteria

□ Extrusion of calcium hydroxide periapically reduces inflammatory reaction by reducing substrate adherence capacity of macrophages

□ Calcium hydroxide has soft tissue dissolving property because of its high pH. Its denaturing effect on the necrotic tissue allows sodium hypochlorite to dissolve remaining tissue more easily

Chlorhexidine gluconate, iodine and potassium iodide are other primary medicaments that can be considered. Use of phenolic medicaments that have an immunologic potential should be avoided to prevent the occurrence of flare-ups.

Medications

□ *Systemic antibiotics:* These are not indicated in the prevention of flare-ups for healthy patients with localized infections. Antibiotics are recommended only in cases of medically compromised patients at high-risk levels and in cases of spreading infection that indicates failure of local host responses to control bacterial irritants. Commonly prescribed antibiotics are penicillin, erythromycin, or cephalosporin. Metronidazole, tinidazole, ornidazole and clindamycin are also used because of their efficacy against anaerobic bacteria

□ *Analgesics:* Nonsteroidal anti-inflammatory drugs (NSAIDs) and acetaminophen are the most commonly used drugs to reduce pain. Treatment with an NSAID before a procedure has shown to reduce postoperative pain. Most commonly used drugs include ibuprofen, diclofenac sodium and ketorolac

Closed Dressing

Leaving a tooth open for drainage is contraindicated as it can cause contaminations from the oral cavity and lead to flare-ups. Tooth is allowed to drain under rubber dam and closed immediately to prevent secondary infection.

Behavioral Management

Providing information about the procedure is an important step in reducing patient anxiety.

Definitive Treatment

Drainage through Coronal Access Opening

First step in relieving pain is to establish drainage through root canal. Sometimes apical trephination may be needed to establish drainage. In patients with periradicular abscess but no drainage through the canal, penetration of the apical foramen with small files may establish drainage that helps in reducing the periapical pressure, thus alleviating the symptoms **(Fig. 21.15)**.

Incision and Drainage

Occasionally, more than one abscess is present in relation to the tooth. One communicates with the apex, while other

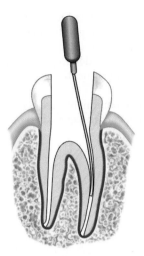

Fig. 21.15 Opening the chamber and placing a small file helps in establishing the drainage and reducing the periapical pressure.

is present in the vestibule. As they do not communicate with one another, flare-up can be best managed through a combination of canal instrumentation and incision and drainage.

Complete Cleaning and Shaping

Under profound local anesthesia, working length should be re-established, apical patency is obtained and thorough chemomechanical preparation is done. This removes the necrotic tissue, microorganisms, and toxic products responsible for causing pain.

Trephination

When drainage through the canal is not possible due to restorative issues, or in case of certain conditions like failing treatments or necessary correction of procedural accidents, surgical trephination can be used as a palliative measure. It involves the surgical perforation of the alveolar cortical plate over the root end to release the accumulated exudates to release pain. However, it is not the first line of treatment because of additional trauma, invasiveness, and questionable beneficial result.

Intracanal Medicaments

Use of corticosteroid–antibiotic combination as an intracanal medicament is recommended to reduce pain, especially in cases of overinstrumentation.

Analgesics and Antibiotics

For most patients, NSAIDs are sufficient to control pain. However, if pain can't be controlled with NSAIDs,

opioid analgesics can be used as supplement to NSAIDs. Commonly used opioids include morphine, codeine, meperidine, tramadol, and propoxyphene. Antibiotics are prescribed for the treatment of flare-ups only when indicated, as discussed before. Use of antihistaminics for treatment of flare-ups has also been suggested.

Preventive methods	Definitive methods
• Accurate diagnosis • Long acting local anesthetics • Determination of proper working length • Complete debridement • Occlusal reduction • Placement of intracanal medicament in multivisit root canal treatment • Medications • Behavioral management	• Drainage through coronal access opening • Incision and drainage • Proper instrumentation • Trephination • Intracanal medicaments • Analgesics and antibiotics (when indicated)

Conclusion

Development of flare-up during endodontic treatment appointment is an extremely undesirable and a challenging problem. Despite judicious and careful treatment procedures, severe pain, swelling, or both may occur. Clinician should employ proper measures and follow appropriate guidelines to prevent these undesirable occurrences. Psychological preparation of the patient, thorough cleaning and shaping of root canal system, use of long acting anesthetic solutions and analgesics may decrease the incidence of flare-ups. Prompt and effective treatment of flare-ups is essential to alleviate patient's symptoms and prevent its recurrence.

Questions

1. Define flare-ups. What are the etiological factors for flare-ups?
2. What is microbiology and immunology of flare-ups?
3. What are the mechanisms responsible for causing a flare-up?
4. How will you manage a case of endodontic flare-up?
5. Describe in detail various conditions associated with flare-ups.
6. Write short notes on:
   • Phoenix abscess.
   • Prevention of flare-ups.

Bibliography

1. Imura N, Zuolo M. Factors associated with endodontic flare-ups: a prospective study. Int Endod J 1995;28:261–5.

2. Imuru N, Zuolo ML. Factors associated with endodontic flare-ups: a prospective study. Int Endod J 1995;28:261–5.
3. Seltzer S, Naidorf IJ. Flare-ups in endodontics: I. Etiological factors. J Endod 2004;30:476–81.
4. Seltzer S, Naidorf IJ. Flare-ups in endodontics: II. Therapeutic factors. J Endod 2004;30:482–7.
5. Siqueira JR. Microbial causes of endodontic flare-ups. Int Endod J 2003;36:453–63.
6. Torabinejad M, Kettering J, McGraw J, et al. Factors associated with endodontic interappointment emergencies of teeth with necrotic pulps. J Endod 1988;14:261–6.
7. Walton R, Fouad A. Endodontic interappointment flare-ups. A prospective study of incidence and related factors. J Endod 1992;18:172–7.
8. Walton R. Interappointment Flare-ups: incidence, related factors, prevention and management. Endod Top 2002;3:67–76.

Endodontic Emergencies

Definition and Classification

Endodontic emergency is defined as any condition leading to an unscheduled visit associated with pain or swelling ensuing from pulpoperiapical pathosis requiring immediate diagnosis and treatment.

True emergency is a condition that requires unscheduled visit with diagnosis and treatment at the same time.

However, **urgency** indicates less severe problem which can be rescheduled for next visit.

Classification of Endodontic Emergencies by P Carrotte

According to P Carrotte, endodontic emergencies can be classified into three types based on their time of occurrence related to endodontic treatment.

Classification of endodontic emergencies (P Carrotte)			
Type	Pretreatment	Intratreatment	Postendodontic
Definition	Patient comes to the clinician for first time with pain, swelling, or injury	Emergency that has occurred during endodontic treatment	Emergency that occurs after the completion of endodontic treatment
Conditions	• Hot tooth • Dentin Hypersensitivity • Acute reversible pulpitis • Acute irreversible pulpitis • Acute apical periodontitis • Acute periapical abscess • Traumatic injury • Cracked tooth Syndrome	• Mid-treatment flare-ups • Exposure of pulp • Fracture of tooth • Recently placed restoration • Periodontal treatment • Hypochlorite accident • Tissue emphysema	• Overextended obturation • Underobturation • Vertical root fracture

Diagnosis of Endodontic Emergencies

Complete history of patient along with clinical examination is basic step for successful management of an endodontic emergency. Following steps are taken for accurate diagnosis.

History of the Patient

Most common component in chief complaint of emergency patient is pain. Initial questions should help establish *two basic components* of pain; *time (chronicity)* and *severity (intensity)*.

Patient should be asked "How painful the tooth is?," "When does it hurt?," "What makes it worse?" etc. A complete history regarding the pain chronology, i.e. mode, periodicity, frequency and duration, pain quality, that is, sharp, dull, recurrent stabbing, throbbing should be taken.

After patient has provided complete history regarding his or her problem, both subjective questioning and objective examination are performed carefully.

Subjective Examination

A patient should be asked questions about history, location, duration, severity, and aggravating factors of pain. For example, if pain occurs on mastication, when teeth are in occlusion, and is localized in nature, it is **periodontal in origin** but if thermal stimuli leads to severe explosive pain and patient is unable to localize, it is **pulpal in origin**.

Objective Examination

In objective examination, tests are done to reproduce the symptoms that mimic what patient reports subjectively. For example, if patient complains of pain to thermal changes and on mastication, same pain can be reproduced by applying cold and pressure, thus identifying the offending tooth. Objective examination includes extraoral examination, intraoral examination, and diagnostic tests for periradicular as well as pulp tissues.

Tests for pulp evaluation	Tests for evaluation of periradicular status
• Thermal tests which include heat and cold test • Electric pulp test • Direct dentin stimulation	• Periodontal probing • Palpation • To check mobility • Selective biting on an object

Radiographic Examination

Good quality intraoral periapical and bitewing radiographs may detect caries, restorations, pulp exposures, root resorption, and periradicular pathologies.

Differential Diagnosis

After all findings and tests, differential diagnosis should be made.

Common features of oral pain			
Source of pain	Associated sign	Useful test	Radiograph
Pulp	Deep caries, previous treatment, extensive restoration	Heat or cold test	Caries, extensive restoration
Periradicular tissue	Swelling, redness, tooth mobility	Percussion, probing, palpation	Caries, sometimes and periradicular signs
Dentin	Caries, defective restoration	Hot, cold test, scratching	Caries, poor restorations
Gingiva	Gingival inflammation	Percussion, visual examination	None

Pretreatment Endodontic Emergencies

Hot Tooth

Hot tooth refers to painful tooth which requires immediate pain relief at first appointment. Most common causes of hot tooth is irreversible pulpitis. Since pulpal tissue has very concentrated sensory nerve supply, particularly in chamber, it becomes more difficult to anaesthetize a hot tooth. Teeth most difficult to anesthetize are the mandibular molars followed by mandibular and maxillary premolars, maxillary molars, mandibular anterior teeth, and maxillary anterior teeth.

Theories

❑ **Hyperalgesia:** Inflammation within the tooth alters the actual nerve (by changing the resting potentials and decreasing excitability threshold) making it more difficult to anaesthetize

❑ **Nervous patient:** In nervous or apprehensive patients, pain threshold further reduces causing difficult to anaesthetize

❑ **Location:** It is assumed that if the area of anesthetic to be administered is away from the target, it becomes difficult to anaesthetize. The anesthetic solution may not penetrate to the sensory nerves that innervate the pulp, especially in mandible

❑ **Local tissue changes because of inflammation:** It states that in area of inflammation, acidic pH of inflamed tissue decreases the amount of base form of anesthetic available to penetrate the nerve membrane causing anesthetic to be less effective. But it can be true only in cases of swelling. This theory fails to explain if injection site is away from the area of inflammation

❑ **Central core theory:** It states that nerves outside of nerve bundle supply molar teeth, whereas nerves on the inside supply anterior teeth, so, anesthetic solution may not penetrate into nerve trunk to make all nerves numb

❑ **Tetrodotoxin-resistant (TTXr) channels:** Special class of sodium channels is present on C-fibers, called TTXr. During inflammation, neuroinflammatory reactions start and sodium channel expression on C-fibers shifts from TTX-sensitive to TTXr causing inflammatory hyperalgesia. These channels have shown to be five times more resistant to anesthetic than TTX-sensitive channels. **Bupivacaine** is more potent than lidocaine in blocking TTXr channels and may be the anesthetic of choice when treating the "hot tooth"

Management

❑ **Explaining patient:** Patient should be informed about the treatment so as to avoid fear of unknown and reducing anxiety
  – Management of anxious patient: It is done by keeping short or no waiting time and use of iatrosedation.

Verbal sedation, talking to the patient, music, hypnosis, and relaxation techniques like deep breathing are helpful

- ❑ Role of premedication:
  - – Prescribe anti-inflammatory to be taken 1 hour before the treatment
  - – Provide time gap between anesthetic injection and starting the procedure. Premedication with lorazepam 1 mg (after checking interaction with other drugs) night before sleep followed by 90 min prior to procedure is helpful
- ❑ Additional anesthetic or supplemental injections are necessary to achieve profound anesthesia. Infiltration, supplemental intraligamentary **(Fig. 22.1)**, or intraosseous injections are most helpful along with pulpal anesthesia. Intraosseous injection **(Fig. 22.2)** allows the anesthetic solution to be deposited directly into

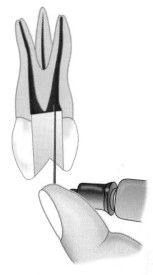

Fig. 22.3 Intrapulpal injection

the cancellous bone around the tooth apices causing better pain relief. Intrapulpal can be painful because here needle is inserted into sensitive and inflamed pulp **(Fig. 22.3).**

Dentin Hypersensitivity

- ❑ Dentin hypersensitivity is defined as "sharp, short pain arising from exposed dentine in response to stimuli typically thermal, chemical, tactile, or osmotic and which cannot be ascribed to any other form of dental defect or pathology"
- ❑ Primary underlying cause for dentin hypersensitivity is exposed dentin tubules. Dentin may become exposed by two processes; either by loss of covering periodontal structures (gingival recession) or by loss of enamel **(Figs. 22.4A and B).**

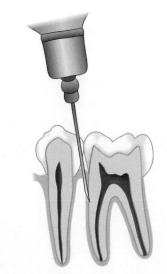

Fig. 22.1 Intraligamentary injection.

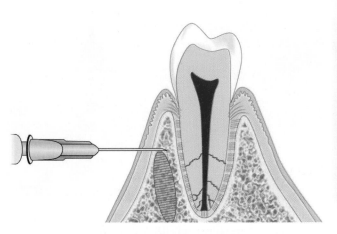

Fig. 22.2 Intraosseous injection.

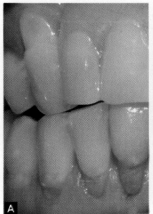
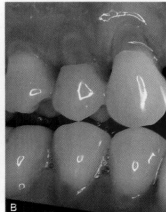

Figs. 22.4A and B Abrasion of teeth may lead to dentin hypersensitivity.

❏ ***Two main principal treatment options*** are plugging the dentinal tubules to prevent the fluid flow and desensitizing the nerve, making it less responsive to stimulation

Acute Reversible Pulpitis

Acute reversible pulpitis is characterized by the following features:
❏ Localized inflammation of the pulp
❏ Lowering of threshold stimulation for Aδ nerve fibers
❏ Exaggerated, nonlingering response to stimuli

Management

❏ Removal of the cause; in case of deep caries, excavate the caries and place restoration.
❏ Recontouring of recently placed restoration which causes pain
❏ Removal of restoration and replacing it with sedative dressing if painful symptoms still persist following tooth preparation

Acute Irreversible Pulpitis

If inflammatory process progresses, irreversible pulpitis can develop. It is characterized by
❏ History of spontaneous pain and exaggerated response to hot or cold that lingers even after removal of stimulus
❏ Extensive restoration or caries involving the pulp
❏ Tooth may be responsive to electrical and thermal tests

Management (Figs. 22.5A to D)

❏ Anesthetize the affected tooth and apply rubber dam
❏ Prepare the access cavity and extirpate the pulp
❏ Thorough irrigation and debridement of the pulp chamber
❏ Determine the working length
❏ Extirpate the pulp followed by cleaning and shaping of the root canal
❏ Thorough irrigation of the root canal system
❏ Drying of the root canal with sterile absorbent points

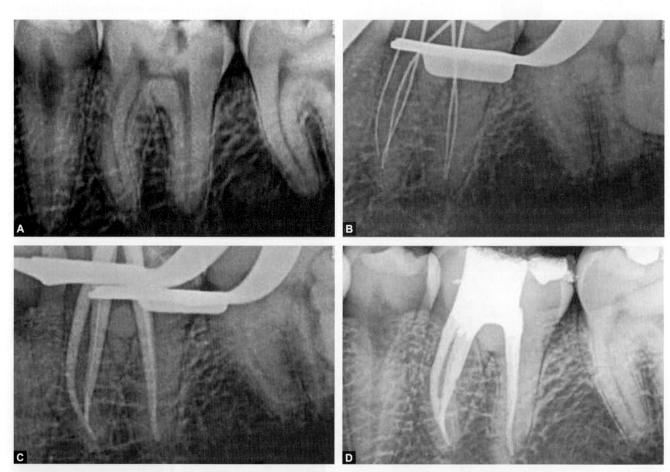

Figs. 22.5A to D Management of mandibular molar with acute irreversible pulpitis: (A) Preoperative radiograph showing mandibular molar with carious exposure of pulp; (B) Working length radiograph; (C) Master cone radiograph; (D) Post obturation radiograph
Courtesy: Jaydev.

- Placement of a dry cotton pellet or pellet moistened with CMCP, formocresol, or eugenol in the pulp chamber and sealing it with the temporary restoration
- Relief of the occlusion
- Appropriate analgesics therapy and antibiotics, if needed

Acute Apical Periodontitis

It is an inflammation of periodontal ligament caused by tissue damage usually from occlusal trauma or extension of pulpal pathology. Pressure on tooth is transmitted to the fluid which pushes on nerve endings in the periodontal ligament. It is characterized by:
- Tooth may be elevated out of its socket because of the increase in fluid pressure in periodontal ligament
- Discomfort on biting or chewing
- Sensitivity to percussion (hallmark diagnostic test)

Management

For vital tooth
Symptomatic treatment and occlusal adjustment if required.

For nonvital teeth
- Anesthetize the involved tooth and prepare the access cavity
- Extirpate the pulp and determine the working length
- Complete the cleaning and shaping of root canal and copiously irrigate
- Place sedative dressing and give temporary restoration
- Relieve the occlusion if indicated
- Prescribe analgesics to reduce the pain

Acute Periapical Abscess

An acute periapical abscess is a severe inflammatory response to microorganisms or their irritants that have been leached into periradicular tissues **(Fig. 22.6)**.

It is characterized by the following features:
- Swelling along with pain and a feeling that tooth is elevated in the socket
- May not have radiographic evidence of bone destruction because fluids rapidly spread away from the tooth
- Systemic features such as fever and malaise may be present
- Mobility may or may not be present

Management
- Biphasic treatment:
  - Pulp debridement
  - Incision and drainage
- Do not leave tooth open between appointments

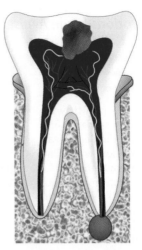

Fig. 22.6 Acute periapical abscess results due to severe inflammatory response to microorganisms and their byproducts which have leached into periradicular tissues

- In case of localized infections, antibiotics provide no additional benefit
- In case of systemic features, antibiotics should be given
- Relieve the tooth out of occlusion in cases of hyperocclusion
- To control postoperative pain, NSAIDs should be prescribed
- Speed of recovery will rely on canal debridement

LA (Local anesthetics) is contraindicated in periapical abscess cases because of the following reasons:
- Pain caused by injection in distended area
- Chances of dissemination of virulent organisms
- Ineffectiveness of local anesthetics

Traumatic Injury

Main objective of the treatment should be immediate relief of pain. Patient with traumatic injury may present; luxation injury, fracture of crown or root, or avulsion of tooth.

In case of **luxation injury**, main aim is to relieve the pain and reposition the dislocated tooth.

In case of **fracture of root or crown**, check the prognosis of fracture and give treatment accordingly.

Avulsion of tooth means complete and total displacement of the tooth out of socket.

Main aim of reimplantation is to preserve maximum number of periodontal ligament cells and prevent them from drying since drying can result in loss of their normal physiology and morphology.

Among various storage media available, order of efficacy is ViaSpan=HBSS>coconut water>milk>green tea>egg white. Water is the least desirable.

Management Options for an Avulsed Tooth

Management of avulsed tooth		
	Mature tooth	*Immature tooth*
Tooth replanted before coming to dental clinic or it is out of socket for less than 15 minutes	• Rinse mouth with water, saline or chlorhexidine and clean the tooth with saline to remove debris • Re-implant the tooth and ask the patient to bite firmly on gauze piece to help stabilize the tooth. • Give flexible splint for 7–10 days	• Clean root surface and socket with saline • Reimplant the tooth gently with firm finger pressure. • Give flexible splint
Extraoral time is less than 60 minutes and has been kept in suitable storage media	• Place tooth in HBSS • Rinse socket with saline to remove debris • Re-implant the tooth • Give flexible splint for 7–10 days	• Soak the tooth in doxycyclin for 5min. • Clean socket with saline • Reimplant the tooth gently with firm finger pressure. • Give flexible splint
Extraoral time is more than 60 minutes or presence of nonviable cells	• Remove periodontal ligament by soaking it in sodium hypochlorite for 10–15 minutes • Soak tooth in 2% stannous fluoride • Start root canal before or after reimplantation • Reimplant the tooth and give flexible splint	• Remove periodontal ligament by soaking it in sodium hypochlorite for 10-15 minutes • Soak tooth in 2% stannous fluoride • Start root canal before or after reimplantation • Reimplant the tooth and give flexible splint

Cracked Tooth Syndrome (Fig. 22.7)

❑ A fracture plane of unknown extent and direction passing through tooth structure may involve pulp and/or periodontal ligament resulting in cracked tooth syndrome.
❑ It is commonly seen in teeth with large and complex restorations
❑ Crack tooth can be diagnosed after taking case history of the patient which includes detailed history regarding

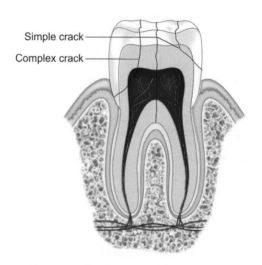

Fig. 22.7 Different types of cracks in teeth.

dietary and parafunctional habits and any previous trauma
❑ During tactile examination, pass the tip of the sharp explorer gently on the tooth surface, so as to locate the crack by catch
❑ Patient can be asked to bite on orangewood stick, rubber wheel, or tooth slooth. Pain during biting, especially upon release of pressure is a classic sign of cracked tooth syndrome

Treatment

Urgent care involves immediate reduction of its occlusal contacts by selective grinding of tooth or its antagonist.

Definitive Treatment

❑ Definitive treatment of the cracked tooth aims to preserve the pulpal vitality by providing full occlusal coverage for cusp protection
❑ Full coverage crown if fracture involves crown portion only
❑ If fracture involves pulp and is superficial to alveolar crest, go for endodontic treatment and restoration of tooth
❑ If fracture of root extends below alveolar crest, extract the tooth

▌Intratreatment Emergencies

Mid-Treatment Flare-ups (Refer Chapter 21)

To summarize, etiology of mid-treatment flare-ups:
❑ Overinstrumentation
❑ Inadequate debridement

- Missed canal
- Hyperocclusion
- Debris extrusion
- Procedural complications

Risk Factors Contributing Interappointment Flare-Ups

- Preoperative pain, percussion, sensitivity, and swelling
- Retreatment
- Apprehension
- History of allergies

Prevention

- Psychological preparation of the patient
- Long-acting anesthetics such as bupivacaine should be preferred
- Complete cleaning and shaping of the root canal
- Analgesics should be prescribed for relief of pain

Treatment

- Reassure patients
- Adjust occlusion
- Complete debridement along with cleaning and shaping of the root canal system
- Prescribe analgesics
- Never leave the tooth open for drainage
- Recall the patient until the painful symptoms subside

Exposure of Pulp

Pulp exposure during tooth preparation can result in severe sharp pain. In these cases, pain can be relieved by complete extirpation of pulp.

Fracture of Tooth

Fracture of tooth can occur during endodontic treatment. It can result in pain due to contamination of root canal. If fracture is vertical extending apical to alveolar crest, one should go for extraction of the tooth; or in case of multi-rooted tooth, one should go for radisection or hemisection.

Recently Placed Restoration

A recently placed restoration may present pain because of many factors like high restoration, microleakage, inadequate pulp protection, galvanism due to dissimilar metal restoration, or chemical irritation from restorative materials or microexposure of the pulp.

Periodontal Treatment

Periodontal treatment can result in exposure of lateral canal which can communicate with periodontal ligament space and cause pain.

Hypochlorite Accident

Hypochlorite accident occurs when sodium hypochlorite gets extruded beyond tooth apex. It manifests a combination of symptoms like severe pain, swelling, and profuse bleeding both through the tooth and interstitial tissues.

Etiology

It can result due to forceful injection of hypochlorite, irrigation of tooth with wide apical foramen, immature apex, or apical resorption.

Clinical Features

Edema, ecchymosis along with tissue necrosis, paresthesia, and secondary injection are commonly seen after hypochlorite accident. Mostly patients recover within 7–10 days, but scarring and paresthesia may take a long time to heal.

Management

- Immediate aspiration and application of icepacks
- Since infection because of tissue destruction can spread, prescribe antibiotics, analgesics, and antihistaminics
- In severe cases, steroids and hospitalization for surgical wound debridement is also indicated
- Home care instructions are given to patients like cold compresses to minimize pain and swelling followed by warm compresses (after 24 h) to encourage healing

Prevention

- Use needles with closed end and lateral vents
- Tip of needle should be 1–2 mm short of the apex
- Never bind the needle in the canal, it should allow back flow of the irrigant
- Oscillate the needle in the canal
- Do not force the irrigant in the canal

Tissue Emphysema

It is defined as collection of gas or air in the tissue spaces or facial planes.

Etiology

❑ During periapical surgery when air from air-rotor is directed toward the exposed soft tissues
❑ When blast of air is directed toward open root canals to dry them
❑ As a complication of fracture involving facial skeleton.

Clinical Features

❑ Development of rapid swelling, erythema and crepitus (crepitus is pathognomonic of tissue emphysema)
❑ Dysphagia and dyspnea, and if emphysema spreads into neck region, it can cause difficulty in breathing and its progression to mediastinum.

Differential Diagnosis

❑ Angioedema
❑ Internal hemorrhage
❑ Anaphylaxis.

Treatment

❑ Antibiotics to prevent risk and spread of infection
❑ Application of moist heat to decrease swelling
❑ If airway or mediastinum is obstructed, immediate medical attention and hospitalization of patient.

Prevention

❑ While using air pressure, blast of air should be directed at horizontal direction against the walls of tooth and not periapically
❑ During surgical procedures, use low-speed or high-speed impact handpiece which do not direct air toward tissues.

▌Postendodontic Emergencies

Following completion of endodontic treatment, patients usually complain of pain, especially on chewing. Incidence of pain after obturation is small and number of visits does not make much difference. Chances of experiencing postoperative discomfort increase if pain is present preoperatively. Painful episodes are caused by pressure exerted by insertion of root canal filling materials or by chemical irritation from ingredients of root canal cements and pastes.

Factors responsible for postobturation pain.

Overextended Obturation

It leads to pain. Periapical inflammation results in firing of proprioceptive nerve fibers in the periodontal ligament. These results are short lived and abate in 24–48 hours. No treatment is usually necessary in these cases.

Under Obturation

Under obturation may result from incomplete cleaning and shaping of the root canal which may cause pain. It may be due to presence of viable pulp tissue left in the canal and failure of resolution of inflammation. In such cases, retreatment is indicated.

Persistent Pain

Persistent pain or sensitivity for longer periods may indicate *failure of resolution of inflammation*. In rare cases, inflamed but *viable pulp tissue may be left in root canal in such cases, retreatment* is indicated.

Vertical Root Fracture

Vertical fracture of crown and/or root can occur:
❑ During obturation due to wedging forces of spreader or plugger
❑ During postplacement in structurally weakened endodontically treated tooth
❑ Due to fracture of coronal restoration because of lack of ferrule effect on remaining root structure.

Diagnosis: Periodontal probing may reveal single isolated narrow pocket adjacent to fracture site. Radiograph may show lateral diffuse widening of periodontal ligament. Surgical exposure of tooth may reveal vertical root fracture (VRF).

Management: Prognosis of VRF is poor and tooth generally undergoes extraction.

High Restoration

It is managed by selective occlusal grinding.

Management of Postobturation Emergencies

Most of the times, there is some discomfort following obturation which subsides in 2–5 days. To manage postobturation endodontic emergencies, the following can be done:
❑ Reassure the patient
❑ Prescribe analgesics
❑ Check occlusion
❑ Do not retreat randomly. Retreatment is done only in cases of persistent untreatable problems.

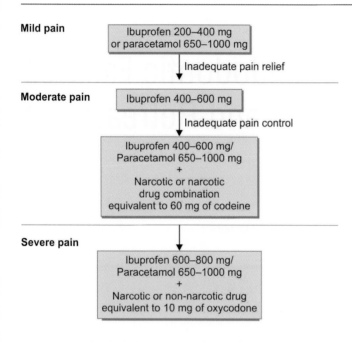

Mild pain

Ibuprofen 200–400 mg
or paracetamol 650–1000 mg

↓ Inadequate pain relief

Moderate pain

Ibuprofen 400–600 mg

↓ Inadequate pain control

Ibuprofen 400–600 mg/
Paracetamol 650–1000 mg
+
Narcotic or narcotic
drug combination
equivalent to 60 mg of codeine

Severe pain

↓

Ibuprofen 600–800 mg/
Paracetamol 650–1000 mg
+
Narcotic or non-narcotic drug
equivalent to 10 mg of oxycodone

Conclusion

One of the greatest challenges in clinical dentistry is managing endodontic emergencies. One should diagnose the emergency and manage it efficiently and under profound pulpal anesthesia.

Reassurance of the patient is the first and foremost step in the treatment of endodontic emergency to control the patient anxiety and overreaction. Sometimes the patient reports severe pain but there is no evidence of acute apical abscess and the root canal treatment has been done properly. These patients are treated with reassurance and analgesics, again the symptoms subside spontaneously. But if apical abscess develops with inadequate root canal treatment, apical surgery may be needed.

Questions

1. Define and classify endodontic emergencies.
2. How will you manage a hot tooth in dental clinic?
3. What are pretreatment endodontic emergencies. Discuss their management?
4. Enumerate postobturation emergencies.

Bibliography

1. Argen E, Danielsson K. Conduction of block analgesia in mandible. Swed Dent J 1981;5:81.
2. Balaban FS, Skidmore AE, Griffin JA. Acute exacerbations following initial treatment of necrotic pulps. J Endod 1984;10:78.
3. Fernandez C, Reader A, Beck M, Nusstein J. A prospective, randomized, double-blind comparison of bupivacaine and lidocaine for inferior alveolar nerve blocks. J Endod 2005;31:499.
4. Hargreaves KM, Berman LH. Cohen's pathways of the pulp. 11th edition .pp. 90–129.
5. Harrington GW, Natkin E. Midtreatment flare-ups. Dent Clin North Am 1992;36:409–23.
6. Malamed S. Handbook of local anaesthesia. 5th edition St Louis: Mosby; 2004.
7. Marshall JG, Liesinger AW. Factors associated with endodontics post-treatment pain. J Endod 1993;19:573.
8. Naidorf IJ. Endodontic flare-ups: bacteriological and immunological mechanisms. J Endod 1985;11:462.
9. Nist R, Reader A, Beck M, Meyers W. An evaluation of the incisive nerve block and combination inferior alveolar and incisive nerve blocks in mandibular anaesthesia. J Endod 1992;18:455.
10. Seltzer S, Naiorf IJ. Flare-ups in endodontics: etiological factors. J Endod 1985;11:472.
11. Vreeland D, Reader A, Beck M, et al. An evaluation of volumes and concentrations in human alveolar nerve block. J Endod 1989;15:6.
12. Walton R, Torabinejad M. Managing local anaesthesia problems in the endodontic patient. J Am Dent Assoc 1992;123:97.
13. Walton R. Managing local anaesthesia problems in the endodontic patient. Endod Pract 1998;1:15.

Endodontic Failures and Retreatment

Many studies have been conducted to determine success and failures of endodontic treatments. Properly executed root canal treatment has shown success in > 95% of the cases.

Endodontic failure cannot be subscribed to any particular criteria of evaluation; instead success or failure following endodontic therapy could be evaluated from a combination of various criteria like clinical, histopathological, and radiographical criteria.

Definitions related to endodontic treatment outcome

Healed: Both clinical and radiographic presentations are normal.

Healing: It is a dynamic process, reduced *radiolucency* combined with normal clinical presentation.

Disease: No change or increase in *radiolucency*, clinical signs may or may not be present or vice versa.

Evaluation of Success of Endodontic Treatment

Evaluation of success of endodontic treatment			
Criteria	Clinical	Radiographic	Histological
Significance	Presence of symptoms indicates the presence of pathology, but absence of symptoms does not confirm absence of a disease	To predict the success or failure, compare the radiographs taken at different times **(Figs. 23.1A and B)**	Check status of periodontal ligament, bone and cementum and inflammation after endodontic therapy
Symptoms	• No tenderness to percussion • Normal tooth mobility • Tooth having normal form function and esthetics • No sign of infection or swelling • No sinus tract minimal to no scarring or discoloration	• Normal or slightly thickened periodontal ligament space • Reduction or elimination of previous rarefaction • No evidence of resorption • Normal lamina dura • A dense three dimensional obturation of canal space	• Absence of inflammation • Regeneration of periodontal ligament fibers • Presence of osseous repair • Repair of cementum • Absence of resorption • Repair of previously resorbed areas

Factors affecting the success or failure of root canal treatment

Factors affecting prognosis in all cases	Factors affecting prognosis in particular case
• Diagnosis and treatment planning • Radiographic interpretation • Anatomy of the tooth and root canal system • Debridement of root canal space • Asepsis of treatment regimen • Quality and extent of apical seal • Quality of postendodontic restoration • Systemic health of patient • Skill of the operator	• Pulpal and periodontal status • Size of periapical radiolucency • Canal anatomy like calcification, presence of accessory or lateral canals, resorption, curvature, etc. • Crown and root fracture • Iatrogenic errors • Occlusal discrepancies, if any • Time of post-treatment evaluation

Factors responsible for endodontic failure

Local	Systemic

1. Infection
2. Excessive hemorrhage
3. Chemical irritants
4. Iatrogenic errors
   i Canal blockage and ledge formation
   ii Incomplete debridement of the root canal system
   iii Overinstrumentation
   iv Separated instruments
   v Perforations
   vi Incompletely filled teeth
   vii Overfilling of root canals
5. Corrosion of root canal fillings
6. Anatomic factors
7. Root fractures
8. Traumatic occlusion
9. Periodontal considerations
	• Nutritional deficiencies
	• Diabetes mellitus
	• Renal failure
	• Blood dyscrasias
	• Hormonal imbalance
	• Autoimmune disorders
	• Opportunistic infections
	• Aging
	• Patients on long-term steroid therapy

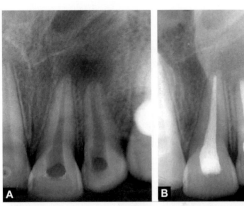

Figs. 23.1A and B Radiographic evaluation of periapical radiolucency in relation to maxillary central incisors: (A) Preoperative radiograph showing periapical radiolucency in relation to maxillary central incisors; (B) Postoperative radiograph 9 months after nonsurgical endodontic treatment showing healed periapical area.

Local Factors Causing Endodontic Failures

Infection

❑ If infected tissue is present, then host parasite relationship, virulence of microorganisms, and ability of infected tissues to heal in the presence of microorganisms are the main factors which influence repair of periapical tissues following endodontic therapy **(Fig. 23.2)**

❑ If apical seal or coronal restorations are not optimal **(Fig. 23.3)**, reinfection of root canal can occur.

Excessive Hemorrhage

Extirpation of pulp and instrumentation beyond periapical tissues lead to excessive hemorrhage. Clump of extravasated blood cells and fluid must be resorbed, otherwise it acts as foreign body and nidus for bacterial growth, especially in the presence of infection.

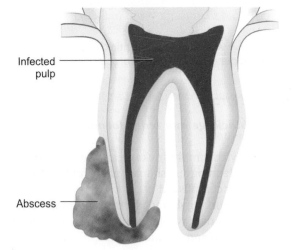

Fig. 23.2 Presence of infected tissue may affect the repair of periapical tissues resulting in endodontic failure.

Chemical Irritants

Chemical irritants in the form of intracanal medicaments and irrigating solution decrease the prognosis of endodontic therapy, if they get extruded in the periapical tissues.

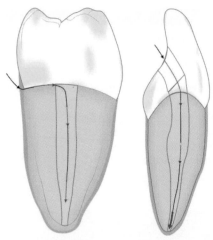

Fig. 23.3 Microleakage because of defective coronal seal can result in endodontic failure.

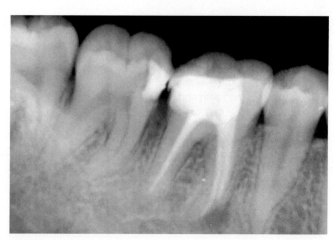

Fig. 23.5 Incomplete obturation of mesiobuccal canal of mandibular first molar due to ledge formation results in periapical radiolucency with respect to mesial root.

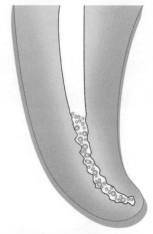

Fig. 23.4 Accumulation of dentin chips and debris cause incomplete instrumentation of apical third of the canal.

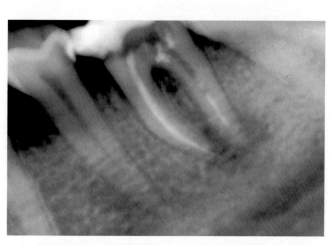

Fig. 23.6 Root canal failure due to inadequate debridement and optimal seal of mandibular first molar.

Iatrogenic Errors

i) Canal blockage and ledge formation (Figs. 23.4 and 23.5)

❑ In cases with canal blockage and ledge formation, complete cleaning and shaping of the root canal system cannot be accomplished

❑ Because of working short of the canal terminus, bacteria and tissue debris may remain in non-instrumented area contributing to endodontic failure.

ii) Incomplete debridement of the root canal system

❑ Presence of infected and necrotic pulp tissue in root canal acts as the main irritant to the periapical tissues (Fig. 23.6)

❑ Poor debridement can cause residual microorganisms, their by-products and tissue debris to recolonize and contribute endodontic failure.

iii) Over instrumentation

Overinstrumentation results in trauma to periodontal ligament and the alveolar bone (Fig. 23.7), thus affecting the success rate.

iv) Instrument separation (Fig. 23.8)

❑ Seltzer et al reported that prognosis of endodontic therapy was not significantly affected in teeth in which vital pulp was present before treatment, but if instrument separation occurred in teeth with pulpal necrosis, prognosis was found to be poor after treatment

❑ Separated instruments impair the mechanical instrumentation of infected root canals apical to instrument, which contribute to endodontic failure.

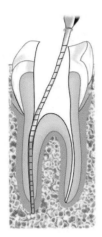

Fig. 23.7 Over instrumentation results in trauma to periodontal tissue and decreases the prognosis of tooth.

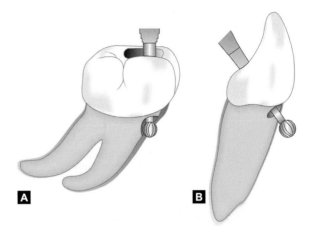

Figs. 23.9A and B Perforation of (A) molar; (B) anterior tooth due to misdirection of bur.

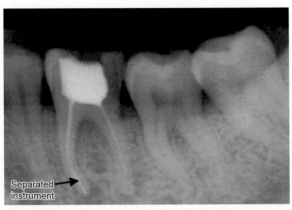

Fig. 23.8 Radiograph showing periapical lesion associated with mesiobuccal canal with separated instrument in mandibular first molar.

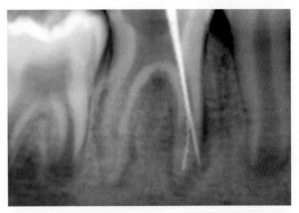

Fig. 23.10 Perforation in mesiobuccal canal of mandibular first molar decreases the prognosis of treatment.

v) Perforation (Figs. 23.9 and 23.10)

❑ Perforation is the mechanical communication between the root canal system and the periodontium
❑ Prognosis of endodontically treated tooth with perforations depends on many factors such as location (its closeness to gingival sulcus), time elapsed before defect is repaired, adequacy of perforation seal, and size of the perforation.

vi) Incompletely filled teeth

❑ Incompletely filled teeth are teeth filled >2 mm short of apex (Fig. 23.11)
❑ Underfilling can occur due to incomplete instrumentation or ledge formation, blockage of canal, and improper measurements of working length
❑ Remaining infected necrotic tissue, microorganism, and their by-products in inadequately instrumented and filled teeth cause continuous irritation to the periradicular tissues and thus endodontic failure (Fig. 23.12).

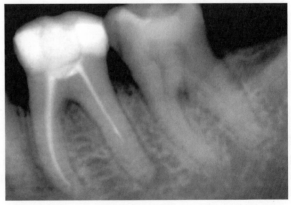

Fig. 23.11 Radiograph showing periapical radiolucency due to underobturated distal canal of mandibular second molar.

vii) Overfilling of root canals (Fig. 23.13)

❑ Overfilling of root canals, that is, obturation of the canal extending >2 mm beyond radiographic apex. Filling material acts as a foreign body which may generate

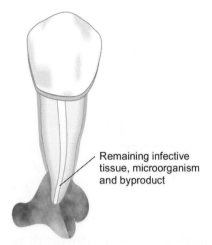

Fig. 23.12 Remaining infective tissue, microorganisms, and their byproducts of incompletely filled space act as constant irritant resulting in endodontic failure.

Remaining infective tissue, microorganism and byproduct

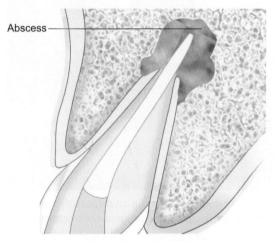

Abscess

Fig. 23.13 Overfilling of canal results in endodontic failure due to constant irritation to periapical tissues.

immunological response and cause continuous irritation of the periapical tissues
❑ Biofilms present on extruded material contain treatment-resistant bacteria resulting in endodontic failure.

Corrosion of Root Canal Fillings

Silver cones show corrosion which is commonly seen in coronal and apical areas due to contact of tissue fluids either periapical exudation or saliva. Corrosion products are cytotoxic and act as tissue irritants causing persistent periapical inflammation.

Anatomic Factors

Presence of curved canals, calcifications, lateral, and accessory canals, bifurcations, aberrant canal anatomy like C- or S-shaped canals may cause inadequate cleaning and

shaping and thereby incomplete obturation, resulting in endodontic failure.

Root Fractures

Partial or complete fractures of the roots can cause endodontic failure.

Traumatic Occlusion

Traumatic occlusion causes endodontic failures because of its effect on periodontium.

Periodontal Considerations (Figs. 23.14 and 23.15)

Recession of attachment apparatus may expose lateral canals to the oral fluids which can lead to reinfection of the root canal system because of percolation of fluids.

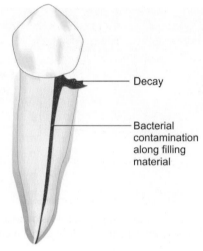

Decay

Bacterial contamination along filling material

Fig. 23.14 Decay at subgingival area below crown can result in contamination of root filling and contribute to endodontic failure.

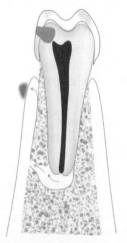

Fig. 23.15 Endodontic periodontal communication results in endodontic failure.

Systemic Factors

Presence of systemic disease (nutritional deficiencies, diabetes mellitus, renal failure, blood dyscrasias, hormonal imbalance, autoimmune disorders, opportunistic infections, aging, and patients on long-term steroid therapy) can intensify the response of periapical tissues to the irritants during endodontic therapy and also impair healing.

Case Selection for Endodontic Retreatment

Retreatment is usually indicated in symptomatic endodontically treated teeth or in asymptomatic teeth with improperly done endodontic therapy to prevent future emergence of the disease.

Before initiating endodontic retreatment, the following factors should be considered:
- When should the treatment be considered, that is, if the patient is asymptomatic even if treatment is not proper, the retreatment should be postponed
- Patient's needs and expectations
- Strategic importance of the tooth
- Periodontal evaluation of the tooth
- Other interdisciplinary evaluation
- Chair time and cost.

Factors affecting prognosis of endodontic treatment
- Presence of any periapical radiolucency
- Quality of the obturation
- Apical extension of the obturation material
- Bacterial status of the canal
- Observation period
- Postendodontic coronal restoration
- Latrogenic complication.

Contraindications of endodontic retreatment
- Unfavorable root anatomy (shape, taper, remaining dentin thickness)
- Presence of untreatable root resorptions or perforations
- Presence of root or bifurcation caries
- Insufficient crown/root ratio

Steps of Retreatment (Figs. 23.16A to F)

Steps of retreatment
- Coronal disassembly
- Establish access to root canal system

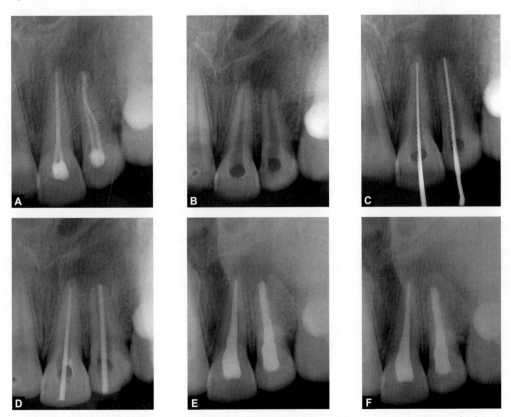

Figs. 23.16A to F Endodontic retreatment in maxillary left central incisor: (A) Preoperative radiograph showing defective root canal of 21; (B) Radiograph after gutta-percha removal; (C) Working length radiograph; (D) Radiograph with master cone in place; (E) Radiograph after obturation; (F) Follow-up after 6 months showing periapical healing.
Courtesy: Manoj Hans.

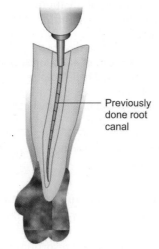

Fig. 23.17 Entry to root canal after coronal dissembly.

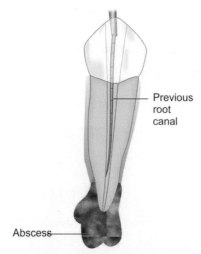

Fig. 23.18 Entry to root canal system through coronal restoration.

❑ Remove canal obstructions and establish patency
❑ Thorough cleaning, shaping, and obturation of the canal.

Coronal Disassembly

Endodontic retreatment procedures require removal of existing coronal restoration (**Fig. 23.17**). Though access can be made through the existing restoration (**Fig. 23.18**), it is removed if it has poor marginal adaptation or secondary caries (**Fig. 23.19**).

Advantages of gaining access through original restoration	Disadvantages of retaining restoration
• Facilitate rubber dam placement • Maintain form, function and esthetics • Reduce cost of replacement	• Reduced visibility and accessibility • Increased risks of irreparable errors • Increased risks of microbial infection if crown margins are poorly adapted

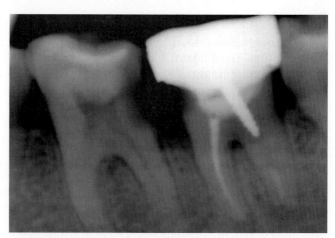

Fig. 23.19 Radiograph showing poor marginal adaptation and secondary caries under coronal restoration. It is advisable to remove such restoration before retreatment.

Establish Access to Root Canal System

In teeth with post and core, post has to be removed for gaining access to the root canal system. **Figs. 23.20A to E** shows endodontic retreatment of mandibular second molar with defective obturation, fractured instrument in mesiobuccal canal associated with periapical radiolucency. Patient complained occasional pain along with sinus tract, which was confirmed by taking radiograph with gutta-percha placed in the sinus tract.

Posts can be removed by the following method:
❑ Weakening the retention of posts by using ultrasonic vibration (**Figs. 23.21A to D**)
❑ Pulling of posts but it increases risk of root fracture
❑ With the help of special pliers using postremoval systems (PRSs)

PRS kit consists of five differently designed trephines and corresponding taps, a torque bar, a transmetal bur, rubber bumpers, and extracting pliers.
❑ Initially, a transmetal bur is used for efficiently dooming of the posthead (**Fig. 23.22A**)
❑ Then a drop of a lubricant like RC Prep is placed on the posthead to further facilitate the machining process
❑ After this, trephine is selected to engage and machine down the coronal 2–3 mm of post (**Fig. 23.22B**)
❑ Subsequently, a microtubular tap is inserted against the posthead and screwed it into post with counterclockwise direction. Before doing this, a rubber bumper is inserted on the tap to act as cushion against forces (**Fig. 23.22C**)
❑ When tubular tap tightly engages the post, rubber bumper is pushed down to the occlusal surface
❑ Mount the postremoval plier on tubular tap by holding it firmly with one hand and engaging it with the other hand by turning screw knob clockwise if post is strongly bonded in the canal, then ultrasonic instrument is vibrated on the

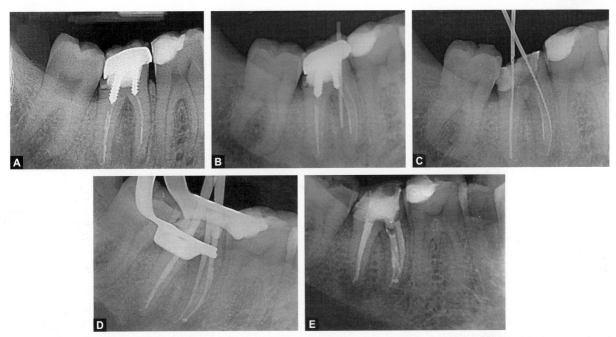

Figs. 23.20A to E Endodontic retreatment of mandibular second molar with post and crown. Patient presented with sinus tract in relation to mandibular molar: (A) Preoperative radiograph showing defective root canal, improper post placement and separated instrument in mesiolingual canal; (B) Sinus tracking radiograph confirmed the offending tooth; (C) Removal of the post and establishing access to the distal and mesiobuccal canals. Separated instrument present in the mesiolingual canal; (D) After removal of instrument, cleaning and shaping, master cone radiograph; (E) Post obturation radiograph.
Courtesy: Viresh.

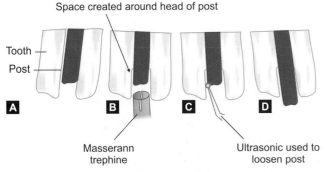

Figs. 23.21A to D Use of ultrasonics to remove post: (A) Post in tooth; (B) Make space; (C) Loosen; (D) Retrieval.

tap or a torque bar is inserted onto the handle to increase the leverage, thereby facilitating its removal (**Fig. 23.22D**)
❑ After that, select an ultrasonic tip and vibrate it on the tubular tap, which casues screwed knob to turn further and thus help in post removal.

Removing Canal Obstructions and Establishing Patency

Patency of canal is regained by removing canal obstructions like silver points, gutta-percha, pastes, sealers, separated instruments and posts, etc.

Silver Point Removal

Silver points can be bypassed or removed depending upon the accessibility and canal anatomy. These can be retrieved from canal by:
❑ Using microsurgical forcep; specially when cone head is sticking up in the chamber (**Fig. 23.23**)
❑ Working ultrasonic file around periphery of the instrument to loosen it (**Fig. 23.24**)
❑ Placing H-files in the canal and working down alongside the silver point (**Fig. 23.25A**). These files are twisted around each other by making clockwise rotation. This rotation will grasp around silver point which then can be removed (**Fig. 23.25B**)
❑ Using hypodermic needle which is made to fit tightly over the silver point on which cyanoacrylate is placed as an adhesive (**Fig. 23.26A**). When it sets, needle is grabbed with pliers (**Fig. 23.26B**)
❑ By tap and thread option using microtubular taps from PRS kit
❑ Using instrument removal system.

Gutta-Percha Removal

Relative difficulty in removing gutta-percha is influenced by length, diameter, curvature, and internal configuration of the canal system.

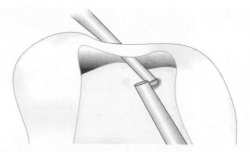

Fig. 23.22A Use of transmetal bur for dooming head of posthead.

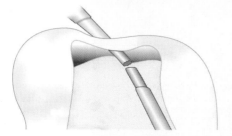

Fig. 23.22B Selection of trephine to engage the 2–3 mm of posthead.

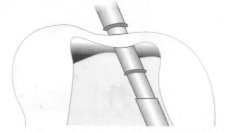

Fig. 23.22C Insert microtubular tap against posthead and move it in counterclockwise direction.

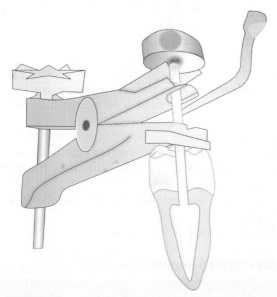

Fig. 23.22D Mount postremoval plier on tubular tap and then vibrate ultrasonic instrument on to the tap to increase leverage.

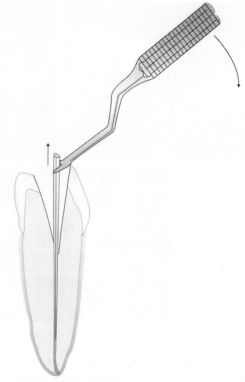

Fig. 23.23 Removal of silver point using microsurgical forcep.

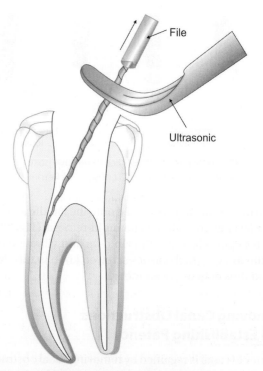

File

Ultrasonic

Fig. 23.24 Ultrasonic file is moved around the silver point to loosen it with vibration.

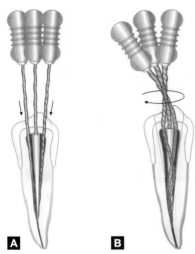

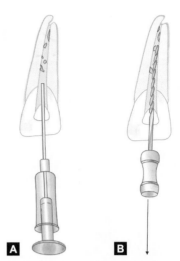

Figs. 23.25A and B (A) Use of hedstroem files to remove silver point; (B) files are twisted around each other by making clockwise rotation to grip the silver point.

Figs. 23.27A and B (A) Use of solvents to dissolve gutta-percha; (B) Removal of dissolved gutta-percha using files.

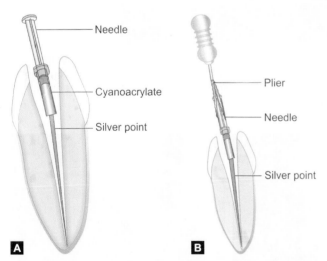

Figs. 23.26A and B (A) Use of hypodermic needle to fit it tightly over silver point over which cyanoacrylate is placed as adhesive; (B) After the cyanoacrylate sets, grab the needle with plier.

The following factors affect gutta-percha removal:
❑ Density of filling
❑ Curvature of canal
❑ Length of canal.
Gutta-percha can be removed by
❑ ***Use of solvents:*** Gutta-percha is soluble in chloroform, methyl chloroform, benzene, xylene, eucalyptol oil, halothane, and rectified white turpentine; it can removed from the canal by dissolving it in these solvents **(Figs. 23.27A and B)**
  • Being highly volatile, chloroform is most effective so commonly used. However, it has shown to be carcinogenic in high concentrations, so excessive filling in pulp chamber should be avoided.

❑ ***Use of hand instruments:*** Hand instruments are mainly used in the apical part of the canal. H-files are used to engage the cones so that they can be pulled out in single piece. Hot file or reamer can also be used to remove the gutta-percha points. With overextended cones, files sometimes have to be extended periapically to avoid separation of the cone at the apical foramen.

Coronal portion of gutta-percha should be explored by Gates-Gliddens to:
❑ Remove gutta-percha quickly
❑ Provide space for solvents
❑ Improve convenience form
❑ ***Use of rotary instrumentation (Figs. 23.28 and 23.29):*** Rotary instruments are safe to be used in straight canals. ProTaper universal system was introduced in 2006, it consists of D_1, D_2, and D_3 to be used at 500–700 rpm **(Fig. 23.30)**

D_1	D_2	D_3
• Removes filling from coronal third • 11 mm handle • 16 mm cutting surface • White ring for identification • ISO 30, active tip for easier penetration of obturation material • 9% taper file	• Removes filling from middle third • 11 mm handle • 18 mm cutting blades • Two white rings for identification • ISO 25, nonactive rounded tip to follow canal path • 8% taper file	• Removes filling from apical third • 11 mm handle • 22 mm cutting blades • Three white rings for identification • ISO 20 nonactive rounded tip to follow canal path • 7% taper file

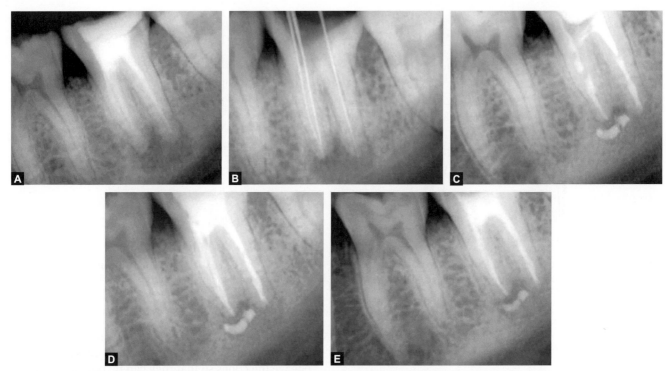

Figs. 23.28A to E Retreatment of mandibular left second molar with periradicular radiolucency treated with D-files, metapex and MTA. (A) Preoperative radiograph showing defective root canal and periapical radiolucency with respect to mandibular second molar; (B) Gutta-percha removed using D-files and working length taken; (C) Metapex placed for periapical healing; (D) After 25 days, obturation done using MTA; (E) Radiograph taken after 3 months, showing healing of periapical area.
Courtesy: Anil Dhingra.

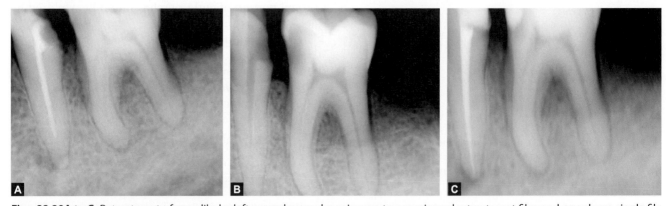

Figs. 23.29A to C Retreatment of mandibular left second premolar using protaper universal retreatment files and one shape single file system: (A) Preoperative radiograph showing defective RCT in 35; (B) Radiograph taken after removal of old gutta-percha using D-files; (C) Postobturation radiograph.
Courtesy: Anil Dhingra.

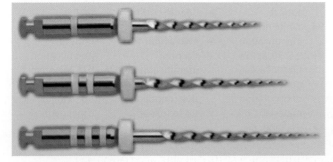

Fig. 23.30 Protaper retreatment files D_1, D_2, and D_3.

❑ *Using microdebriders:* These are small files constructed with 90° bends and are used to remove any remaining gutta-percha on the sides of canal walls or isthmuses after repreparation.

Removal of Resilon

Resilon can be removed using combination of hand and rotary instruments similar to gutta-percha. For effective removal of resilon, combination of chloroform dissolution and rotary instrumentation is recommended. For removal of resilon sealer, use of Gates-Glidden drills and H-files is recommended.

Carrier Based Gutta-Percha Removal

❏ Grasp the carrier with pliers and try to remove it using fulcrum mechanism rather than straight pulling it from the tooth
❏ Use ultrasonics along the side of the carrier and thermosoften the gutta-percha. Then move ultrasonics apically and displace the carrier coronally
❏ Use solvents to chemically soften the gutta-percha and then use hand files to loosen the carrier
❏ Use rotary instruments to remove plastic carrier from the canal
❏ Use instrument removal system to remove carrier especially if it is metal carrier.

Removal of Paste

Soft setting pastes can be removed using the normal endodontic instruments preferably using crown-down technique **(Fig. 23.31)**
Hard setting cements like resin cements can be first softened using solvents like xylene, eucalyptol, etc. and then removed using endodontic files. Ultrasonic endodontic devices can also be used to breakdown the pastes by vibrations and facilitate their removal **(Fig. 23.32)**.

The following methods can be employed to remove pastes for retreatment cases:
❏ Heat is employed for some resin pastes for softening them
❏ Ultrasonic energy is employed to remove brick hard resin type pastes
❏ Chemicals like Endosolve "R" and Endosolve "E" are employed for softening hard paste (R denotes resin-based and E denotes eugenol-based pastes)
❏ Microdebriders are used to remove remnants of paste material. These are available in 16 mm length with Hedstroem type cutting blades and tip diameter of 0.2 and 0.3 mm in 2% taper

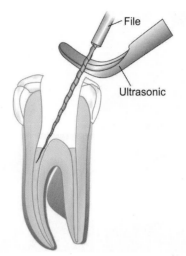

Fig. 23.32 Use of ultrasonic vibration for paste removal.

❏ End cutting NiTi rotary instruments are used to penetrate paste. But to avoid iatrogenic errors, they should be used with caution.

Separated Instruments and Foreign Objects

❏ Primary requirement for removal of broken instruments or foreign objects is their accessibility and visibility
❏ if root canal is obstructed by foreign object in coronal-third, then attempt retrieval, in middle-third, attempt retrieval or bypass and if it is in apical third leave it or treat surgically **(Figs. 23.33 to 23.35)**
❏ If overpreparation of canal compromises the dentin thickness, leave the instrument in place rather than compromising the coronal dentin

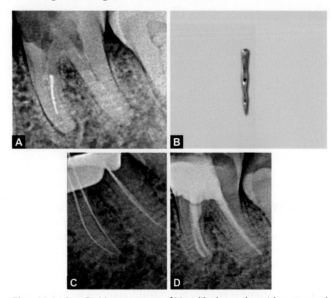

Figs. 23.33A to D Management of Mandibular molar with separated instrument: (A) Preoperative radiograph showing separated instrument present in mesiolingual canal of mandibular first molar; (B) Separated instrument; (C) Working length radiograph after removal of instrument; (D) Post obturation radiograph.
Courtesy: Jaydev.

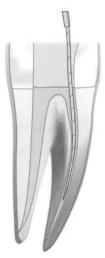

Fig. 23.31 Removal of soft setting paste using normal endodontic instrument in crown down technique.

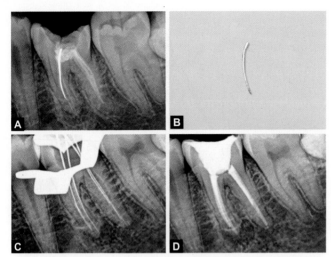

Figs. 23.34A to D Management of mandibular first molar with separated instrument: (A) Preoperative radiograph showing separated instrument present in mesiobuccal canal of Mandibular first molar; (B) Separated instrument removed; (C) Working length radiograph after removal of instrument; (D) Post obturation radiograph. *Courtesy* - Jaydev.

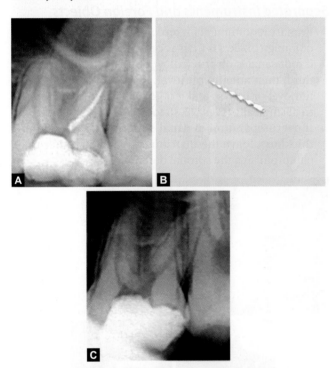

Figs. 23.35A to C Management of maxillary first molar with separated instrument: (A) Preoperative radiograph showing separated instrument present in distobuccal canal of maxillary first molar; (B) Separated instrument removed using ultrasonic vibration; (C) Radiograph after removal of instrument.

❑ If instrument is readily accessible, remove it by holding with instruments like Stieglitz pliers and Massermann extractor. Massermann extractor comprises a tube with

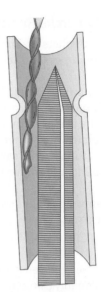

Fig. 23.36 Use of Massermann extractor for removal of separated instrument.

a constriction into which a stylet is introduced to grasp the fractured instrument **(Fig. 23.36)**
❑ Ultrasonics can also be used to remove the instrument by vibration effect **(Figs. 23.37A to D)**
❑ Modified Gates-Glidden bur can also be used. It creates a staging platform before using an ultrasonic tip to rotate around the file in a counterclockwise direction so to remove it
❑ When it is not possible to remove the foreign objects, attempts should be made to bypass it and complete biomechanical preparation of the canal system
❑ Bypassing of instrument can be done by using hand instruments like reamers and files. These instruments are inserted alongside the broken instrument to soften its cementation and thus facilitate its removal. While making efforts to the bypass the instrument, copious irrigation is needed. Irrigation with sodium hypochlorite, hydrogen peroxide, and RC Prep may float the object coronally through the effervescence they create
❑ Use of ultrasonic K-file no. 15 or 20 with vibration and copious irrigation may also pull the instrument coronally.

Completion of the Retreatment

After gaining access to the root canal system, with its thorough cleaning and shaping and managing other complications, the treatment is completed using the routine procedures. It is difficult to retreat a case nonsurgically especially if:
❑ Access is to be made through previously placed restoration
❑ Postremoval is impossible

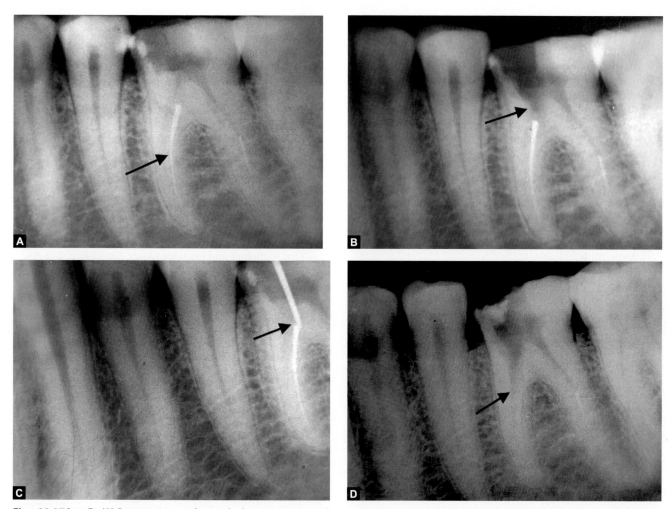

Figs. 23.37A to D (A) Preoperative radiograph showing separated instrument in mesiobuccal canal of mandibular first molar; (B) Groove made for ultrasonic tip to reach the file head; (C) Usltrasonic tip checked for its path till it reaches file; (D) Postoperative radiograph showing after file retrival.
Courtesy: Poonam Bogra.

❑ Gutta-percha is extended periapically
❑ There is presence of foreign objects, or hard setting pastes which are amenable to remove nonsurgically.

Outcome of Retreatment

Outcome of retreatment can be short-term and long-term. *Short-term outcome* is associated with postoperative discomfort including pain and swelling. *Long-term outcome* of retreatment depends on regaining the canal patency and obturation of root canal system.

Conclusion

One should attempt primary endodontic treatement if tooth can be saved successfully with endodontic therapy, but due to some factors, if it fails, nonsurgical endodontic retreatment should be considered before going for surgical intervention or extraction of the tooth. Non surgical endodontic retreatment is a predictable procedure that allows patients to maintain their teeth. But, as with any procedure, the correct diagnosis to understand indications and limitations helps proper treatment planning.

Questions

1. What are different criteria used for evaluation of endodontic treatment?
2. What is etiology of endodontic failures?
3. What are criteria of case selection for endodontic retreatment? Enumerate different steps of retreatment
4. Write short note on:
   • Gutta-percha removal
   • Silver point removal.

▍Bibliography

1. Friedman S, Abitbol S, Lawrence HP. Treatment outcome in endodontics: the Toronto study. Phase 1: initial treatment. Journal of Endodontics. 2003;29(12):787-93.
2. Imura N, Pinheiro ET, Gomes BPFA, Zaia AA, Ferraz CCR, Souza-Filho FJ. The outcome of endodontic treatment: a retrospective study of 2000 cases performed by a specialist. Journal of Endodontics. 2007;33(11):1278-82.
3. Kerekes K, Tronstad L. Long-term results of endodontic treatment performed with a standardized technique. Journal of Endodontics. 1979;5(3):83-90.
4. Mounce R. Current concepts in gutta-percha removal in endodontic retreatment. NY State Dent J. 2004;70(7):32-5.
5. Mounce R. Endodontic retreatment possibilities: evaluation, limitations, and considerations Compend Contin Educ Dent. 2004;25(5):364-8.
6. Paik S, Sechrist C, Torabinejad M. Levels of evidence for the outcome of endodontic retreatment. J Endod. 2004; 30(11):745-50.
7. Ruddle CJ. Nonsurgical retreatment. J Endod. 2004;30(12): 827-45.
8. Sae-Lim V, Rajamanickam I, Lim BK, et al. Effectiveness of ProFile .04 taper rotary instruments in endodontic retreatment. J Endod. 2000;26(2):100-4.
9. Sjögren U, Hägglund B, Sundqvist G. Factors affecting the long-term results of endodontic treatment. Journal of Endodontics. 1990;16(10):498-504.
10. Wong R. Conventional endodontic failure and retreatment. Dent Clin North Am. 2004;48(1):265-89.
11. Caliskan MK. Nonsurgical retreatment of teeth with periapical lesions previously managed by either endodontic or surgical intervention. Oral Surgery, Oral Medicine, Oral Pathology, Oral Radiology and Endodontology. 2005;100(2):242-8.

Procedural Accidents

Like any other field of dentistry, a clinician may face unwanted situations during root canal treatment which can affect the prognosis of endodontic therapy. These procedural accidents are collectively termed ***endodontic mishaps.***

Accurate diagnosis, proper case selection, and adherence to basic principles of endodontic therapy may prevent occurrence of procedural accidents. But if any endodontic mishap occurs, inform the patient about:

- ❑ Incidence and nature of mishap
- ❑ Procedures to correct it
- ❑ Alternative treatment options
- ❑ Prognosis of the affected tooth.

Endodontic mishaps may have dentolegal consequences. Thus, their prevention is the best option, both for patient as well as dentist. Knowledge of etiological factors involved in endodontic mishaps is mandatory for their prevention. Recognition of a procedural accident is the first step in its management.

Endodontic mishaps
- Inadequately cleaned and shaped root canal system
  - Loss of working length
  - Canal blockage
  - Ledge formation
  - Missed canals
- Instrument separation
- Deviation from normal canal anatomy
  - Zipping
  - Stripping or lateral wall perforation
  - Canal transportation

- Inadequate canal preparation
  - Overinstrumentation
  - Overpreparation
  - Underpreparation
- Perforations
  - Coronal perforations
  - Root perforations
    - Cervical canal perforations
    - Mid-root perforations
    - Apical perforations
  - Postspace perforations
- Obturation related
  - Over obturation
  - Under obturation
- Vertical root fracture
- Instrument aspiration

Inadequately Cleaned and Shaped Root Canal System

Main objective of cleaning and shaping is to remove pulp tissue, debris, bacteria and to shape the canal for obturation. Errors that most often occur during canal preparation include:

Loss of Working Length

Loss of working length during cleaning and shaping is a common procedural error. It is noted only on the master cone radiograph or when the master apical file is short of established working length **(Fig. 24.1)**.

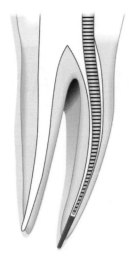

Fig. 24.1 Master apical file short of working length.

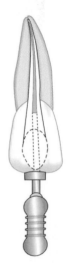

Fig. 24.3 Use of sound reference point.

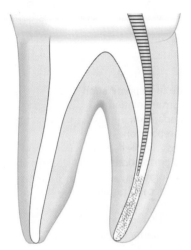

Fig. 24.2 Accumulation of dentinal debris in apical third because of loss of working length.

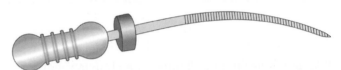

Fig. 24.4 Precurve the instrument before using it in a curved canal.

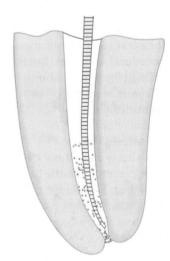

Fig. 24.5 Recapitulation is done with smaller number file to remove the debris.

Etiology

❑ Secondary to other endodontic procedural errors, like blockages, ledge formation, and fractured instruments
❑ Rapid increase in file size
❑ Accumulation of dentinal debris in apical third of the canal (Fig. 24.2)
❑ Lack of attention to details, like malpositioned instrument stops, variations in reference points, poor radiographic technique, and improper use of instruments.

Prevention

❑ Use sound and reproducible reference points (Fig. 24.3)
❑ Precurve all instruments for use in curved canals (Fig. 24.4)
❑ Use directional instrument stops

❑ When verifying the instrument position radiographically, use consistent radiographic angles
❑ Always maintain the original preoperative shape of the canal
❑ Copious irrigation and recapitulation throughout cleaning and shaping procedures (Fig. 24.5)
❑ Always use sequential file sizes.

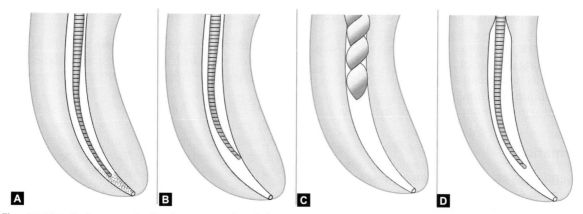

Figs. 24.6A to D Reasons why file does not reach to full working length: (A) Dentin chips; (B) Wrong angulation of instrument; (C) Larger instrument than canal diameter; (D) Restriction to instrument making it short of apex.

Canal Blockage

A blockage is obstruction in a previously patent canal system that prevents access to the apical constriction or apical stop. It is confirmed by taking radiograph which shows that file is not reaching up to its established working length.

Etiology (Figs. 24.6A to D)

- ❑ Common causes of canal blockage can be packed dentinal chips, tissue debris, cotton pellets, restorative materials, or presence of fractured instruments
- ❑ If tip of the instrument used is wider than canal diameter.

Treatment

- ❑ When a blockage occurs, place a small amount of EDTA lubricant on a fine instrument and introduce into the canal. Use a gentle watch winding motion along with copious irrigation of the canal to remove the dentin chips or tissue debris
- ❑ If this does not solve the problem, endosonics may be used to dislodge the dentin chips by the action of acoustic streaming
- ❑ Whatever happens, do not force the instrument into the blockage as it may further pack the dentinal debris and worsen the condition. Moreover, forcing instruments may cause perforation of the canal.

Prevention

- ❑ Remove all caries, unsupported tooth structure, restorations before completion of access cavity preparation **(Fig. 24.7)**
- ❑ Keep pulp chamber filled with an irrigant during canal preparation
- ❑ There should be a straight line access to the canal apex **(Fig. 24.8)**

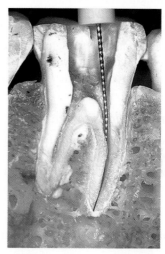

Fig. 24.7 Gain straight line access to canal orifices by removing all caries, restoration and unsupported tooth structure.

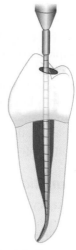

Fig. 24.8 Straight line access to canal apex.

- ❑ Carry out copious irrigation during cleaning and shaping
- ❑ Intracanal instruments must always be wiped clean before reinserting into the canal system
- ❑ Use instruments in sequential order
- ❑ Recapitulate during instrumentation
- ❑ Avoid excessive pressure and rotation of instruments.

Ledge Formation

Ledge is an artificially created deviation of root canal wall which prevents an endodontic instrument to established working length in an otherwise patent canal.

Etiology

- ❑ By forcing straight instruments short of working length in a curved canal **(Fig. 24.9)**
- ❑ Rotating the file at working length causes deviation from the natural canal pathway, straightening of the canal and creation of ledge in dentinal wall **(Fig. 24.10)**
- ❑ Rapid advancement in file sizes or skipping file sizes.

Identification of Ledge Formation

One may get suspicious that ledge has been formed when there is
- ❑ Loss of tactile sensation at the tip of the instrument
- ❑ Loose feeling instead of binding at the apex
- ❑ Instrument can no longer reach its estimated working length
- ❑ When in doubt, take a radiograph with instrument placed in canal.

Treatment

- ❑ To negotiate a ledge, choose a smaller number file, usually No. 10 or 15
- ❑ Give a small bend at tip of the instrument **(Figs. 24.11A and B)** and penetrate the file carefully into the canal
- ❑ Once the tip of the file is apical to ledge, it is moved in and out of the canal utilizing ultrashort push–pull movements with emphasis on staying apical to the defect
- ❑ When file moves freely, it may be turned clockwise upon withdrawal to rasp, reduce, smooth, or eliminate the ledge. When ledge is bypassed, then efforts are directed towards establishing the apical patency with a No. 10 file.

Prevention of Ledge Formation

- ❑ Use of stainless steel patency files to determine canal curvature
- ❑ Accurate evaluation of radiograph and tooth anatomy
- ❑ Precurving the instruments for curved canals
- ❑ Use of flexible NiTi files

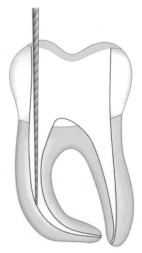

Fig. 24.9 Ledge is formed by forcing uncurved instruments apically short of working length in a curved canal.

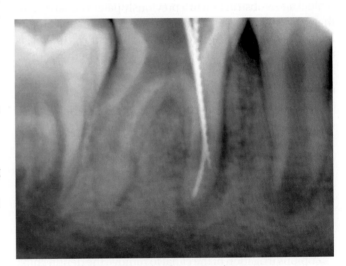

Fig. 24.10 Ledge formation due to use of straight files in curved canal.

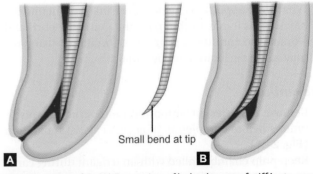

Small bend at tip

Figs. 24.11A and B (A) Formation of ledge by use of stiff instrument in curved canal; (B) Correction of ledge; ledge is bypassed by making a small bend at tip of instrument. Bent instrument is passed along canal wall to locate original canal.

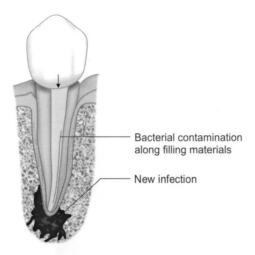

Fig. 24.12 Missed canal leading to root canal failure.

- ❑ Use of safe-ended instruments with noncutting tips
- ❑ Use of sequential filing. Avoid skipping instrument sizes
- ❑ Frequent irrigation and recapitulation during biomechanical preparation.

Missed Canal

Missed canal can contribute to endodontic failure because it holds the tissue debris, bacteria and other irritants **(Fig. 24.12)**. Thus, a tooth should be retreated first conservatively if endodontic failure exists, before going for endodontic surgery procedure.

Etiology

- ❑ Lack of thorough knowledge of root canal anatomy and its variations
- ❑ Inadequate access cavity preparation.

Common Sites for Missed Canals

- ❑ During canal exploration, if canal is not centered in the root, one should look for presence of extracanal
- ❑ There are several teeth which have predisposition for extracanal which might be missed if not explored accurately while treatment. For example,
  - Maxillary premolars may have three canals (mesiobuccal, distobuccal, and palatal) **(Figs. 24.13A to C)**
  - Maxillary first molars usually have four canals
  - Mandibular incisors usually have two canals **(Fig. 24.14)**
  - Mandibular premolars often have complex root anatomy **(Fig. 24.15)**
  - Mandibular molars may have extramesial and/or distal canal in some cases **(Fig. 24.16)**.

Missed canals can be located by
- ❑ Taking radiographs **(Fig. 24.17)**
- ❑ Use of magnifying loupes or endomicroscope
- ❑ Accurate access cavity preparation
- ❑ Use of ultrasonics

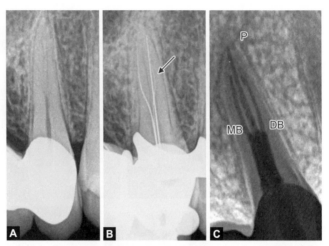

Figs. 24.13A to C Radiograph showing fast break in maxillary first premolar, i.e. one main canal almost becomes untraceable as we go apically: (A) Preoperative radiograph; (B) Working length radiograph; (C) Post obturation radiograph.
Courtesy: Jaydev.

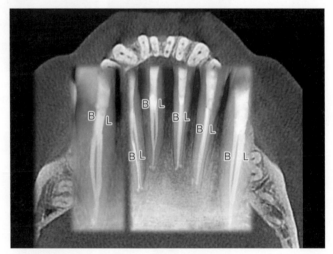

Fig. 24.14 Mandibular anterior teeth showing two canals (one buccal and one lingual in each). Cross section of CBCT showing presence of two canals.

- ❑ Use of dyes such as methylene blue
- ❑ *Use of sodium hypochlorite:* After thorough cleaning and shaping, pulp chamber is filled with sodium hypochlorite. If bubbles appear in, it indicates either there is residual tissue present in a missed canal or residual chelator in the prepared canal. This is called **Champagne test**.

Prevention of Missed Canal

- ❑ Good radiographs taken at different horizontal angulations
- ❑ Good illumination and magnification
- ❑ Adequate access cavity preparation
- ❑ Clinician should always look for an additional canal in every tooth being treated.

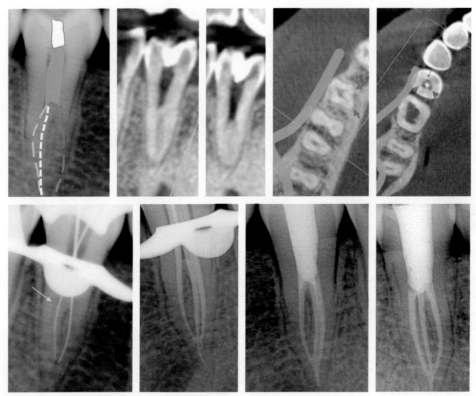

Fig. 24.15 Endodontic treatment of mandibular premolar with split canals. Presence of three canals confirmed with CBCT.
Courtesy: Jaydev.

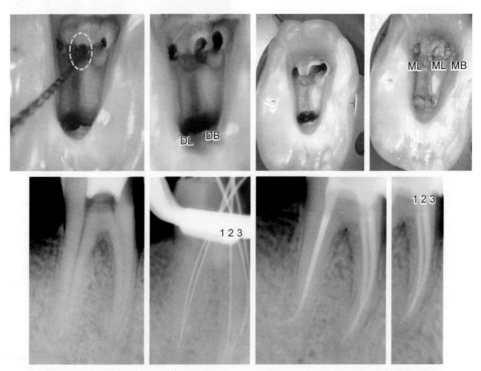

Fig. 24.16 Endodontic treatment of mandibular molar with five canals, i.e. mesiobuccal,
middle mesial, mesiolingual, distobuccal and distolingual.
Courtesy: Jaydev.

Instrument Separation

Instrument seperation is a common and frustrating problem in endodontic treatment which occurs due to improper or overuse of instruments especially while working in curved, narrow, or tortuous canals (**Figs. 24.18A to G**).

Etiology

- ❑ Variation from normal root canal anatomy
- ❑ Overuse of damaged instruments
- ❑ Overuse of dull instruments

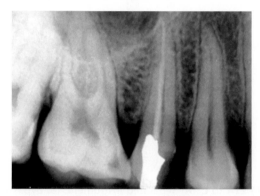

Fig. 24.17 Radiograph showing missed canal in maxillary second premolar.

- ❑ Inadequate irrigation
- ❑ Use of excessive pressure while inserting in canal
- ❑ Improper access cavity preparation.

Management

When an instrument fracture occurs, take a radiograph to evaluate (Figs. 24.19 and 24.20):
- Curvature and length of canal
- Accessibility of instrument
- Location of separated instrument
- Amount of dentin present around the instrument

File Bypass Technique

- ❑ Key to bypass a file is to establish straight line access and patency with No. 6 or 8 file (**Figs. 24.21A to C**)
- ❑ In order to get past the broken instrument fragment, a small sharp bend should be given at the end of the instrument
- ❑ Insert the file slowly and carefully into the canal. When negotiation occurs past the fragment, one will find a catch. Do not remove file at this point. Use small in and out movements along with copious irrigation of canal

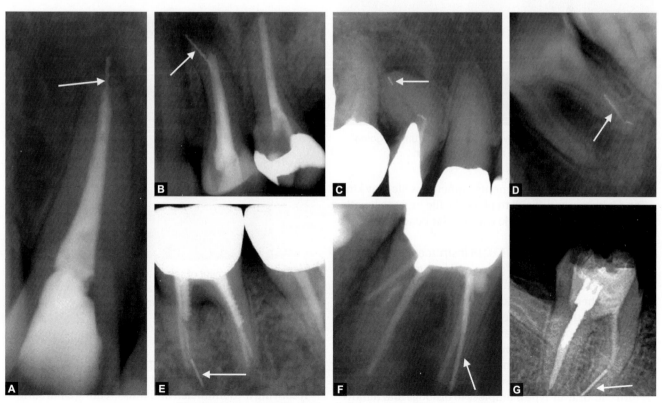

Figs. 24.18A to G Radiographs showing separated instruments.
Courtesy: Yoshitsugu Terauchi

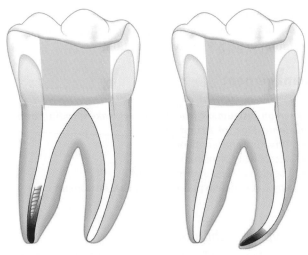

Fig. 24.19 Radiograph helps to see curvature of canal and location of separated instrument.

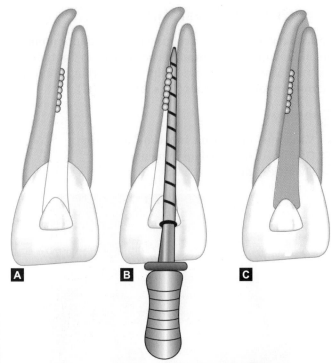

Figs. 24.21A to C (A) Separated instrument; (B) Bypassing the separated instrument; (C) incorporating separated file in final obturation.

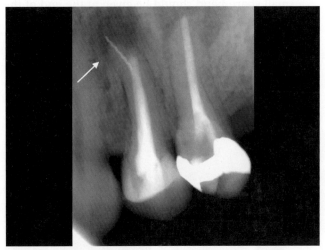

Fig. 24.20 Radiograph showing fractured instrument going beyond apex in maxillary premolar.

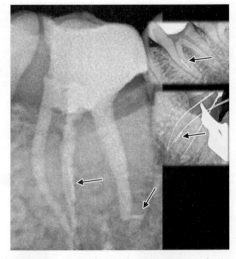

Fig. 24.22 Management of separated instrument by instrument bypass technique and incorporating it in final obturation. *Courtesy:* Jaydev.

❑ While doing these movements, sometimes file may kink and it becomes difficult to place the file to same length. In such cases, use new file with similar bend and repeat the above procedure

❑ Once the patency with a No. 15 instrument is achieved, shift to K reamers. Use "place pull/rotate/withdrawal" movement rather than a filing motion. Every time reamer rotates, there will be a "clicking" sound as the flutes brush up against the file fragment

❑ One must avoid placing an instrument directly on top of the broken file. This can push it deeper resulting in loss of patency. If the file is visible at this point, it is possible to use a small-tipped ultrasonic instrument or one-fourth turn withdrawal-type handpiece to dislodge and remove it. **Figures 24.22** and **24.23** show management of separated instrument by bypass technique and incorporating the separated instrument in final obturation of the canal.

Instrument Retrieval

❑ To remove separated file, expose it first. It can be done by modified Gates-Glidden drills. GG is modified by removing its bottom half and thus creating a flat surface

❑ Perform crown down technique with Gates-Glidden drills. Then use modified Gates-Glidden to enlarge the canal to a point where instrument is located; this way a

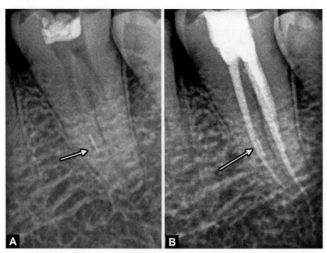

Figs. 24.23 (A) Preoperative radiograph showing separated instrument; (B) Postoperative radiograph showing separated instrument incorporated in final obturation.

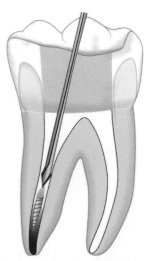

Fig. 24.24 Modified Gates-Glidden modified to form a platform which enables to visualize broken fragment.

platform is created which enables to visualize the broken fragment **(Fig. 24.24)**. It creates a flat area of dentin surrounding the file fragment

❑ Thereafter, a small tipped ultrasonic instrument is used in a counter-clockwise motion to loosen the file **(Fig. 24.25)**

❑ Irrigation combined with ultrasonics can frequently flush the file out.

Special instruments used for retrieval of separated instrument are

❑ Masserann kit
❑ Endoextractor
❑ Instrument removal system
❑ Wire-loop technique
❑ Surgical removal of broken instrument.

Masserann Kit

In Masserann kit, an extractor is present into which the instrument to be retrieved is locked. It has assorted end cutting trepan burs which are large and rigid meant to be used only in coronal portion of straight canals.

Steps for retrieving instruments using Masserann kit

❑ Enlarge the canal orifice using a round bur
❑ Gain a straight line access to fractured instrument using Gates-Glidden drills
❑ Move end cutting trepan burs slowly in anticlockwise direction so as to free 4 mm of the fragment. These burs can be used by hand or with reduction gear contra-angle handpiece at the speed of 300–600 rpm
❑ Take extractor and slide it over free end of the fragment
❑ Firmly hold the extractor in place and rotate the screw head until the fragment is gripped
❑ Once gripped tightly, move extractor in anticlockwise direction for removal of all cutting root canal instruments and in clockwise direction for removing instrument.

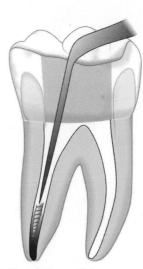

Fig. 24.25 Use of ultrasonic instrument to remove fractured instrument.

Use of Endoextractor

In endoextractor, cyanoacrylate adhesive is placed on it so as to lock the object into the extractor. Technique for removal is the same as that for Masserann extractor.

Instrument Removal System (Fig. 24.26)

Instrument removal system consists of different size of microtubes and insert wedge which fit into separated instrument. Microtube has 45° beveled end and a handle.

Technique of using IRS (Figs. 24.27A to E)

❑ Gain straight line access to the canal
❑ Select a microtube and insert it into the canal
❑ After this guide, the head of the separated instruments into the lumen of the microtube

- Place an insert wedge through the open end of microtube till it comes in contact with separated instrument
- Turn the insert wedge clockwise to engage the instrument

- Finally move the microtube out of canal to retrieve the separated instrument.

Wire Loop Technique

It consists of burs, ultrasonic tips, and loop device for removal of broken instrument (**Fig. 24.28**).

Before removal of fractured instrument, the canal should be enlarged and so as to gain straight line access and exposure of the instrument. For this Gates-Glidden drills or greater taper files can be used.

Once the file is exposed, remove it using loop device (**Figs. 24.29A to C**).

Surgical Management for Removal of Separated Instrument

It is indicated when
- Broken file is behind the curve
- File fragment is not visible because of the curved root
- Instrument is in the apical part of the canal and is difficult to retrieve (**Figs. 24.30A to C**)
- Much of the dentin has to be removed to allow file removal.

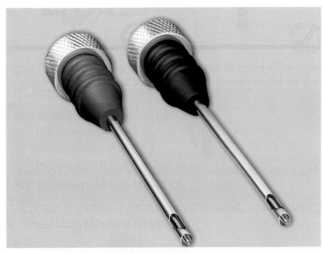

Fig. 24.26 Microtubes of instrument removal system.

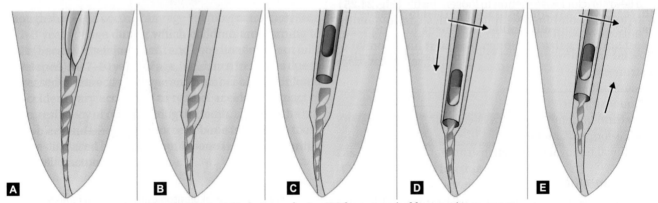

Figs. 24.27A to E Technique of using IRS for removal of fractured instrument.

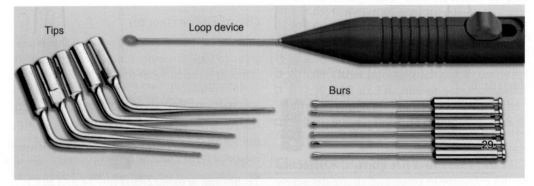

Fig. 24.28 Components of wire loop instrument removal system
Courtesy: Yoshitsugu Terauchi

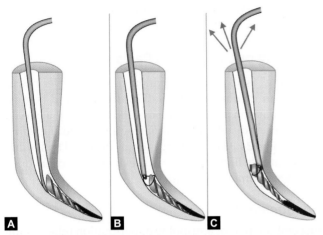

Figs. 24.29A to C (A) Straight line access to the fractured instrument; (B) Use of loop to remove the instrument; (C) Removal of instrument.

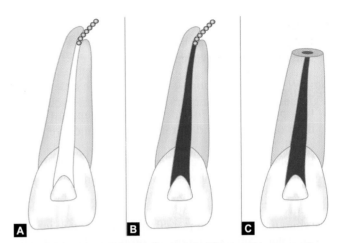

Figs. 24.30A to C Surgical removal of fractured instrument.

Prognosis

Prognosis of separated instrument depends upon the following factors:
- Timing of separation
- Status of pulp tissue
- Position of separated instrument
- Ability to retrieve or by pass the instrument.

Separated instrument are not the prime cause of endodontic failure but they impede mechanical instrumentation of the canal, which may cause endodontic failure. Studies have shown that if instrument separates at later stages of instrumentation and close to apex, prognosis is better than if it separates in undebrided canals, short of the apex, or beyond apical foramen.

Prevention

- Examine each instrument before placing it into the canal. Always discard the instrument when there is
  - Bending of instruments
  - Corrosion of instrument
  - Unwinding of flutes
  - Excessive heating of instrument
  - Dulling of the instrument
- Instead of using carbon steel, use stainless steel files
- Use smaller size of instruments only once
- Always use instruments in sequential order
- Never force the instrument into canal
- Canals should be copiously irrigated during cleaning and shaping procedure
- Never use instruments in dry canals
- Always clean the instrument before placing it into the canal. Debris collected between the flutes retard the

cutting efficiency and increase the frictional torque between the instrument and canal wall
- Do not give excessive rotation to instrument while working with it.

Deviation from Normal Canal Anatomy

Zipping

Zipping is defined as transposition of the apical portion of the canal due to improper shaping technique **(Fig. 24.31)**. Terms given to describe this shape are "hour glass shape," "foraminal rip," or "tear drop shape."

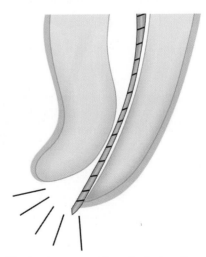

Fig. 24.31 Zipping is transposition of apical portion of the canal.

Etiology

❑ Failure to precurve the files
❑ Forcing instruments in curved canal.

Features

❑ In zipping, apical foramen tends to become a tear drop or elliptical and is transported from curve of the canal
❑ File placed in curved canal cuts more on the outer portion of the canal wall at its apical extent and inner most portion of the canal wall at the coronal third causing an uneven reduction of the dentin
❑ When a file is rotated in a curved canal a biomechanical defect, "elbow" is formed coronal to the elliptically shaped apical seat. This is the narrowest portion of the canal (**Fig. 24.32**)
❑ In many cases, the obturating material terminates at the elbow leaving an unfilled zipped canal apical to elbow. This is the common occurrence with laterally compacted gutta-percha technique. Use of vertical compaction of warm gutta-percha or thermoplasticized gutta-percha is ideal in these cases to compact a solid core material into the apical preparation without using excessive amount of sealer.

Prevention

❑ Use of precurved files
❑ Use of incremental filing technique
❑ Use of flexible files
❑ Remove flutes of file at certain areas, for example, file portion which makes contact with outer dentinal wall at the apex and portion which makes contact with inner dentinal wall especially in the mid-root area

❑ By over curving in apical part of the file, especially when working for severely curved canals.

Stripping or Lateral Wall Perforation

"Stripping" is a lateral perforation caused by overinstrumentation through a thin wall in the root and is most likely to happen on the inside or concave wall of a curved canal such as distal wall of mesial roots in mandibular first molars (**Fig. 24.33**). Stripping is easily detected by sudden appearance of hemorrhage in a previously dry canal or by a sudden complaint by patient.

Management

Successful repair of a stripping or perforation relies on the adequacy of the seal established by repair material.

Access to mid-root perforation is most often difficult and repair is not predictable. Mineral trioxide aggregate (MTA) or calcium hydroxide can be used as a biological barrier against which obturating material is packed.

Prevention

❑ Use of precurved files for curved canals
❑ Use of modified files for curved canals. A file can be modified by removing flutes of file at certain areas, for example, file portion which makes contact with outer dentinal wall at the apex and portion which makes contact with inner dentinal wall especially in the mid-root area (**Fig. 24.33**)
❑ Using anticurvature filing, that is, more filing pressure is placed on tooth structure away from the direction of root curvature and away from the invagination, thereby preventing root thinning and perforation of the root structure (**Fig. 24.34**).

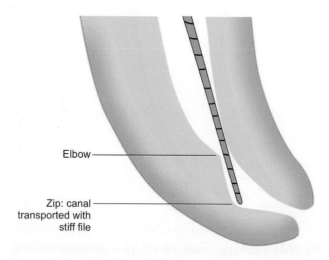

Fig. 24.32 Elbow formed in a curved canal.

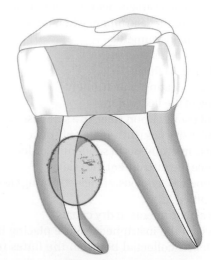

Fig. 24.33 Strip perforation occurs more commonly on inner side of curve.

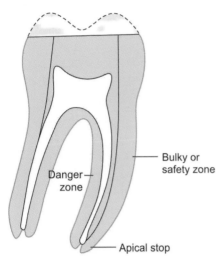

Fig. 24.34 Schematic representation of danger zone in curved canal. In anticurvature filing, more pressure is applied in the area away from the curvature to avoid strip perforation.

Elbow

It is the narrowest portion of the zipped canal. It is usually formed in middle of the curve in canal with 30° curvature. This type of preparation results in insufficient taper and flow which further makes cleaning, shaping, and obturation difficult (*see* **Fig. 24.32**).

Canal Transportation

"Apical canal transportation is moving the position of canal's normal anatomic foramen to a new location on external root surface" (**Figs. 24.35A to C**).

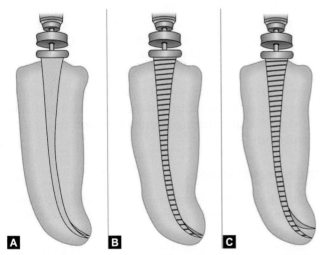

Figs. 24.35A to C Type I, II and III canal transportation: (A) Minor movement of apical foramen (Type I); (B) Moderate movement of apical foramen (Type II); (C) Severe movement of apical foramen (Type III).

Classification

Type I: It is minor movement of physiologic foramen. In such cases, if sufficient residual dentin can be maintained, one can try to create positive apical canal architecture to improve the prognosis of the tooth (**Fig. 24.35A**).

Type II: Apical transportations of Type II show moderate movement of the physiologic foramen to a new location (**Fig. 24.35B**). Such cases compromise the prognosis and are difficult to treat. Biocompatible materials like MTA can be used to provide barrier against which obturation material can be packed.

Type III: Apical transportation of Type III shows severe movement of physiological foramen (**Fig. 24.35C**). In Type III prognosis is poorest when compared to Type I and Type II. A three-dimensional obturation is difficult in this case. This requires surgical intervention for correction, otherwise tooth is indicated for extraction.

▌Inadequate Canal Preparation

Overinstrumentation

- ❑ Excessive instrumentation beyond the apical constriction violates the periodontal ligament and alveolar bone
- ❑ Loss of apical constriction creates an open apex with an increased risk of overfilling, lack of an adequate apical seal (**Fig. 24.36**), pain and discomfort for the patient
- ❑ Overinstrumentation is recognized when hemorrhage is evident in the apical portion of canal with or without patient discomfort (**Fig. 24.37A**) and when tactile resistance of the boundaries of canal space is lost. It can be confirmed by taking a radiograph and inserting paper point in the canal (**Fig. 24.37B**).

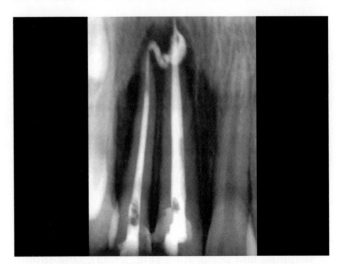

Fig. 24.36 Overfilling of the canal causing irritation to periapical area.

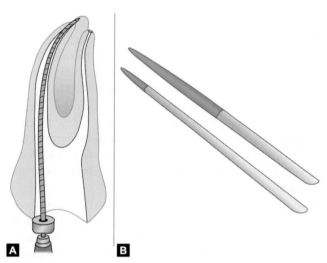

Figs. 24.37A and B (A) Excessive instrumentation; (B) Paper point showing hemorrhage at the tip.

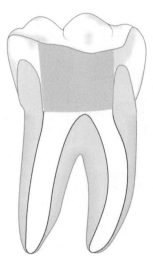

Fig. 24.38 Overpreparation of canal causes excessive removal of root dentin.

Treatment

- Re-establish the working length and carefully obturate the canal so as to prevent extrusion of the filling beyond apex
- Another technique to prevent overextrusion of the filling is developing an apical barrier. Materials used for this include dentin chips, calcium hydroxide powder, hydroxyapatite (HA) and MTA.

Prevention

- Using good radiographic techniques
- Accurately determining the apical constriction of the root canal
- Using sound reference points
- Using stable instrument stops
- Maintaining all instruments within the confines of the canal system
- Occlusal alterations before determination of the working length
- Intermittent radiographic confirmation of the working length
- Confirming the integrity of the apical stop with paper points.

Overpreparation

- Overpreparation is excessive removal of tooth structure in mesiodistal and buccolingual direction **(Fig. 24.38)**
- During biomechanical preparation of the canal, size of apical preparation should correspond to size, shape, and curvature of the root
- Excessive canal flaring increases the chances of stripping and perforation **(Fig. 24.39)**. One should

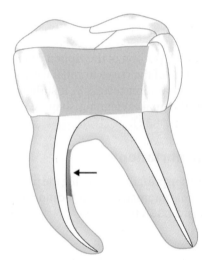

Fig. 24.39 Overpreparation increases the chances of strip perforation (arrow) especially on inner side of a curved canal.

avoid excessive removal of tooth structure because overprepared canals are potentially weaker and subject to fracture during compaction and restorative procedures.

Underpreparation

- Underpreparation is the failure to remove pulp tissue, dentinal debris, and microorganisms from the root canal system
- Sometimes, canal system is inadequately shaped which prevents three-dimensional obturation of the root canal space **(Fig. 24.40)**.

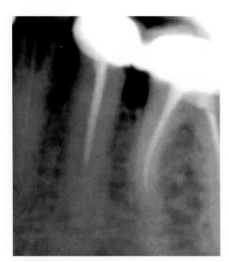

Fig. 24.40 Inadequately shaped canal prevents three-dimensional obturation of root canals.

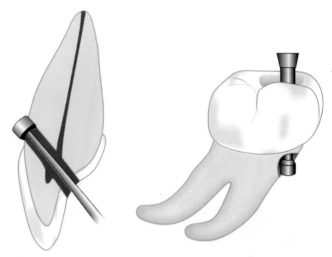

Fig. 24.41 Perforation caused during access cavity preparation.

Etiology

- Insufficient preparation of the apical dentin matrix
- Insufficient use of irrigants to dissolve tissues and debris
- Inadequate canal shaping, which prevents depth of spreader or plugger penetration during compaction
- Establishing the working length short of the apical constriction
- Creation of ledges and blockages that prevent complete cleaning and shaping.

Prevention

- Underprepared canals are best managed by strictly following the principles of working length determination and biomechanical preparation
- Copious irrigation and recapitulation during instrumentation ensure a properly cleaned canal.

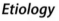 Perforation

According to glossary of endodontic terms (by AAE), *perforation is defined as "the mechanical or pathological communication between root canal system and the external tooth surface."* It can be cervical, mid-root, or apical levels depending upon site of the perforation.

Coronal perforation occurs during access cavity preparation **(Fig. 24.41)**. If the perforation is above the periodontal attachment, leakage of saliva into cavity or sodium hypochlorite in mouth is the main sign. But if perforation occurs into the periodontal ligament, bleeding is the hallmark feature.

Root canal perforation can occur at three levels:
1. *Cervical canal perforation:* It commonly occurs while locating the canal orifice and flaring of the coronal third

of the root canal. Sudden appearance of blood from canal is the first sign of perforation
2. *Mid-root perforation:* It commonly occurs due to over-instrumentation and over-preparation of thin wall of root or concave side of the curved canals. Sudden appearance of bleeding is the pathognomonic feature
3. *Apical root perforation:* It occurs if when instrument goes beyond the confines of the root canal and by overuse of chelating agents along with straight and stiffer large-sized instruments to negotiate ledge, canal blockage, or zipping, etc. **(Figs. 24.42A and B)**.

Management

Occurrence of a perforation can be recognized by:
- Placing an instrument into the opening and taking a radiograph
- Using paper point
- Sudden appearance of bleeding
- Complain of pain by patient when instrument touches periodontal tissue.

Factors Affecting Prognosis of Perforation Repair

- **Location:** If perforation is located at alveolar crest or coronal to it, prognosis is poor because of epithelial migration and periodontal pocket formation. Perforation in the furcation area has a poor prognosis. Perforation occurring in mid-root and apical part of root does not have communication with oral cavity and thus has good prognosis
- **Size**: A smaller perforation has less tissue destruction and inflammation, thus having better prognosis than larger sized perforation

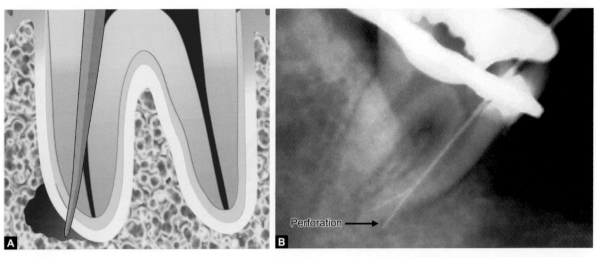

Figs. 24.42A and B (A) Perforation caused by use of stiff instruments in a curved canal; (B) Perforation of mesial root of mandibular second molar.

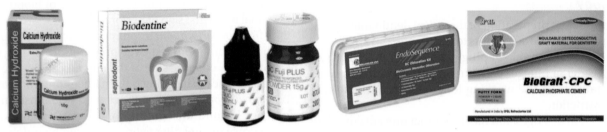

Fig. 24.43 Photograph showing materials used for perforation repair.

- *Visibility and accessibility* also affects the perforation repair
- *Time* Perforation should be repaired as soon as possible to discourage further loss of attachment and prevent sulcular breakdown
- *Associated periodontal condition*: If attachment apparatus is intact without pocket formation, nonsurgical repair is recommended, whereas in the case of loss of attachment, surgical treatment should be planned
- *Esthetics* influence the perforation repair and material to be used for repair of the perforation.

Materials Used for Perforation Repair (Fig. 24.43)

An ideal material for perforation repair should
- Adhere to preparation walls of the cavity and seal the root canal system.
- Be nontoxic
- Be easy to handle
- Be radiopaque
- Be dimensionally stable
- Be well tolerated by periradicular tissue
- Be nonabsorbable
- Not corrode
- Not to be affected by moisture
- Not stain periradicular tissues

Indium foil: It was used as a perforation repair material but it has shown greater bone resorption as compared to other materials.

Zinc oxide eugenol (ZOE): Studies have shown that ZOE can cause severe inflammatory reactions and resorption of alveolar crest when used for perforation repair.

Intermediate restorative material (IRM): It is reinforced ZOE cement. If used without an internal matrix, it shows leakage, so it should be used only with matrix.

Cavit: It produces superior seal when compared to ZOE cement, zinc phosphate cement, and amalgam.

Glass ionomer cement: It shows greater sealing potential than ZOE, zinc phosphate cement, and amalgam due to its adhesion property.

Amalgam: It has been used since ages but produces inflammatory changes.

Plaster of Paris: It is biocompatible with rate of resorption equaling the rate of new bone growing into the tissue. It has been used as a bone substitute for filling defects.

Calcium hydroxide: It consists of a base paste and catalyst paste. It is a biocompatible material which has shown positive results.

Dentin chips: These are used as matrix in repair of perforation defects.

Hydroxyapatite (HA): It is used as an internal matrix and for perforation repair material.

Decalcified freeze–dried bone: These chips are biocompatible, inexpensive, easy to obtain, easy to use and degradable during the repair process and acts as an excellent barrier against which filling material could be placed. When packed into the bony defect, it mixes with the blood and fuses together into a solid mass and fills the defect.

Calcium phosphate cement: It is a mixture of two calcium phosphate compounds; one is acidic [dicalcium phosphate dehydrate or anhydrous dicalcium phosphate and other is basic (tetracalcium phosphate)]. When mixed with water, HA is formed as end product. It is biocompatible and is replaced by bone via osteoconduction and simultaneous cement absorption.

Portland cement: It consists of tricalcium silicate, dicalcium silicate, tricalcium aluminate, tetracalcium alumino ferrate, and hydrated calcium sulfate. It induces bone and cementum formation but does not provide a fluid tight seal.

Mineral trioxide aggregate (MTA): It is a osseoconductive, inductive, and biocompatible material which was introduced by Dr. Torabinejad in 1993. It is available as gray and white MTA. It mainly consists of Portland cement (75%), bismuth oxide 20%, and gypsum. MTA has advantages of being hygroscopic so requires moisture for setting, biocompatible, radiopaque, with excellent sealing ability. Problems with MTA include are difficult handling characteristics due to sandy nature, long setting time, and discoloration by grey MTA.

Biodentine: It is a calcium silicate-based bioactive material. It is easy to handle and manipulate. High-alkaline pH and its biocompatibility make it the material of choice for perforation repair.

Bioaggregate: It is a bioceramic material composed of tricalcium silicate, dicalcium silicate, calcium phosphate monobasic, amorphous silicon dioxide, and tantalumpent oxide. It induces mineralized tissue formation and precipitation of apatite crystals that become larger with increasing immersion time.

EndoSequence: It is a bioceramic material consisting of calcium silicates, zirconium oxide, calcium phosphate monobasic, and filler agents. It is produced with nanosphere particles that allow the material to enter into the dentinal tubules and interact with the moisture present in the dentin. This creates a mechanical bond on setting and provides dimensional stability, biocompatibility due to its high pH. It simulates tissue fluid, phosphate buffered saline resulting in precipitation of apatite crystals that become larger with increasing immersion times due to its being bioactive.

Management of the Coronal Third Perforations

❑ Anterior teeth where esthetics is the main concern, calcium sulfate barrier along with composites, glass ionomer cements and white MTA can be used for perforations repair
❑ Posterior teeth where esthetics is not the main criteria, super EBA, amalgam, MTA can be tried **(Figs. 24.44 to 24.47)**.

Management of Perforation in Mid-Root Level

In these cases, success of perforation repair depends on hemostasis, accessibility, visibility, and selection of material for repair.

If the defect is small and hemostasis can be achieved, perforation can be sealed and repaired during three dimensional obturation of the root canal. But in case the perforation defect is large and moisture control is difficult, then one should prepare the canal before going for perforation repair.

Lemon in 1992 gave the internal matrix concept for the repair of inaccessible strip perforations using microsurgical technique. Rationale behind this concept was that a matrix (HA) controls the material and prevents overfilling of repair material into the periradicular tissues. Material to be used as matrix should be biocompatible and able to stimulate osteogenesis.

Technique of placement of matrix (Figs. 24.48A to C)

❑ Attain the hemostasis and place file, silver cones, or gutta-percha point in the canals to maintain their patency
❑ HA particles are wetted with saline to make a clump, then placed into perforation and condensed with pluggers
❑ Excess material is removed with excavator to the level of periodontal ligament
❑ After that, a bur is used to prepare the perforation site to receive the material. Using a flat instrument, apply restorative material like amalgam or GIC to repair the perforation.

Management of Perforation in Apical Third of the Root Canal

These types of perforations can be repaired both surgically as well as nonsurgically. But one should attempt nonsurgical repair before going for surgery. MTA is a choice of material for perforation repair.

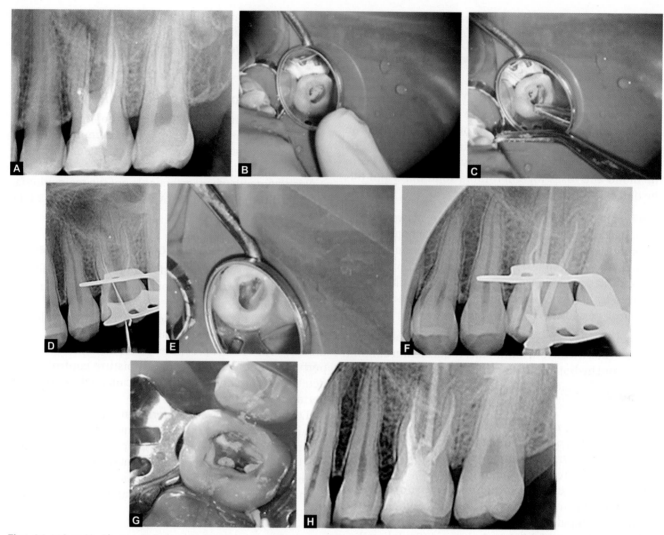

Figs. 24.44A to H: Photographs A to H showing management of perforation with MTA and gutta percha: (A) Preoperative radiograph showing gutta-percha in furcation area but not in mesial root; (B) Photograph showing gutta-percha in perforation site; (C) Removal of gutta-percha from perforation site; (D) Negotiating MB1 and MB2 canals; (E) Photograph showing 4th canal; (F) Master cone radiograph; (G) Obturation with MTA in mesiobuccal canal; (H) Post operative radiograph.
Courtesy: Viresh.

Technique

❑ Dry the root canal with paper points and isolate the perforation site
❑ Prepare the MTA material and condense it into perforation site using pluggers or paper points
❑ During MTA placement, file is placed into the canal to maintain its patency and moved up and down till MTA sets. It is done to avoid file getting frozen in MTA. Place the temporary restoration to seal chamber. In next appointment, obturation is done.

Precautions to Prevent Perforation

❑ Evaluate the anatomy of the tooth before starting endodontic therapy
❑ Use smaller, flexible files for curved canals
❑ Do not skip the file sizes
❑ Recapitulate with smaller files between sizes
❑ Confirm the working length and maintain instruments within confines of the working length
❑ Use anticurvature filling technique in curved canals to selectively remove the dentin

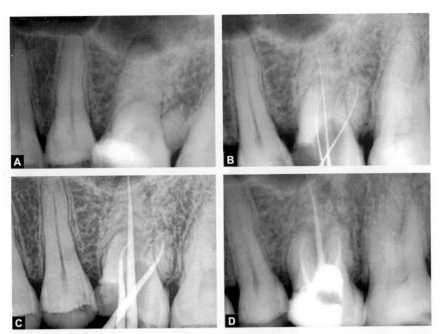

Figs. 24.45A to D Perforation management in maxillary right first molar using MTA: (A) Preoperative radiograph; (B) Working length determination; (C) Master cone; (D) Postobturation using MTA as sealer and perforation repair.
Courtesy: Anil Dhingra.

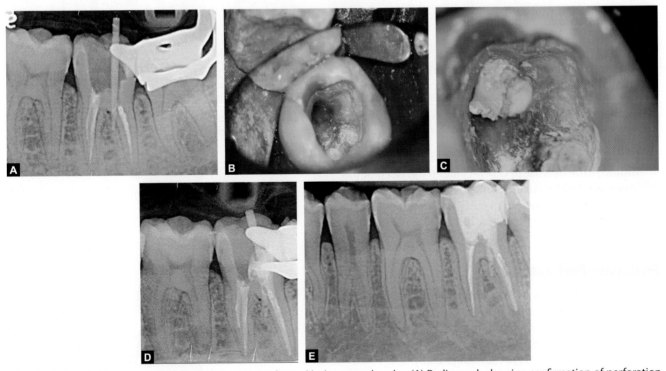

Figs. 24.46A to E Management of perforation repair of mandibular second molar: (A) Radiograph showing confirmation of perforation using gutta-percha; (B) Obturation of mesial canals; (C) Coronal part of distal canal sealed with gutta-percha to avoid MTA blocking the canal. MTA placed at perforation site; (D) Distal master cone radiograph after MTA placement at perforation site; (E) Postobturation radiograph.

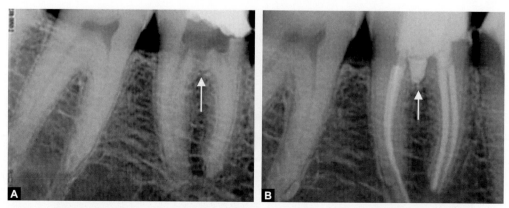

Figs. 24.47A and B Perforation repair of mandibular first molar using MTA: (A) Preoperative radiograph; (B) Postoperative radiograph.

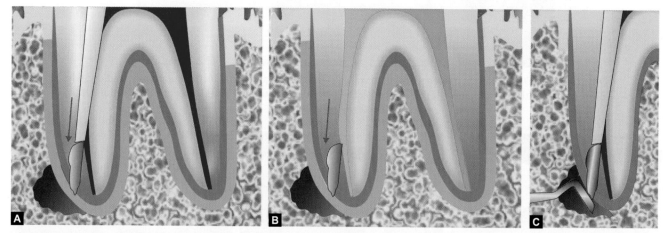

Figs. 24.48A to C (A) Hydroxyapatite crystals are packed and condensed in perforation using pluggers; (B) Complete packing of HA crystals in canal with perforation; (C) A flat instrument is used to pack the restorative material outside the tooth at the site of defect.

❑ Minimize the overuse of Gates-Glidden too deep or too large especially in curved canals
❑ Avoid overuse of chelating agents, larger stiff files in an attempt to negotiate procedural errors like ledges, canal blockages, etc.

Postspace Perforation

Iatrogenic perforations during postspace preparations are usually caused by poor clinical judgment and improper orientation of the postpreparation drills **(Figs. 24.49 and 24.50)**. Perforation can be recognized by sudden appearance of blood in the canal or radiographically.

Treatment of postspace perforation involves the same principles as for repair of other perforations. Materials like dental amalgam, calcium hydroxide, glass ionomer, composite resins, freeze–dried bone and tricalcium phosphate are used to repair the perforation.

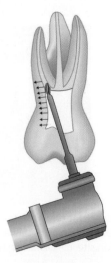

Fig. 24.49 Postspace perforation caused by misdirection of postpreparing drills.

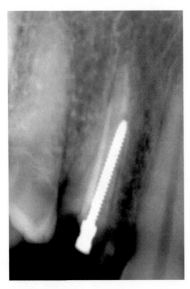

Fig. 24.50 Improper postplacement due to improper direction of drill.

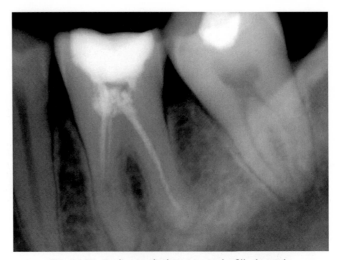

Fig. 24.51 Radiograph showing underfilled canals.

Prevention

- Evaluate the root anatomy and its variations
- Avoid excessive use of Gates-Glidden or Peeso reamers to cut the dentin.

▌Obturation Related

Underfilling/Incompletely Filled Root Canals

Underfilling is obturation of root canal >2 mm short of radiographic apex (**Fig. 24.51**).

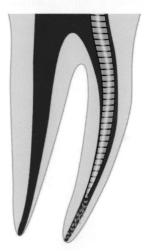

Fig. 24.52 Accumulation of dentin chips and tissue debris resulting in incomplete instrumentation.

Etiology

- Inaccurate working length determination
- Inadequate irrigation and recapitulation during biomechanical preparation which can lead to accumulation of dentin chips and tissue debris and thus canal blockage (**Fig. 24.52**)
- Presence of ledge

Significance (Figs. 24.53 and 24.54)

Inadequate removal of infected necrotic tissue in the apical portion of root canal results in persistent bacterial infection and thus initiation or perpetuation of existing periapical pathosis (**Fig. 24.55**).

Prevention of Underfilling

- Obtaining straight line access to apex
- Precurving the files before using in curved canals
- Copious irrigation and recapitulation of the canal
- Attaining apical patency
- Using the files in sequential manner.

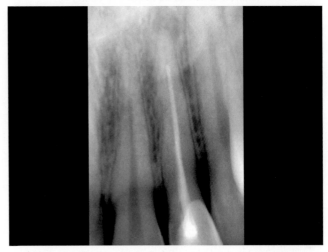

Fig. 24.53 Radiograph showing incomplete obturation (short of the apex).

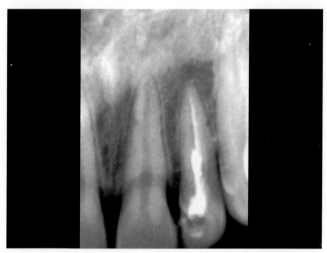

Fig. 24.54 Radiograph showing inadequate obturation and periapical radiolucency in relation to left maxillary lateral incisor

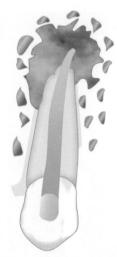

Fig. 24.56 Overfilling of canal causes irritation of periapical tissues.

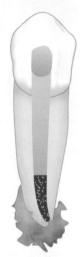

Fig. 24.55 Persistent bacterial infection in root canal with filling short of apex causes treatment failure.

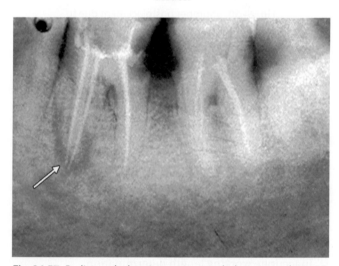

Fig. 24.57 Radiograph showing over-extended gutta-percha in 36.

Overfilling of the Root Canals

Overfilling of the root canals is filling >2 mm beyond the radiographic apex **(Fig. 24.56)**.

Etiology

- Overinstrumentation of the root canal
- Inadequate determination of working length
- Incompletely formed root apex
- Inflammatory apical root resorption
- Improper use of reference points for measuring working length.

Significance

- Overinstrumentation often precedes overfilling which inevitably poses risk of forcing infected root canal

contents into the periradicular tissues, thereby impairing the healing process **(Fig. 24.57)**
- Overfilling may cause foreign giant call reaction and may act as a foreign body which may support the formation of biofilms.

▌Vertical Root Fracture

Vertical root fracture can occur at any phase of root canal treatment. It results from wedging forces within the canal. These excessive forces exceed the binding strength of existing dentin causing fatigue and fracture **(Fig. 24.58)**.

Clinical Features

- It commonly occurs in faciolingual plane
- Sudden crunching sound accompanied by pain is the pathognomonic of root fracture

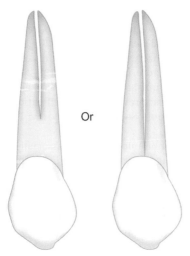

Fig. 24.58 Vertical root fracture.

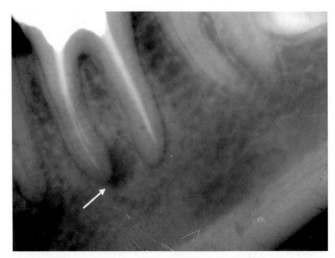

Fig. 24.59 Radiograph showing J-shaped radiolucency around mesial root of mandibular molar with vertical root fracture.

□ Fracture begins along the canal wall and grows outwards to the root surface
□ Certain root shapes and sizes are more susceptible to vertical root fracture, for example roots which are deep facially and lingually but narrow mesially and distally
□ Susceptibility of root fracture increases by excessive dentin removal during canal preparation and excessive condensation forces during compaction of gutta-percha
□ Radiographically vertical root fracture may vary from no significant changes to extensive resorption patterns. In chronic cases, they may show hanging drop radiolucent appearance. According to Cohen, it can be seen radiographically as "J" shaped radiolucency or may appear as a halo-shaped defect around the involved root **(Fig. 24.59)**.

Treatment of vertical root fracture involves extraction in most of the cases. In multirooted teeth root resection or hemisection can be tried.

Prevention of Root Fracture

Main *principles* to prevent root fracture are to
□ Avoid weakening of the canal wall
□ Minimize the internal wedging forces.
To avoid occurrence of vertical root fracture:
□ Avoid over preparation of the canal
□ Use less tapered and more flexible compacting instruments to control condensation forces while obturation
□ Posts should not be used unless they are necessary to retain a tooth.

▌Instrument Aspiration

Aspiration of instruments can occur during endodontic therapy if accidentally dropped in the mouth. It occurs especially if rubber dam is not applied. High-volume suction

tips, hemostats, or cotton pliers can be helpful only in some cases, when the objects are readily accessible in throat, otherwise medical care is needed. Patient must be provided medical care for examination which includes radiograph of chest and abdomen.

This accident can be prevented by using rubber dam and tying up the rubber dam clamp or endodontic instrument with floss.

▌Conclusion

Endodontic treatment presents a great challenge to a clinician owing to difficult and variable root canal anatomy. Endodontic mishap can occur at any stage of the treatment which can be avoided with thorough knowledge of complications, variations in root canal anatomy, good clinical skills and excellent training. The advent of magnification and contemporary instruments decreases the frequency of procedural accidents. Our ethical obligation towards the patient is met if we can provide treatment to prevent the loss of the tooth.

▌Questions

1. Classify different procedural accidents. Write in detail about instrument separation.
2. Define perforation. How will you manage a case of mid-root perforation?
3. Discuss the sequelae and the treatment of a defective root canal filling.
4. Write short notes on:
   • Ledging
   • Perforation repair
   • Instrument separation
   • Zipping

- Canal transportation
- Failures in endodontically restored tooth
- Rotary instruments used in retreatodontics
- Criteria used for evaluation of endodontic treatment
- Local factors responsible for endodontic failures
- Systemic factors responsible for endodontic failures
- Silver point retrieval
- Gutta-percha retrieval
- Success and failures in endodontics

Bibliography

1. Bahcall JK, Carp S, Miner M, Skidmore L. The causes, prevention, and clinical management of broken endodontic rotary files. Dent Today. 2005;24(11):74, 76.
2. Cohen S, Burns RC. Pathways of the pulp. 8th edition. St Louis, MO: Mosby; 2002. p. 94, 242–52, 530, 870, 910–6.
3. Cohen SJ, Glassman G, Mounce R. Rips, strips and broken tips: handling the endodontic mishap. Part I: The separated instrument. Oral Health 2005. pp.10–20.
4. Di Fiore P. A dozen ways to prevent nickel-titanium rotary instrument fracture. JADA 2007;138:196–201.
5. Gutmann JL, Dumsha TC, Lovdahl PE, et al. Problem solving in endodontics: prevention, identification and management. 3rd edition. St Louis, MO: Mosby; 1997. pp. 96–100, 117.
6. Kapalas A, Lambrianidis T. Factors associated with root canal ledging during instrumentation. Endod Dent Traumatol 2000;16:229–31.
7. Walton RE, Torabinejad M. Principles and practice of endodontics. 3rd edition. Philadelphia, PA: WB Saunders; 2002. p. 184, 222–223, 319–320.
8. West JD. Cleaning and shaping the root canal system. In: Cohen S, Burns RC (editors). Pathways of the pulp. 7th edition. St Louis, MO: Mosby; 1998. p. 242.

Surgical Endodontics

Introduction

Root canal treatment has more than 95% of success rate but it fails if infection remains within the root canal. To treat endodontic failure, one should attempt nonsurgical endodontic retreatment but if it is not possible, then endodontic surgery is performed to save the tooth. After case evaluation, surgical success mainly depends on careful management of hard and soft tissues, complete removal of pathognomic tissues and final sealing of root canal. To check the success of surgical procedure, a radiograph should be exposed following treatment for comparison with future radiographs to assess healing.

Definition

Endodontic surgery is defined as *"removal of tissues other than the contents of root canal to retain a tooth with pulpal or periapical involvement."* Surgical intervention is required for cases where retreatment has failed or is not an option and the tooth is to be retained rather than extracted.

First case of endodontic surgery was performed by *Abulcasis* in the *11th century*. A root-end resection procedure to manage a tooth with a necrotic pulp and an alveolar abscess was documented in 1871 and root-end resection with retrograde cavity preparation and filling with amalgam in the 1890s. Endodontic surgery was often considered as an alternative to root canal treatment and indications for surgery were proposed first in the 1930s. Over past decade, periradicular surgery has continued to evolve into a precise, biologically based adjunct to nonsurgical root canal therapy.

Rationale

Rationale of surgical endodontics is to remove the diseased tissue present in canal and around the apex and retrofill the root canal space with biologically inert material so as to achieve a fluid tight seal.

Objectives

- Removal of diseased periapical tissue like granuloma, cyst, overfilled material, etc.
- Root inspection for knowing etiology of endodontic failure, fracture, accessory canals, etc.
- To provide fluid tight seal at apical end by retrograde preparation and obturation

❑ To eliminate apical ramifications by root resections so as to completely remove the cause of failure for endodontic treatment.

Indications

❑ Need for surgical drainage
❑ Failed nonsurgical treatment:
  • Irretrievable root canal filling material
  • Irretrievable intraradicular post
  • Continuous postoperative discomfort
  • Recurring exacerbations of nonsurgical endodontic treatment
❑ Calcific metamorphosis of the pulp space
❑ Horizontal fracture at the root tip with associated periapical disease
❑ Procedural errors:
  • Instrument separation
  • Non-negotiable ledging
  • Root perforation
  • Severe apical transportations
  • Symptomatic over filling
❑ Anatomic variations
  • Root dilacerations
  • Apical root fenestrations
  • Non-negotiable root curvatures
❑ Biopsy
❑ Corrective surgery
  • Root resorptive defects
  • Root caries
  • Root resection
  • Hemisection
  • Bicuspidization
❑ Replacement surgery
  • Intentional replantation
  • Post-traumatic replantation
❑ Implant surgery
  • Endodontic implants
  • Osseointegrated implants.
❑ Exploratory surgery.

Contraindications

❑ *Periodontal health of the tooth:* Tooth mobility and periodontal pockets are two main factors affecting the treatment plan
❑ *Patients health considerations:*
  • Leukemia or neutropenia in active state leading to more chances of infection after surgery and impaired healing
  • *Uncontrolled diabetes mellitus:* Defective leukocyte function, defective wound healing commonly occurs in severe diabetic patients
  • Recent serious cardiac or cancer surgery
  • *Very old patients:* Old age is usually associated with complications like cardiovascular or pulmonary

disorders, decreased kidney functions and liver functions
  • Uncontrolled hypertension
  • Uncontrolled bleeding disorders
  • Immunocompromised patients
  • Recent myocardial infarction or patient taking anticoagulants
  • Patients who have undergone radiation treatment of face because in such cases incidence of osteoradionecrosis and impaired healing is high
  • *Patient in first trimester of pregnancy:* It is during this period, the fetus is susceptible to insult, injury and environmental influences that may result in postpartum disorders
❑ *Patient's mental or psychological status:*
  • Patient does not desire surgery
  • Very apprehensive patient
  • Patient unable to handle stress for long complicated procedures
❑ *Surgeon's skill and ability:* Clinician must be completely honest about their surgical skill and knowledge. Beyond their abilities, case must be referred to endodontist or oral surgeon
❑ Anatomic considerations such as in mandibular second molar area:
  • Roots are inclined lingually
  • Root apices are much closer to mandibular canal
  • Presence of too thick buccal plate
  • Restricted access to the root tip
❑ Short root length in which removal of root apex further compromises the prognosis
❑ *Proximity to nasal floor and maxillary sinus:* A careful surgical procedure is required to avoid surgical perforation of sinus
❑ Miscellaneous
  • Nonrestorable teeth
  • Poor periodontal prognosis
  • Vertically fractured teeth
  • Nonstrategic teeth.

Classification

❑ Surgical drainage
  • Incision and drainage (I and D)
  • Cortical trephination (fistula surgery)
❑ Periradicular surgery
  • Curettage
  • Biopsy
  • Root-end resection
  • Root-end preparation filling
  • Corrective surgery
    – Perforation repair
      ▪ Mechanical (iatrogenic)
      ▪ Resorptive (internal and external)
    – Root resection
    – Hemisection

- ❑ Replacement surgery
- ❑ Implant surgery
  - Endodontic implants
  - Root-form osseointegrated implants.

Classification of Endodontic Microsurgical Cases (Fig. 25.1)

Given by Richard Rubenstein and Kim according to assessment of root form osseous integrated implant treatment outcome.

Class A: Absence of periradicular lesion but persistent symptoms after nonsurgical treatments.

Class B: Presence of small periapical lesion and no periodontal pockets.

Class C: Presence of large periapical lesion progressing coronally but no periodontal pockets.

Class D: Any of Class B or C lesion with periodontal pocket.

Class E: Periapical lesion with endodontic and periodontal communication but no root fracture.

Class F: Tooth with periapical lesion and complete denudation of buccal plate.

▌Presurgical Considerations

Before initiating the surgical procedure, clinician should evaluate the following factors which affect the treatment outcome:
- ❑ Success of surgical treatment versus nonsurgical retreatment

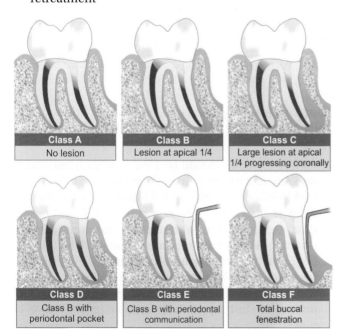

Fig. 25.1 Classification of endodontic microsurgical cases.

- ❑ Review of medical history of the patient and consultation with physician if required
- ❑ Patient motivation
- ❑ Aesthetic considerations like scarring
- ❑ Evaluation of anatomic factors by taking radiographs at different angles
- ❑ Periodontal evaluation
- ❑ Presurgical preparation
- ❑ Taking informed consent.

Protocol of treatment
- Intraoral and localized swelling—only incision and drainage
- Diffuse swelling or it has spread into extraoral facial tissues or spaces—surgical drainage and systemic antibiotics
  - Hard, indurated and diffuse swelling—allow it to localize, become soft and fluctuant before incision and drainage

▌Incision and Drainage

Surgical Drainage

Surgical drainage is indicated when purulent and/or hemorrhagic exudates forms within the soft tissue or the alveolar bone as a result of symptomatic periradicular abscess **(Fig. 25.2)**.

Steps

- ❑ Give local anesthesia
- ❑ Give incision to the most dependent part of swelling with scalpel blade, No. 11 or No. 12. Place horizontal incision at dependent base of the fluctuant area for effective drainage to occur **(Figs. 25.3A to D)**.

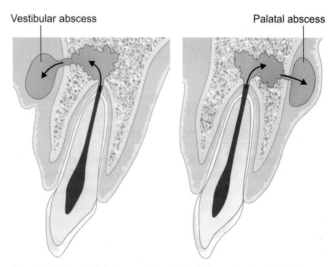

Fig. 25.2 Surgical drainage is indicated if purulent exudate forms within the soft tissue or the alveolar bone.

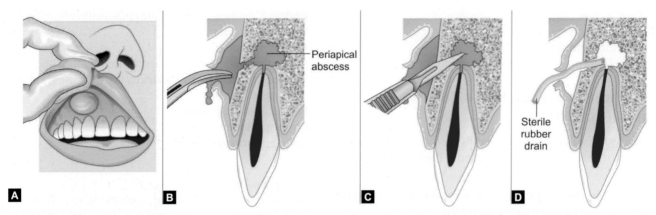

Figs. 25.3A to D (A) Large vestibular abscess; (B) Vestibular abscess is formed due to large periradicular abscess; (C) Incision given at most dependent part of the lesion; (D) Drainage tube to drain the purulent exudates.

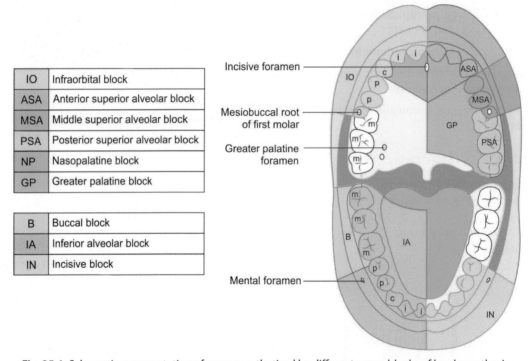

IO	Infraorbital block
ASA	Anterior superior alveolar block
MSA	Middle superior alveolar block
PSA	Posterior superior alveolar block
NP	Nasopalatine block
GP	Greater palatine block

B	Buccal block
IA	Inferior alveolar block
IN	Incisive block

Fig. 25.4 Schematic representation of areas anasthetised by different nerve blocks of local anesthesia.

Periradicular Surgery

Local Anesthesia and Hemostasis

❑ Lidocaine with adrenaline is local anesthesia of choice to obtain profound anesthesia and optimal hemostasis. If amide is contraindicated, then ester agent, that is, procaine, propoxicaine with levonordefrin, is indicated

❑ For nerve blocks, 2% lidocaine with 1:100,000 or 1:200,000 adrenaline is used. But for obtaining hemostasis, adrenaline concentration should be 1:50,000 **(Fig. 25.4)**

❑ Rate of injection should be 1 mL/min with maximum safe rate of 2 mL/min. Rapid injection produces localized pooling of solution in the injected site resulting in delayed and limited diffusion into the adjacent tissue, thus surface contact with microvasculature reduces, resulting in reduced hemostasis. Hemostasis is clinically indicated by blanching of soft tissues

❑ Submucosal infiltration for hemostasis should be given with 30 gauge needle with the bevel toward bone and penetration just superficial to periosteum at the level of root apices.

Receptor and mechanism of hemostasis

- Gage demonstrated that the action of a vasopressor drug on microvasculature depends on predominant receptor type:
  - α-Receptors—Stimulation of α-receptors (mainly in oral mucosa and gingiva) causes vasoconstriction, thus decrease in the blood flow
  - β-Receptors—Stimulation of β-receptors (skeletal muscles) causes vasodilatation

Reactive hyperemia: rebound phenomenon

- In reactive hyperemia, concentration of vasoconstrictor decreases so it does not cause α adrenergic response but after some time blood flow increases more than normal leading to reactive hyperemia. It occurs due to rebound from an α to β response
- Rebound phenomenon is because of localized tissue hypoxia and acidosis caused by prolonged vasoconstriction
- Once this reactive hyperemia occurs, it is impossible to re-establish hemostasis by additional injections

Flap Designs and Incisions

Principles and Guidelines for Flap Designs

- ❑ Avoid horizontal and severely angled vertical incisions, because
  - Gingival blood supply occurs from supraperiosteal vessels and these follow vertical course parallel to long axis of teeth **(Fig. 25.5)**

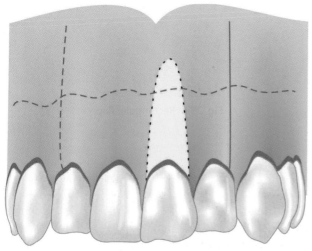

Fig. 25.5 Avoid horizontal and severely angled vertical incisions, because supraperiosteal vessels follow vertical course parallel to long axis of teeth

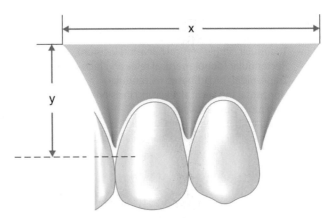

Fig. 25.6 Base of flap > free margin to preserve an adequate blood supply.

- Collagen fibers of gingiva and alveolar mucosa form attachments for crestal bone and supracrestal cementum to the gingiva and periosteum of radicular bone
- ❑ Avoid incisions over radicular eminences (e.g., in canines and maxillary first premolars)
- ❑ Incisions should be placed such that flap is repositioned over solid bone
- ❑ Base of flap should be more than free margin to preserve an adequate blood supply **(Fig. 25.6)**
- ❑ Incisions should never be placed over areas of periodontal bone loss or periradicular lesions
- ❑ *Hooley and Whitacre* suggested that minimum 5 mm of bone should exist between edge of a bony defect and incision line
- ❑ Extent of vertical incisions should be sufficient to allow the tissue retractor to seat on solid bone, thereby leaving the root apex well exposed
- ❑ Extent of horizontal incision should be adequate to provide visual and operative access with minimal soft tissue trauma
- ❑ Avoid incisions in the mucogingival junction
- ❑ Junction of horizontal sulcular and vertical incisions should either include or exclude the involved interdental papilla
- ❑ When submarginal incision is used, there must be a minimum of 2 mm of attached gingiva around each tooth to be flapped.

Functions of a Flap

- ❑ Raise the soft tissue to give the best possible view and exposure of the surgical site
- ❑ To provide healthy tissue that will cover the area of surgery, decrease pain by eliminating bone exposure and aid in obtaining optimal healing.

Classification
- Full mucoperiosteal flaps
  - Triangular (single vertical releasing incision)
  - Rectangular (double vertical releasing incision)
  - Trapezoidal (broad-based rectangular)
  - Horizontal (no vertical releasing incision)
- Limited mucoperiosteal flaps
  - Submarginal curved (semilunar)
  - Submarginal scalloped rectangular (Luebke-Ochsenbein)

Full Mucoperiosteal Flaps

In this, the entire soft tissue overlying the cortical plate in the surgical site is reflected. Major advantage of this type of flap is that supraperiosteal vessels are maintained intact. But disadvantages are postsurgical flap dislodgement, loss of soft tissue attachment level and crestal bone height.

Triangular Flap (*Fischer* in 1940)

It is a full thickness most commonly used flap in endodontics **(Fig. 25.7)**.

Indications
- Maxillary incisor region
- Maxillary and mandibular posterior teeth
- It is the only recommended flap design for posterior mandible region.

Contraindications
- Teeth with long roots (maxillary canine)
- Mandibular anteriors because of lingual inclination of their roots.

Advantages
- Enhanced rapid wound healing
- Ease of wound closure.

Disadvantage
Limited surgical access.

Rectangular Flap

It is extension of triangular flap. Here two vertical releasing incisions and horizontal intrasulcular incision is given **(Fig. 25.8)**.

Indications
- Mandibular anteriors
- Maxillary canines
- Multiple teeth.

This flap is not recommended for mandibular posterior teeth.

Advantages
- Enhanced surgical access
- Easier apical orientation
- Excellent wound healing potential.

Disadvantages
- Wound closure as flap reapproximation and postsurgical stabilization are more difficult than triangular flap
- Potential for flap dislodgement is greater.

Trapezoidal Flap

It was described by *Neumann and Eikan in 1940*. Trapezoidal flap is formed by two releasing incisions which join a horizontal intrasulcular incision at obtuse angles **(Fig. 25.9)**.

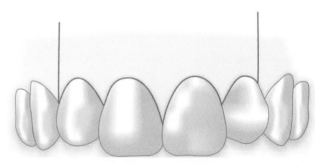

Fig. 25.8 Rectangular flap.

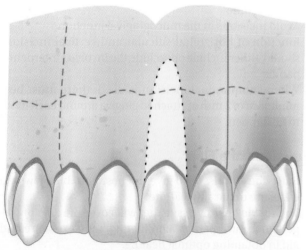

Fig. 25.7 Triangular flap.

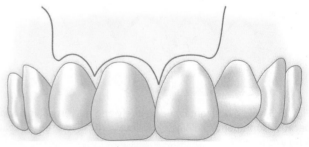

Fig. 25.9 Trapezoidal flap.

Disadvantages

- Wound healing by secondary intention
- Pocketing or clefting of soft tissue
- Compromise in blood supply
- Contraindicated in periradicular surgery.

Envelope Flap

It is formed by a single horizontal intrasulcular incision and is usually recommended for corrective endodontic surgery.

Indications

- For repair of perforation defects
- For root resections
- In cases of hemisections.

Advantages

- Improved wound healing
- Easiness of wound closure and postsurgical stabilization.

Disadvantages

- Extremely limited surgical access
- Essentially impractical for periradicular surgery, but-some use it for palatal surgery.

▊ Limited Mucoperiosteal Flaps

Semilunar Flap

- It was first given by *Partsch,* also known as *Partsch incision*
- It is formed by a single curved incision. It is called as semilunar flap because horizontal incision is modified to have a dip toward incisal aspect in center of the flap, giving resemblance to the half-moon **(Fig. 25.10)**.

Advantages

- Fast and easy to reflect
- No involvement of marginal and interdental gingiva.

Disadvantages

- Limited surgical access
- Difficult wound closure
- Poor apical orientation

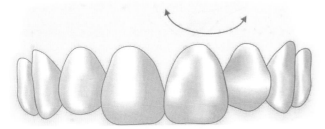

Fig. 25.10 Semilunar flap.

- Potential for postsurgical soft tissue defects by incising through tissues unsupported by bone
- Maximum disruption of blood supply to unflapped tissues.

Ochsenbein-Luebke Flap/Submarginal Scalloped Rectangular Flap

- Ochsenbein-Luebke flap was developed by an endodontist and periodontist
- It is modification of rectangular flap **(Fig. 25.11)**
- In this, scalloped horizontal incision is given in the attached gingival which forms two vertical incisions made on each side of surgical site **(Fig. 25.12)**.

Indications

- In presence of gingivitis or periodontitis associated with fixed prosthesis
- Where bony dehiscence is suspected.

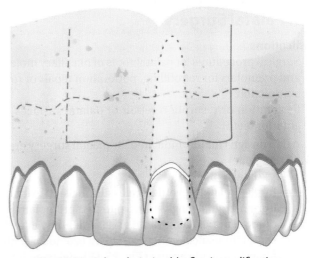

Fig. 25.11 Ochsenbein-Luebke flap is modification of rectangular flap

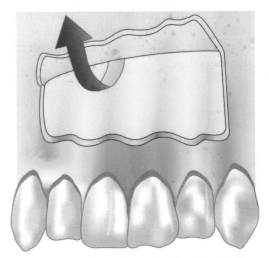

Fig. 25.12 Flap design for Ochsenbein-Luebke flap.

Advantages
- Marginal and interdental gingiva are not involved
- Unaltered soft tissue attachment level
- Crestal bone is not exposed
- Adequate surgical access
- Good wound healing potential—as compared to semi-lunar flap.

Disadvantages
- Disruption of blood supply to unflapped tissues
- Flap shrinkage
- Difficult flap reapproximation and wound closure
- Untoward postsurgical sequelae
- Healing with scar formation
- Limited apical orientation
- Limited or no use in mandibular surgery.

Flap Design Consideration in Palatal Surgery

Indications
- Surgical procedures for palatal roots of maxillary molars and premolars for retrofilling, perforation repair or root amputation
- Perforation or resorption repair of palatal surfaces of anterior teeth.

Two flap designs mainly indicated for palatal surgery are:
1. Triangular
2. Horizontal
   - In triangular flap, vertical releasing incision extends from marginal gingiva mesial to first premolar to a point near palatal midline and is joined by a horizontal intrasulcular incision which extends distally far as to provide access (**Fig. 25.13**). Relaxing incisions are given between first premolar and canine to decrease the chances for severance of blood vessels
   - Posterior part of palate is pebblier which makes it difficult area during elevation. Here, scalpel can be used to partially dissect the tissues for modified thickness flap.

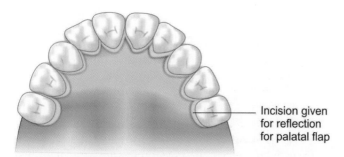

Fig. 25.13 Flap for palatal surgery.

Incision given for reflection for palatal flap

Flap Reflection and Retraction

- Reflection of a flap is the process of separating the soft tissues (gingiva, mucosa and periosteum) from surface of alveolar bone
- It should begin in the vertical incision a few millimeters apical to the junction of horizontal and vertical incisions (**Fig. 25.14**)
- Once these tissues are lifted from cortical plate, periosteal elevator is placed between tissue and bone. It is moved coronally to separate marginal and interdental gingiva from underlying bone and opposing incisional wound edge without direct application of dissectional forces. This elevation is continued until the attached gingival is lifted from underlying bone to the full extent of horizontal incision (**Fig. 25.15**).

Flap Retraction

Retraction of the tissues provides access to the periradicular area. For this, retractor should rest on cortical bone with light but firm pressure directed against the bone. If retractor rests on the base of reflected tissues, it can result in damage to microvasculature of alveolar mucosa and thus delayed healing.

Time of Retraction

Longer the flap is retracted, greater are the complications of the following surgery because
- Vascular flow is reduced during retraction
- Tissue hypoxia may result causing delayed wound healing

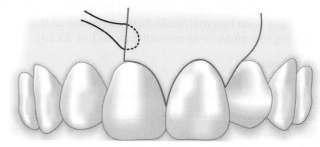

Fig. 25.14 Flap reflection begins in the vertical incision, apical to junction of horizontal and vertical incision.

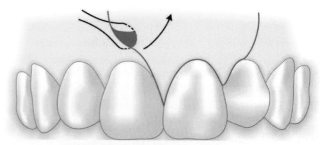

Fig. 25.15 Lifting of mucoperiosteum.

❏ During retraction, flap should be irrigated with normal saline to prevent dehydration of periosteal surface of the flap. Because of severance of the vertically oriented supraperiosteal vessels, limited mucoperiosteal flaps are more susceptible to dehydration and thus require more frequent irrigation than full mucoperiosteal flaps.

Hard Tissue Management

After reflection of flap, root apices are approached by making an access through cortical plates. In case, radiolucency is present around root apex, osseous tissue need not be removed surgically. But when radiolucency is not present periapically, osseous cutting is required to gain access to the root apex.

Tissue Response to Bone Removal

Bone in surgical site has temporary decrease in blood supply because of local anesthesia. This causes bone to become more heat sensitive and less resistant to injury. So, any small changes during bone removal can affect bone physiology and viability.

Speed of Cutting

❏ *At 8,000 rpm:* Almost similar tissue response are seen when irrigation is done with or without a coolant or with a mixture of blood and saliva or water
❏ *At high speed (up to 300,000 rpm):* Favorable tissue response is noted when other parameters (coolant, pressure, type of bur) are controlled.

Use of Coolant

Coolant (water, saline) should be used to dissipate heat generated during cutting osseous tissue and keep the cutting flutes of instrument free of debris there by reducing friction and using cutting efficacy of bur.

Types of Bur for Cutting

No. 6 or No. 8 round bur causes less inflammation and produces smoother cut surface than produced by fissure or diamond bur. It also reduces the healing time. Cutting bone with a diamond stone is the most inefficient as defects produced by these burs heal at very slow rate.

Principles of Surgical Access to Root Structure

Normally, when radiolucent area is present periapically, root is visible through cortical plate. But if periapical radiolucency is not present, then bone is to be removed to gain access to the root. Guidelines to be strictly followed for determining location of root apex are
❏ Assess angulation of crown to the root
❏ Measure entire tooth to root length
❏ Locate root from coronal to apex where bone covering root is thinner. Once it is located, then remove the covering bone with light brush strokes working in apical direction
❏ Expose radiographs from different angles
❏ Probe the apical region using endodontic explorer or straight curette to know whether a small defect is present or not
❏ If a small defect is present in the bone, then place a small piece of lead sheet, gutta-percha point, or plug of alloy to know the position of apex.

POINTS TO REMEMBER

Barnes gave some features which are helpful in differentiating root surface from surrounding osseous tissue:
• Root structure is yellowish in color
• Texture of root is smooth and hard while that of bone is porous and granular
• Root doesn't bleed when probed
• Root is surrounded by periodontal ligament which can identified using methylene blue dye

---

Periradicular Curettage

It is a *surgical procedure to remove diseased tissue from the alveolar bone in the apical or lateral region surrounding a pulpless tooth* (**Figs. 25.16A to F**).

Indications

❏ Access to the root structure for additional surgical procedures
❏ For removing the infected tissue from the bone surrounding the root
❏ For removing overextended fillings
❏ For removing necrotic cementum
❏ For removing a long standing persistent lesion especially when a cyst is suspected
❏ To assist in rapid healing and repair of the periradicular tissues.

Surgical Technique

❏ Give local anesthesia, design flap and expose the surgical site
❏ Use bone curette to remove the pathologic tissue surrounding the root. Insert curette between soft tissue and bone, apply pressure against the bone
❏ After removing the tissue from bony area, grasp the soft tissue with the help of tissue forceps and send it for histopathological examination.

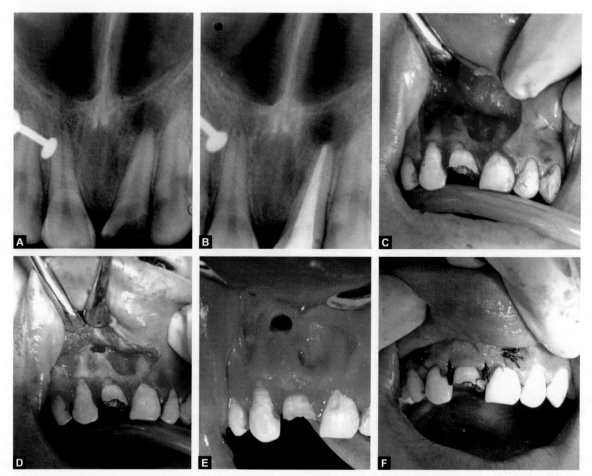

Figs. 25.16A to F Management of right maxillary central incisor with periapical radiolucency by periapical curettage: (A) Preoperative radiograph; (B) Obturation; (C) Mucoperiosteal flap raised; (D) Window preparation in 11; (E) Periapical curettage; (F) Sutures placed. *Courtesy:* Jaidev Dhillon.

Root-End Resection (Apicoectomy, Apicectomy)

Apicoectomy is the surgical resection of a tooth and its removal together with pathological periapical tissue **(Figs. 25.17 to 25.20)**.

Indications
- Inability to perform nonsurgical endodontic therapy due to anatomical, pathological and iatrogenic defects in root canal
- Persistent infections after conventional endodontic treatment
- Need for biopsy
- Need to evaluate the resected root surface for any additional canals or fracture
- Medical reasons
- Lack of time
- For removal of iatrogenic errors like ledges, fractured instruments and perforation which are causing treatment failure
- For evaluation of apical seal
- Blockage of the root canal due to calcific metamorphosis or radicular restoration.

Factors to be Considered before Root-end Resection

Instrumentation

High-speed handpiece with surgical length fissure bur is preferred because round bur may result in gouging of root surface. Nowadays, use of Er:YAG laser for root-end resection is recommended as it produces clean and smooth root surface, decreases permeability of root surface, reduces postoperative pain and discomfort.

Extent of Resection

According to Cohen et al., length of root tip resection depends upon frequency of lateral canals and apical

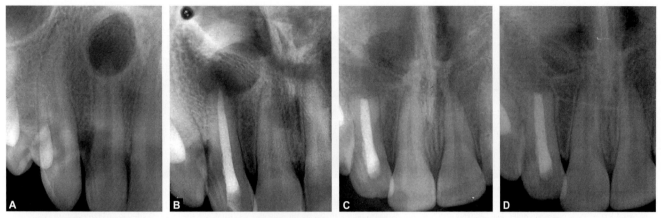

Figs. 25.17A to D Surgical treatment of maxillary right lateral incisor with periapical lesion: (A) Preoperative radiograph; (B) Post obturation radiograph; (C) Radiograph after periapical surgery and root resection; (D) Follow-up after 12 months showing decrease in size of periapical radiolucency.
Courtesy: Manoj Hans.

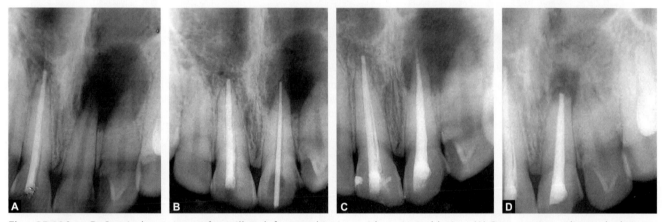

Figs. 25.18A to D Surgical treatment of maxillary left central incisor with periapical lesion: (A) Preoperative radiograph showing periapical radiolucency; (B) Radiograph after obturation; (C) Follow-up 6 months after surgery; (D) Follow-up 12 months after surgery.
Courtesy: Manoj Hans.

ramifications at root end. It was found that when apical 3 mm is resected, lateral canals are reduced by 93% and apical ramifications 98% **(Fig. 25.21)**.

Angle of Root-End Resection

Earlier it was thought that root-end resection at 30–45° from long axis of root facing buccally or facially provides improved accessibility and visibility of resected root end. But studies have shown that beveling of root end results in opening of dentinal tubules on the resected root surface which communicate with root canal space, causing apical leakage even after retrofilling is done **(Figs. 25.22A and B)**. So, a bevel of 0–10° is recommended for resection because
- It allows inclusion of lingual anatomy with less reduction
- If multiple canals are present, increase in bevel causes increase in distance between them

- With short bevel, its easier to keep instruments within long axis of the tooth (so to avoid unnecessary removal of radicular dentin) than with long bevel
- Long bevel exposes more dentinal tubules to oral environment resulting in microleakage over a period of time

▌ Root-End Preparation

Main objective of root-end preparation is to create a cavity to receive root-end filling. Root-end preparation should accept filling materials so as to seal off the root canal system from periradicular tissues.

Car and Bentkover defined an ideal root-end preparation as "a class I preparation at least 3.0 mm into root dentine with walls parallel to a coincident with the anatomic outline of the pulp space".

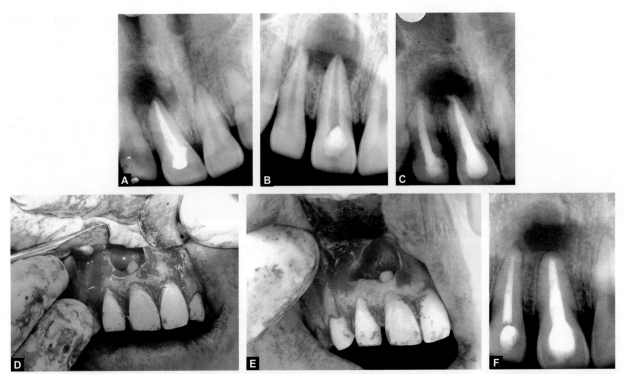

Figs. 25.19A to F Surgical management of periapical cyst in relation to 21: (A) Preoperative radiograph; (B) After removal of previous root canal filling; (C) Postobturation radiograph; (D) After elevation of flap; (E) After cyst enucleation and root-end resection.
Courtesy: Jaidev Dhillon.

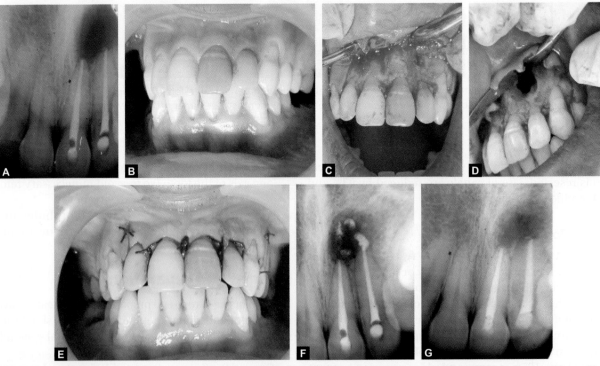

Figs. 25.20A to G Surgical management of periapical lesion: (A) Radiograph showing obturation of maxillary central and lateral incisor; (B) Preoperative photograph; (C) Raising the flap; (D) Curettage of the periapical lesion; (E) Postoperative photograph; (F) Postoperative radiograph; (G) Follow-up radiograph after 3 months.
Courtesy: Jaidev Dhillon.

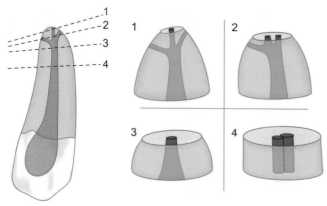

Fig. 25.21 Diagram showing root resection at different levels. Figure shows that root resection of 3 mm at 0° bevel, eliminates most of the anatomic features.

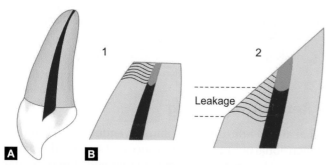

Figs. 25.22A and B (A) Zero degree bevel exposes less of dentinal tubules to oral environment; (B) Beveling results in opening of dentinal tubules on resected tooth surface, which communicate with root canal space, and result in apical leakage.

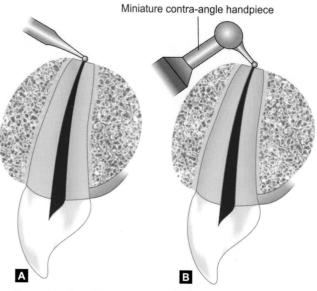

Figs. 25.23A and B (A) Root-end preparation using straight handpiece; (B) Root-end preparation using handpiece.

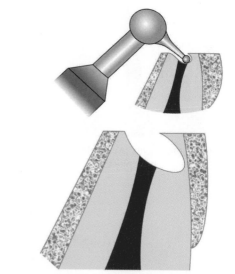

Fig. 25.24 Perforation of root caused by misdirection of handpiece.

Five requirements suggested for a root-end preparation to fulfill:
1. Apical 3 mm of root canal must be cleaned and shaped
2. Preparation must be parallel to anatomic outline of the pulp cavity
3. Creation of an adequate retention form
4. Removal of all isthmus tissue if present
5. Remaining dentine walls should not be weakened

Traditional Root-End Cavity Preparation

Miniature contra-angle or straight handpiece with a small round or inverted cone bur is used to prepare a class I cavity at the root end within confines of the root canal **(Figs. 25.23 A and B)**. Though, these preparations seem to be placed along long axis of the tooth, but they are directed palatally causing perforations **(Fig. 25.24)**.

Ultrasonic Root-End Preparation

It was developed to resolve the main shortfalls of bur preparation. In this, specially designed ultrasonic root-end preparation instruments are developed which result in smaller preparation size with minimal bevel, parallel walls for better retention and less debris and smear layer than those prepared with a bur **(Figs. 25.25 and 25.26)**.

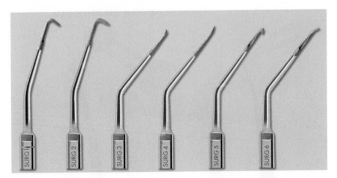

Fig. 25.25 Ultrasonic tip for root-end preparation.

Difference between traditional and microsurgery		
Procedure	*Traditional*	*Microsurgery*
• Apex identification	Difficult	Precise
• Osteotomy	Large (8–10 mm)	Small (3–4 mm)
• Angle of bevel	45–60°	Less than 10°
• Identification of isthmus	Almost impossible	Easy
• Root surface inspection	None	Always
• Retropreparation	Approximate	Precise
• Root-end filling	Imprecise	Precise
• Root-end preparation	Sometimes inside canal	Always in the canal
• Suture material (silk suture)	3–0 or 4–0	5–0 or 6–0
• Suture removal (postoperative)	After 1 week	After 2–3 day
• Healing	Slow	Fast

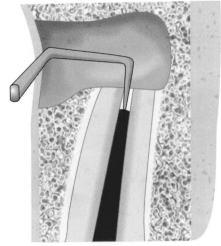

Fig. 25.26 Retrograde cavity preparation using ultrasonic handpiece.

Retrograde Filling

Main aim of nonsurgical or surgical endodontics is three-dimensional obturation of the root canal system. Therefore, after apical surgery, placement of a root-end filling material is an equally important step. To place a material in the retropreparation, it is mixed in the desired consistency, placed into the retropreparation (**Fig. 25.27A**) and compacted with the help of burnisher. After it is set, excess is removed with carver or periodontal curette (**Fig. 25.27B**). Finally, the

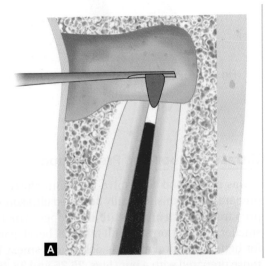

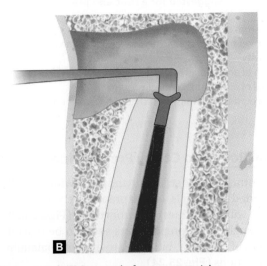

Figs. 25.27A and B (A) Placement of restorative material; (B) Removal of excess material.

root-end filling is finished with carbide finishing bur and a radiograph is taken to confirm the correct placement of the filling.

Root-End Filling Materials

An ideal root-end filling material should
- ❑ Be well tolerated by periapical tissues
- ❑ Adhere to tooth surface
- ❑ Be dimensionally stable
- ❑ Resist dissolution
- ❑ Promote cementogenesis
- ❑ Be bactericidal or bacteriostatic
- ❑ Be noncorrosive and electrochemically inactive
- ❑ Not stain tooth or periradicular tissue
- ❑ Be readily available and easy to handle
- ❑ Allow adequate working time, then set quickly
- ❑ Be radiopaque.

Commonly used root-end filling materials
- Amalgam
- Gutta-percha
- Gold foil
- Titanium screws
- Glass ionomers
- Zinc oxide eugenol
- Cavit
- Composite resins
- Polycarboxylate cement
- Poly HEMA
- Super ethoxybenzoic acid (EBA)
- Mineral trioxide aggregate (MTA)

Amalgam

It is one of the most popular and widely used retrograde filling materials since the last century.

Advantages	Disadvantages
• Easy to manipulate	• Slow setting
• Readily available	• Dimensionally unstable
• Well tolerated by soft tissues	• It shows leakage
• Radiopaque	• Stains overlying soft tissues, resulting in formation of tattoo
• Initially provides tight apical seal	• More cytotoxic than IRM, super EBA, or MTA

Abbreviations: IRM, intermediate restorative material; MTA, mineral trioxide aggregate.

Zinc Oxide Eugenol Cement

Unmodified ZOE cement is weak and has long setting time and high water solubility. On contact with moisture, it releases free eugenol which is responsible for most of the effects caused by zinc oxide eugenol cement.

Intermediate Restorative Material

Intermediate restorative material is a ZOE cement reinforced by addition of 20% polymethacrylate by weight to zinc oxide powder. It shows low water solubility, milder reaction than unmodified ZOE cements.

Super Ethoxybenzoic Acid

It is a ZOE cement modified with EBA to alter the setting time and increase the strength of mixture.

Advantages	Disadvantages
• Low solubility and nonresorbable	• Difficult to manipulate because setting time is short and greatly affected by humidity
• Radiopaque	
• Strongest and least soluble of all ZOE formulations	• Tends to adhere to all surfaces so difficult to place
• Yield high compressive and tensional strength	

Mineral Trioxide Aggregate

- ❑ Mineral trioxide aggregate (MTA) is composed of tricalcium silicate, tricalcium aluminate, tricalcium oxide, bismuth oxide and silicate oxide
- ❑ Its pH is 2.5 (when set) and setting time is 2 h 45 min.

MTA Placement Technique

Mix MTA powder and liquid and carry it to cavity with amalgam carrier or messing gun **(Fig. 25.28)** compact it

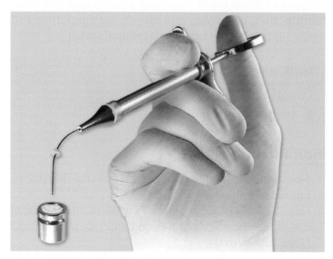

Fig. 25.28 Carrying MTA with messing gun or amalgam carrier.

using micropluggers and clean the surface with damp cotton pellet

Advantages	Disadvantages
• Excellent biocompatibility, in contact with periradicular tissues, it forms cementum • Hydrophilic so not adversely affected by blood or moisture • Radiopaque	• More difficult to manipulate • Longer setting time • Expensive

Composite Resins

Though composite resins have shown superior physical properties but they are very technique sensitive. Since it is very difficult to obtain a total dry field, their use is not encouraged as root-end filling material.

Reapproximation of the Soft Tissue

Following surgery, final inspection of the root-end filling and cleaning of the surgical site is done and a radiograph is taken to assess presence of any root fragments or surplus root-end filling material.

Repositioning of the Flap

Flap is replaced in the original position with the incision lines approximated as close as possible. Now flap is compacted by applying light yet firm pressure for 2–5 min with the help of damp surgical gauze. This compression helps in approximation of the wound edges and their initial adhesion.

Replantation

Grossman, in 1982, defined intentional replantation as "the act of deliberately removing a tooth and following examination, diagnosis, endodontic manipulation and repair—returning the tooth to its original socket."

Classification
It can be of two types:
1. Intentional replantation
2. Unintentional replantation

Indications

❑ Nonsurgical endodontic treatment not possible due to limited month opening
❑ Calcifications, posts, or separated instruments present in canals making nonsurgical endodontics therapy difficult **(Figs. 25.29A to D)**
❑ Persistent infection even after root canal treatment
❑ Inaccessibility for surgical approach due to anatomic factors

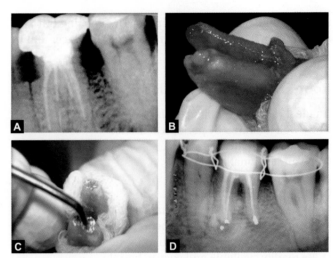

Figs. 25.29A to D Management of separated instrument in mandibular first molar by intentional replantation: (A) Separated fragment in the mesiolingual canal of mandibular first molar; (B) Radicular view after extraction; (C) Placement of retrograde filling material; (D) Post operative radiograph.

❑ Perforations in inaccessible areas where for surgery excessive bone loss in required
❑ Accidental avulsion, that is, unintentional replantation
❑ For thorough examination of root defects like crack or perforation.

Contraindications

❑ Curved and flared canals
❑ Nonrestorable tooth
❑ Moderate-to-severe periodontal disease
❑ Missing interseptal bone
❑ Presence of vertical root fractures.

Precautions to be taken during replantation procedure:
• Root surface (with PDL cells) should be kept moist with Hanks balanced salt solution or saline during the time tooth is out of socket
• Out of socket, time should be shortest possible
• One should take care not to damage PDL cells and cementum. Avoid touching forceps' beaks on cementum

Technique

❑ Extract the tooth with minimal trauma to tooth and socket
❑ Incise periodontal fibers using No. 15 scalpel blade
❑ Gently elevate the tooth using forceps in rocking motion until grade I mobility is achieved. Forceps should be placed away from the cementum so as to avoid damage to periodontal ligament **(Fig. 25.30)**
❑ Keep the root surface moist by wrapping it with gauge soaked in a physiologic solution such as Hanks balanced salt solution

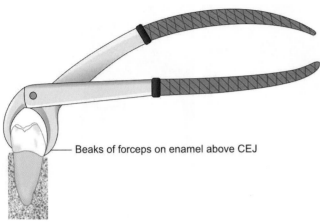

Fig. 25.30 Beaks of forcep should rest above cementoenamel junction so as to avoid injury to periodontal tissue.

Beaks of forceps on enamel above CEJ

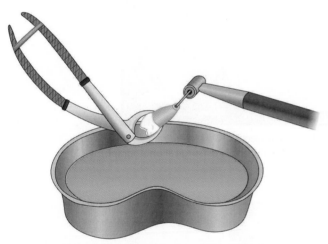

Fig. 25.31 Any repair or procedure should be done as quickly as possible in the bath of normal saline or HBSS solution to prevent desiccation.

❑ Thoroughly examine the roots for defects or fractures and repair the defects if indicated. Any repair or procedure should be done quickly in the bath of normal saline or HBSS solution so as to prevent desiccation **(Fig. 25.31)**
❑ Irrigate the extraction socket using normal saline
❑ Gently place the tooth back in the socket and place a rolled gauze piece on occlusal surface. Ask the patient to bite on it for at least 5–10 min. This will help in seating the tooth into socket
❑ Stabilize the tooth using periopak, sutures, or splints. Recall the patient after 7–14 days so as to remove the stabilization and to evaluate the mobility
❑ Follow-up should be done after 2, 6, 9 and 12 months of surgery.

Prognosis

It depends on preventing trauma to the PDL and cementum during extraction and minimizing extraoral time.

Causes of Failure of Reimplantation

❑ Extended extraoral time resulting in damage to periodontal cells
❑ Contamination during procedure—resulting in infection and resorption
❑ Undetected fracture of tooth
❑ Mishandling of tooth during reimplantation procedure.

▌Transplantation

It is the procedure of replacement of a tooth in a socket other than the one from which it had been extracted from.

▌Hemisection/Root Resection/ ▌Root Amputation

Hemisection is defined as removal of a unrestorable root which may be affected by periodontal, structural (cracks) and caries. Hemisection is independent of bicuspidization. Hemisection includes splitting of the tooth, extraction of one half, followed by a bridge whereas bicuspidization involves retaining of both the split sections of the tooth and then restoring them with crowns **(Figs. 25.32 and 25.33)**.

Indications

❑ Extensive bone loss in relation to root where periodontal therapy cannot correct it
❑ Severely curved canal which cannot be treated
❑ Extensive calcifications in root
❑ Fracture of one root, which does not involve other root
❑ Resorption, caries, or perforation involving one root.

Contraindications for Root Resections

❑ Fused roots
❑ Root in close proximity to each other
❑ Uncooperative patient
❑ Lack of optimal bone support for remaining root/roots
❑ Endodontically incompatible remaining root/roots.

Technique

Before root resection, carryout endodontic treatment in roots to be retained. After this, carry out root resection. There are basically two approaches for root resections:

1. *Vertical:* Here complete root is resected along with its associated portion of crown. This procedure also called as hemisection or trisection. It is done from mesial to distal in maxillary molars and buccal to lingual in mandibular molars

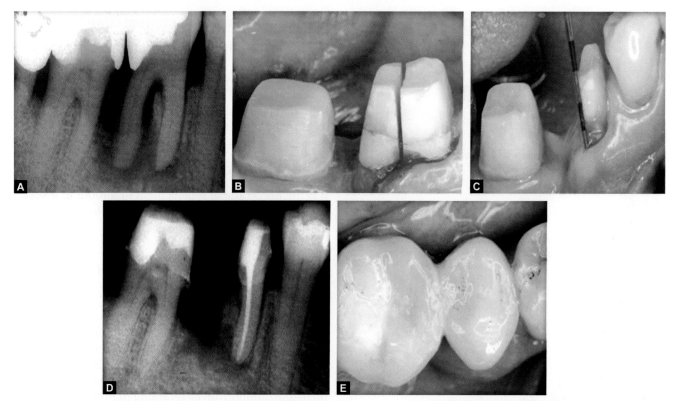

Figs. 25.32A to E Management of mandibular first molar by hemisection: (A) Pre-Operative radiograph; (B and C) Hemisection of first molar; (D) Post-surgical radiograph; (E) Postsurgical photograph.

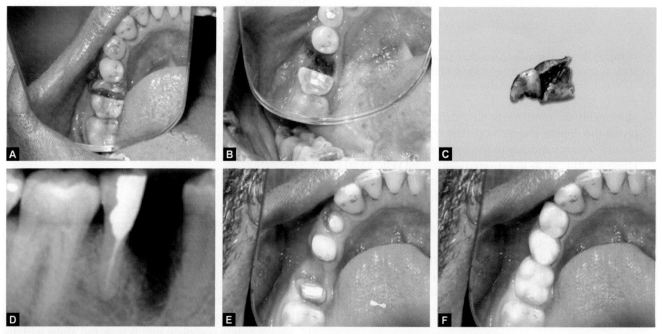

Figs. 25.33A to F Management of mandibular first molar by hemisection: (A) Preoperative photograph showing cut for hemisection; (B) Hemisection; (C) Ressected piece of tooth; (D) Postsurgical radiograph; (E) Photograph showing tooth preparation; (F) Postsurgical photograph.
Courtesy: Jaidev Dhillon.

2. *Horizontal/oblique:* In this, root is resected at the point where it joins to the crown. It is also called as root resection.

Presurgical Crown Contouring

This method involves trimming the portion of crown over the root to be amputated so as to gain access **(Fig. 25.34)**. Before carrying out this technique, roots should be obturated with gutta-percha. Tapered fissure bur is moved so as to trim the crown portion present to the level of cementoenamel junction.

Bicuspidization/Bisection

It is defined as surgical separation of a multirooted tooth into two halves and restoring each root with a separate crown. It is exclusively carried out in mandibular molars where mesial and distal roots are separated with their respective crown portions. Their separation eliminates existence of furcation making the area easy to clean.

Indications

- □ When periodontal disease involves the furcation area. Periodontal treatment does not improve the condition of tooth
- □ Furcation is transferred to make interproximal space which makes the area more manageable by the patient.

Contraindications

- □ Fused roots
- □ Lack of osseous support for separate segments
- □ Uncooperative patient.

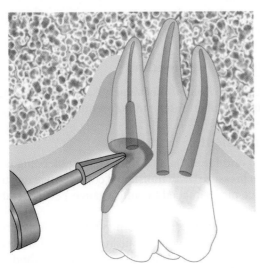

Fig. 25.34 In presurgical contouring, crown which is present over root to be amputated is trimmed with bur up to the level of cementoenamel junction.

Endodontic Implants

Endodontic implants are used for providing stabilization of teeth in which alveolar support is lost due to endodontic and periodontal disease. It enhances root anchorage by extension of artificial material beyond alveolar socket but within range of alveolar bone **(Fig. 25.35)**.

Case Selection for Endodontic Implants

- □ Teeth with straight canals
- □ Presence of sufficient alveolar height
- □ Absence of systemic disease
- □ Absence of any anatomic complications
- □ Absence of any calcifications in canals.

Indications

- □ Horizontal root fracture
- □ Unaffordable root crown ratio
- □ Periodontally involved teeth
- □ Endodontically involved teeth with short roots.

Contraindications

- □ Presence of calcifications in roots
- □ Proximity of anatomic structures
- □ Patient suffering from systemic disease
- □ Presence of curved canals.

Material Used for Implants

- □ Titanium
- □ Chrome cobalt alloys.

Technique

- □ Give local anesthesia and isolate the tooth
- □ Extirpate the pulp and take working length radiograph
- □ Add 2–3 mm to the estimated working length so that instrument goes periapically with a minimal preparation of ISO size 60

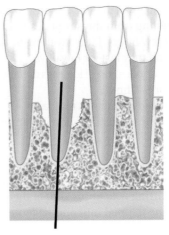

Fig. 25.35 Endodontic implant.

- Start intraosseous preparation using 40 mm long reamers
- Ream the bone about 10 mm beyond the apex with sequentially increased sizes so as to achieve round apical preparation
- Complete the preparation till at least ISO No. 70, or until apex is reamed round
- Dry the canal and check the fitting of implant. If tugback is there at working length, cut 1 mm of apical end of implant so as to avoid its butting against bone
- Irrigate and dry the canal, take care not to disturb the apical clot
- Fit the canal and cut it at the point below gingival level using carborundum disk. One should take care that cement is applied only to the part of implant with in confines of the canal
- Seal the implant using gutta-percha
- Do coronal restoration using crown, or composite restoration.

Reasons for Failure of Endodontic Implants

- Extrusion of cementing media
- Inadequate seal at junction of implant and the apex
- Wrong technique of placement.

Postsurgical Care

It includes providing genuine expression of concern and reassurance to patient, good patient communication regarding the expected and normal postsurgical sequelae as well as detailed home care instructions.

Instructions

- No difficult activity or work for the rest of day
- No alcohol or any tobacco for next 3 days
- Good nutritious diet. Drink lot of liquids for first few days after surgery
- Do not lift up lip or pull back cheek to look at where surgery was done. It may pull the stitches loose and cause bleeding
- A little bleeding from the surgical site is normal and it can last for few hours. Little swelling or bruising of face is normal and may last for few days
- Intermittent application of ice bags on face where surgery was done for 6–8 hours
- Take prescribed medicines regularly
- Remove suture and make follow-up appointment.

Suturing

A suture is strand of material used to close the wound. Purpose of suturing is to approximate incised tissues and also stabilize the flapped mucoperiosteum until reattachment occurs.

Classification of sutures	
According to absorbency	*According to physical property*
• Absorbable • Nonabsorbable	• Monofilament • Multifilament • Twisted or braided

Principles of Suturing

- Needle should enter the mucosal skin perpendicular to surface of tissue
- Needle should always pass from free tissue to fixed tissue
- Needle should always be inserted at an equal depth and distance from incision line on both sides
- Tissue should not be closed under tension
- Sutures should be spaced evenly
- Suture should not be too tight. If sutures are too tight, there will be local ischemia underneath the suture tracks
- Suture knot should never lie on the incision line
- After tying, knot should be left to one side.

Postsurgical Complications

Postoperative Swelling

Postoperative swelling usually reaches maximum after 24 or 48 hours and resolves within a week. Proper compression of surgical flap both before and after suturing reduces postoperative swelling.

Management

- Inform the patient earlier as it reduces the anxiety
- Application of ice packs is recommended for next 6–8 hours
- Warm saline rinses two to three times a day is recommended after 24 hours.

Postoperative Bleeding

Slight oozing of blood after surgery is normal, but significant bleeding is uncommon and may require attention.

Management

- First and foremost step in managing bleeding is apply firm pressure (with moistened cotton gauge or a tea bag or ice pieces placed in cotton gauge) over the area for 10–20 min
- If bleeding still continues, then remove the sutures and search for blood vessels causing bleeding. Cauterize the blood vessel using thermal or electrical method
- Place local hemostatics if required
- If bleeding is still unmanageable, hospitalize the patient.

Extraoral Ecchymosis (Extraoral Discoloration)

Discoloration/ecchymosis usually results when blood has leaked into the surrounding tissues. This condition is self-limiting in nature and lasts up to 2 weeks and does not affect the prognosis.

Management

Application of moist heat for 2 weeks is helpful as heat promotes fluid exchange and speeds up resorption of discoloring agents from tissues.

Pain

Postoperative pain usually maximum on the day of surgery and it decreases thereafter.

Management

❏ Prescribe NSAIDs
❏ If pain is severe, opioid analgesics may be combined with NSAIDs
❏ Give long acting anesthetics like bupivacaine in severe cases.

Infection

Postoperative infection usually occurs due to inadequate aseptic technique and improper soft tissue handling, approximation and stabilization. Symptoms appear 36–48 hours after surgery. Suppuration, elevated temperature and lymphadenopathy are seen in some cases.

Management

Prescribe systemic antibiotics. Antibiotic of choice in these cases is penicillin. If person is allergic to penicillin, then clindamycin should be given (initial dose—600 mg, maintenance 150–300 mg).

Miscellaneous

❏ Maxillary sinusitis
❏ Paresthesia.

▌Conclusion

Success of surgical endodontics varies between 30% and 80%. The preservation of natural teeth should be our ultimate goal, because natural teeth are always far better than any man-made replacement. Endodontic surgery is considered as last resort to save a tooth with endodontic failure. With advent of magnification, microinstruments, ultrasonic tips and biologically acceptable root end filling materials, the success rate of surgical endodontics has shown to increase upto 92% along with favorable patient response.

▌Questions

1. Classify various endodontic surgical procedures.
2. What are indications and contraindications of endodontic surgery?
3. What are indications and technique of root-end resection?
4. Write in detail about factors to be considered before root-end resection.
5. What are different materials used for root-end restoration?
6. How do you manage lower right first molar having periapical abscess with furcation involvement?
7. Write short notes on
   • Incision and drainage
   • Ochsenbein-Luebke flap.
   • Semilunar flap
   • Hemisection
   • Reimplantation
   • Endodontic implants

▌Bibliography

1. Cohen S, Burns RC. Pathways of the pulp. 8th edition. St Louis, MO: CV Mosby; 2002.
2. Cohen S, Hargreaves KM. Pathways of the Pulp. 9th edition. St Louis, MO: Mosby; 2006.
3. Dorn SO, Gartner AH. Retrograde filling materials: a retrospective success-failure study of amalgam, EBA and IRM. J Endod 1990;16:391-3.
4. Grossman I, Oliet S, Del Rio C. Endodontic practice. 11th edition. Varghese Publication; 1991.
5. Grossman LI. A brief history of endodontics. J Endod 1982;8:536.
6. Gutmann JL, Harrison JW. Posterior endodontic surgery. Anatomical considerations and clinical techniques. Int Endod J 1985;18:8-34.
7. Gutmann JL, Pitt Ford TR. Management of the resected root end: a clinical review. Int Endod J 1993;233:273-83.
8. Harty FJ, Parkins BJ, Wengraf AM. The success rate of apicectomy. Br Dnet J 1970;129:407-13.
9. Kim S. Principles of endodontic microsurgery. Dent Clin North Am 1997;47:481-97.
10. Luebke RG. Surgical endodontics. Dent Clin North Am 1974;18:379-91.
11. Peters LB, Wesselink PR. Soft tissue management in endodontic surgery. Dent Clin North Am 1997;41:513-25.
12. Siqueira Jr JF. Aetiology of root canal failure: why well treated can fail. Int Endod J 2001;34:1-10.
13. Weine FS. Endodontic therapy. 5th edition. St Louis, MO: Mosby; 1998.

CHAPTER
26

Endodontic Periodontal Lesions

Chapter Outline

- ❑ Definition
- ❑ Pathways of Communication between Pulp and Periodontium
- ❑ Impact of Pulpal Diseases on the Periodontium
- ❑ Impact of Periodontal Disease on Pulpal Tissue
- ❑ Etiology of Endodontic–periodontal Lesions
- ❑ Classification of Endodontic–periodontal Lesions
- ❑ Diagnosis of Endodontic–periodontal Lesions
- ❑ Primary Endodontic Lesions

- ❑ Primary Endodontic Lesion with Secondary Periodontal Involvement
- ❑ Primary Periodontal Lesions
- ❑ Primary Periodontal Lesions with Secondary Endodontic Involvement
- ❑ Independent Endodontic and Periodontal Lesions which do not Communicate
- ❑ True Combined Endo–perio Lesions

Health of periodontium is important for normal physiology of the tooth. Periodontium is anatomically inter-related with pulp by virtue of apical foramina and lateral canals which create pathways for exchange of noxious agents between these two tissues (**Fig. 26.1**). Not only the interaction between periodontium and pulp produces or aggravates the existing lesion, but it also presents challenges in deciding the direct cause of an inflammatory condition. So a correct diagnosis should be made after careful history taking and clinical examination.

▌ Definition

An endo–perio lesion is one where both pulp and periodontal tissues are affected by the disease progress.

Pathways of communication between pulp and periodontium (Fig. 26.2)

Physiological	Pathological	Miscellaneous

• Apical foramen
 • Lateral and accessory canals
 • Atypical ana-tomical factors:
   – Palatogingival groove
   – Cervical enamel projection
   – Dentinal tubules
	• Perforation
	 • Vertical root fracture
	 • Loss of cementum
	 • Pathological exposures of lateral canals (in case of infrabony pockets and bone loss at furcation area)
	 • Trauma from occlusion-crown fracture
		• Iatrogenic
		   – Perforation during endodontic therapy
		   – Root fracture during root canal therapy
		   – Exposure of dentinal tubules during root planning
		 • Systemic
		 • Systemic disease like diabetes mellitus can be a cause of com-bined lesions

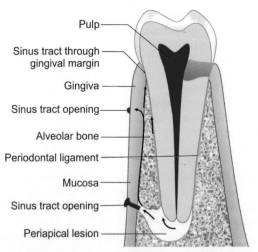

Fig. 26.1 Pathway for exchange of noxious agents between endodontic and periodontal tissue.

Pulp ——

Sinus tract through gingival margin ——

Gingiva ——

Sinus tract opening ——

Alveolar bone ——

Periodontal ligament ——

Mucosa ——

Sinus tract opening ——

Periapical lesion ——

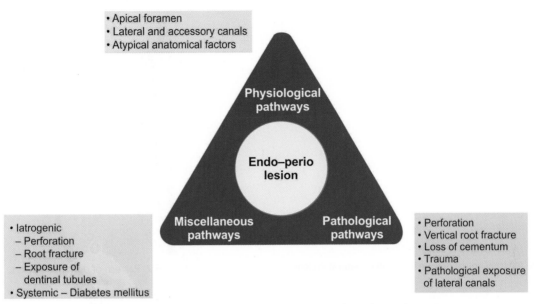

Fig. 26.2 Pathways of communication between pulp and periodontium.

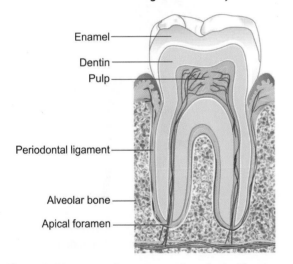

Fig. 26.3 Diagrammatic representation of apical foramen.

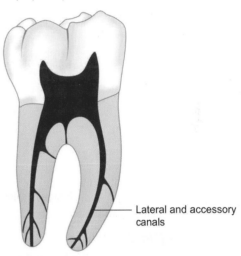

Fig. 26.4 Lateral and accessory canals can exist anywhere on the root surface.

Pathways of Communication between Pulp and Periodontium

Physiological Pathways

Apical Foramen (Fig. 26.3)

It is one of the major pathways of communication between dental pulp and periodontium. Inflammatory factors exit through apical foramen and irritate periodontium.

Lateral or Accessory Canals (Fig. 26.4)

Majority of lateral or accessory canals are found in apical third and furcation area of the root. As periodontal disease progresses down the root surface, accessory and lateral canals get exposed to oral cavity. It is difficult to identify lateral canals on radiographs. These can be identified by isolated defects on the lateral surface of roots or by postobturation radiographs showing sealer puffs.

Palatogingival Groove (Fig. 26.5)

It is developmental anomaly commonly seen in maxillary lateral incisor. Groove begins in the central fossa, crosses the cingulum and extends apically at varying distance.

Cervical Enamel Projections (Fig. 26.6)

These are flat, ectopic extensions of enamel that extend beyond normal contours of cementoenamel junction (CEJ). They interfere with the attachment apparatus and are important in initiating the periodontal lesions.

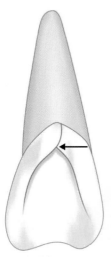

Fig. 26.5 Palatogingival groove in maxillary lateral incisor.

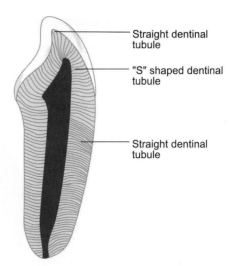

Straight dentinal tubule

"S" shaped dentinal tubule

Straight dentinal tubule

Fig. 26.7 Pattern of dentinal tubules.

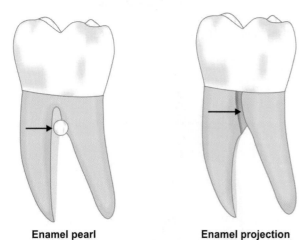

Enamel pearl   **Enamel projection**

Fig. 26.6 Enamel pearl and projections.

Dentinal Tubules (Fig. 26.7)

Dentinal tubules traverse from pulpodentinal junction to cementodentinal or dentinoenamel junction. Cementum acts as protective barrier to the dentin but because of periodontal disease, periodontal therapy, etc., if cementum is damaged, a direct communication between dentinal tubules and the oral cavity may occur.

Pathological Pathways

Perforation of the Root (Fig. 26.8)

Perforation creates an artificial communication between the root canal system and periodontium. Closer is the perforation to gingival sulcus, greater is the chances of apical migration of gingival epithelium in initiating a periodontal lesion.

Vertical Root Fracture (Fig. 26.9)

Vertical root fracture forms a communication between root canal system and periodontium

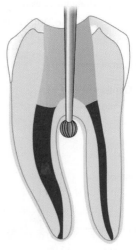

Fig. 26.8 Perforation of root creates communication between root canal system and periodontium.

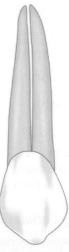

Fig. 26.9 A communication can form between root canal system and periodontium via vertical root fracture.

Loss of Cementum (Fig. 26.10)

Loss of cementum can occur due to gingival recession, presence of inadequate attached gingiva, abrasion, periodontal surgery, overzealous tooth cleansing habits, etc.

Pathological Exposure of Lateral Canals

Infrabony pocket or furcation bone loss can result in pulp exposure by exposing the lateral canals to the oral environment.

Miscellaneous Pathways

Iatrogenic

Perforation during endodontic therapy (Fig. 26.11): It produces mechanical or pathological communication between root canal system and external tooth surface.

Root fracture during root canal therapy: Root fracture can occur due to excessive dentin removal during biomechanical preparation and weakening of tooth during postspace preparation. Fracture site provides entry for bacteria and their toxic products from root canal system to the surrounding periodontium.

Exposure of dentinal tubules during root planning: It can result in communication between pulpal and periodontal space.

Impact of Pulpal Diseases on the Periodontium (Fig. 26.12)

Pulpal infection may cause a tissue destructive process which may progress from apical region to the gingival margin, termed as ***retrograde periodontitis*** **(Fig. 26.13)**. Restorative procedures and traumatic injuries cause inflammatory changes in the pulp, though it is still vital. Though a vital pulp does not affect the periodontium, necrosed pulp is seen associated with periodontal problem. Inflammatory lesions may develop from a root canal infection through lateral and accessory canals.

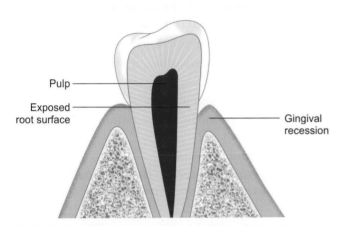

Fig. 26.10 Loss of cementum can occur because of gingival recession.

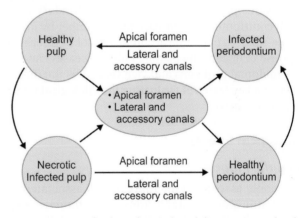

Fig. 26.12 Impact of pulp and periodontal diseases on each other.

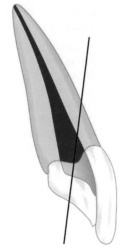

Fig. 26.11 Perforation during endodontic treatment can result in endo-perio lesion.

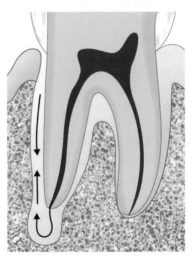

Fig. 26.13 In retrograde periodontitis, pulpal infection progresses from apical region to the gingival margin.

Impact of Periodontal Disease on Pulpal Tissue (Fig. 26.12)

Pathogenic bacteria and inflammatory products of periodontal diseases may enter into the root canal system via accessory canals, lateral canals, apical foramen, dentinal tubules resulting in **retrograde pulpitis**. As periodontal disease extends from gingival sulcus toward apex, the auxiliary canals get affected which results in pulpal inflammation. It becomes more serious if these canals get exposed to oral cavity because of loss of periodontal tissues by extensive pocket depth.

Periodontal therapy using ultrasonic scalers, vibrators, curettes and chemicals may harm the pulp specially if remaining dentin thickness is <2 mm.

Etiology of Endodontic-Periodontal Lesions

Primary etiologic agent in periodontitis is bacterial plaque. Besides this primary factor, there are secondary factors which contribute to the disease process either by increasing the chances of plaque accumulation or by altering the response of host to the plaque. Pulpal diseases can result in periodontal problems and vice versa. It is the duration which is a key factor in evaluating the etiological effect of a particular factor.

Etiological Effects

Bacterial Plaque

Commonly associated microorganisms associated with endodontic–periodontal lesions are *Actinomyces* spp., *F. nucleatum*, *P. intermedia*, *P. gingivalis*, and *Treponema* spp. Sometimes *C. albicans*, viruses like herpes simplex, cytomegalovirus and EBV have also shown to play an important role in periapical lesions.

Foreign Bodies

Foreign bodies like amalgam filling, root canal filling material, dentin or cementum chips, and calculus deposits can irritate pulp and periodontium.

Contributing Factors Resulting in Combined Endodontic–Periodontal Lesions

❏ Malpositioned teeth causing trauma
❏ Presence of additional canals in teeth
❏ Cervical enamel projects into furcation of multirooted teeth
❏ Large number of accessory and lateral canals
❏ Trauma combined with gingival inflammation
❏ Vertical root fracture
❏ Crown fracture
❏ Root resorption
❏ Perforations
❏ Systemic factors such as diabetes

Classification of Endodontic-Periodontal Lesions

According to Weine: Based on etiology and treatment plan:

Class I: Tooth which clinically and radiographically simulates the periodontal involvement but it is due to pulpal inflammation or necrosis.

Class II: Tooth has both pulpal and periodontal disease occurring concomitantly.

Class III: Tooth has no pulpal problem but requires endodontic therapy plus root amputation for periodontal healing.

Class IV: Tooth that clinically and radiographically simulates pulpal or periapical disease but has periodontal disease.

According to Simon et al.: Based on etiology, diagnosis, prognosis and treatment (Figs. 26.14A to E).

Type I: Primary endodontic lesion.

Type II: Primary endodontic lesion with secondary periodontal involvement.

Type III: Primary periodontal lesions.

Type IV: Primary periodontal lesion with secondary endodontic involvement.

Type V: True combined lesion.

According to Grossman et al.: Oliet and Pollock's classification based on treatment protocol

Type I	Type II	Type III
Lesions requiring endodontic treatment only	Lesion that require periodontal treatment only	Lesions that require combined endodontic and periodontal treatment
• Tooth with necrotic pulp reaching periodontium • Root perforations • Root fractures • Chronic periapical abscess with sinus tract • Replants • Transplants • Teeth requiring hemisection	• Occlusal trauma causing reversible pulpitis • Suprabony or infrabony pockets caused during periodontal treatment resulting in pulpal inflammation • Occlusal trauma and gingival inflammation resulting in pocket formation	• Any lesion of type I which result in irreversible reaction to periodontium requiring periodontal treatment • Any lesion of type II which results in irreversible damage to pulp tissue requiring endodontic therapy

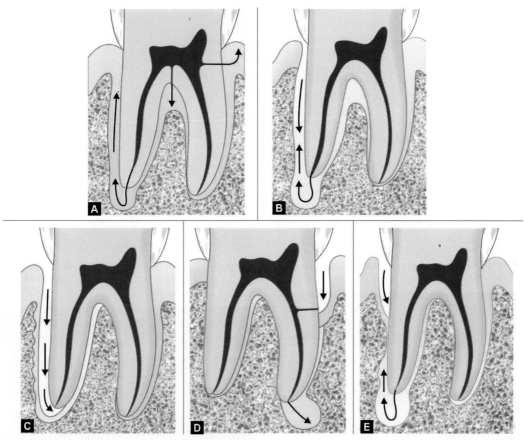

Figs. 26.14A to E (A) Primary endodontic lesion; (B) Primary endodontic lesion with secondary periodontal involvement; (C) Primary periodontal lesions; (D) Primary periodontal lesion with secondary endodontic involvement; (E) True combined lesion.

Diagnosis of Endodontic–Periodontal Lesions

Diagnosis of a combined endodontic and periodontal lesion is often multifaceted and exasperating. A growing periapical lesion with secondary involvement of the periodontal tissue may have the similar radiographic appearance as a chronic periodontal lesion which has reached to the apex. Thus, a careful history taking, visual examination, diagnostic tests involving both pulpal and periodontal testing, and radiographic examination are needed to diagnose such lesions.

Tooth with combined endodontic–periodontal lesion must fulfill following criteria:
- Tooth involved should be nonvital
- There should be destruction of the periodontal attachment which can be diagnosed by probing from gingival sulcus to either apex of the tooth or to the level of involved lateral canal
- Both endodontic therapy and periodontal therapies are required to resolve the lesion completely

Chief Complaint of Patient

Patient may tell the pain indicating pulpal or periodontal type. History of patient may reveal previous pulpal exposure or any periodontal treatment. Pulpal condition is usually acute, whereas periodontal or secondary pulpal or combined lesions are usually chronic in nature.

Associated Etiology

For pulpal disease, caries, trauma, or pulp exposure is common etiology, whereas for periodontal disease is associated with plaque/calculus, history of bleeding gums, or bad odor.

Clinical Tests

Different signs and symptoms can be assessed by visual examination, palpation, and percussion **(Fig. 26.15)**. presence of carious tooth, recession, swelling of gingiva, plaque/calculus, or increased pocket depth may indicate endo–perio lesion **(Fig. 26.16)**. Mobility tells the integrity of attachment apparatus or extent of inflammation in periodontal ligament.

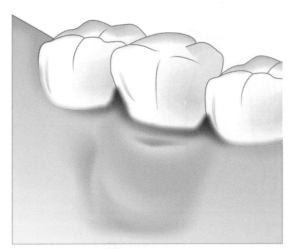

Fig. 26.15 Clinical picture of periodontal abscess.

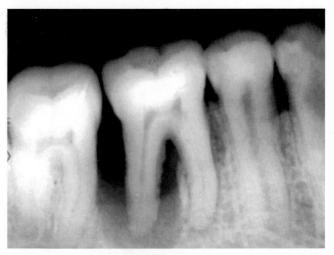

Fig. 26.17 Radiograph showing endo–perio lesion with bone resorption in right mandibular molar.

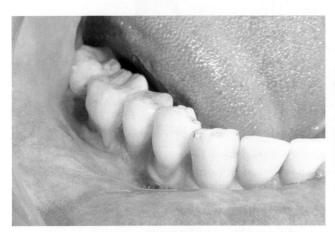

Fig. 26.16 Presence of carious tooth, recession, swelling of gingiva indicate endo–perio lesion.

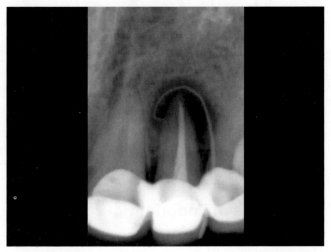

Fig. 26.18 Tracking a sinus tract using gutta-percha and then taking radiograph.

Radiographs

Radiographs help in diagnosing caries, extensive restorations, previous root canal treatment, root form, root resorption, root fracture, root canal obliteration, thickened periodontal ligament space and any changes in the alveolar bone (Fig. 26.17).

Pulp Vitality Tests

Any abnormal response of pulp may indicate degenerative changes occurring in the pulp. Cases associated with non-vital pulp have pulpal pathology, whereas teeth associated with vital pulp usually have periodontal disease. Commonly used pulp vitality tests are cold test, electric test, blood flow test, and cavity test.

Tracking Sinus or Fistula

Gutta-percha is inserted slowly through the sinus and X-ray is taken to track it. Being radiopaque, gutta-percha helps

in determining and differentiating the source of infection (Fig. 26.18).

Pocket Probing

Pocket probing helps to know the location and depth of pocket and furcation involvement, if any (Fig. 26.19).

Microbiological Examination

Microbiological analysis provides important information regarding the main source of the problem.

Distribution

Pulpal pathology is usually localized in nature, whereas periodontal condition is generalized.

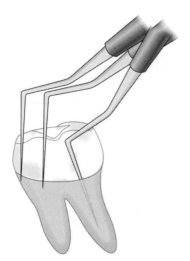

Fig. 26.19 Probing of tooth helps in knowing extent of pockets.

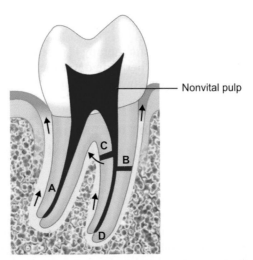

Nonvital pulp

Fig. 26.20 Spread of infection can occur—A. from apical foramen to gingival sulcus via periodontium, B. from lateral canal to pocket, C. from lateral canal to furcation; D. from apex to furcation.

Bone Loss

In pulpal disease, bone loss is generally localized and wider apically. It is not associated with vertical bone loss. In periodontal disease, bone loss is generalized which is wider coronally. It may be associated with vertical bone loss.

Pain

Pain in pulpal pathology is acute and sharp and patient cannot identify the offending tooth. In periodontal pathology, pain is dull in nature and patient can identify the offending tooth (because of presence of proprioceptive nerve fibers in periodontal ligament).

Swelling

If swelling is seen on the apical region, it is usually associated with pulpal disease. If it is seen around the margins or lateral surface of teeth, swelling is usually associated with periodontal disease.

Treatment and Prognosis

Treatment planning and prognosis depends mainly on diagnosis of the specific endodontic and/or periodontal disease. In teeth with combined endodontic—periodontal lesions, the prognosis depends on extent of destruction caused by periodontal disease. If lesion is of endodontic origin, an adequate endodontic treatment has good prognosis. Thus in combined disease, prognosis depends on efficacy of periodontal therapy.

▌Primary Endodontic Lesions (Fig. 26.20)

Sometimes an acute exacerbation of chronic apical lesion in a nonvital tooth may drain coronally through periodontal ligament into the gingival sulcus, thus resembling clinical picture of periodontal abscess. The lesion presents as an isolated pocket or the swelling on the side of the tooth.

Etiology

- ❑ Dental caries
- ❑ Deep restorations close to pulp
- ❑ Traumatic injury
- ❑ Poor root canal treatment

Clinical Features

- ❑ Patient is usually asymptomatic, but history of acute exacerbation may be present
- ❑ Since tooth is associated with necrotic pulp, pulp does not show response to vitality tests
- ❑ Sinus tract may be seen from apical foramen, lateral canals, or the furcation area
- ❑ Probing shows true pockets. Pocket is associated with minimal plaque or calculus. Significant sign of this lesion is that patient does not have periodontal disease in other areas of oral cavity

Diagnosis

- ❑ Necrotic pulp draining through periodontal ligament into gingival sulcus
- ❑ Isolated pocket on side of tooth
- ❑ Pocket associated with minimal amount of plaque or calculus
- ❑ Patient asymptomatic with history of acute exacerbations

Treatment

- ❑ Root canal therapy
- ❑ Good prognosis

Prognosis

Prognosis after endodontic therapy is excellent. In fact, if periodontal therapy is performed without considering pulpal problem, prognosis becomes poor.

Primary Endodontic Lesion with Secondary Periodontal Involvement (Fig. 26.21)

This lesion appears if primary endodontic lesion is not treated. In such case, the endodontic disease continues, resulting in destruction of periapical alveolar bone, progression into the inter-radicular area and finally causing breakdown of surrounding hard and soft tissues. As drainage persists through periodontal ligament space, accumulation of irritants results in periodontal disease and further apical migration of attachment.

Clinical Features

- Isolated deep pockets are seen though there may be the presence of generalized periodontal disease
- In such cases, endodontic treatment will heal part of the lesion but complete repair will require periodontal therapy.

Diagnosis

- Continuous irritation of periodontium from necrotic pulp or from failed root canal treatment
- Isolated deep pockets
- Periodontal breakdown in the pocket.

Treatment

- Root canal treatment to remove irritants from pulp space
- Retreatment of failed root canal therapy
- Concomitant periodontal therapy
- Extraction of teeth with vertical root fracture if prognosis is poor
- Good prognosis.

Prognosis

In case vertical root fracture is causing the endo–perio lesions, tooth is extracted, otherwise the prognosis is good.

Primary Periodontal Lesions (Fig. 26.22)

Primarily these lesions are caused by periodontal disease. In these lesions, periodontal breakdown slowly advances down to the root surface until apex is reached. Pulp may be normal in most of the cases but as disease progress, pulp may become affected.

Etiology

- Plaque
- Calculus
- Trauma.

Clinical Features

- Periodontal probing may show presence of plaque and calculus within the periodontal pocket
- Due to attachment loss, tooth may become mobile
- Usually generalized periodontal involvement is present

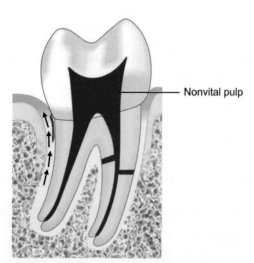

Fig. 26.21 Primary endodontic lesion with secondary periodontal involvement.

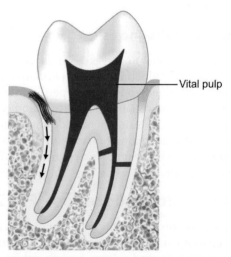

Fig. 26.22 Primary periodontal lesion.

Diagnosis

- Periodontal destruction associated with plaque or calculus
- Patient experiencing periodontal pain
- Pulp may be normal in most of the cases.

Treatment

- Oral prophylaxis and oral hygiene instructions
- Scaling and root planning
- Periodontal surgery, root amputation may be required in advanced cases.

Prognosis

Prognosis becomes poor as the disease advances.

Primary Periodontal Lesions with Secondary Endodontic Involvement (Figs. 26.23 to 26.25)

Periodontal disease affects pulp via lateral and accessory canals, apical foramen, dentinal tubules, or during iatrogenic errors. Once pulp gets secondarily affected, it can in turn affect the primary periodontal lesion.

Etiology

Periodontal procedures such as scaling, root planning and curettage may open up lateral canals and dentinal tubules to the oral environment, resulting in pulpal inflammation. Here, patient complains of sensitivity or inflammation after periodontal therapy.

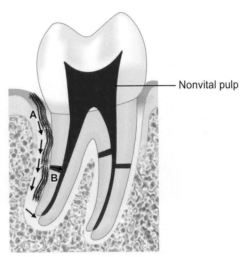

Nonvital pulp

Fig. 26.23 Spread of periodontal lesion into endodontic space via: A. periodontium into apex; B. lateral canals.

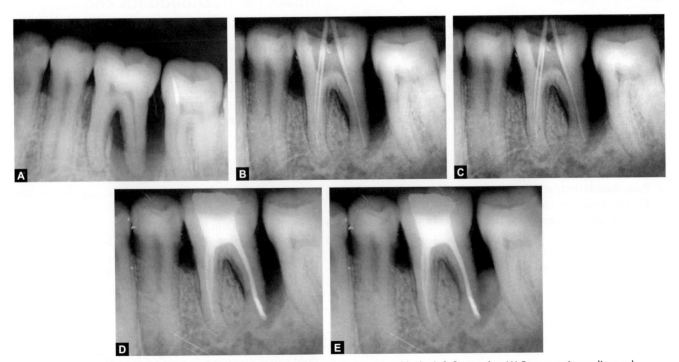

Figs. 26.24A to E Management of endodontic-periodontal lesion in mandibular left first molar: (A) Preoperative radiograph; (B) Working length radiograph; (C) Master cone radiograph; (D) Radiograph after obturation; (E) Follow-up after 3 months.
Courtesy: Manoj Hans.

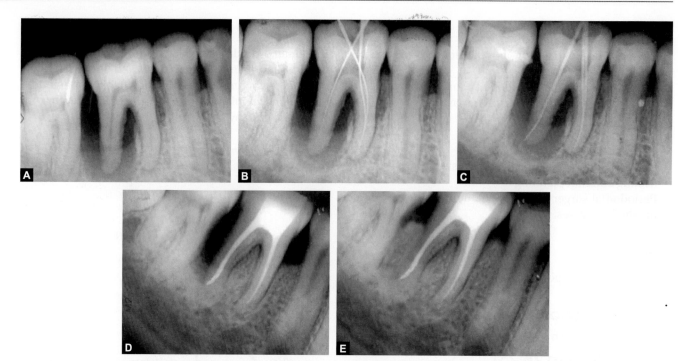

Figs. 26.25A to E Management of endodontic-periodontic lesion in mandibular right first molar. (A) Preoperative radiograph; (B) working length radiograph; (C) master cone radiograph; (D) radiograph after obturation; (E) follow-up after 6 months.
Courtesy: Manoj Hans.

Clinical Features

- ❑ Oral examination of patient reveals presence of generalized periodontal disease
- ❑ Tooth is usually mobile when palpated
- ❑ If severe periodontal destruction exposes the root surface, irreversible pulpal damage can result
- ❑ Radiographically, these lesions become indistinguishable from primary endodontic lesions with secondary periodontal involvement.

Diagnosis

- ❑ Periodontal destruction associated with nonvital tooth
- ❑ Generalized periodontal disease present
- ❑ Patient may complain sensitivity after routine periodontal therapy
- ❑ Usually the tooth is mobile
- ❑ Pocket may show discharge on palpation.

Treatment

- ❑ Root canal treatment
- ❑ Periodontal surgery in some cases (**Fig. 26.26**).

Prognosis

Prognosis depends on the periodontal problem.

Independent Endodontic and Periodontal Lesions which do not Communicate

One may commonly see a tooth associated with pulpal and periodontal disease as separate and distinct entities. Both the disease states exist but with different etiological factors and with no evidence that either of disease has impact on the other.

Clinical Features

- ❑ Periodontal examination may show periodontal pocket associated with plaque or calculus
- ❑ Tooth is usually nonvital
- ❑ Though both periodontal and endodontic lesions are present concomitantly, they cannot be designated as true combined endo–perio lesions because there is no demonstrable communication between these two lesions.

Treatment

- ❑ Root canal treatment is needed for treating pulp space infection
- ❑ Periodontal therapy is required for periodontal problem

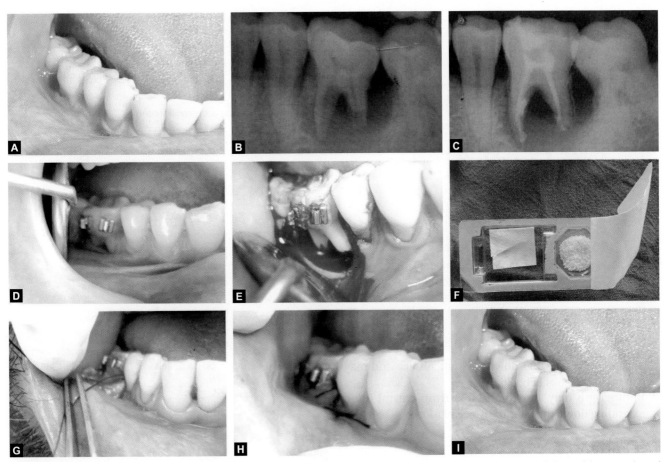

Figs. 26.26A to I Management of an endo–perio lesion in mandibular first molar by endodontic treatment followed by periodontal surgery: (A) Preoperative photograph; (B) Preoperative radiograph; (C) Obturation with MTA; (D) Buccal tubes bonded to the tooth; (E) Flap retracted after giving primary and secondary incisions; (F) Graft material (Equinox Ossifi); (G) After placement of the graft and barrier membrane; (H) Flap placed coronally; (I) 1 month follow-up showing better periodontal status and decreased tooth mobility.
Courtesy: Jaidev Dhillon.

Prognosis

Prognosis of the tooth depends on the periodontal prognosis.

True Combined Endo–Perio Lesions (Fig. 26.27)

True combined lesions are produced when one of these lesion (pulpal or periodontal) which are present in and around the same tooth coalesce and become clinically indistinguishable. These are difficult to diagnose and treat.

Clinical Features

❑ Periodontal probing reveals conical periodontal type of probing and at base of the periodontal lesion the probe

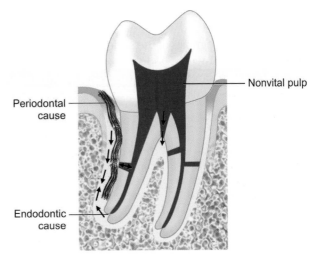

Fig. 26.27 True combined endo–perio lesion

Nonvital pulp

Periodontal cause

Endodontic cause

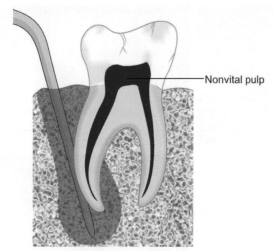
Nonvital pulp

Fig. 26.28 In true combined endodontic-periodontal lesion at the base of periodontal lesion the probe abruptly drops farther down the root and extend to tooth apex.

abruptly drops farther down the root surface and may extend to the apex **(Fig. 26.28)**

❑ Radiograph may show bone loss from crestal bone extending down the lateral surface of root

Treatment

❑ First see whether periodontal condition is treatable, if promising and then go for endodontic therapy. Endodontic therapy is completed before initiation of definitive periodontal therapy

❑ After completion of endodontic treatment, periodontal therapy is started which may include scaling, root planning, and surgery along with oral hygiene instructions

Prognosis

It depends upon prognosis of the periodontal disease.

Different between combined lesions and concomitant lesion	
Combined lesions	Concomitant lesion
• Chronic and generalized in nature	Acute and localized in nature
• There is communication between pulpal and periodontal lesion when seen clinically or radiographically	There may not be communication between pulpal and periodontal lesion when seen clinically and radiographically

Differential diagnosis between pulpal and periodontal disease		
Features	Periodontal	Pulpal
Etiology	Periodontal infection	Pulpal infection
Plaque and calculus	Commonly seen	No relation
Tooth vitality	Tooth is vital	Nonvital
Restorations	No relation	Usually show deep and extensive restoration
Periodontal destruction	Usually present and generalized	If present single, isolated
Gingiva and epithelial attachment	Recession of gingival with apical migration of attachment	Normal
Pattern of disease	Generalized	Localized
Radiolucency	Usually not related	Periapical radiolucency
Inflammatory and granulation tissue	Usually present on coronal part of tooth	Commonly seen on apical part of tooth
Treatment	Periodontal therapy	Root canal therapy
Microbial	Complex	Few
Bone loss	Wider coronally	Wider apically
Pattern	Generalized	Localized
Gingiva	Some recession	Normal
pH of saliva	Often alkaline	Often acidic

▌Conclusion

Endodontic periodontal lesions present a diagnostic and treatment dilemma which can have a diverse pathogenesis ranging from quite simple to complex. To reach at correct diagnosis, the operator should have a thorough understanding and scientific knowledge of these lesions. Treatment of combined endodontic and periodontal lesions does not differ from the treatment given when the two disorders occur separately.

Even though dentistry is divided into the multiple fields of specialization, to achieve the best outcome for endo–perio lesions, a multi-disciplinary approach should be involved, though some cases may require only endodontic therapy or periodontal treatment and others may require the combined approach.

Questions

1. What are etiological factors for endodontic–periodontal lesions? How will you diagnose a case of endodontic–periodontal lesion?
2. Classify endodontic–periodontal lesions.
3. Write in detail about primary endodontic lesion with secondary periodontal involvement.
4. Write short notes on
   - Classification of endodontic–periodontal lesions
   - Differential diagnosis of pulpal and periodontal lesion
   - True-combined endodontic–periodontal lesion.

Bibliography

1. Abbott P. Endodontic management of combined endodontic-periodontal lesions. J N Z Soc Periodontol 1998;83:15–28.
2. Grossman LI, Oliet SM, Del Rio CE. Endodontic–periodontic inter-relationship. Endodontic practice. 11th edition Philadelphia, PA: Lea and Febiger; 1988
3. Harrington GW, Steiner DR, Ammons WF. The periodontal-endodontic controversy. Periodontol 2000 2002;30:123–30.
4. Harrington GW. The perio-endo question: differential diagnosis. Dent Clin North Am 1979;23:673–90
5. Langeland K, Rodrigues H, Dowden W. Periodontal disease, bacteria, and pulpal histopathology. Oral Surg Oral Med Oral Pathol 1974;37:257–70.
6. Rotstein I, Simon JH. Diagnosis, prognosis and decision making in the treatment of combined periodontal-endodontic lesions. Periodontol 2004;34:265–303.
7. Simon JH, Glick DH, Frank AL. The relationship of endodonticperiodontic lesions. J Clin Periodontol 1972;43:202.
8. Stock C, Gulabivala K, Walker R. Perio-endo lesions. Endodontics. 3rd edition St. Louis, MO: Mosby, 2004
9. Torabinejad M, Kiger RD. A histologic evaluation of dental pulp tissue of a patient with periodontal disease. Oral Surg Oral Med Oral Pathol 1985;59:198–200
10. Wang HL, Glickman GN. Endodontic and periodontic inter-relationships. In: Cohen S, Burns RC, editors. Pathways of the Pulp. 8 th edition St Louis: C. V. Mosby; 2002. pp. 651–64.

Restoration of Endodontically Treated Teeth

Introduction

Long-term success of endodontically treated teeth depends upon the skilled integration of endodontic and restorative procedures. Postendodontic restoration is necessary to prevent fracture of the remaining tooth structure, reinfection of the root canal and to replace the missing tooth structure.

Importance of Coronal Restoration (Fig. 27.1)

Postendodontic coronal restoration is important to prevent ingress of microorganisms into coronal pulp. To prevent coronal leakage, the clinician should
❑ Temporarily seal the tooth during or after the treatment
❑ Provide adequate coronal restoration after treatment
❑ Do long-term follow-up so as to evaluate the integrity of restoration

But, even a properly done endodontic treatment can fail due to following reasons:
❑ Poor quality of temporary restoration
❑ Delay in permanent restoration after completion of endodontic treatment
❑ Poor marginal integrity of final restoration
❑ Fractured tooth

Therefore, it is very important to seal the root canal system during or after the endodontic treatment. Commonly used materials for temporary restoration are IRM and Cavit.

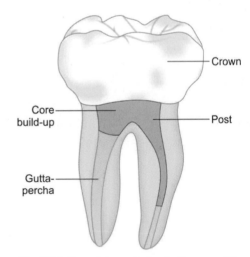

Fig. 27.1 Complete endodontic therapy with postendodontic restoration.

Factors Making Endodontically Treated Teeth Different from Vital Teeth

Endodontically treated teeth are more susceptible to fracture than unrestored vital teeth and also lack a lifelike translucency, thus requiring a specialized restorative treatment.

Differences between endodontically treated and vital tooth are
- Structural changes/architectural changes
- Changes in the dentin physical characteristics/moisture loss
- Change in esthetics

Structural Changes/Architectural Changes

Fracture resistance of the tooth decreases as more tooth structure is lost due to decay, dental procedures and endodontic therapy **(Figs. 27.2 and 27.3)**. A tooth does not become more brittle due to endodontic treatment, but it is loss of structural integrity (provided by dome-shaped roof of pulp chamber at the time of endodontic access cavity preparation) which leads to increased risk of tooth fracture. This compromised structural integrity makes the tooth insufficient to perform its function because of loss of

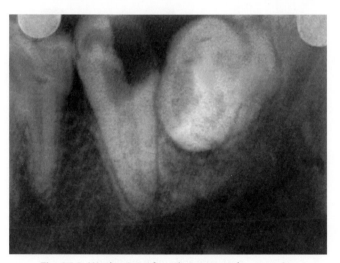

Fig. 27.2 Weakening of tooth structure due to caries.

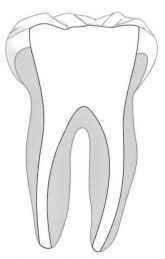

Fig. 27.3 Excessive removal of radicular dentin may result in weakening of roots.

occlusion with its antagonist and adjacent teeth. In addition, the excessive removal of radicular dentin during canal preparation compromises the root.

Changes in the Dentin Physical Characteristics/Moisture Loss

Dehydration and loss of collagen intermolecular cross-linking causes irreversible altered physical properties of endodontically treated teeth. A decrease in 14% strength and toughness of dentin has been observed in endodontically treated teeth.

Clinical implication: Cementation of the active post can induce mechanical stresses that may result in root fracture and failure of postendodontic restorations.

Esthetic Consideration (Fig. 27.4)

Nonvital teeth show loss of translucency and discoloration due to various reasons like necrotic pulp, endodontic procedures, and root canal filling materials. Loss of tooth structure due to fracture or caries also requires further esthetic consideration for restoration of endodontically treated teeth.

Biomechanical Changes

Proprioceptive feedback mechanism is lost after endodontic treatment. This might subject endodontically treated tooth to greater loads than a vital tooth. Tidmarish showed that a normal tooth is hollow laminated structure which deforms under load but complete elastic recovery occurs after physiological loading.

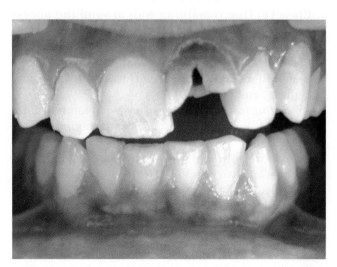

Fig. 27.4 A decrease in tooth structure due to caries requires esthetic consideration using crown.

Restorative Treatment Planning for Endodontically Treated Teeth

Following factors should be taken into consideration before planning restoration for endodontically treated teeth:

❑ Amount of the tooth structure present
❑ Occlusal forces and the anatomic position of the tooth
❑ Restorative requirements
❑ Esthetic requirements.

Amount of the Tooth Structure

This is the most important factor that dictates the choice of restoration and is not under the control of clinician. The resistance form of an endodontically treated tooth depends on amount of radicular dentin and coronal tooth structure present. Loss of tooth structure in endodontically treated teeth can vary from minimal access cavity to an extensively damaged tooth. Restorative treatment decision depends upon amount of remaining tooth structure present.

Ingrid Peroz et al. (2005) classified the restoration plan of endodontically treated teeth depending upon number of walls remaining around the access cavity preparation.

❑ **Class I: Four remaining walls around the access cavity preparation**: If all axial walls of the cavity remain with a thickness >1 mm, then only intracoronal restoration of access cavity if sufficient, provided the tooth is not subjected to undue occlusal forces

❑ **Classes II and III: Two or three remaining walls around access cavity preparation (Fig. 27.5)**: In these cases, core followed by a crown is indicated

❑ **Class IV: One remaining wall around the access cavity preparation (Fig. 27.6)**: In such cases, post is indicated

❑ **Class V: No remaining wall around the access cavity preparation (Fig. 27.7)**: Placement of post is mandatory in these cases.

According to Cohen, choice of postendodontic restoration depends upon the amount of the remaining coronal tooth structure.

❑ Tooth with minimal loss of structure is inherently stronger and can be restored with only coronal restoration **(Fig. 27.8)**

❑ Tooth with >50% of remaining coronal structure can be restored with crown

❑ Tooth with 25–50% of remaining coronal structure can be restored with nonrigid post

❑ Tooth with <25% of remaining coronal structure, or <3–4 mm of cervical tooth structure must be restored with rigid posts.

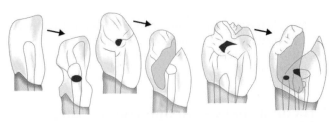

Fig. 27.5 If two to four cavity walls are present around access cavity preparation, post is not required. Only restoration or core build up followed by crown is indicated.

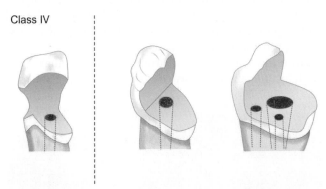

Class IV

Fig. 27.6 If only one wall is present around the access preparation, the use of post followed by crown is indicated.

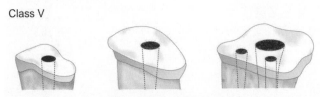

Class V

Fig. 27.7 If no cavity walls remain around the access preparation, post, core and crown are given.

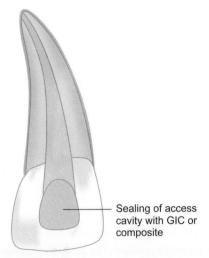

Sealing of access cavity with GIC or composite

Fig. 27.8 In anterior tooth with most of healthy structure remaining, access preparation can be sealed with GIC or composite.

Structurally compromised teeth are prone to
- Root fracture
- Dislodgement of the prosthesis
- Recurrent caries
- Endodontic failure as a result of coronal–apical leakage
- Invasion of biologic width causing periodontal injury

Occlusal Forces and the Anatomic Position of the Tooth

❏ Anterior teeth with minimal loss of tooth structure can be restored with coronal restoration. If tooth is discolored, bleaching and veneer should be considered (**Fig. 27.9**). Anterior teeth with heavy horizontal forces should be restored with stronger restorative components

❏ Posterior tooth with considerable structure requires restoration with onlay or crown to protect it against fracture (**Fig. 27.10**). In case of extensive tooth damage, post/core followed by crown is indicated (**Fig. 27.11**)

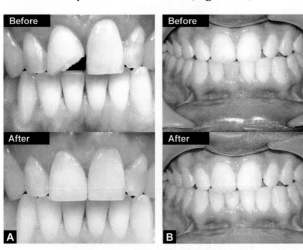

Figs. 27.9A and B If there is minimal loss of tooth structure, esthetics can be restored with (A) direct composite restoration; (B) bleaching of discolored tooth.

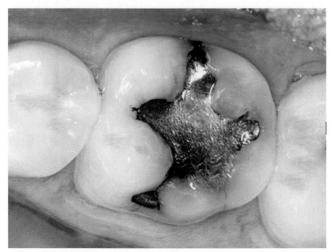

Fig. 27.10 Molar with sufficient tooth structure can be restored using crown.

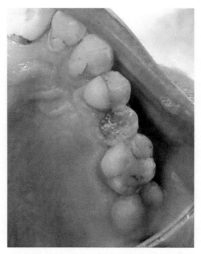

Fig. 27.11 Grossly carious maxillary second premolar is indicated for post and core followed by crown.

Restorative Requirements

Teeth included as abutments in the fixed or partial dentures undergo more forces and thus need additional retention and protection against fracture and caries due to leakage.

Esthetic Requirements

Loss of translucency and discoloration in endodontically treated teeth especially in esthetic zone require restorative materials like tooth-colored posts, composites or ceramic cores and ceramic crowns.

Requirements of a Tooth to Accept a Post and Core

❏ Optimal apical seal
❏ Absence of fistula or exudate
❏ Absence of active inflammation
❏ No sensitivity to percussion
❏ Absence of associated periodontal disease
❏ Sufficient bone support around the root
❏ Sound tooth structure coronal to alveolar crest
❏ Absence of any fracture of root

Contraindications of Placing Post

❏ Presence of signs of endodontic failures like poor apical seal, active inflammation, presence of fistula or sinus and tenderness on percussion (**Figs. 27.12 and 27.13**)
❏ If adequate retention of core can be achieved by natural undercuts of crown
❏ If there are horizontal cracks in coronal portion of the teeth
❏ When tooth is subjected to excursive occlusal stresses like lateral stresses of bruxism or heavy incisal guidance

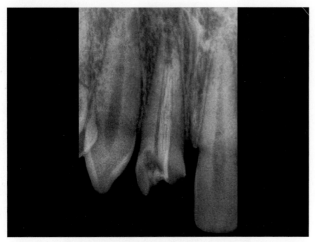

Fig. 27.12 A tooth with poor apical seal and poor quality obturation is not indicated for post and core.

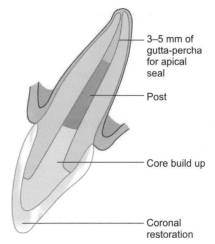

Fig. 27.14 Components of post and core.

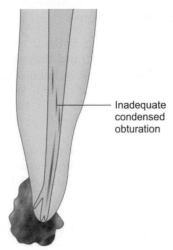

Fig. 27.13 A tooth with endodontic failure due to poor quality obturation is not indicated for post and core.

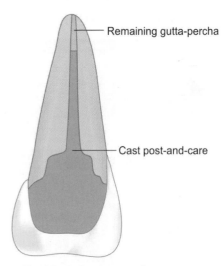

Fig. 27.15 Cast post-and-core system.

Components of the Restored Tooth (Fig. 27.14)

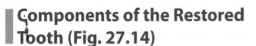

Components of the restored tooth
Parts of fully restored tooth:
- Residual tooth structure
- Restorative components:
  - Post
  - Core
  - Luting agent

Residual Tooth Structure

Prognosis of endodontically treated tooth depends on amount of remaining coronal tooth structure present above the marginal gingiva. A minimum of 1.5–2 mm of the axial wall height of the tooth structure with a thickness of ≥1 mm is shown to significantly reduce the incidence of fracture in nonvital teeth. This is referred to as the ferrule effect (for details please see page number 445).

Restorative Components

Post

It is a relatively rigid, restorative material placed in the root of nonvital teeth for retention of the core and to transmit the forces on the core to the root (*Cohen*). Traditionally, endodontically treated teeth received a post to reinforce them and a crown to protect them **(Fig. 27.15)**.

Purpose of using post

❏ It helps to retain the core
❏ It helps to distribute the stresses through the radicular dentin to the root apex

Earlier, it was believed that post strengthens or reinforces the tooth but it has been shown by various studies that posts actually weakens the tooth and increases the risk of root fracture. Therefore, a post should be used only when there is insufficient tooth structure remaining to support the final restoration.

Ideal requirements of a post
A post should
• Provide maximum protection of the root to resist root fractures
• Provide maximum retention of the core and crown
• Be easy to place
• Be less technique sensitive
• Have high strength and fatigue resistance
• Be visible radiographically
• Be biocompatible
• Be easily retrievable when required
• Be esthetic
• Be easily available and not expensive

Classification of Posts

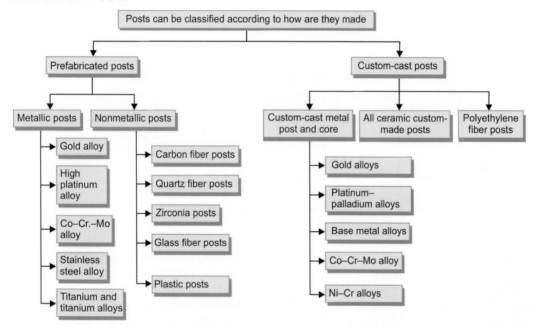

According to shape (Fig. 27.16)

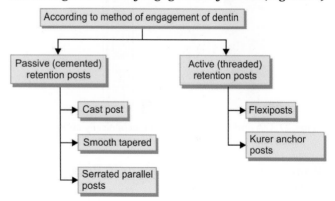

According to method of engagement of dentin (Fig. 27.17)

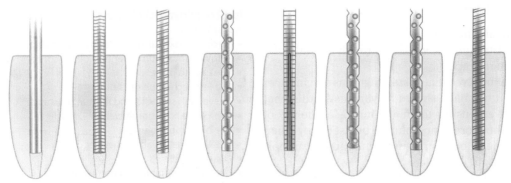

Fig. 27.16 Different types of posts designs like smooth, serrated, parallel, tapered, or combination.

According to material of the post

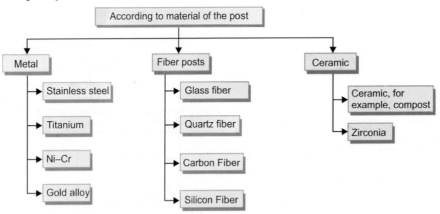

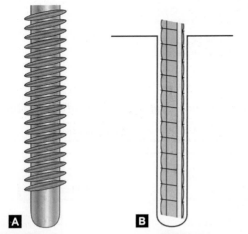

Figs. 27.17A and B (A) Active post mechanically engages the canal walls; (B) Cemented post.

Biomechanical Considerations in Post and Core-Treated Teeth

❑ The normal tooth under functional forces experiences bending stresses, with compressive stress on one side and tensile stress on the other

❑ In tooth restored with post and core, stress distribution pattern is different because post–core–tooth system bends as a single unit

❑ The difference in the stress distribution predisposes the tooth structure to increased stresses and fracture

❑ Tensile stresses from post are transmitted to the tooth with characteristic pattern depending on the modulus of elasticity (MOE) of post. MOE of the post should be as near as possible to that of dentin for the best stress distribution

❑ If a post has higher modulus than the tooth, the stress concentration is near the apical end of the post. This is evident in cases of rigid post where root fracture originates at the apex of the post

❑ When modulus of the post is similar to that of dentin, stress concentration is near the top of the post resulting in stress concentration near the cervical end. Thus nonrigid posts result in loss of marginal seal

Stresses produced in
- Tapered post > Parallel post
- Active posts > Passive post
- Shorter post > Longer post

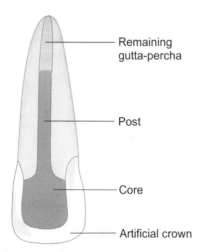

Fig. 27.18 Custom-made post and core.

Parallel post	Tapered post
• More retentive	• Less retentive
• Induce less stresses because of less wedging effects	• Causes more stresses because of wedging effects
• Less likely to cause root fracture	• Causes increased chances of root fracture
• Require more dentin removal	• Require less dentin removal

Custom-Cast Metal Post (Fig. 27.18)

The custom-fabricated cast gold post and core has been used for decades as foundation restoration. Custom-cast metal post is post of choice for single-rooted teeth, especially when remaining coronal tooth structure supporting the artificial crown is minimal (**Figs. 27.19 to 27.21**). In such case, post must be capable of resisting the rotation which can be better achieved by custom-cast posts.

Advantages

- ❑ Adaptable to large irregularly shaped canals
- ❑ Better core retention because core is an inherent part of the post
- ❑ In multirooted teeth, they are cost-effective
- ❑ Better choice for small teeth
- ❑ Beneficial in cases where angle of the core must be changed in relation to the post (**Figs. 27.22A and B**)

Disadvantages

- ❑ Requires more chair side time
- ❑ Very rigid so lead to greater stress concentration in root causing root or post fracture

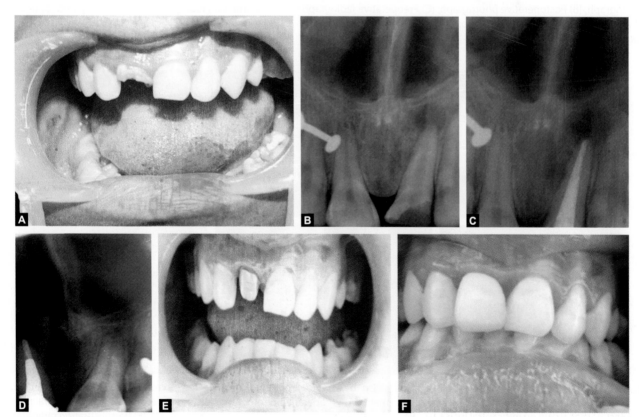

Figs. 27.19A to F Restoration of grossly carious 11 using cast post and core: (A) Preoperative photograph; (B) preoperative radiograph showing grossly carious 11; (C) Postobturation radiograph; (D) Canal space prepared cast and core post-cemented; (E) Trial fit of cast post and core; (F) Postoperative photograph.
Courtesy: Jaidev Dhillon.

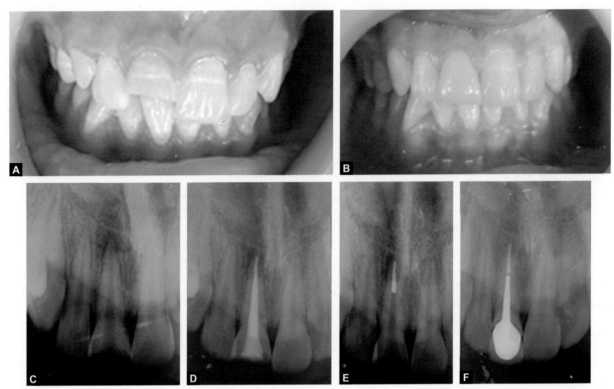

Figs. 27.20A to F Restoration of right maxillary central incisor using cast post and core followed by crown placement: (A) Preoperative photograph; (B) Postoperative photograph; (C) Preoperative radiograph; (D) Postobturation radiograph; (E) Space prepared for post; (F) Postoperative radiograph after cast post and core cementation.
Courtesy: Jaidev Dhillon.

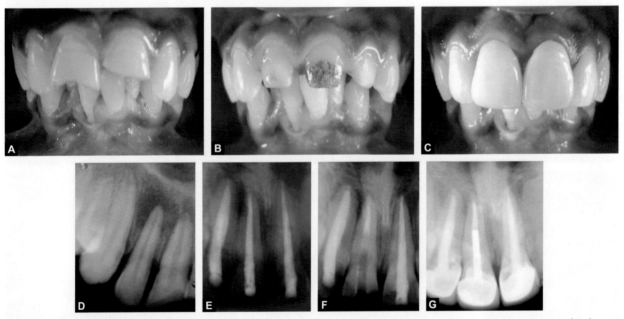

Figs. 27.21A to G Restoration of left maxillary central incisor by using cast post and core followed by crown placement and right central incisor by tooth preparation followed by crown placement: (A) Preoperative photograph; (B) Tooth preparation of right central incisor and cast post and core on left central incisor; (C) Postoperative photograph; (D) Preoperative radiograph; (E) Postobturation radiograph; (F) Space prepared for post; (G) Postoperative radiograph after cast post and core cementation.
Courtesy: Jaidev Dhillon.

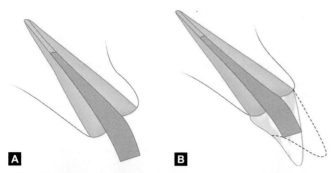

Figs. 27.22A and B Advantage of custom cast metal post when angle of core is to be changed in relation to post.

- Poor esthetics
- Require temporization
- Prone to corrosion
- Risk of casting inaccuracy
- Difficult retrieval
- Hypersensitivity in some cases because of Ni–Cr ions

All Ceramic Post and Cores

Advantages

- Excellent esthetics
- Biocompatibility
- Good radiopacity.

Disadvantages

- Brittle, so not indicated in high-stress conditions like bruxism
- Very rigid, so more risk of root or post fracture.

Prefabricated Posts (Figs. 27.23)

Indications of Prefabricated Posts

- Sufficient width and length of root structure is present
- Roots are of circular cross section, for example, roots of maxillary premolars
- Gross undercuts in root canals make pattern fabrication for cast posts difficult.

Prefabricated Metal Posts

These have been widely used for the past 20 years. They are available in various metal alloys and can be available in active or passive forms.

Advantages

- Simple to use
- Less time consuming
- Easy retrieval (of passive posts)
- Available in various shapes and sizes

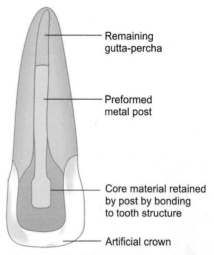

- Remaining gutta-percha
- Preformed metal post
- Core material retained by post by bonding to tooth structure
- Artificial crown

Fig. 27.23 Prefabricated post and core.

- Retentive with in the root especially serrated and parallel-sided posts
- Radiopaque
- Cost-effective.

Disadvantages

- Not conservative because root is designed to accept the post
- Cannot be placed in tortuous canals
- Poor esthetics
- Very rigid
- Difficult retrieval of active posts
- Prone to corrosion
- Tapered posts can have wedging effect in the canal.

Carbon Fiber Posts

Carbon fiber posts were introduced by Duret et al. in 1996 based on the carbon fiber reinforcement principle. Carbon fiber post consists of bundle of stretched carbon fibers embedded into an epoxy matrix. This was the first nonmetallic post introduced to the dentistry. The original form of carbon post was black and unesthetic.

Advantages

- Clinical procedure is less time consuming
- Strong but low stiffness and strength than ceramic and metal posts
- Easily retrievable
- Less chair side time
- Modulus of elasticity similar to dentin
- Biocompatible
- Good retention.

Disadvantages

- Black in color, so unaesthetic
- Radiolucent, so difficult to detect radiographically
- Flexural strength decreases by 50% by moisture contamination
- On repeated loading show reduced modulus of elasticity

Glass Fiber Post (Figs. 27.24 and 27.25)

It was introduced in 1992. It consists of unidirectional glass fibers embedded in a resin matrix which strengthens the dowel without compromising the modulus of elasticity.

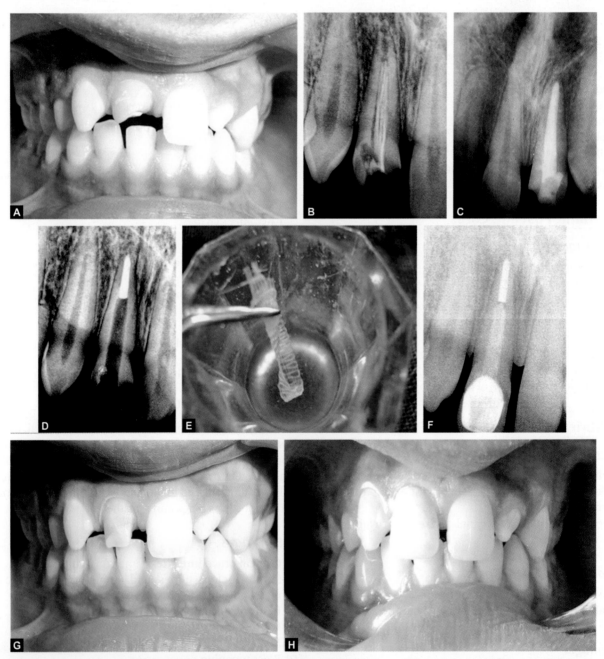

Figs. 27.24A to H Esthetic rehabilitation of a fractured right maxillary central incisor with custom-made fiber post: (A) Preoperative photograph; (B) Preoperative radiograph; (C) Postobturation radiograph; (D) Postspace preparation; (E) Customizing fiber post; (F) Radiograph after post cementation; (G) After tooth preparation; (H) Postoperative photograph.
Courtesy: Jaidev Dhillon.

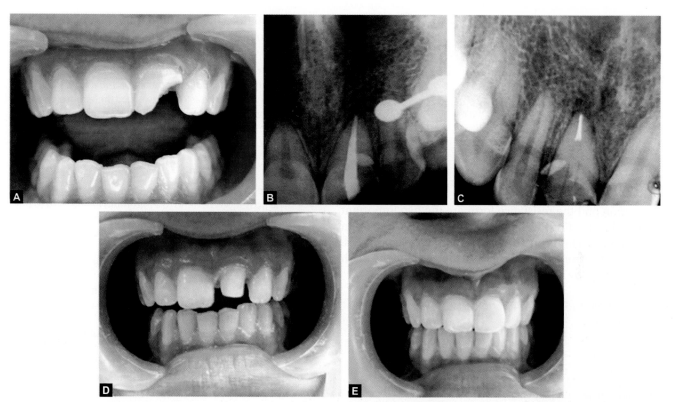

Figs. 27.25A to E Restoration of right maxillary central incisor using fiber post followed by crown: (A) Preoperative photograph; (B) Postobturation radiograph; (C) Radiograph after fiber post placement; (D) Composite core build up; (E) Postoperative photograph.
Courtesy: Jaidev Dhillon.

Advantages

- Esthetically acceptable
- Modulus of elasticity similar to dentin
- Biocompatible
- Distributes stresses over a broad surface area, thus increasing the load threshold
- Easy to handle and place
- Less time consuming
- Favorable retention in conjunction with adhesive bonding technique
- High resistance to fracture
- Easy retrieval

Disadvantages

- Poor radiographic visibility
- Expensive
- Technique sensitive

Zirconia Post

These were introduced in dentistry in the late 1980 by Christel et al. They are made from fine grained tetragonal zirconium polycrystals (TZP).

They possess high flexural strength and fracture toughness.

Advantages

- For teeth with severe coronal destruction, zirconia posts provide adequate strength
- Smaller zirconia posts can be used for an all ceramic post and core construction for narrower canals
- Combination of glass ceramic and zirconia ceramic can be used because of their similarity in coefficient of thermal expansion

Disadvantages

- Adhesion to tooth and composite is compromised which becomes a problem for retreatment
- They are brittle with high modulus of elasticity
- When used with direct composite resin buildup, high stresses and functional forces may lead to microleakage and their deformation because of high polymerization shrinkage and high coefficient of thermal expansion of composites
- Expensive

Factors to be Considered while Planning Post and Core (Fig. 27.26)

Following factors are considered while planning posts:
- ❑ Retention and resistance form
- ❑ Preservation of tooth structure
- ❑ Ferrule effect
- ❑ Mode of failure
- ❑ Retrievability

Retention and the Resistance Form

Retention and the resistance form are the two important properties affecting the longevity of the post. Postretention refers to the ability of post to resist vertical dislodging forces. Postresistance refers to the ability of the post and the tooth to withstand the lateral and rotational forces.

Factors affecting post retention	Factors affecting post resistance
• Post length	• Ferrule
• Post diameter	• Rigidity
• Post taper and design	• Post length
• Luting agent	• Antirotational groove
• Luting method	
• Canal shape	
• Position of the tooth in the arch	

Post Length

The length of the post is one of the most important factors affecting the longevity of the post. As the length of the post

increases, so does the retention. About 5% of the failures occur due to the loosening of the post.

Guidelines regarding post length (Figs. 27.27)
- *For metal posts (nonadhesive cementation):*
  - The post should be as long as two third the length of the canal
  - The length of the post should be at least the coronal length of the core
  - The post should be at least half the length of root in the bone

- *For fiber posts (adhesive cementation):*
  - The post should extend to a maximum of one third to one half the length of the canal
  - The length of the post should be at least the coronal length of the core

Other important factors to be considered in the selection of the post length include
- The post should be as long as possible without disturbing the apical seal. At least 3–5 mm of the apical gutta-percha should be retained
- To decrease the dentinal stress, the post should extend ≥4 mm apical to the bone crest
- Molar posts should not extend >7 mm apical to the canal orifice so as to avoid the risk of perforation of the root canal

Post Diameter

It has been seen that post diameter has little difference in the retention of post, but increase in post diameter increases the resistance form but it also increases the risk of root fracture **(Figs. 27.28A to C)**.

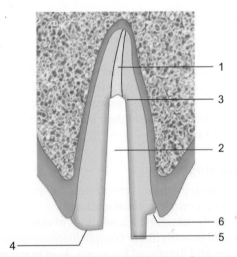

Fig. 27.26 Features of successful design of post and core. 1. Adequate apical seal, 2. Minimum canal enlargement,3. Adequate post length, 4. Positive horizontal stop, 5. Vertical wall to prevent rotation, 6. Extension of the final restoration margin onto sound tooth structure.

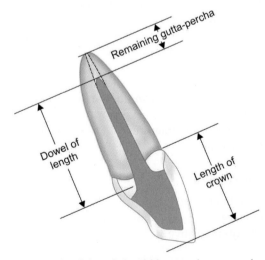

Fig. 27.27 Length of dowel should be equal to crown length or two-thirds the length of the root. The length of the remaining gutta-percha should be at least 3–5 mm.

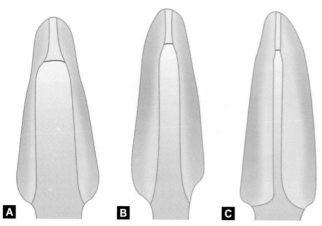

Figs. 27.28A to C (A) Too wide diameter of post space; (B) Optimum diameter of post space; (C) Too narrow diameter of post space.

Presently, there are three different theories regarding the post diameter in literature. These are

1. ***Conservationist (Fig. 27.29A):*** It suggests the narrowest diameter that allows the fabrication of a post to the desired length. It allows minimal instrumentation of the canal for post-space preparation. According to this, teeth with smaller dowels exhibit greater resistance to fracture
2. ***Preservationist (Fig. 27.29B):*** It advocates that ≥1 mm of sound dentin should be maintained circumferentially to resist the fracture

3. ***Proportionist (Fig. 27.29C):*** This advocates that post width should not exceed one third of the root width at its narrowest dimensions to resist fracture. The guideline for determining appropriate diameter of post involves mesiodistal width of the roots.

Post Taper and Design (Figs. 27.30A to G)
- ❑ Parallel-sided posts may distribute stress more evenly than tapered posts, which may have a wedging effect
- ❑ The parallel posts generate the highest stress at the apex
- ❑ High stresses can be generated during insertion, particularly with parallel-sided smooth post with no vent
- ❑ Threaded posts produce the high stress during insertion and loading.

Luting Agents (Figs. 27.31A to D)
The post is retained in the prepared post channel with dental cement. The factors that influence the durability of the bond of the post to the root are compressive strength, tensile strength and adhesive qualities of the cement, cement's potential for plastic deformation, microleakage and water imbibition.

The most common luting cements are zinc phosphate, polycarboxylate, glass ionomer, resin modified glass ionomer and resin-based cements. The primary disadvantage of zinc phosphate cement is solubility in oral fluids and lack of true adhesion. Resin modified glass ionomer cement is not

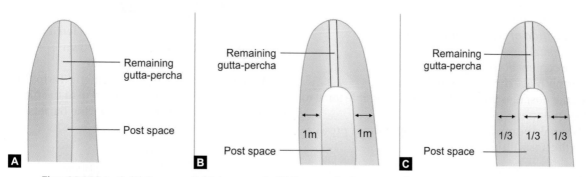

Figs. 27.29A to C (A) Conservationist approach; (B) Preservationist approach; (C) Proportionist approach.

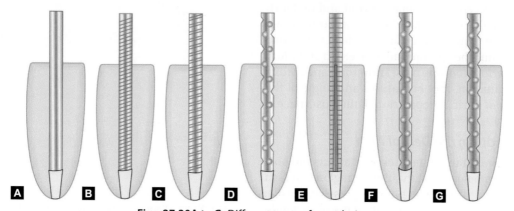

Figs. 27.30A to G Different types of post designs.

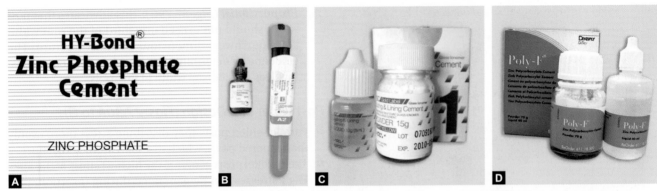

Figs. 27.31A to D (A) Zinc phosphate cement; (B) Resin cement; (C) Glass ionomer cement (luting); (D) Polycarboxylate cement.

indicated for post cementation, because of its hygroscopic expansion. Currently, trend is shifting toward the use of adhesive cements. The rationale for using these cements is that adhesive bonding to root canal dentin has strengthening effect on the tooth in addition to retention of the restoration. Disadvantage of resin cement is technique sensitivity. The bonding to root canal dentin can be compromised due to use of various irrigants and eugenol-based sealers. Eugenol can prevent or stop polymerization reaction and can interfere with bonding.

Luting Method

Luting method also affects the retention of post. Since luting agents are susceptible to moisture present in the canal, so canal should be absolute dry.

Optimal method of cementation of posts is

❑ Dry the canal
❑ Mix the cement according to instructions
❑ Uniformly place the cement in the canal
❑ Place the post into the canal with least possible force to reduce the stress
❑ Vents should be made to release the hydrostatic pressure when the posts thrust back

Canal Shape

The most common shape of canal is ovoid and prefabricated posts usually come parallel in shape, so these are unlikely to adapt along their entire interface with canal walls. To determine the appropriate post length and width to avoid root perforation, one must know root taper, proximal root invagination, root curvatures and angle of the crown to the root during preparation of the post space.

Position of Tooth in the Dental Arch

Location of the tooth in dental arch also affects the post retention. For example, maxillary anterior region is at high risk for failure because of effect of compressive, tensile, shearing and torquing forces especially at the post–dentin

interface. If all factors are equal, then post of posterior teeth tends to be more retentive than anterior ones.

Preservation of the Tooth Structure

One should try to preserve maximum of the coronal and radicular tooth structure whenever possible. Minimal removal of radicular dentin for post-space preparation should be the criteria. Further enlargement of posts only weakens the tooth. Various studies have shown use of bonded posts, but their strengthening effect degrades with time because of weakening of resin dentin bond as the tooth is exposed to functional stress.

Ferrule Effect (Fig. 27.32)

Ferrule is derived from a Latin word ferrum means iron, variola means bracelet, that is crown bracing against remaining supragingival tooth tissue.

As per "The Glossary of Prosthetic Terms" Ferrule is defined as "a metal ring/band used to fit the root or crown of a tooth. It can be correlated to wine barrels. The metal

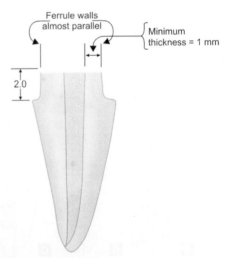

Fig. 27.32 Diagrammatic representation of ferrule effect.

band, which encompasses the wooden barrel, gives support when barrel is full."

According to Sorensen and Engelman, ferrule is defined as "360° metal collar of the crown surrounding the parallel walls of the dentin extending coronal to the shoulder of the preparation" **(Figs. 27.33A and B)**.

It has been seen that a ferrule with 1–2 mm of vertical tooth structure doubles the resistance to fracture than in teeth without any ferrule effect. This is called as crown ferrule that is, crown ferrule is ferrule created by overlying crown engaging the tooth structure. Core ferrule is part of cast metal.

Height of ferrule may vary according to different functional occlusal loading. For example, maxillary incisor needs longer ferrule on palatal aspect and mandibular incisor needs longer ferrule on labial aspect.

Sometimes when adequate tooth structure is not present, crown lengthening or orthodontic eruption is needed of a tooth to provide an adequate ferrule.

Requirements of the Ferrule

- ❑ The axial wall height of the ferrule must be ≥1–2 mm
- ❑ The ferrule should consist of parallel axial walls
- ❑ The margins of the preparation should rest on the sound tooth structure
- ❑ Restoration should completely encircle the tooth
- ❑ The restoration should not completely encroach on the biological width. A minimum of 4–5 mm of suprabony tooth structure should be available to accommodate for the restoration and attachment apparatus
- ❑ A ferrule with minimum thickness of 1 mm is needed to be effective

Functions of Ferrule

Sorensen and Engelman (1990) found that 1.5–2 mm of ferrule reduces the fracture resistance of endodontically treated teeth. They showed that protective effect of ferrule is because

- ❑ It dissipates the forces that concentrate at cervical area of clinical crown **(Fig. 27.34)**. Lack of ferrule may result in fracture because of forcing core, post and root to high-function stresses
- ❑ It protects integrity of root by bracing action **(Fig. 27.35)**
- ❑ It reduces the lateral forces exerted during post insertion
- ❑ It resists the wedging effect of the tapered posts
- ❑ It resists the functional lever forces

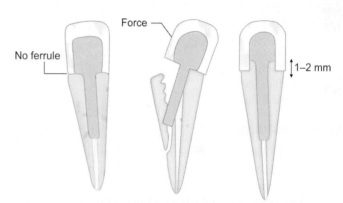

Fig. 27.34 Ferrule dissipates the forces that concentrate at the cervical area of tooth, thus it prevents fracture of tooth.

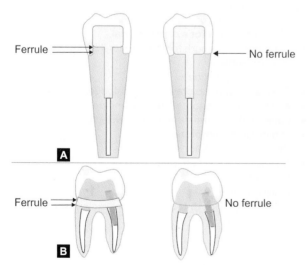

Figs. 27.33A and B Schematic representation of ferrule effect of (A) Anterior teeth; (B) Posterior teeth.

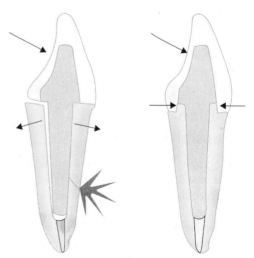

Fig. 27.35 Ferrule protects the integrity of root by bracing action.

Secondary Ferrule/Core Ferrule

Sometimes a contra bevel is given on a tooth being prepared for cast post with collar of metal which encircles the tooth. This serves as secondary ferrule independent of ferrule provide by cast crown.

Mode of Failure

All post systems show some percentage of failure but with variable range. Post failures are higher in cases of nonrestorable teeth.

Factors affecting clinical longevity of post and core

❏ Magnitude and direction of force
❏ Tooth type
❏ Thickness of remaining dentin
❏ Post selection
❏ Quality of cement layer

Failures of posts and core can occur in form of (Figs. 27.36A to E)

❏ Post fracture
❏ Root fracture
❏ Core fracture
❏ Post dislodgement
❏ Esthetic failures

Retrievability

Ideally, a post system selected should be such that if an endodontic treatment fails, or failure of post and core occurs, it should be retrievable.

Metal posts especially the cast post and core system is difficult to remove. Fiber posts are easy to retrieve, whereas zirconium and ceramic posts are difficult to remove.

Posts can be removed by
• Use of rotary instruments and solvents
• Use of ultrasonic
• Using special kits like Masserann kit, post-removal system and endodontic extractors

Preparation of the Canal Space and the Tooth

❏ Take radiograph and assess the case for length and diameter of the post according to the tooth type. Remove the gutta-percha filling from the root canal while maintaining the apical seal
❏ Prepare the canal space using Gates-Glidden drills or Peeso reamers (**Fig. 27.37**). The canal space enlargement depends on type of the post. If it is custom made, the main requirement is minimal space preparation without undercuts. For prefabricated post, generally specific penetration drills for each system are supplied for canal preparation
  • Various errors can occur during root canal preparation for post-space-like periapical extrusion of obturation material (**Fig. 27.38A**), disturbance of apical seal (**Fig. 27.38B**), overenlargement of the canal space (**Fig. 27.38C**) and perforation (**Figs. 27.38D and E**)
❏ Following the preparation of canal space, preparation of coronal tooth structure should be prepared in the same manner as if an intact crown irrespective of the remaining tooth structure (**Fig. 27.39**)
❏ Remove all the unsupported tooth structure (**Fig. 27.40**)
❏ Place an antirotational notch with the help of cylindrical diamond or carbide bur. This is done to provide the antirotational stability (**Fig. 27.41**)
❏ Ferrule effect is provided thereafter. The remaining coronal tooth structure is sloped to buccal and lingual surfaces so as to provide a collar around the occlusal circumference of the preparation (**Fig. 27.42**). This gives rise to 360° ferrule effect. Ferrule ensures that the final restoration encircles the tooth apical to the core and rests on sound tooth structure. It also presents the vertical root fracture by posts
❏ Finally, eliminate all the sharp angles, undercuts and establish a smooth finish line (**Fig. 27.43**)

Core

Core is the supragingival portion that replaces the missing coronal tooth structure and forms the center of new restoration. Basically, it acts as a miniature crown.

Core build-up materials available are
• Dental amalgam
• Resin modified glass ionomers
• Composite resin
• Reinforced glass ionomers cement

Ideal requirements for a core material
• Compressive strength to resist intraoral forces
• Biocompatibility
• Ease of manipulation
• Flexural strength to present core dislodgement
• Ability to bond to tooth structure and post
• Coefficient of thermal expansion similar to dentin
• Minimal water absorption
• Dimensionally stable
• No reaction with chemicals
• Low cost
• Easily available
• Contrasting color to tooth structure except when used for anterior teeth

Composite Resins

Composite resin is the most popular core material and has some characteristics of an ideal build-up material.

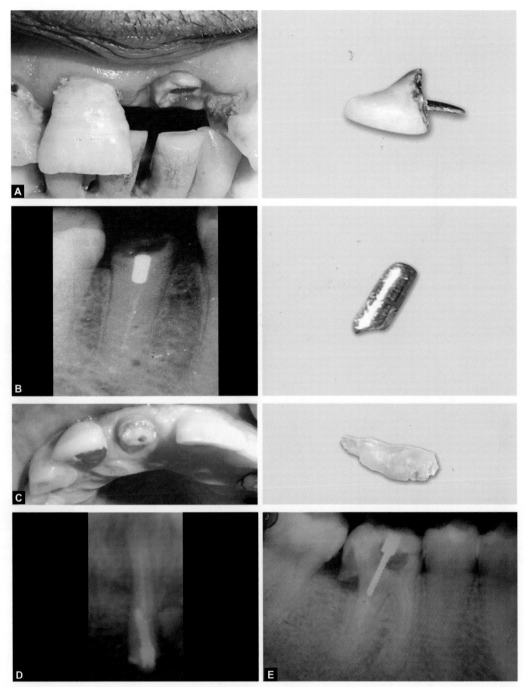

Figs. 27.36A to E Failures of post and core can occur in form of: (A) Dislodged post with crown in maxillary central incisor; (B) Fracture of cast post in mandibular premolar; (C) Fracture fiber post in maxillary lateral incisor; (D) Perforation of root with post in maxillary premolar; (E) Fracture tooth of mandibular molar with threaded screw post.
Courtesy: Vijay S Babloo.

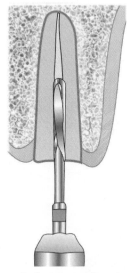

Fig. 27.37 Removal of gutta-percha using peeso reamer.

Advantages
- Bonded to many of the current posts and to the remaining tooth structure to increase retention
- High tensile strength and the tooth can be prepared for a crown immediately after polymerization
- It has fracture resistance comparable to amalgam and cast post and cores, with more favorable fracture pattern when they fail. It is tooth colored and can be used under translucent restorations without affecting the esthetic result

Disadvantages
- Composite shrinks during polymerization, causing gap formation in the areas in which adhesion is weakest. It absorbs water after polymerization, causing it to swell and undergoes plastic deformation under repeated loads
- Adhesion to dentin on the pulpal floor is generally not as strong or reliable as to coronal dentin. Strict isolation is an absolute requirement. If the dentin surface is contaminated with blood or saliva during bonding procedures, the adhesion is greatly reduced. Although composite resin is far from ideal, it is currently the most widely used build-up material

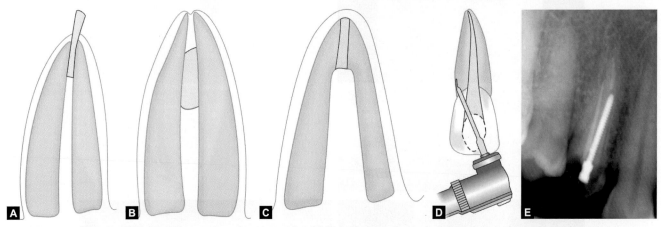

Figs. 27.38A to E (A) Periapical extrusion of gutta-percha; (B) Disturbance of apical seal; (C) Over enlargement of canal space; (D) Perforation due to misdirection of drill; (E) Perforation of root space due to misdirection of drills while preparing post space.

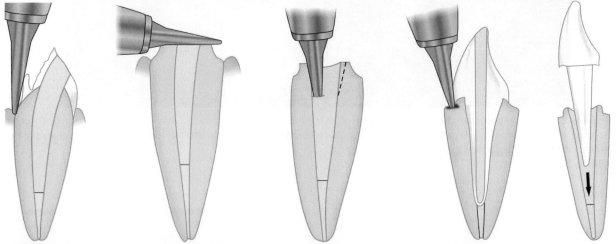

Fig. 27.39 Preparation of tooth structure.   **Fig. 27.40** Removal of unsupported tooth structure.   **Fig. 27.41** Place antirotational notch with the help of cylindrical diamond bur.   **Fig. 27.42** Preparation of ferrule effect.   **Fig. 27.43** Establish smooth finish line and remove all undercuts.

Cast Core

The core is an integral extension of the post and it does not depend upon the mechanical means of retention on the post. It prevents dislodgement of the core and the crown from the post. But sometimes valuable tooth structure must be removed to create path of withdrawal. Procedure is time consuming and expensive.

Amalgam Core

- ❏ Amalgam has been used as a build-up material, with well-recognized strengths and limitations. It has good physical and mechanical properties and works well in high-stress area
- ❏ In many cases, it requires the addition of pins or other methods to provide retention and resistance to rotation. Placement can be clumsy when there is minimal coronal tooth structure and the crown preparation must

be delayed to permit the material time to set. Moreover, amalgam can cause esthetic problems with ceramic crowns, it makes the gingiva look dark. There is a risk of tattooing the cervical gingiva with amalgam particles during the crown preparation.

- ❏ For these reasons and potential concern about mercury, it is no longer widely used as a build-up material. Amalgam has no natural adhesive properties and should be used with an adhesive system for buildup

Glass Ionomer Cements

The glass ionomer materials, including resin-modified glass ionomer, lack adequate strength and fracture toughness as a build-up material and should not be used in teeth with extensive loss of tooth structure. It is also soluble and sensitive to moisture. When there is minimal loss of tooth structure and a post is not needed, GIC works well for block out such as after removal of an MOD restoration.

S. No.		Advantages	Disadvantages	Indication	Precautions
1.	Amalgam	• Conservation of tooth structure • Easy	• Poor tensile strength • Corrosion	• Posterior teeth with adequate coronal structure	• Not used in anteriors
2.	Glass ionomer	• Conservation of tooth structure • Easy	• Low strength	• Teeth with adequate coronal structure	• Not used in teeth under lateral load
3.	Composite resin	• Conservation of tooth structure	• Low strength • Polymerization shrinkage	• Teeth with adequate coronal structure	• Not used in teeth under lateral load
4.	Custom-cast post	• High strength • Better fit	• Time consuming • Complex procedure	• For flared and elliptical canals	
5.	Parallel-sided prefabricated post	• Good retention • High strength	• Less conservation of tooth structure • Corrosion of stainless steel	• Circular canals	
6.	Tapered prefabricated post	• High strength and stiffness • Conservation of tooth structure	• Less retentive	• Circular canals	• Not used in flared canals
7.	Threaded post	• High retention	• Stress generation is more • Not conservation of tooth structure	• Only when more retention is required	

Biomechanical criteria for evaluation of core materials

Bonding (maximum to least)
Resin composites > glass ionomers> amalgam

Strength
Amalgam > resin composite > glass ionomers

Ease of use
Resin composites > amalgam > glass ionomers

Setting time
Resin composite > glass ionomers> amalgam

Dimensional stability
Amalgam > glass ionomers> composite resins

Custom-Made Post

A custom-made post can be cast from a direct pattern fabricated in the patient's mouth, or an indirect pattern can be fabricated in the dental laboratory.

Direct Procedure

- Lightly lubricate the canal and notch a loose fitting plastic dowel. It should extend to the full depth of the prepared canal. Use the bead-brush technique to add resin to the dowel and seat it in the prepared canal
- Do not allow the resin to harden fully with in the canal. Loosen and reseat it several times while it is still rubbery
- Once the resin has polymerize, remove the pattern
- Form the apical part of the post by adding additional resin and reseating and removing the post, taking care not to lock it in the canal
- Identify any undercuts that can be trimmed away carefully with scalpel

The post pattern is complete when it can be inserted and removed easily without binding in the canal. Once the pattern has been made, additional resin is added for the core.

Indirect Procedure

- Any elastomeric material will make an accurate impression of the root canal if a wire reinforcement is placed to prevent distortion
- Cut pieces of orthodontic wire to length and shape them like the letter J. Verify the fit of the wire in each canal. It should fit loosely and extend to the full depth of the post space. If the fit is too tight, the impression material will strip away from the wire when the impression is removed
- Coat the wire with tray adhesive. If subgingival margins are present, tissue displacement may be helpful. Lubricate the canals to facilitate removed of the impression without distortion
- Using a lentulo spiral, fill the canals with elastomeric impression material. Before loading the impression

syringe, verify that the lentulo will spiral material in an apical direction (clockwise). Pick-up a small amount of material with the largest lentulo spiral that fits into the post space
- Insert the lentulo with handpiece set at low rotational speed to slowly carry material into the apical portion of the post space. Then increase handpiece speed and slowly withdraw the lentulo from the post space
- This technique prevents the impression material from being dragged out. Repeat until the post space is filled
- Then insert the impression tray. Remove the impression, evaluate it and pour the working cast. In the laboratory, roughen a loose-fitting plastic post and, using the impression as a guide, make sure that it extends into the entire depth of the canal
- Apply a thin coat of sticky wax to the plastic post and, after lubricating the stone cast, add soft inlay wax in increments. Start from the most apical and make sure that the post is correctly oriented as it is seated to adapt the wax. When this post pattern has been fabricated, the wax core can be added and shaped

Core Fabrication

- The core of a post-and-core restoration replaces missing coronal tooth structure and thereby forms the shape of the tooth preparation. It can be shaped in resin or wax and added to the post pattern before the assembly is cast in metal. This prevents possible failure at the post–core interface
- The core can also be cast onto most prefabricated post systems (although there is then some concern that the casting process may unfavorably affect the physical properties of wrought metal posts)
- A third alternative is to make the core from a plastic restorative material such as amalgam, glass ionomer, or composite resin

Investing and Casting

- A cast post-and-core should fit somewhat loosely in the canal. A tight fit may cause root fractures
- The casting should be slightly undersized, which can be accomplished by restricting expansion of the investment (i.e., by omitting the usual ring liner or casting at a lower mold temperature)
- The casting alloy should have suitable physical properties. Extrahard denture gold (ADA Type IV) or nickel chromium alloys have high moduli of elasticity and are suitable for cast posts
- A sound casting technique is essential because any detected porosity could lead to a weakened casting that might fail in function. Casting a core onto a prefabricated post avoids problems of porosity

Evaluation

The practitioner must be particularly careful that casting defects do not interfere with seating of the post; otherwise, root fracture will result. Post-and-cores should be inserted with gentle pressure. However, the marginal fit of a cast foundation is not as critical as that of other cast restorations, because the margins will be covered by the final casting. The shape of the foundation is evaluated and adjusted as necessary. No adjustments should be made immediately after cementation because vibration from the bur could fracture the setting cement and cause premature failure.

Cementation

The luting agent must fill all dead space within the root canal system. Voids may be a cause of periodontal inflammation via the lateral canals. A rotary (lentulo) paste filler or cement tube is used to fill the canal with cement. The post-and-core is inserted gently to reduce hydrostatic pressure, which could cause root fracture. If a parallel-sided post is being used, a groove should be placed along the side of the post to allow excess cement to escape.

Conclusion

Following the endodontic treatment, it is necessary to restore the original morphology and function of the tooth which can be achieved by restoration of the endodontically treated teeth. The restoration should begin at the earliest possible because tooth exposed to oral conditions without optimal restoration cannot resist the occlusal forces and oral bacteria for a long period which can result in the treatment failure. Restoration of endodontically treated tooth begins with understanding of its physical and biomechanical properties and anatomy. Though various new materials have become available for past many years, yet the basic concepts of restoring endodontically treated teeth remains the same. Most post systems can be used successfully if basic principles are followed. After selection of the post system, finally it is the choice of core material and final restoration which increases the longevity of the treated tooth. Selection of post should be made by keeping in mind its strength, modulus of elasticity, biocompatibility, retrievability, esthetics and cost.

Questions

1. Enumerate various changes in a tooth caused by endodontic treatment.
2. Define post and core. What are indications and contraindications of post and core restoration?
3. Classify post. What are advantages and disadvantages of various posts?
4. Enumerate different core materials with their advantages and disadvantages.
5. What are the principles governing restoration for endodontically treated teeth? Describe the restorations given for endodontically treated teeth.
6. Define and classify post and core in detail.
7. Describe core materials, with their advantages and disadvantages.
8. Discuss in detail procedures of restoring a badly damaged endodontically treated posterior tooth.
9. Write short notes on:
   - Retention and resistance form of a post
   - Preparation of post space
   - Ferrule effect
   - Changes in tooth caused by endodontic treatment
   - Postendodontic restorations
   - Post and core
   - Core materials
   - Ferrule effect
   - Factors to be considered during post-selection
   - Carbon fiber post
   - Restoring endodontically treated tooth
   - Requirements of a post
   - Preparation of post space
   - Requirements of a tooth to accept post and core
   - Biomechanics of post retained restoration
   - Retention and resistance form of post
   - Ideal characteristics of a dowel
   - Glass fiber post
   - Zirconia post
   - Custom-made posts
   - Prefabricated posts.

Bibliography

1. Bakland I. Endodontics. 4th edition Malvern: Williams and Wilkins; 1994.
2. Block PL. Restorative margins and periodontal health: a new look at an old perspective. J Prosthet Dent 1987;57:683–9.
3. Burns C. Pathways to the pulp. 8th edition St Louis, MO: Mosby; 2002.
4. Caputo AA, Standlee JP. Pins and posts-why, when and how. Dent Clin North Am 1976;20:299–311.
5. Fernandes A, Rodrigues S, SarDessai G, Mehta A. Retention of endodontic post: a review. Endodontology 2001;13:11–18.
6. Freedman GA. Esthetic post and core treatment. Dent Clin North Am 2001;45:103–16.
7. Verissimo DM, Vale MS. Methodologies for assessment of apical and coronal leakage of endodontic filling materials a critical review. J Oral Sci 2006;48:93–8.
8. Vire DE. Failure of endodontically treated teeth: classification and evaluation. J Endod 1991;17:338–42.
9. Weine FS. Endodontic therapy. 6th edition St Louis, MO: Mosby; 2004.

Management of Traumatic Injuries

Dental traumatic injuries can manifest in many forms but cracked and chipped teeth are seen most commonly. Though these can occur at any age but most commonly seen at 1–3 years of age during which children are learning to walk (because their judgment and coordination is not fully developed). At 7–10 years of age, incidence increases due to increased sports activity. Type and number of teeth injured in accident vary according to type of accident, impact of force, resiliency of object hitting the tooth, shape of the hitting object and direction of force. If bone is resilient, tooth will be displaced by trauma but if bone is thick and brittle tooth will fracture.

Etiology of traumatic injuries
- **A**utomobile injury
- **B**attered child
- **C**hild abuse
- **D**rug abuse
- **E**pilepsy
- **F**all from height
- **S**ports-related injuries

   Risk factor for injuries is higher in the case of Angle's class II div 1 malocclusion and predisposing factors are high overjet, protrusion of maxillary incisors and insufficient lip closure.

Extent of trauma depends on (Hallet, 1954)
1. *Energy of impact:* Hitting object with more mass or high velocity creates more impact (energy = mass × velocity)
2. *Direction of impacting force*
3. *Shape* (sharp or blunt) *of impacting object*
4. *Resilience* (*hardness or softness*) *of impacting objec*t

▌Classification of Dentofacial Injuries

Purpose of classifying dental injuries is to provide description of specific condition allowing the clinician to identify and treat that condition using specific treatment remedies.

WHO Classification

WHO gave the following classification in 1978 with code no. corresponding to International Classification of Diseases.
- 873.60: Enamel fracture
- 873.61: Crown fracture involving enamel, dentin without pulpal involvement
- 873.62: Crown fracture with pulpal involvement
- 873.63: Root fracture
- 873.64: Crown root fracture
- 873.66: Luxation
- 873.67: Intrusion or extrusion
- 873.68: Avulsion
- 873.69: Other injuries such as soft tissue lacerations
- 802.20, 802.40: Fracture or communication of alveolar process which may or may not involve the tooth
- 802.21, 802.41: Fracture of boy of maxilla or mandible

Classification by Andreasen (1981)

Injuries to Hard Dental Tissues and Pulp

- Crown infarction N873.60: Incomplete fracture of enamel without loss of tooth substance

- Uncomplicated crown fracture N873.61: Fracture of enamel and dentin but not involving pulp
- Complicated crown fracture N873.62: Fracture of enamel and dentin exposing the pulp
- Uncomplicated crown root fracture N873.63: Fracture of enamel, dentin and cementum but not involving pulp
- Uncomplicated crown root fracture N873.64: Fracture of enamel, dentin and cementum and exposing pulp
- Root fracture N873: Fracture involving dentin, cementum and pulp.

Injuries to the Periodontal Tissues

- Concussion N873.66: An injury to tooth supporting structure without loosening or displacement of tooth but marked reaction to percussion
- Subluxation N873.66: An injury to tooth supporting with abnormal loosening but without displacement of tooth
- Intrusive luxation 873.66: Displacement of tooth into the alveolar bone. It is usually accompanied by fracture of alveolar socket
- Extrusive luxation 873.66: Partial displacement of tooth out of its socket
- Lateral luxation 873.66: Displacement of tooth in a direction other than axially. It is usually accompanied by fracture of alveolar socket
- Exarticulation 873.68: Complete displacement of tooth out of its socket

Injuries of Supporting Bone

- Communication of alveolar socket (mandible N802.20, maxilla 802.40): Crushing and compression of alveolar socket. This is normally found with intrusive and lateral luxation
- Fracture of alveolar socket wall (mandible N802.20, maxilla 802.40): Fracture contained to facial or lingual socket wall
- Fracture of alveolar process (mandible N802.20, maxilla 802.40): Fracture of alveolar process which may or may not involve socket
- Fracture of mandible and maxilla (mandible N802.20, maxilla 802.40): A fracture involving base of maxilla or mandible and alveolar process. Fracture may or may not involve alveolar socket

Injuries to Gingival or Oral Mucosa

- Laceration of gingiva or oral mucosa N873.69: Wound in mucosa resulting from tear and is normally produced by sharp object

- Contusion of gingiva or oral mucosa N902.00: Bruise resulting from impact of a blunt object and not associated with break in continuity in mucosa causing submucosal hemorrhage
- Abrasion of gingiva or oral mucosa N910:00: Wound resulting from rubbing or scraping of mucosa leaving a raw bleeding surface

Ingle's Classification

Soft Tissue Injury

- Laceration
- Abrasion
- Contusion

Luxation Injury

- Concussion
- Intrusive luxation
- Lateral luxation
- Extrusive luxation
- Avulsion

Tooth Fractures

- Enamel fractures
- Uncomplicated crown fracture
- Complicated crown fracture
- Crown root fracture
- Root fracture

Facial Skeletal Injury

- Alveolar process
- Body of mandible
- TMJ

Ellis and Davey's Classifications (1970) (Fig 28.1)

- Class I: Crown fracture involving enamel
- Class II: Crown fracture without involving the pulp
- Class III: Crown fracture involving pulp
- Class IV: Traumatized tooth becomes nonvital (with or without loss of crown structure)
- Class V: Tooth lost due to trauma
- Class VI: Fracture of root with or without fracture of crown
- Class VII: Displacement of tooth without crown or root fracture
- Class VIII: Fracture of crown en masse
- Class IX: Fracture of deciduous teeth

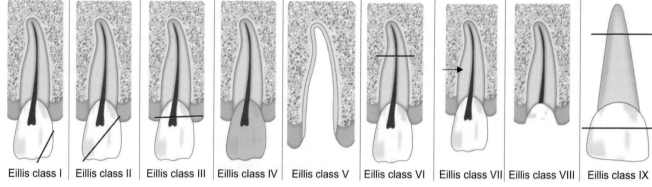

| Eillis class I | Eillis class II | Eillis class III | Eillis class IV | Eillis class V | Eillis class VI | Eillis class VII | Eillis class VIII | Eillis class IX |

Fig. 28.1 Schematic representation of Ellis and Davey's classification of dental traumatic injuries.

Classification by Heithersay and Morile

Heithersay and Morile recommended a classification of subgingival fracture based on level of fracture in relation to horizontal planes of periodontium as follows:

Class I: Fracture line does not extend below level of attached gingivae

Class II: Fracture line extends below attached gingivae but not below level of alveolar crest

Class III: Fracture line extends below level of alveolar crest

Class IV: Fracture line is within coronal third of root but below level of alveolar crest

History and Examination of Traumatic Injuries

A history of the injury followed by a thorough examination should be completed in any traumatic injury.

Dental History

Patient should be asked for pain and other symptoms and listed in order of importance to the patient.

- ❑ When did injury occur?: Time interval between injury and treatment affects the prognosis of injuries like avulsions, crown fractures (complicated or uncomplicated) and dentoalveolar fractures
- ❑ Where did injury occur?: This indicates the need for tetanus prophylaxis
- ❑ How did injury occur?: Nature of trauma can suggest type of injury expected
- ❑ Is there any lost teeth/fragments?: If there is loss of a tooth or fractured piece with history of loss of consciousness, a chest radiograph should be taken to exclude inhalation

- ❑ Previous dental history: Previous trauma can affect pulpal vitality tests and repair ability of the pulp. It can also affect attitude of the patient toward choice of treatment

Medical History

Patient should be asked for
- ❑ Allergic reaction to medication
- ❑ Disorders like bleeding problems, diabetes, epilepsy, etc.
- ❑ Any current medication patient is taking
- ❑ **Condition of tetanus immunization**—In case of contaminated wound, booster dose should be given if more than 5 years have elapsed since last dose. But for clean wounds, no booster dose needed, if time elapsed between last dose is less than 10 years

Extraoral Examination

If severe injury is seen, one should look for signs of shock (pallor, hypotension and irregular pulse). One should check for facial swelling, discoloration, or lacerations which may suggest injury to underlying bone and multiple tooth injury **(Fig. 28.2)**. Limited or deviated mandibular movements indicate jaw fracture or dislocation.

Intraoral Examination

A thorough systematic intraoral examination should be carried out.
- ❑ Laceration, hemorrhage and swelling of gingiva should be examined for tooth fragments etc.
- ❑ Look for abnormalities in occlusion, fractured crowns, or displacement of teeth

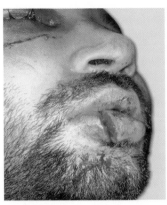

Fig. 28.2 Facial swelling, discoloration, or lacerations may suggest underlying bony and tooth injury.

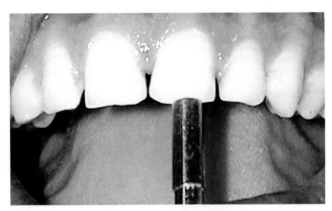

Fig. 28.4 Percussion to check integrity of periodontal ligament.

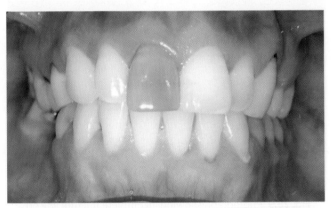

Fig. 28.3 Discolored maxillary right central incisor with history of trauma indicates its nonvital status.

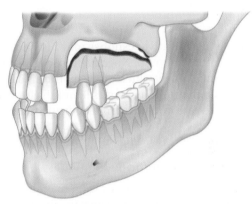

Fig. 28.5 Abnormalities in occlusion may indicate fracture of alveolar process or jaw.

- Color of tooth should be noted as it shows vitality of the pulp **(Fig. 28.3)**
- Reaction to percussion should be compared with a contralateral normal tooth (a dull sound indicates root fracture) **(Fig. 28.4)**
- Mobility should be tested in a horizontal and vertical direction. If multiple teeth move together, one should suspect fracture of the alveolar process **(Fig. 28.5)**. In case of excessive mobility, one should consider root fracture or tooth displacement **(Fig. 28.6)**
- Pulp vitality tests: Vitality tests should be performed at the time of initial examination and recorded to establish a baseline for comparison with subsequent repeated tests in future. One should not assume that teeth which give a positive response at initial examination will continue to give positive response and vice versa. A tooth with positive response may show

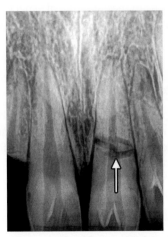

Fig. 28.6 If an isolated tooth shows excessive mobility, one should suspect root fracture. Radiograph showing root fracture of maxillary central incisor.

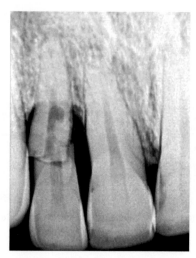

Fig. 28.7 Radiograph showing root fracture in maxillary incisor.

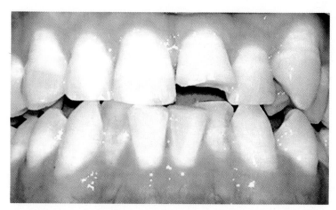

Fig. 28.8 Clinical photograph can be used as documentation for legal purpose.

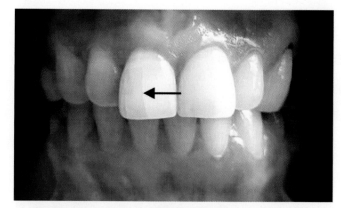

Fig. 28.9 Photograph showing incomplete fracture line on maxillary right central incisor.

necrosis and a negative response may not necessarily indicate a nonvital pulp. Negative response is due to a "shock-wave" effect which damages the apical nerve supply. Pulp may take as long as 9 months for normal blood flow to return to the coronal pulp of traumatized tooth.

Radiographic Examination

An occlusal exposure of anterior region may show lateral luxation, root fracture, or discrepancy in alveolar region. Periapical radiographs can assess crown and root fracture **(Fig. 28.7)**.

Three angulations recommended by *International Association of Dental Traumatology (IADT) are*
1. Occlusal view
2. Lateral view from mesial or distal aspect of the tooth
3. 90° horizontal angle with central beam through the tooth.

Clinical Photographs (Fig. 28.8)

Clinical photographs are helpful for establishing clinical record and monitoring treatment progress. They also help as additional means of documenting injuries for legal purposes and insurance.

▋ Crown Infraction

A crown infraction is incomplete fracture of enamel without loss of tooth structure **(Fig. 28.9)**. This type of injury is very common but often unnoticed. It results from traumatic impact to enamel and appears as craze line running parallel with direction of enamel rods and ending at dentinoenamel junction.

Biological Consequences

❑ Fracture lines are the weak points through which bacteria and their products can travel to pulp
❑ Crown infraction can occur alone or can be a sign of a concomitant attachment injury where force taken up by attachment injury leaves enough force to crack the enamel.

Diagnosis

❑ Tooth sustaining fracture is usually vital
❑ Easily recognized by viewing long axis of tooth from incisal edge

□ Examined by exposing it to fiber optic light source, resin curing light, indirect light, or by transillumination.

Treatment

Infracted tooth does not require treatment but vitality tests are necessary to determine extent of pulp damage.
□ Smoothening of rough edges by selectively grinding of enamel **(Figs. 28.10A and B)**
□ Repairing fractured tooth surface by composite if needed for cosmetic purposes **(Figs. 28.11A and B)**
□ Regular pulp testing should be done and recorded for future reference
□ Follow-up of patient at 3, 6 and 12 months interval is done

Prognosis

Prognosis is good for infraction cases.

█ Uncomplicated Crown Fracture

Crown fracture involving enamel and dentin but not pulp is called uncomplicated crown fracture **(Figs. 28.12 and 28.13)**. It occurs more frequently than the complicated crown fracture. This type of fracture is usually not associated with pain and it does not require urgent care.

Incidence

It accounts 26–92% of all traumatic injuries of teeth.

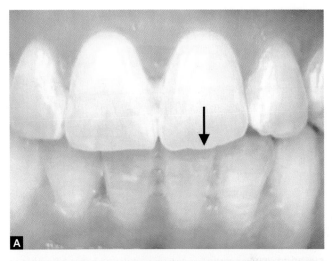

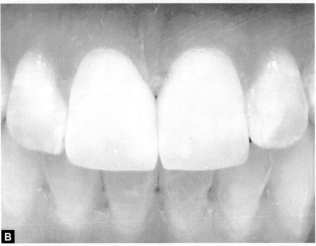

Figs. 28.11A and B Photograph showing: (A) Chipped off maxillary left central incisor; (B) smoothening and repair of incisor.

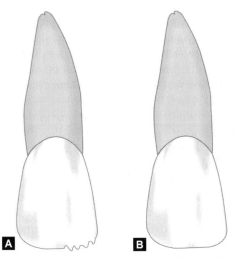

Figs. 28.10A and B Smoothening of rough edges by selective grinding of enamel: (A) Central incisor with ragged margins; (B) Smoothening of rough edges.

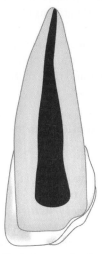

Fig. 28.12 Uncomplicated crown fracture involving enamel and dentin.

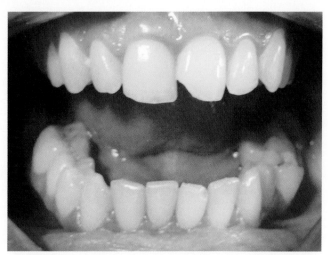

Fig. 28.13 Photograph showing uncomplicated crown fracture of maxillary left central incisor involving enamel and dentin.

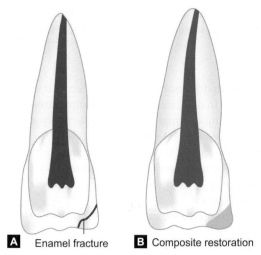

A Enamel fracture   B Composite restoration

Figs. 28.14A and B Repairing of fractured tooth surface by composite.

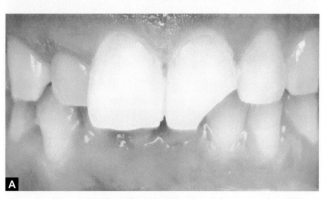

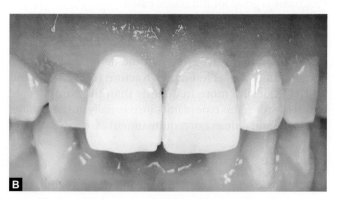

Figs. 28.15A and B (A) Ellis Class II fracture of maxillary left central incisor; (B) Composite buildup of fractured tooth.

Biological Consequences

- Minimal consequences are seen if only enamel is fractured but if dentin is exposed, a direct pathway for various irritants to pass through dentinal tubules to underlying pulp is formed
- Pulp may remain normal or get chronically inflamed depending upon proximity of fracture to the pulp, size of dentinal tubules and time of the treatment provided

Diagnosis

If dentin is exposed, sensitivity to thermal changes is seen.

Treatment

- Main objective of treatment is to protect the pulp by obliterating dentinal tubules
- *In the case of enamel fracture*, selective grinding of incisal edge is done to remove sharp edges and prevent injury to lips, tongue, etc.
- For esthetic reasons, composite restoration is done (**Figs. 28.14 to 28.16**)

If both enamel and dentin are involved, a restoration is done to seal the dentinal tubules and restore the esthetics.

Dentinal tubules can be sealed using calcium hydroxide, zinc oxide eugenol cement, glass ionomer cement, or dentin bonding agent. But eugenol cement should not be used where composite restoration is to be placed because eugenol may interfere with polymerization of composites.

If the fracture fragment of crown is available, reattach it (Figs. 28.17 A to C).

Following modifications are made for reattachment of fractured fragment:

- *Beveling of enamel:* Beveling helps to increase retention of fragment by increasing area for bonding and altering enamel prism orientation
- *Internal dentinal groove:* Internal dentinal groove is used as reinforcement for fragment but it compromises the esthetics because of internal resin composite
- *Internal enamel groove:* Here V-shaped retention groove is placed in enamel to which fragment is attached. But due to limited thickness of enamel, this procedure is difficult to perform

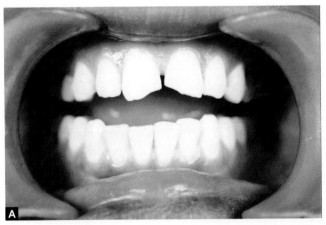
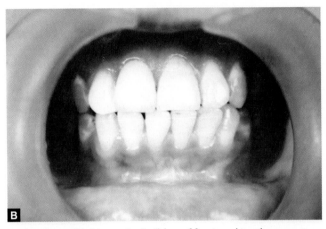

Figs. 28.16A and B (A) Ellis Class II fracture of maxillary central incisors; (B) Composite buildup of fractured teeth.

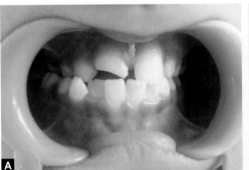
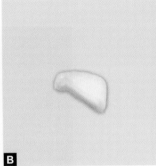
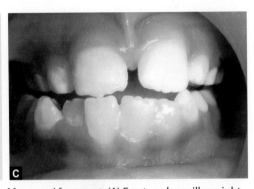

Figs. 28.17A to C Management of maxillary right central incisor by reattachment of fractured fragment: (A) Fractured maxillary right central incisor; (B) Fracture segment; (C) Reattachment of the fractured segment with composite.

❑ ***Overcontouring:*** This technique is used when fracture line is still noticeable after reattachment. Here, after joining the fractured fragment, a composite layer of 0.3 mm is placed superficially on buccal surface. But composite can show abrasion and discoloration with time

❑ ***Simple reattachment:*** In this, fragment is reattached using bonding agent without any additional preparation

Prognosis

Patient should be recalled and sensitivity testing is done at regular interval of 3, 6 and 12 months. Prognosis is good.

Complicated Crown Fracture

Crown fracture involving enamel, dentin and pulp is called complicated crown fracture (**Figs. 28.18 and 28.19**).

Incidence

This type of fracture occurs in 2–13 % of all dental injuries.

Biological Consequences

❑ Extent of fracture helps to determine the pulpal treatment and restorative needs
❑ Degree of pulp involvement may vary from pin point exposure to total uncovering of the pulp chamber
❑ If left untreated, it can lead to pulp necrosis

Diagnosis

Diagnosis is made by clinically evaluating the fracture, pulp status and radiographs (**Fig. 28.20**).

Treatment

❑ Factors like extent of fracture, stage of root maturation are imperative in deciding the treatment plan for complicated root fracture. Maintaining the pulp vitality is the main concern of treatment

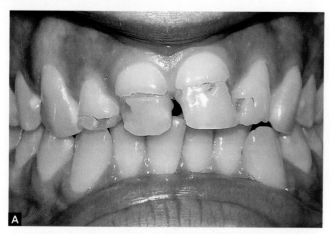
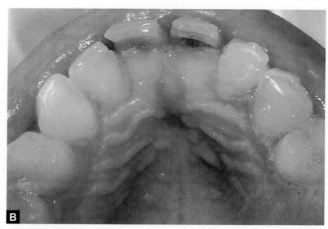

Figs. 28.18A and B Fracture of maxillary central incisors showing Ellis Class III fracture involving enamel, dentin and pulp.

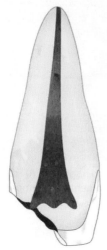

Fig. 28.19 Complicated tooth fracture involving enamel, dentin and pulp.

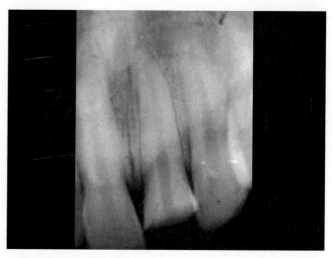

Fig. 28.20 Radiograph showing complicated tooth fracture.

❑ In the case of immature teeth, apexogenesis, which is normal process of root development, will occur only if pulp is vital

❑ Roots of immature teeth become thin and fragile near the apex. The goal of treatment is to allow the apex to mature and dentin walls to thicken sufficiently to permit successful root canal therapy

Factors Affecting Pulpal Survival

Optimal blood circulation is necessary to nourish the pulp and keep it healthy. Type of injury, stage of root development and degree of infection are the factors that affect circulation to the injured area and pulp vitality.

Pulp Capping and Pulpotomy

Pulp capping and pulpotomy are the measures that permit apexogenesis to take place and may avoid the need for root canal therapy. Choice between pulp capping and pulpotomy depends on

❑ Size of the exposure

❑ Presence of hemorrhage

❑ Time elapsed since injury

Pulp Capping

Pulp capping implies placing the dressing directly onto the pulp exposed (**Figs. 28.21A and B**).

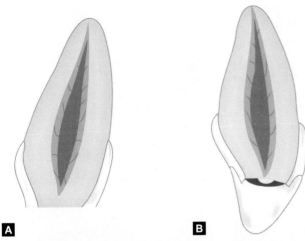

Figs. 28.21A and B Pulp capping is done by placing the dressing directly on to the pulp

Indications

It is indicated in case of very recent exposure (<24 h) with simple restorative plan

Technique

- ☐ After adequate anesthesia, apply rubber dam
- ☐ Rinse the exposed dentinal surface with saline followed by disinfection with 0.12% chlorhexidine or betadine
- ☐ Place calcium hydroxide or MTA over the exposed pulp
- ☐ Restore the tooth with permanent restoration.

Follow-up

Vitality tests, palpation tests, percussion tests and radiographs should be carried out at 3 weeks; 3, 6 and 12 months; and every 12 months subsequently to see continued root development.

Prognosis

Prognosis is up to 80% and it depends on:
- ☐ Ability of calcium hydroxide to disinfect the superficial pulp and dentin and to necrose the zone of superficially inflamed pulp
- ☐ Quality of bacterial tight seal provided by restoration.

Pulpotomy

Pulpotomy refers to coronal extirpation of vital pulp tissue. Two types:
1. Partial pulpotomy
2. Full (cervical) pulpotomy

Partial Pulpotomy/Cvek Pulpotomy

Partial pulpotomy implies the removal of the coronal pulp tissue to the level of healthy pulp **(Figs. 28.22 and 28.23)**.

Indications

It is indicated in vital, traumatically exposed, young permanent teeth with incomplete root formation. Objective is that remaining pulp tissue continues to be vital after partial pulpotomy.

Technique

- ☐ After anesthetizing the area, apply the rubber dam
- ☐ Prepare 1–2 mm deep cavity into the pulp using a diamond bur
- ☐ Use a wet cotton pellet to impede hemorrhage
- ☐ Place a thin coating of calcium hydroxide mixed with saline solution or anesthetic solution over it
- ☐ Seal the access cavity with hard setting cement like IRM

Follow-up

Satisfactory results and evaluation following pulpotomy should show
- ☐ Absence of signs or symptoms
- ☐ Absence of resorption, either internal or external
- ☐ Evidence of continued root formation in developing teeth

Prognosis

Prognosis is good (94–96%).

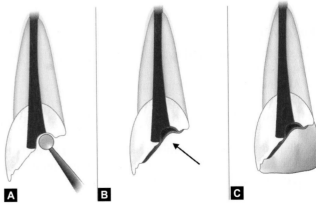

Figs. 28.22A to C (A) Removal of coronal pulp with round bur; (B) Placement of Ca(OH)$_2$ dressing over it and (C) Restoration of tooth using hard setting cement.

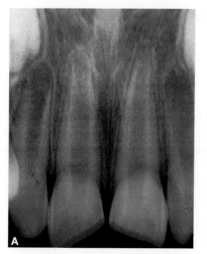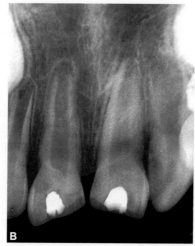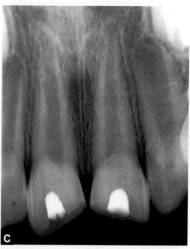

Figs. 28.23A to C Partial pulpotomy of maxillary traumatized central incisors with vital pulp allowing apexogenesis: (A) Preoperative radiograph; (B) Partial pulpotomy using calcium hydroxide; (C) Radiograph showing continuous development of root.

Cervical Pulpotomy/Deep Pulpotomy

Cervical pulpotomy involves removal of entire coronal pulp to the level of root orifices **(Fig. 28.24)**.

Indications

- When the gap between traumatic exposure and the treatment provided is >24 h
- When pulp is inflamed to deeper levels of coronal pulp

Technique

Coronal pulp is removed in the same way as in partial pulpotomy except that it is up to the level of root orifice.

Follow-up

Satisfactory results and evaluation following pulpotomy should show
- Absence of signs or symptoms
- Absence of resorption, either internal or external
- Evidence of continued root formation in developing teeth
- Main disadvantage of this treatment is that sensitivity tests cannot be done because of loss of coronal pulp. Thus radiographic examination is important for follow-up

Prognosis

80–95% success rate is reported.

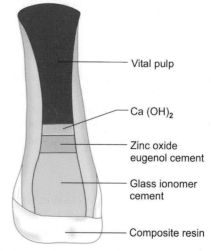

Fig. 28.24 Deep pulpotomy involves removal of entire coronal pulp, placement of $Ca(OH)_2$ dressing and restoration of the tooth.

Prerequisites for Success

Vital pulp therapy has an extremely high success rate if clinician strictly adheres to following requirements:
- *Treatment of a noninflamed pulp:*
  - Treatment of a noninflamed pulp is found to be better than the inflamed pulp. Therefore, optimal time for treatment is first 24 h when pulp inflammation is superficial
- *Pulp dressing:*
  - Calcium hydroxide is dressing of choice. It causes necrosis of superficial layers of pulp, which results in

mild irritation to adjacent vital pulp tissue. This irritation initiates an inflammatory response resulting in formation of hard tissue barrier
- Bioceramics like mineral trioxide aggregate (MTA), biodentine produce optimal results
- ❑ ***Bacterial tight seal:*** It is the most significant factor for successful treatment, because introduction of bacteria during the healing phase can cause failure.

Apexification

Apexification is a method of inducing calcific barrier at the apex of a nonvital tooth with incomplete root formation **(Fig. 28.25)**.
- ❑ Apexification using calcium hydroxide: After cleaning the canals, pack calcium hydroxide in to the canal till apical third. Place a cotton pledget and seal the coronal surface with IRM **(Fig. 28.26)**. When completion of hard tissue is suspected (after 3–6 months), remove calcium hydroxide and take radiograph. If formation of hard tissue is found satisfactory, obturate the canal using softened gutta-percha technique **(Fig. 28.27)**. One should avoid excessive lateral forces during obturation because of thin walls of the root
- ❑ Apexification using MTA: MTA is preferred over calcium hydroxide for apexification. After cleaning the canal, place calcium hydroxide for 1 week. After 1 week, remove the calcium hydroxide and fill apical 3–5 mm with MTA. Place a moist cotton pledget and temporary restoration over it. After 24 hours, root canal is obturated coronal to MTA using thermoplasticized gutta-percha

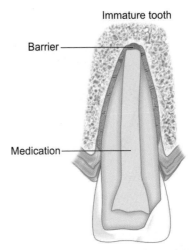

Fig. 28.26 Apexification using calcium hydroxide.

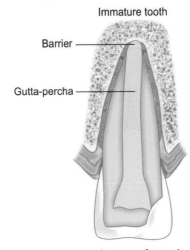

Fig. 28.27 If hard tissue barrier is formed, root canal can be filled using gutta-percha.

▌ Crown Root Fracture

Crown root fracture involves enamel, dentin and cementum with or without the involvement of pulp **(Fig. 28.28)**. It is usually oblique in nature involving both crown and root **(Fig. 28.29)**. This type of injury is considered as more complex type of injury because of its greater severity and involvement of the pulp **(Figs. 28.30 and 28.31)**.

Incidence

It contributes 5% of total dental injuries. In anterior teeth, it occurs by direct trauma causing chisel type fracture

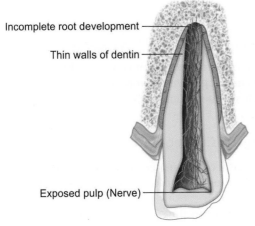

Fig. 28.25 Apexification stimulates hard tissue barrier across the apex.

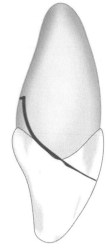

Fig. 28.28 Crown root fracture.

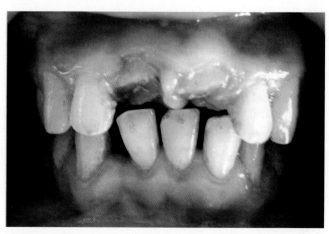

Fig. 28.31 Photograph showing complicated crown fracture in maxillary right central incisor and crown root fracture in left central incisor.

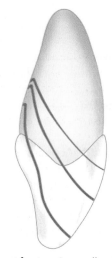

Fig. 28.29 Crown root fracture is usually oblique in nature.

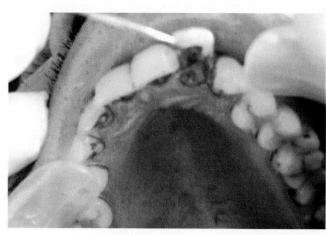

Fig. 28.32 Chisel-shaped fracture of 22 splitting crown and root.

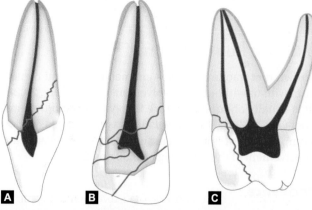

Figs. 28.30A to C Oblique type of fracture is considered as more complex because of its severity and pulp involvement.

which splits crown and root **(Fig. 28.32)**. In posterior teeth, fracture is rarely seen but it can occur because of indirect trauma like large-sized restorations, pin placements, high-speed instrumentation, etc.

Biological Consequences

❑ Biological consequences are similar to as that of complicated or uncomplicated fracture depending upon pulp involvement
❑ In addition to these, periodontal complications are also present because of encroachment of attachment apparatus

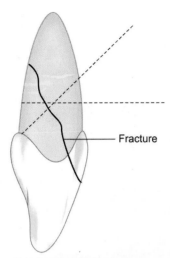

Fig. 28.33 Radiographs taken at more than one angle can show the extent of fracture.

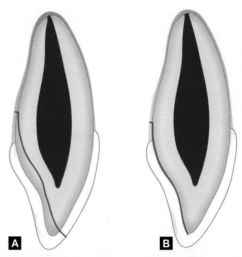

Figs. 28.34A and B Crown root fracture without pulp involvement can be treated by removing the coronal segment and restoring it with composite.

Diagnosis

Crown root fractures are complex injuries which are difficult both to diagnose and treat. A tooth with crown root fracture exhibits the following features:

- Coronal fragment is usually mobile. Patient may complain of pain on mastication due to movement of coronal portion
- Inflammatory changes in pulp and periodontal ligament are seen due to plaque accumulation in the line of fracture
- Patient may complain of sensitivity to hot and cold
- Radiographs are taken at different angles to assess the extent of fracture **(Fig. 28.33)**
- Indirect light and transillumination can also be used to diagnose this type of fracture

Treatment

Primary goal of treatment is the elimination of pain which is mainly because of mobile crown fragment. It can be done by applying bonding agents to bond the loose fragments together, temporary crown placement, or by using glass ionomer cement.

Objectives of treating crown root fracture are to:
- Allow subgingival portion of the fracture to heal
- Restoration of the coronal portion

Depending upon extent of fracture, the following should be considered while managing crown root fracture:
- If there is no pulp exposure, fragment can be treated by bonding alone or by removing the coronal structure and then restoring it with composites **(Figs. 28.34A and B)**
- If pulp exposure has occurred, pulpotomy or root canal treatment is indicated depending upon condition of the tooth
- When remaining tooth structure is adequate for retention, endodontic therapy followed by crown is done. If fractured fragment is available, one should attempt to reattach it **(Figs. 28.35A to H)**
- When root portion is long enough to accommodate a postretained crown, then surgical removal of the coronal fragment followed by surgical extrusion of the root segment is done **(Figs. 28.36A and B)**
- To accommodate a postretained crown, after removal of the crown portion, orthodontic extrusion of root can also be done **(Figs. 28.37A and B)**
- When the fracture extends below the alveolar crest level, the surgical repositioning of tissues by gingivectomy, osteotomy, etc. should be done to expose the level of fracture and subsequently restore it

Prognosis

If pulp is not involved, condition should be evaluated from time to time. Long-term prognosis depends on quality of coronal restoration. Otherwise the prognosis is similar to complicated or uncomplicated fracture.

▌ Root Fracture

These are uncommon injuries but represent a complex healing pattern due to involvement of dentin, cementum, pulp and periodontal ligament **(Figs. 28.38 and 28.39)**.

Incidence

- Root fracture form only 3% of the total dental injuries
- These fractures commonly result from a horizontal impact and are transverse to oblique in nature
- These are most commonly seen in mature roots and least common in incomplete roots

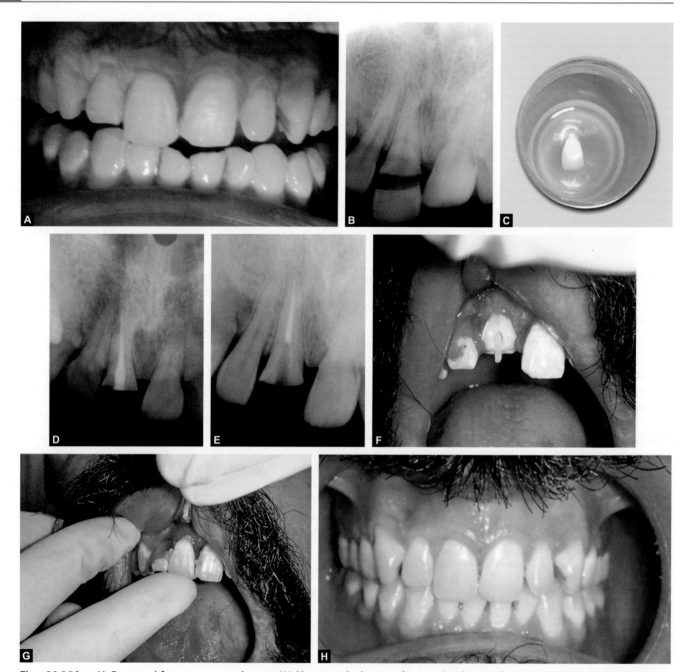

Figs. 28.35A to H Fractured fragment reattachment: (A) Photograph showing fractured right maxillary central incisor; (B) Radiograph showing oblique fracture in middle third of crown; (C) Fractured fragment removed and preserved in saline; (D) Postobturation radiograph of fractured tooth; (E) Post-space preparation; (F) Fiber post cementation; (G) Reattachment of fractured fragment; (H) Postoperative photograph.

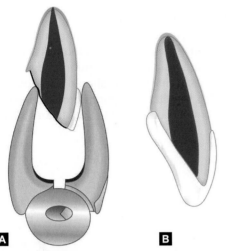

Figs. 28.36A and B When root portion is long enough to accommodate post-supported crown, remove the coronal segment, extrude root fragment, and perform endodontic therapy.

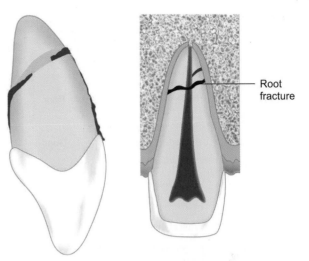

Root fracture

Fig. 28.38 Root fracture involves dentin, cementum, and periodontal ligament.

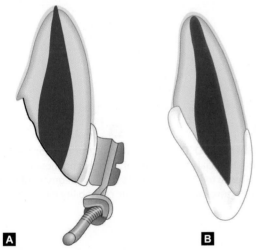

Figs. 28.37A and B (A) Orthodontic extrusion of root; (B) Restoration of tooth after endodontic therapy.

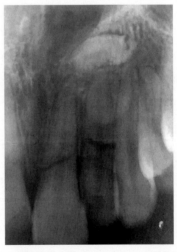

Fig. 28.39 Root fracture at cervical third.

Classification of Root Fracture (Fig. 28.40)

Biological Consequences

When root fractures occur horizontally, coronal segment is displaced to varying degrees. If vasculature of apical segment is not affected, it rarely becomes necrotic.

Diagnosis

❑ Displacement of coronal segment usually reflects the location of fracture **(Figs. 28.41A to D)**

❑ Radiographs at varying angles (usually at 45°, 90° and 110°) are mandatory for diagnosing root fractures **(Figs. 28.42A and B)**

Treatment of Root Fractures

Prognosis of root fracture depends upon
- *Amount of dislocation and degree of mobility of coronal segment*: More is the dislocation, poorer is the prognosis
- *Stage of tooth development*: More immature the tooth, better the ability of pulp to recover from trauma

			Prognosis
Type	Horizontal		Good
	Vertical		Poor
Extension	Partial		Good
	Complete		Poor
Location	Apical third		Good
	Middle third		Good
	Cervical third		Poor
Number	Simple		Good
	Multiple		Poor
Position of root fragments	Fragments not displaced		Good
	Fragments displacement		Poor

Fig. 28.40 Classification of root fracture and prognosis.

Apical Third Fracture

- ❏ Prognosis is good if fracture is at apical third level provided there is no mobility and tooth is asymptomatic
- ❏ To facilitate pulpal and periodontal ligament healing, displaced coronal portion should be repositioned accurately. It is stabilized by splinting for 2–3 weeks and tooth is kept out of occlusion (**Figs. 28.43 and 28.44**)

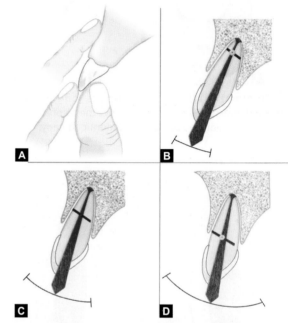

Figs. 28.41A to D Diagnosis of location of root fracture: (A) Palpating the facial mucosa with one finger and moving crown with other finger; (B to D) Arc of mobility of incisal segment of tooth with root. As fracture moves incisally, arc of mobility increases.

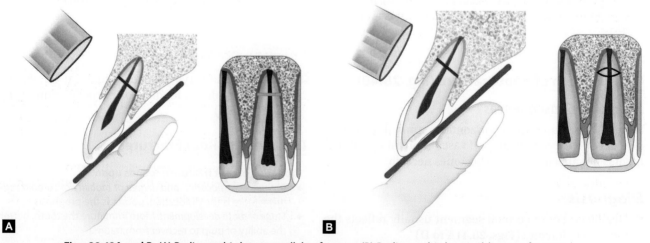

Figs. 28.42A and B (A) Radiographic beam parallel to fracture; (B) Radiographic beam oblique to fracture.

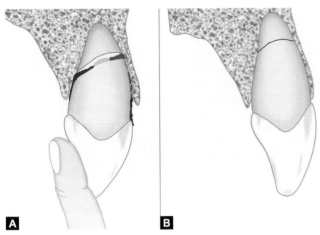

Figs. 28.43A and B If there is no mobility and tooth is asymptomatic with only apical third involvement (A), the displaced coronal segment is repositioned accurately (B) and stabilized.

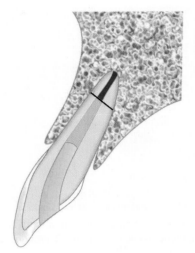

Fig. 28.45 Endodontic treatment of coronal segment only when apical segment contains vital pulp.

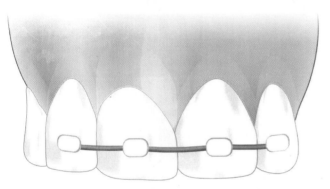

Fig. 28.44 Splinting of teeth.

❑ Since apical third has vital pulp, prognosis is good. If pulp in coronal third is also vital and tooth is made stable, no additional treatment is needed
❑ If pulp in coronal portion is nonvital, then root canal therapy of coronal segment and no treatment of apical segment is suggested **(Fig. 28.45)**
❑ If tooth fails to recover, surgical removal of apical segment is suggested **(Fig. 28.46)**

Mid-Root Fracture

Treatment plan and prognosis of mid-root fracture depend upon
❑ Mobility of coronal segment
❑ Location of fracture line
❑ Status of pulp
❑ Position of tooth after fracture

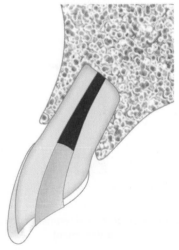

Fig. 28.46 Endodontic treatment of coronal segment with surgical removal of apical part.

Various treatment options are
❑ Root canal therapy for both coronal and apical segment, when they are not separated **(Figs. 28.47A to D)**
❑ Root canal therapy for coronal segment and surgical removal of apical third if apical segment is separated
❑ Apexification procedure of coronal segment, i.e. inducing hard tissue barrier at exit of coronal root canal and no treatment of apical segment. Other method is to use MTA for creating apical barrier in coronal segment. This is the most commonly used procedure nowadays **(Fig. 28.48)**

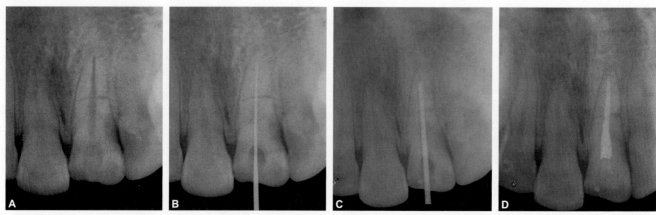

Figs. 28.47A to D Root canal treatment of both apical and coronal portion done in the case of root fracture of left maxillary central incisor. (A) Preoperative radiograph; (B) Working length radiograph; (C) Master cone radiograph; (D) Postobturation radiograph.

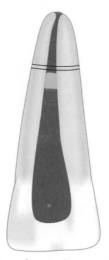

Fig. 28.48 Apexification of coronal segment and no treatment of apical segment.

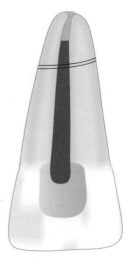

Fig. 28.49 Treatment of root fracture involves repositioning of tooth and intraradicular splinting.

❑ Intraradicular splint in which rigid type of post is used to stabilize the two root segments **(Fig. 28.49)**
❑ Endodontic implants, here, the apical portion of implant replaces the surgically removed apical root segment **(Fig. 28.50)**

Coronal Third–Root Fracture

❑ Prognosis is poor because it is difficult to immobilize the tooth
❑ Because of constant movement of tooth, repair does not take place

❑ If fracture level is at or near the alveolar crest, root extrusion is indicated. Here coronal segment is removed and apical segment is extruded orthodontically to allow restoration of missing coronal tooth structure **(Fig. 28.51)**

Healing of Root Fracture

According to the Andreasen and Hjorting-Hansen, root fracture can show healing in the following ways:
❑ Healing with calcified tissue in which fractured fragments are in close contact **(Fig. 28.52A)**

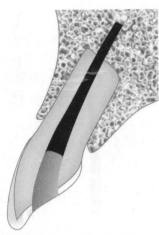

Fig. 28.50 Endodontic implant replaces the surgically removed apical portion of the root.

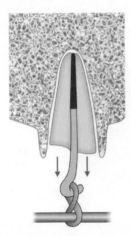

Fig. 28.51 Orthodontic extrusion of apical segment.

□ Healing with interproximal connective tissue in which radiographically fragments appear separated by a radiolucent line **(Fig. 28.52B)**

□ Healing with interproximal bone and connective tissues. Here fractured fragments are seen separated by a distinct bony bridge radiographically **(Fig. 28.52C)**

□ Interproximal inflammatory tissue without healing, radiographically it shows widening of fracture line **(Fig. 28.52D).**

Follow-up Procedure

□ Pulp testing and radiographic examination should be performed at 3 weeks, 6 weeks, 6 and 12 months after the injury

□ Radiographs are taken to predict healing of root fracture. Resorption within the root canal originating at fracture line indicates healing following pulpal damage after trauma. But resorption within the bone at the level of fracture line indicates pulp necrosis which requires endodontic therapy.

▌Luxation Injuries

Luxation injuries cause trauma to supporting structures of teeth ranging from minor crushing of periodontal ligament and neurovascular supply of pulp to total displacement of teeth. These are caused by sudden impact such as blow, fall, or striking a hard object.

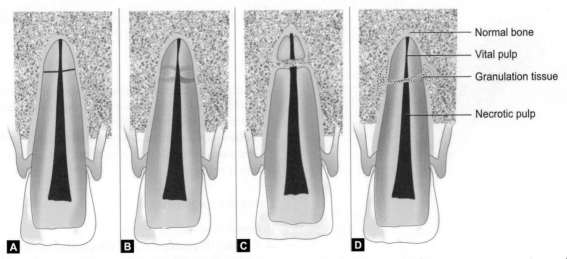

— Normal bone
— Vital pulp
— Granulation tissue
— Necrotic pulp

Figs. 28.52A to D Healing of root fracture can occur by: (A) Calcified tissue; (B) Interproximal inflammatory tissue seen in root fracture; (C) Interproximal bone; (D) Formation of connective tissue between the segments.

Incidence

Luxation injuries account for 30–40% of all dental injuries.

Types of luxation injuries:
- Concussion
- Subluxation
- Lateral luxation
- Extrusive luxation
- Intrusive luxation

Concussion

In concussion (**Fig. 28.53**):
- Tooth is not displaced
- Mobility is not present
- Tooth is tender to percussion because of edema and hemorrhage in the periodontal ligament
- Pulp may respond normal to testing.

Subluxation

In subluxation
- Teeth are sensitive to percussion and have some mobility
- Sulcular bleeding is seen showing damage and rupture of the periodontal ligament fibers (**Fig. 28.54**)
- Pulp responds normal to testing
- Tooth is not displaced.

Treatment of Concussion and Subluxation

- Rule out the root fracture by taking radiographs
- Relieve the occlusion by selective grinding of opposing teeth (**Figs. 28.55A and B**)
- Immobilize the injured teeth.

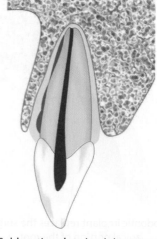

Fig. 28.54 Subluxation showing injury to periodontium.

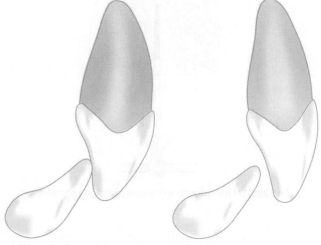

Figs. 28.55A and B Treatment of injury by selective grinding of tooth.

- Endodontic therapy should not be carried out at first visit because both negative testing results and crown discoloration can be reversible

  Follow-up is done at 3 weeks, 3, 6 and 12 months

  Prognosis there is only a minimal risk of pulp necrosis and root resorption

Lateral Luxation

In lateral luxation:
- Trauma displaces the tooth lingually, buccally, mesially, or distally, in other words out of its normal position away from its long axis (**Fig. 28.56**)

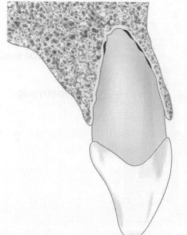

Fig. 28.53 Concussion.

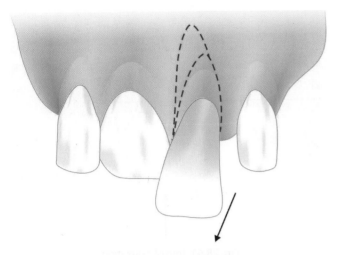

Fig. 28.56 Lateral luxation.

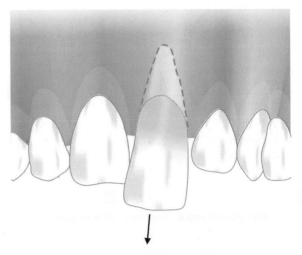

Fig. 28.58 Extrusive luxation.

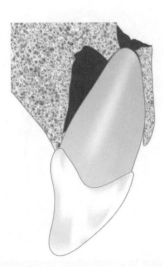

Fig. 28.57 Lateral luxation resulting in injury to periodontium.

□ Sulcular bleeding is present indicating rupture of periodontal ligament (PDL) fibers (Fig. 28.57)
□ Tooth is sensitive to percussion
□ Clinically, crown of laterally luxated tooth is usually displaced horizontally with tooth locked firmly in the new position. Here percussion may elicit metallic tone indicating that root has forced into the alveolar bone.

Extrusive Luxation

In extrusive luxation:
□ Tooth is displaced from the socket along its long axis (Fig. 28.58)
□ Tooth is very mobile
□ Radiograph shows the displacement of tooth.

Treatment of Lateral and Extrusive Luxation

Treatments of these injuries consist of atraumatic repositioning and fixation of teeth which prevents excessive movement during healing.

Repositioning of laterally luxated teeth require minimal force for repositioning. Before repositioning laterally luxated teeth, anesthesia should be administrated. Tooth must be dislodged from the labial cortical plate by moving it coronally and then apically. Thus tooth is first moved coronally out of the buccal plate of bone and then fitted into its original position (Figs. 28.59A and B).

For repositioning of extruded tooth, a slow and steady pressure is required to displace the coagulum formed between root apex and floor of the socket (Figs. 28.60A and B). After, this tooth is immobilized, stabilized and splinted for approximately 2 weeks. Local anesthesia is not needed while doing this.

Follow-up: Splint is removed 2 weeks after extrusion. If tooth has become nonvital, inflammatory root resorption can occur, requiring immediate endodontic therapy.

Pulp testing should be performed on regular intervals.

Prognosis

It depends on stage of root development at the time of injury. Commonly seen sequelae of luxation injuries are pulp necrosis, root canal obliteration and root resorption.

Intrusive Luxation

In intrusive luxation:
□ Tooth is forced into its socket in an apical direction (Fig. 28.61)
□ It is the most damaging injury to a tooth. In other words, it results in maximum damage to pulp and the supporting structures (Fig. 28.62)

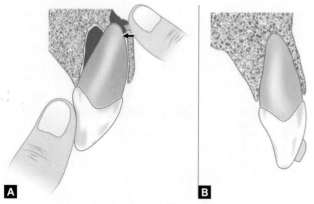

Figs. 28.59A and B Treatment of lateral luxation.

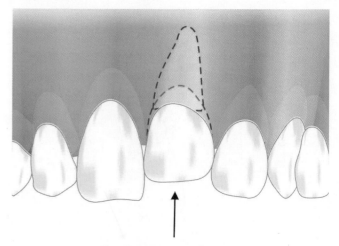

Fig. 28.61 Intrusive luxation.

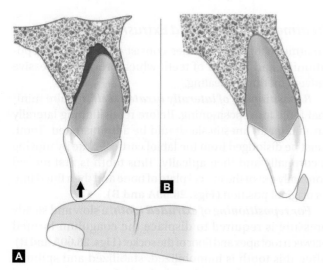

Figs. 28.60A and B Treatment of extrusive luxation.

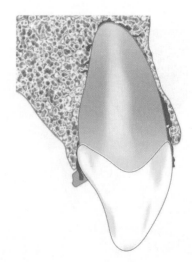

Fig. 28.62 Damage to periodontium by intrusive luxation.

❑ When examined clinically, the tooth is in infraocclusion
❑ Tooth presents with clinical presentation of ankylosis because of being firm in socket
❑ On percussion metallic sound is heard
❑ In mixed dentition, diagnosis is more difficult as intrusion can mimic a tooth undergoing eruption
❑ Radiographic evaluation is needed to know the position of tooth

Treatment

Healing following the intrusive luxation is complicated because intensive injury to the PDL can lead to replacement resorption and further dentoalveolar ankylosis. Pulp is also affected by this type of injury. So the main objective of treatment is to reduce the extent of these complications. Treatment mainly depends upon stage of root development.

In immature teeth, spontaneous re-eruption is usually seen. If re-eruption stops before normal occlusion is attained, orthodontic movement is initiated before tooth gets ankylosed **(Fig. 28.63)**.

If tooth is severely intruded, surgical access is made to the tooth to attach orthodontic appliances and extrude the tooth.

Tooth can also be repositioned by loosening the tooth surgically and aligning it with the adjacent teeth.

Follow-up

Regular clinical and radiographic evaluation is needed in this case because of frequent occurrence of pulpal and periodontal healing complications.

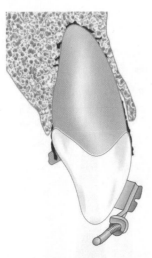

Fig. 28.63 Orthodontic extrusion of intruded tooth.

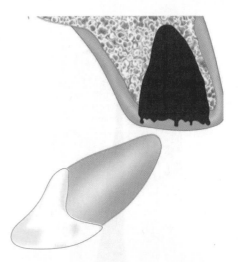

Fig. 28.65 Periodontium of avulsed tooth.

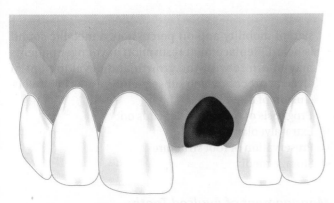

Fig. 28.64 Avulsion of tooth.

Consequences of trauma to primary teeth	Consequences of injury to permanent teeth
• Infection	• Infection
• Abscess	• Abscess
• Loss of space in the dental arch	• Loss of space in the dental arch
• Ankylosis	• Ankylosis
• Failure to continue eruption	• Resorption of root structure
• Color changes	• Abnormal root development
• Injury to the permanent teeth	• Color changes

Avulsion/Exarticulation/Total Luxation

It is defined as complete and total displacement of the tooth out of socket **(Fig. 28.64)**. Common cause is a directed force sufficient to overcome the bond between the affected tooth and the periodontal ligament within the alveolar socket **(Fig. 28.65)**.

Incidence

❏ It usually occurs in age group of 7–10 years
❏ 1–16% of all traumatic injuries occurring to permanent dentition
❏ Sports, fall from height and automobile accidents are most frequent causes

Biologic Consequences

Following are the predominant consequences of avulsion injury to teeth:
❏ *Pulpal necrosis:* It occurs due to disruption of blood supply to the tooth. Pulp testing and frequent monitoring of pulp vitality should be done at regular intervals
❏ *Surface resorption:* In this, small superficial resorption cavities occur within cementum and the outer dentin **(Fig. 28.66)**. It is repair process of physical damage to calcified tissue by recruitment of cells following removal of damaged tissues by macrophages
❏ *Inflammatory resorption:* It occurs as a result of necrotic pulp becoming infected in presence of severely damaged cementum. This infected pulp allows bacterial toxins to migrate out through the dentinal tubules into the periodontal ligament

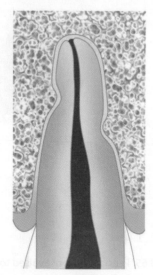

Fig. 28.66 Surface resorption.

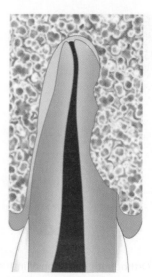

Fig. 28.68 Ankylosis with direct union of bone and tooth.

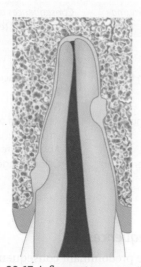

Fig. 28.67 Inflammatory resorption.

causing resorption of both root and adjacent bone **(Fig. 28.67)**

❏ *Replacement resorption:* It occurs when there is extensive damage to periodontal ligament and cementum. Healing occurs from alveolar side creating a union between tooth and bone. It is incorporation of the root into normal remodeling process of alveolus with gradual replacement by bone. As a result, the root is ultimately replaced by bone **(Fig. 28.68)**. Radiographically, there is absence of lamina dura and root assumes a moth-eaten appearance as dentin is replaced by bone. Clinically the tooth will not show any

sign of mobility and on percussion, a metallic sound is heard. Replacement resorption in younger patients may interfere with the growth and development of alveolar process which subsequently results in infraocclusion of that tooth

Prognosis of treatment depends on
❏ Extra-alveolar time
❏ Preservation of root structure
❏ Storage media

Management of Avulsed Tooth

Main aim of reimplantation is to preserve maximum number of periodontal ligament cells which have capability to regenerate and repair the injured root surface. Periodontal ligament cells should be prevented from drying since drying can result in loss of their normal physiology and morphology. If it is not possible to maintain the viable cells of PDL, aim of the treatment should be directed to slow down the resorption process. Lesser is the time lapse between avulsion and replantation, better is the prognosis. If it is not possible to reimplant the tooth immediately, it should be placed in an adequate storage media.

Ideal storage media should
❏ Be capable of preserving vitality of periodontal ligament cells
❏ Be nontoxic
❏ Have osmolality of 290–330 mOsm/L
❏ Have pH of 6.7–7.8

Classification of storage media	
Natural	*Synthetic*
• Milk • Coconut milk • Egg white • Water • Saliva • Green tea extract • Honey milk • Aloe vera • Pomegranate juice	• HBSS • Normal saline • ViaSpan • Contact lens solution • ORS • Probiotics • Gatorade

Milk: It has shown to maintain vitality of periodontal ligament cells for 3–4 hours. It is relatively bacteria-free with pH and osmolality compatible with vital cells.

Coconut water: Electrolyte composition of coconut water is similar to intracellular fluid. It consists of vitamins, minerals, amino acids and antioxidants. It preserves vitality up to 8 hours. It has advantage of easy availability, economical and sterile nature.

Egg white: It consists of proteins, minerals and ovalbumin. Its advantage is being free from contamination and can store the tooth up to 8 hours.

Water: This is the least desirable transport medium because it results in hypotonic rapid cell lysis.

Saliva: It has advantage that it is a biological fluid. Tooth is kept in buccal vestibule or in a container with saliva. It provides 2 hours of storage time for an avulsed tooth. However, it is not ideal because of incompatible osmolality, pH and presence of bacteria.

Green tea extract: It is antioxidant and anti-inflammatory which provides storage up to 24 hours.

Honey milk: It consists of essential amino acids, vitamins and minerals. It can preserve cells up to 8 hours. It maintains vitality of cells and is bacteriostatic in nature.

Aloe vera: It consists of vitamins, enzymes, minerals and amino acids. It increases fibroblasts which increases collagen proliferation. Tooth can be stored for up to 2 h.

Pomegranate juice: It consists of polyphenolic flavonoids and ellagic acids which have antioxidant properties and promote healing. It can store the tooth from 6–24 h.

Hank's balanced solution (Save-A-Tooth): HBSS is biocompatible to periodontal ligament cells and can keep them viable for up to 72 h because of its ideal pH and osmolality. It contains sodium chloride, potassium chloride, glucose, calcium chloride, magnesium chloride, sodium bicarbonate, and sodium phosphate.

Saline: It is isotonic and sterile and thus can be used as tooth carrier solution. It provides storage up to 30 min.

ViaSpan: It has pH of 7.4 and osmolarity of 320 Osm/L. These properties are advantageous for cell growth. It can preserve the viability of fibroblasts for 24 h.

Probiotics: It contains microorganism Lactobacillus reuteri. It provides viability of periodontal ligament cells similar to HBSS.

Order of efficacy of different storage media:
ViaSpan=HBSS>Coconut water>Milk>green tea>egg white

Management Options for an Avulsed Tooth

Closed apex	Open apex
Tooth replanted before coming to dental clinic or it is out of socket for <15 min	Tooth replanted before coming to dental clinic or it is out of socket for <15 min
Extraoral time is <60 min and has been kept in suitable storage media	Extraoral time is <60 min and has been kept in suitable storage media
Extraoral time is >60 min or presence of nonviable cells	Extraoral time is >60 min or presence of nonviable cells

Tooth replanted before coming to dental clinic or it is out of socket for <15 min

Closed apex

❑ Hold the tooth by the crown
❑ Tell patient to rinse mouth with water, saline, or chlorhexidine
❑ Reimplant the tooth gently with firm finger pressure. Ask the patient to bite firmly on gauze piece to help stabilize the tooth. If possible, splint the tooth with adjacent teeth using wire for 7–10 days, arch bars, or a temporary periodontal pack
❑ Put the patient on a soft diet and instruct to do chlorhexidine mouth rinses twice a day for 1–2 weeks
❑ Prescribe systemic antibiotics preferably tetracycline and plan next dental appointment. In patient <12 years of age, the preferred antibiotic is phenoxymethyl penicillin. RCT is started after 1 week. Place calcium hydroxide medicament for 1 month followed by obturation of the tooth. Remove the splint and take radiographs after 1, 3, 6, and 12 months for follow-up.

Tooth with open apex

❑ Goal of the replanting immature tooth is to allow revascularization of the pulp, if it does not occur, RCT is indicated
❑ Clean the root surface with saline
❑ Examine alveolar socket after cleaning it with saline
❑ Cover the root surface with minocycline hydrochloride microspheres before reimplantation to kill the bacteria which could enter the immature apex and form an abscess

- ❑ Reimplant the tooth gently with firm finger pressure. Ask the patient to bite firmly on gauze piece to stablize the tooth
- ❑ After evaluating the occlusion, give flexible splint for not >7–10 days
- ❑ RCT should be avoided unless there is clinical or radiographic evidence of pulp necrosis
- ❑ Take radiographs after 1, 3, 6, and 12 months for follow-up

Extraoral time is <60 min and has been kept in suitable storage media

Tooth with closed apex
- ❑ Clean the root surface with saline
- ❑ Do not touch a viable root with hands, forceps, gauze, or anything, or try to scrub or clean it to avoid injury to the periodontal ligament which makes it difficult to revascularize the reimplanted tooth
- ❑ Examine alveolar socket after cleaning it with saline. Do not overlook fracture of tooth and alveolar ridge

- ❑ Reimplant the tooth gently with firm finger pressure. Ask the patient to bite firmly on gauze piece to stabilize the tooth **(Fig. 28.69A to C)**
- ❑ After evaluating the occlusion, give flexible splint for not >7–10 days
- ❑ RCT is started after 1 week. Place calcium hydroxide medicament for 1 month followed by obturation of the tooth. Remove the splint and take radiographs after 1, 3, 6, and 12 months for follow-up

Tooth with open apex
- ❑ Goal of the replanting immature tooth is to allow revascularization of the pulp, if it does not occur, RCT is indicated
- ❑ Clean the root surface with saline
- ❑ Examine alveolar socket after cleaning it with saline
- ❑ Cover the root surface with minocyclin hydrochloride microspheres before reimplantation to increase the chances of revascularization of the pulp. Soaking the tooth in 2% sodium fluoride for 20 min slow down the process of replacement resorption

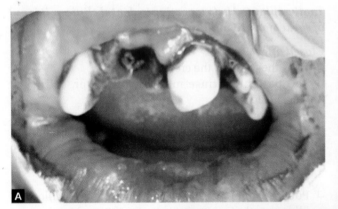
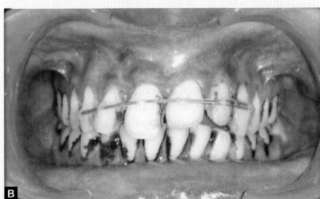
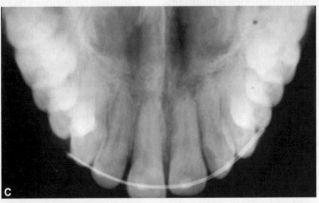

Figs. 28.69A to C Management of case with avulsed right maxillary central incisor: (A) Photograph showing avulsed central incisor; (B) Tooth repositioned and splinting done; (C) Radiograph showing positioning and stabilization of teeth.

□ Reimplant the tooth gently with firm finger pressure. Ask the patient to bite firmly on gauze piece to stabilize the tooth

□ After evaluating the occlusion, give flexible splint for not >7–10 days

□ RCT should be avoided unless there is clinical or radiographic evidence of pulp necrosis

□ Take radiographs after 1, 3, 6, and 12 months for follow-up

Extraoral time is >60 min or presence of nonviable cells.

Tooth with closed apex:

□ If the tooth was out over 2 h, periodontal ligament becomes dead and should be removed along with the pulp. Goal of delayed replantation is to promote alveolar bone growth to encapsulate the tooth

□ Local anesthesia will probably be needed before reimplanting as above

□ Tooth should be soaked for 20 min in 2.4% stannous fluoride, or sodium hypochlorite for 5 min to remove all remaining dead periodontal ligament cells that may initiate the resorption process on replantation

□ Endodontic treatment is done either before replantation or 7–10 days after replantation

□ Replant the tooth gently with firm finger pressure. Ask the patient to bite down firmly on a piece of gauze to help stabilize the tooth

□ Verify the position of replanted tooth on radiograph

□ Stabilize it for 4 weeks

□ Administer systemic antibiotics

After completion of endodontic treatment, take follow-up radiographs after 1, 3, 6, 9 and 12 months.

Tooth with open apex:

□ Periodontal ligament is dead and is not expected to heal. Goal of delayed replantation is to preserve the alveolar ridge contour

□ Tooth should be soaked for 20 min in 2.4% stannous fluoride and 5 min in doxycycline to slow down the replacement resorption of the tooth

□ RCT can be started prior to or after replantation

□ Replant the tooth gently with firm finger pressure. Ask the patient to bite down firmly on a piece of gauze to help stabilize the tooth

□ Verify the position of replanted tooth on radiograph

□ Stabilize it for 4 weeks

□ Administer systemic antibiotics

□ After completion of endodontic treatment, take follow-up radiographs after 1, 3, 6, 9 and 12 months

□ Replanted primary tooth heals by ankylosis which can cause

• Cosmetic deformity because an ankylosed tooth will not grow at same rate as rest of dentofacial complex

• Interference with eruption of permanent tooth

Types of Splints (Figs. 28.70A to F)

Composite Splint

It is a rigid splint, here composite is applied to the surfaces of teeth. Composite resin is applied on the labial or interproximal surfaces of the teeth for splinting mobile tooth to the adjacent teeth.

Composite and Wire Splint

It is the most commonly used flexible splint. Here, wire having diameter of 0.3–0.4 mm is used with composite resin.

Orthodontic Wire and Bracket Splint

This splint uses orthodontic brackets bonded to the teeth and connected with a light 0.014 NiTi flexible wire. It can be irritating to the lips when compared to composite and wire splints and titanium trauma splints; this can be solved by applying wax.

Fiber Splint

It uses a polyethylene fiber mesh and is attached with an unfilled resin and/or with composite resin. Commercially available materials are Fiber-Splint, Ribbond, or EverStick.

Titanium Trauma Splints

The titanium trauma splint is a flexible splint made of titanium approximately 0.2 mm thick and 2.8 mm wide. It has a rhomboid mesh structure which is fixed to the flowable composite resin.

Arch Bar Splint

Here a metal bar is bent into the shape of the arch and fixed with ligature wires. It is a rigid splint and may cause gingival irritation.

Wire Ligature Splint

It is a rigid splint and may impinge on the gingival tissues causing inflammation.

Flexible Splint

Composite and wire splints, orthodontic wire and bracket splints and titanium trauma splint are types of flexible splints. These allow physiologic movement to the tooth during healing phase reducing the chances of ankylosis. The IADT guidelines recommend a flexible splint for all injury classifications except for alveolar fracture where no recommendation is given.

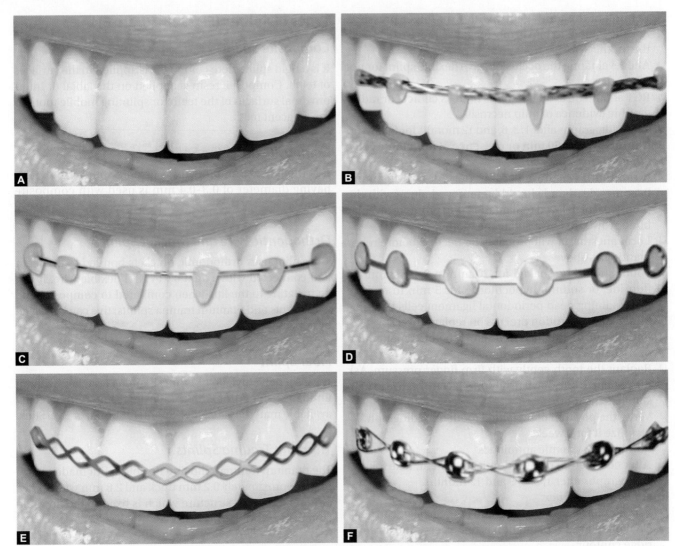

Figs. 28.70A to F Different types of splints for teeth: (A) Composite used interdentally to bond with adjacent teeth; (B); Wire composite splint-splint is made with three stranded orthodontic wire with composite (C) Wire composite splint-splint is made by using orthodontic wire and fixed with composite; (D) Commercially available trauma splint bonded with composite; (E) Titanium trauma splint bonded with composite resin; (F) Bracket splint; here brackets are connected using soft wire around buttons.

IADT recommendation of splinting times and type according to injury		
Type of injury	*Splint type*	*Splinting time*
Subluxation	flexible splint	2 weeks
Extrusion	flexible splint	2 weeks
Intrusion	flexible splint	4 weeks
Lateral luxation	flexible splint	4 weeks
Middle third root fracture	flexible splint	4 weeks
Cervical third root fracture	flexible splint	4 weeks
Alveolar fracture	no recommendation	4 weeks
Avulsion	flexible splint	2 weeks
Avulsion	flexible splint	4 weeks
>60 min extraoral time		

Contraindications of replantation:
- Compromised medical status of the patient
- Extensive damage to supporting tissues of the tooth
- Child's stage of dental development in which there are chances of ankylosis are more

Legal consequences:
- Delaying reimplantation
- Improper handling and transportation of the tooth
- Reimplanting a primary tooth
- Not providing the tetanus prophylaxis
- Incomplete examination of the surrounding traumatized tissue for tooth fragments
- Failure to warn patients that any trauma to teeth may disrupt the neurovascular supply and lead to long-term pulp necrosis or root resorption.

Assessment of Traumatic Injuries

Patient's History

- ❑ Medical
- ❑ Dental
- ❑ Injury
  - How injury occurred
  - Where injury occurred
  - When injury occurred.

Check if Present and Describe

- ❑ Loss of consciousness
- ❑ Orientation to person, place and time
- ❑ Hemorrhage/bleeding from nose/ears/oral cavity
- ❑ Nausea
- ❑ Vomiting
- ❑ Headache
- ❑ Amnesia
- ❑ Spontaneous dental pain
- ❑ Pain on medication

Extraoral Examination

- ❑ Abrasions/contusions/lacerations/ecchymosis
- ❑ Asymmetry
- ❑ Bones
  - Mobility
  - Crepitus
  - Tenderness
- ❑ Swelling
- ❑ Hemorrhage
- ❑ Presence of foreign bodies
- ❑ Check whether any injury to lips, cheeks, nose, ear and eyes

TMJ Assessment

- ❑ Deviation
- ❑ Tender on palpation
- ❑ Intraoral opening whether restricted or not
- ❑ Deflection
- ❑ Pain on opening

Intraoral Examination (Check Any Injury Present)

- ❑ Buccal mucosa
- ❑ Gingiva
- ❑ Tongue
- ❑ Floor of the mouth
- ❑ Palate
- ❑ Periodontal status

Occlusion

- ❑ Classification
- ❑ Molar
- ❑ Canine
  - Overjet
  - Overbite
- ❑ Crossbite; deviation

Teeth

- ❑ Color
- ❑ Mobility (mm)
- ❑ Pain
  - On percussion
  - Response to cold
  - On biting
- ❑ Pulp testing
  - Electrical
  - Thermal
- ❑ Pulp exposure
- ❑ Size
- ❑ Appearance
- ❑ Infraction
- ❑ Crown fracture/root fracture
- ❑ Luxation
  - Direction
  - Extent
- ❑ Avulsion
  - Extraoral time
  - Storage medium
- ❑ Carries/previous restorations

Radiograph

- ❑ Pulp size
- ❑ Periodontal ligament space
- ❑ Crown/root fracture
- ❑ Periapical pathology
- ❑ Alveolar fracture
- ❑ Foreign body

Photographs

Treatment

- ❑ Repositioning and stabilization
- ❑ Soft tissue management
- ❑ Pulp therapy
- ❑ Medications
- ❑ Instructions
  - Follow-up
  - Diet

- Medicines
- Complications

Prevention of Traumatic Injuries

Children with untreated trauma to permanent teeth often exhibit greater impacts on their daily living than those without any traumatic injury. Incidence of dental and orofacial trauma is more in sports affecting upper lip, maxilla and maxillary incisors. Use of mouth guard may protect the upper incisors. However, studies have shown that even with mouth guard in place, 25% of dentoalveolar injuries still occur.

A dental expert may be able to alter certain risk factors such as patient's dental anatomy and occlusion. The frequency for dental trauma is significantly higher for children with increased overjet and insufficient lip coverage. Instigating preventive orthodontic treatment in early to mixed dentition of patients with an overjet >3 mm has shown to prevent traumatic injuries to permanent incisors. Although some sports-related traumatic injuries are unavoidable, most can be prevented by means of helmets, face masks and mouth guards. These appliances reduce both the frequency and severity of dental and orofacial trauma. The mouth guard has been used as a protective device in sports like boxing, soccer, wrestling and basketball.

The mouth guard, also referred to as gum shield or mouth protector, is "a resilient device or appliance placed inside the mouth to reduce oral injuries, particularly to teeth and surrounding structures."

Mouth guard can be classified into three categories (given by the American Society for Testing and Materials).

1. **Type I**
   a. Stock mouth guards are purchased over the counter
   b. Designed to use without any modification
2. **Type II**
   a. Mouth-formed, made from thermoplastic material adapted to the mouth by finger tongue and biting pressure after immersing the appliance in hot water
   b. Commonly used by athletes
3. **Type III**
   a. Custom-fabricated mouth guards
   b. Produced on a dental model by either vacuum forming or heat pressure lamination technique
   c. Should be fabricated for maxillary class I and class II occlusions and mandibular class III occlusions
   d. Best in performance

Functions of Mouth Guard

- Protect the lips and intraoral structures from bruising and laceration
- Act as cushion and distribute forces so that crown fractures, root fractures, luxation and avulsions are avoided
- Protect jaw from fracture and dislocation of the mandible
- Protect against neck injuries
- Provide support for edentulous space
- Prevent the teeth in opposing arches from violent contact

Questions

1. Classify traumatic injuries. How will you diagnose a case with traumatic injury?
2. How will you manage a case of root fracture? How does healing takes place for a root fracture?
3. Define exarticulation/avulsion. How will you manage if patient comes with avulsed tooth in your clinic?
4. Classify injuries to anterior teeth. Discuss management of injury with exposure of pulp at the age of 8.5 years.
5. Give classification of traumatized teeth? Discuss in detail the treatment of avulsed right central maxillary incisor in a 10-year-old boy who reports within 20 min of injury.
6. Discuss management of right central incisor avulsed due to an accident.
7. Discuss treatment modalities for 1-week-old class III fracture in an 8-year-old male patient.
8. Write short notes on
   - Crown fracture
   - Crown root fracture
   - Luxation injuries
   - Biological consequences of avulsion
   - Complicated crown fracture

Bibliography

1. Anderson JO, Anderson FM, Anderson L. Textbook and color Atlas of traumatic injuries to the teeth. 4th edition Copenhagen: Blackwell Publishing; 2007.
2. Andreasen FM. Pulpal healing after luxation injuries and root fracture in the permanent dentition. Endod Dent Traumatol 1989;5:111.
3. Andreason JO, Andreasen FM. Textbook and colour atlas of traumatic injuries to the teeth. 3rd edition Copenhagen: Munksgaard; 1994.
4. Barret EJ, Kenny DJ. Avulsed permanent teeth review of literature and treatment guidelines. Endod Dent Traumatol 1997;13:153-63.
5. Cavalleri G, Zerman N. Traumatic crown fractures in permanent incisors with immature roots: a follow-up study. Endod Dent Traumatol 1995;11:294-6.
6. DCNA. Traumatic injuries to the teeth. 1993. p. 39.
7. Duggal MS, Toumba KJ, Russell JL, Paterson SA. Replantation of avulsed permanent teeth with avital periodontal ligaments. Endod Dent Traumatol 1994;10:282-5.
8. Finn SB. Clinical pedodontics. 4th edition 1988.

9. Flores MT, Anderson JO. Guidelines for the management of traumatic dental injuries, Part II. Avulsion of permanent teeth. Dent Traumatol 2007;23:130–6.

10. Gopikrishna V, Thomas T, Kandaswamy D. Quantitative analysis of coconut water; a new storage media for avulsed tooth. OOOE 2008;15:61–5.

11. Kahler B, Hu JY, Smith Marriot CS. Splinting of teeth following trauma: a review and a new splinting recommendations. Aust Dental J 2016;61:59–73.

12. McDonald F. Dentistry of child and adolescent. 5th edition Mosby, Harwurt Asia; 1987.

13. Oulis C, Vadiakas G, Siskos G. Management of intrusive luxation injuries. Endod Dent Traumtol 1996;12:113–9.

14. Pagadala S, Tadikonda DC. An overview of classification of dental trauma. IAIM 2015;2:157–64.

15. Pagadala S, Tadikonda DC. An overview of classification of dental trauma. IAIM 2015;2:157–64.

16. Schatz JP, Joho JP. A retrospective study of dento-alveolar injuries. Endod Dent Traumatol 1994;10:11–4.

Pulpal Response to Caries and Dental Procedure

Introduction

Dental pulp performs formative, nutritive and defensive functions throughout it's life. The dentine-pulp complex shows a broad spectrum of responses to caries and other operative procedures ranging from summation of injury, defense and repair events. These responses can occur if pulp is vital and to preserve the pulp viability and functions, utmost care should be taken to avoid or reduce the potentially injurious effects of tooth preparation, conditioning and restorative materials.

Response of Pulp to Dental Caries

Pulp gets affected by caries directly or indirectly from the bacteria, acids and other toxic substances which penetrate through the dentinal tubules. Depending upon the caries progression, pulp shows different types of defense mechanisms **(Figs. 29.1 and 29.2)**.

Factors Affecting Carries Progression on Pulp Dentin Complex

1. **Type of decay:** In case of chronic decay, pulp shows better defense as compared to acute decay.
2. **Speed of caries progression:** Chronic decay leads to repair whereas acute decay causes destruction of pulp.

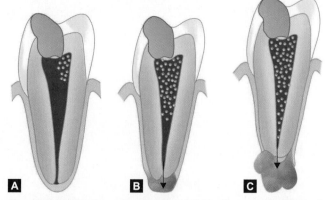

Figs. 29.1A to C Sequelae of caries: (A) Small number of bacteria close to pulp; (B) As caries progress close to pulp, inflammation starts with more of plasma cells, macrophages and lymphocytes; (C) Exposure of pulp by caries. Site of exposure shows small abscess consisting of dead inflammatory cells and other cells.

3. **Extent of caries:** Even with more depth, chronic caries may show repair whereas acute caries cause pulp exposure.
4. **Tooth resistance factors:** The greater the remaining dentin thickness, the lesser the pulpal damage. The more the permeability and solubility of dentin, the more the pulpal damage.
5. **Individual factors:** As the age increases, vascularity of the pulp decreases; this further reduces the repair capability of the pulp.

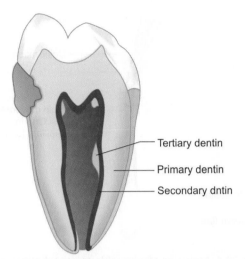

Fig. 29.2 Various defense reactions which take place in a carious tooth to protect pulp.

The following defense reactions take place in a carious tooth to protect the pulp:

Decrease in Dentin Permeability

❑ It is the first and the fastest defense to caries in the form of dentin sclerosis.
❑ In this, there is increase in deposition of mineral crystals in dentinal tubules causing narrowing of the tubules and thus decrease in permeability of dentin.

Tertiary Dentin Formation

❑ Formation of tertiary dentin occurs after a mild injury (mild-to-moderate carious lesion), in which odontoblasts survive after the stimuli. Here, acidic products of carious process degrade the dentine matrix and release bioactive molecules which resume their role of dentin formation.

More intense injury leads to odontoblast death which is followed by formation of reparative dentine. Here, healing takes place by recruitment of stem or progenitor cells from pulpal origin which differentiate to odontoblast-like cells. These cells perform secretory activity and tissue mineralization resulting in reparative dentin formation. Rate of reparative dentin formation is related to rate of carious attack. More reparative dentin is formed in response to slow chronic caries than acute caries.

Inflammatory and Immunological Reactions

Bacterial toxins, enzymes, organic acids and the products of tissue destruction show inflammatory response in the pulp. Degree of pulpal inflammation depends on remaining dentin thickness (RDT). Pulp underlying reparative dentin remains relatively normal until the carious process comes close to it. Bacteria are seldom seen in unexposed pulp. When pulp is exposed, bacteria penetrate the infected dentinal tubule and cause beginning of inflammation of the pulp **(Figs. 29.3A and B)**.

❑ The early evidence of pulpal reaction to caries is seen in the underlying odontoblastic layer. There is reduction in number and size of odontoblast cells bodies, change in the shape of odontoblasts, that is, from tall and columnar to flat and cuboidal before any inflammatory changes seen in pulp
❑ Concomitant with the changes in odontoblastic layer, hyperchromatic line may develop along the pulpal margin of the dentin, which indicates disturbance in normal equilibrium of the odontoblasts
❑ In addition to dentinal changes, antibodies are also produced by the pulp. Immunoglobulins, IgG, IgM, IgA, complement components, etc. found in the odontoblasts and adjacent pulp cells are capable of reacting against invading microorganisms

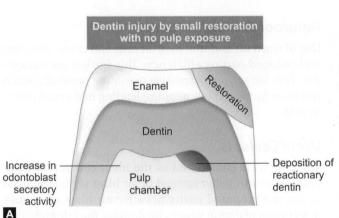

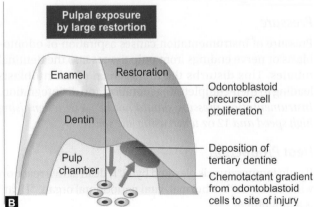

Figs. 29.3A and B Schematic representation of defense mechanism of pulp to dental caries/restoration: (A) Slight tooth injury small restoration, without pulp exposure; (B) Severe tooth injury, extensive restoration, with pulp exposure.

- Presence of bacterial antigens and immunoglobulins emphasize the involvement of specific immunologic reactions during carious process
- Persistence of dental caries provides a continuous stimulus for an inflammatory response in dental pulp
- Pulp reacts at site of exposure with infiltration of inflammatory cells. In the region of exposure, small abscess develops consisting of dead inflammatory cells and other cells. The remainder of the pulp may be uninflamed or if the exposure is present for long time, the pulp gets converted into granulation tissue
- Chronic inflammation can be partial or complete, depending upon the extent and amount of pulp tissue involved
- As the exposure progresses, partial necrosis of pulp may be followed by total pulp necrosis

Response of Pulp to Tooth Preparation

Pulpal inflammation resulting from the operative procedures is often termed **dentistogenic pulpitis**. Pulpal reaction depends on
- Degree of pulpal inflammation before treatment
- Degree of physical, chemical and biological irritation
- Proximity of restorative procedure to pulp

Degree of Pulpal Inflammation before Treatment

In case of symptoms of pulpal exposure, clinician cannot determine the degree of preoperative inflammation but if pulp is healthy, every effort should be made to minimize the irritation to dental pulp.

Degree of Physical, Chemical and Biological Irritation

Pressure

Pressure of instrumentation causes aspiration of odontoblasts or nerve endings from pulp tissues into the dentinal tubules. This disturbs the metabolism of odontoblasts leading to their complete degeneration and disintegration. *Instrumentation pressure should not be >4 oz when using high speed and 12 oz when using low speed.*

Heat Production

If pulp temperature is elevated by 11°F, destructive reaction will occur even in a normal, vital periodontal organ. "Heat" is a function of
- **RPM,** that is, more the RPM greater is the heat production
- **Pressure:** It is directly proportional to heat generation

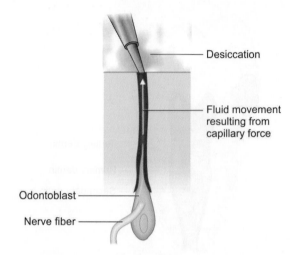

Fig. 29.4 Aspiration of odontoblasts into tubules due to desiccation.

- **Surface area of contact:** The more the contact between tooth structure and revolving tool, the greater heat generation
- **Desiccation:** It causes aspiration of odontoblasts into tubules **(Fig. 29.4)**. Subsequent disturbances in their metabolism may lead to the complete degeneration of odontoblasts

Vibrations

Vibrations are measured by their amplitude or their frequency (the number/unit time). Vibrations are an indication of eccentricity in rotary instruments. Higher the amplitude, more destructive is the pulp response.

Speed of Rotation

Ultrahigh speed should be used for removal of enamel and superficial dentin. A speed of 3,000–30,000 rpm without coolant can cause pulpal damage.

Nature of Cutting Instrument

Use of worn off and dull instruments can cause vibration and reduced cutting efficiency. This further encourages the clinician to apply excessive operating pressure, which results in increased temperature leading to thermal injury to pulp.

Use of Coolants

Water spray is considered as the ideal coolant. In deep cavities, cotton pellet instead of air blast should be used to dry the prepared cavity because air blast can cause desiccation of dentin which can damage the odontoblasts. Commonly used coolants are air spray, water jet, air and water.

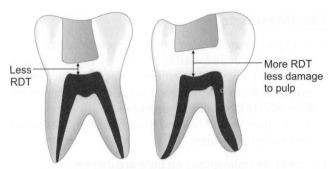

Fig. 29.5 As the remaining dentin thickness decreases, the pulp response increases.

Proximity of Restorative Procedure to Pulp

Remaining Dentin Thickness

Remaining dentin thickness (RDT) is the dentin present between floor of the tooth preparation and pulp chamber. This measurement differs from the depth of tooth preparation since the pulpal floor in deeper preparation on larger teeth may be far from the pulp than that in shallow preparations on smaller teeth.

Generally, 2 mm of dentin thickness between floor of the tooth preparation and the pulp will provide an adequate insulting barrier against irritants. As dentin thickness decreases, the pulpal response increases (**Fig. 29.5**). Studies have shown that 0.5 mm of remaining dentin thickness reduces the effect of toxic substances on pulp by

75% whereas 1.00 mm of thickness of dentin reduces it by 90%. If remaining dentin thickness is more than 2 mm or more, a little or none pulpal reaction is seen. This helps us to make the decision regarding use of liners and bases (**Flowchart 29.1**).

Response of Pulp to Local Anesthetics

❏ Vasoconstrictors are added to local anesthesia for prolonging the anesthetic effect by reducing the blood flow in the area where anesthetics is administered. Most commonly used vasoconstrictor is epinephrine
❏ Epinephrine causes decrease in pulpal blood flow which is directly related to concentration of epinephrine
❏ Low oxygen consumption in the pulp helps the healthy pulp to withstand a period of low blood flow when a vasoconstrictor is administered to it
❏ Reduction in blood flow during a restorative procedure can cause an increase in concentration of irritants accumulating within the pulp
❏ However, prolonged reduction in oxygen transport could interfere with cellular metabolism and alter response of pulp to injury
❏ Intrapulpal anesthesia is achieved by injecting the anesthetic solution into the pulpal tissue under pressure. Here anesthesia occurs due to pharmacologic action of anesthetic on nerve cell membrane and circulatory interference from the mechanical pressure of injection.

Flowchart 29.1 Effect of remaining dentin thickness on tooth.

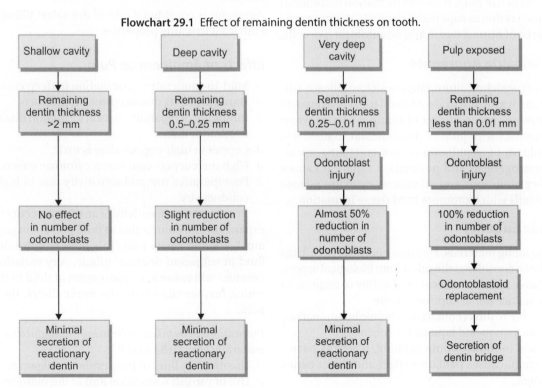

□ Though pulp can withstand decreased blood flow, when blood flow is completely arrested or decreased for prolonged time, the accumulation of the vasoactive agents occurs into the extracellular compartment of pulp which can cause permanent damage to pulp.

Dentin Sterilizing Agents

□ *Silver nitrate:* Silver salts diffuse rapidly through the dentinal tubules and reach the pulp tissue, causing an inflammatory reaction in the pulp
□ *Phenol:* Phenol causes increase in dentin permeability which may further result in greater pulp damage
□ *Camphorated parachlorophenol and penicillin:* A combination of parachlorophenol and penicillin was found to be an effective sterilizing agent for deep cavities. But studies have shown that this combination produces the pulpal inflammation.

Response of Pulp to Restorative Materials

Calcium Hydroxide

Calcium hydroxide has been used in dentistry for past many years. It inhibits bacterial enzymes and activates tissue enzymes like alkaline phosphatase. It is used in pulp capping and pulpotomy procedures. Due to its high pH, it causes inflammation, necrosis and dystrophic calcifications of the pulp. It causes formation of dentinal bridges which is due to superficial necrosis, deeply staining zone, area of fibrous tissue and odontoblast like cells.

Mineral Trioxide Aggregate

It consists of tricalcium aluminate, tricalcium silicate, silicate oxide and tricalcium oxide. Mineral trioxide aggregate (MTA) promotes regeneration of original tissues when placed in contact with pulp or periradicular tissues. It is used for pulp capping, pulpotomy, root-end filling, apexification, apexogenesis and perforation repair. It causes release of calcium ions and stimulates cytokine release from bone cells which promote hard tissue formation.

Zinc Oxide Eugenol

□ Of all the filling materials, zinc oxide eugenol (ZOE) has always been considered the safest from biological aspect. The sedative effects are because of ability of eugenol to block or reduce nerve impulse activity
□ Its effects due to direct contact are chronic inflammation, abscess formation and liquefaction necrosis
□ When used in indirect pulp capping, it acts as bactericidal agent, causes palliative effect and arrest caries progression.

Zinc Phosphate

□ Zinc phosphate cement can cause severe pulpal damage because of its irritating properties. Toxicity is more pronounced when the cement is placed in deep cavity preparations so it should not be used without intervening liner of ZOE or calcium hydroxide
□ Thick mixes should be used to minimize pulp irritation and marginal leakage.

Effects of zinc phosphate on pulp are due to:
□ Components of zinc phosphate
□ Acidic nature
□ Heat produced during setting
□ Marginal leakage.

Zinc Polycarboxylate Cement

Zinc polycarboxylate cement contains modified zinc oxide powder and an aqueous solution of polyacrylic acid. It is well tolerated by the pulp, being roughly equivalent to ZOE cement in this respect.

Glass Ionomer Cement

□ It possesses anticariogenic properties and is well tolerated by the pulp
□ Toxicity diminishes with setting time. Its pH at mixing is 2.33 and after 24 hours, it is 5.67.

Amalgam

Amalgam is considered one of the safest filling materials with least irritating properties.

Effects of Amalgam on Pulp

□ Mild-to-moderate inflammation in deep caries
□ Harmful effects due to corrosion products
□ Inhibition of reparative dentin formation due to damage to odontoblasts
□ Copper in high-copper alloy is toxic
□ High mercury content exerts cytotoxic effects on pulp
□ Postoperative thermal sensitivity due to high thermal conductivity

Postoperative sensitivity of amalgam occurs because of expansion and contraction of fluid present in gap between amalgam and cavity wall. This fluid communicates with fluid in subjacent dentinal tubule. Any variation in temperature will cause axial movement of fluid in the tubules which further stimulates the nerve fibers, thus causing pain.

Precautions to be taken while using amalgam as a restorative material (Figs. 29.6A and B)
□ Use of cavity liner or base under amalgam restoration
□ Use of varnish restoration and at the margins

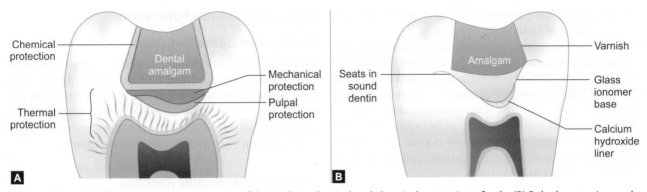

Figs. 29.6A and B (A) Schematic representation of thermal, mechanical and chemical protection of pulp; (B) Pulpal protection under amalgam is provided by applying liner and base at floor of the cavity and varnish at the walls.

Restorative Resins

❏ Restorative resins have been used in dentistry for past many years. Despite of having several advantages, they are not considered best materials because of their high coefficient of thermal expansion and polymerization shrinkage, which results in marginal leakage, subsequently the recurrent caries and pulp damage
❏ Monomer present in composite resins acts as an irritant to the pulp
❏ Use of cavity-liner-like calcium hydroxide is advocated under composite restoration to protect the pulp

Acid Etchants

Acid etching is done with 37% phosphoric acid. By etching, mineralized peritubular dentin is dissolved causing exposure of collagen fibrils into which resin monomer infiltrates. If preparation is too dry, collagen fibrils collapse, so it is always recommended to hydrate the dentin prior to bonding so as to keep collagen fibrils patent.

▌Effects of Pin Insertion

Pins are used in amalgam restoration for building up badly broken tooth or to support amalgam restoration. Pin insertion results:
❏ Dentinal fractures and unnoticed pulp exposure **(Fig. 29.7)**
❏ Increases the pulp irritation of already stressed pulp (inflammation of pulp directly proportioned to depth, extensiveness of decay)
❏ Cements used for pins, add more irritation to the pulp.

▌Impression Material

❏ Impression taking for inlay and crown fabrication exposes the pulp to serious hazards
❏ Seltzer et al. showed that pulpal trauma can occur when more pressure is applied while taking impression

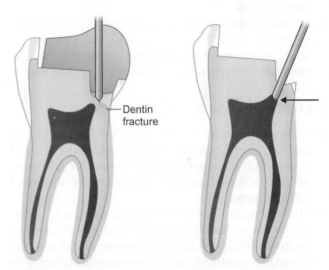

Fig. 29.7 Dentinal fracture or pulpal exposure can occur due to pin placement.

❏ When the modeling compound is applied to the cavity or full crown preparation, a pressure is exerted on pulp. Also a negative pressure is created while removing an impression, which may cause odontoblastic aspiration.

▌Effects of Radiations on Pulp

❏ Basic cellular effect of ionizing radiation is interference with cell division
❏ Radiation damage to teeth depends on dose, source, type of radiation, exposure factors and stage of tooth development at the time of irradiation
❏ In developing human teeth, extent of damage depends on amount of radiation and stage of tooth development. Heavy doses at the earliest stage of development can cause complete failure of the tooth to develop; mild doses can result in root-end distortions and dilacerations. Circulatory disturbances in the tooth germ are also

manifested by the presence of dilated vessels, hemorrhages and endothelial cells swelling

- Odontoblasts fail to function normally and may elaborate abnormal dentin and amelogenesis is retarded or ceases. In later stages, fibrosis or atrophy of the pulp may occur
- Pulps of fully formed human teeth also get affected in irradiated teeth. Though mature odontoblasts appear to be extremely radioresistant, pulp cells exposed to the ionizing radiation may become necrotic. The effects appear to be related to vascular damage and interference with mitosis of cells.

Effect of Heat from Electrosurgery

- Heat may be delivered to the pulp by electrosurgical gingivoplasty
- Contact of activated electrode with gingival restorations to no more than 0.2–0.4 s is compatible with clinical usage. However, longer periods of exposure to the electrosurgical currents produced severe pulpal damage

Effect of Lasers on Pulp

- Commonly used lasers in operative dentistry are Nd:YAG and CO_2 laser. Larger doses of laser can cause damage to pulp. Pulp damage can be manifested by coagulation necrosis of the odontoblast, edema and inflammatory cell infiltration
- Mode of action in hypersensitivity teeth is by altering dentin surface, blocking dentinal tubules and by melting and glazing dentin. It may be also due to the transient anesthesia due to permanent damage to sensory nerves

Defense Mechanism of Pulp

Tubular Sclerosis

Peritubular dentin becomes wider gradually filling the tubules with calcified material progressing with the dentinoenamel junction pulpally. These areas are harder, denser, less sensitive and more protective to the pulp against subsequent irritation. Sclerosis resulting from aging is physiological dentin sclerosis and resulting from mild irritation is reactive dentin sclerosis.

Smear Layer

Smear layer is an amorphous debris layer consisting of both organic and inorganic constituents caused iatrogenically during operative procedures. It decreases both sensitivity and permeability of dentinal tubules.

Reparative Dentin Formation

Healthy Reparative Reaction

This is the most favorable response and it consists of stimulating the periodontal organ to form sclerotic dentin. These are followed by normal secondary dentin containing dentinal tubules. Secondary dentin is different from primary dentin, in that the tubules of secondary dentin are slightly deviated from the tubules of the primary dentin.

Unhealthy Reparative Reaction

This response begins with degeneration of odontoblasts, followed by formation of dead tract in the dentin and complete cessation in formation of secondary dentin. Unhealthy reparative response is accompanied by mild pathological and clinical changes of a reversible nature in the pulp tissues, resulting in the formation of an irregular type of tertiary dentin. The tertiary dentin formation is considered to be the function of the pulp tissue proper. However, tertiary dentin has certain limitations. It is not completely impervious like the calcific barrier. Also, the rapid formation of tertiary dentin can occupy part of a pulp chamber with tissues other than those normally responsible for repair, metabolism and innervations. Thus, tertiary dentin is said to "age the pulp," reducing its capacity for further defensive action against irritation. This is very important clinically, because if this reaction occurs as a result of a carious process, the restoration of this tooth may not be favorable, received by the periodontal organ.

Destructive Reaction

This is the most unfavorable pulpal response to irritation. It begins with the loss of odontoblasts and the outer protective layer of the pulp which ultimately involves the pulp tissue proper exceeding its reparative capacity. The resulting tissue reaction will be inflammation, which may progress to abscess formation, chronic inflammation and finally, complete necrosis of the pulp. In any event, the pulp tissues cannot recover from these pathologic changes and removal of these tissues or the whole tooth becomes necessary.

Defense mechanism of the pulp
- Tubular sclerosis
- Smear layer
- Reparative dentin formation:
  - Healthy reparative reaction
  - Unhealthy reparative reaction
  - Destructive reaction

Prevention of Pulpal Damage Due to Operative Procedure

To preserve integrity of the pulp, the following measures should be taken:

Irritant/procedure	Method to prevent pulpal injury
Tooth preparation	• Effective cooling • High-speed ratio • Intermittent cutting
Restorative material	• Use material after considering physical and biological properties according to tooth preparation
Marginal leakage	• Pulp protection using liners and bases • Use of bonding agents
While insertion	• Avoid application of excessive forces of restoration
While polishing	• Effective cooling to avoid heat generation during polishing
Irritants to dentin	• Avoid application of any irritant, desiccant on freshly cut dentin

How Does Pulp Recover?

❑ As tissue pressure increases from increased blood flow, arteriovenous anastomoses (AVAs) open and shunt blood before it reaches an inflamed region, thus preventing a further increase in blood flow and tissue pressure
❑ Increase in tissue pressure pushes macromolecules back into blood stream via venules in the adjacent healthy pulp
❑ Once macromolecules and excess fluid leave the extracellular tissue space via venule, tissue pressure decreases and normal blood flow is restored

Questions

1. What is defense mechanism of pulp to various irritants?
2. Write short notes on:
   • Pulpal response to caries
   • Effect of tooth preparation on pulp
   • Pulp response to restorative procedures
   • Pulp response to restorative materials
   • Pulp reaction to different esthetic filling materials
   • Defense mechanism of pulp to various irritants.

Bibliography

1. Bergenholtz G, Cox CF, Loesche WJ, Syed SA. Bacterial leakage around dental restorations: its effect on the dental pulp. J Oral Pathol 1982;11:439–50.
2. Costa CAS, Hebling J, Hanks CT. Current status of pulp capping with dentin adhesive systems: a review. Dent Mater 2000;16:188–97.
3. Kitamura C, Ogawa Y, Morotomi T, Terashita M. Differential induction of apoptosis by capping agent during pulp wound healing. J Endod 2003;29:41–3.
4. Pereira JC, Segala AD, Costa CAS. Human pulpal response to direct pulp capping with an adhesive system. Am J Dent 2000;13:139–47.
5. Pittford TR. Pulpal response to a calcium hydroxide material for capping exposures. Oral Surg Oral Med Oral Pathol Oral Radiol Endod 1985;59:194–7.
6. Schöder U. Effects of calcium hydroxide-containing pulp capping agents on pulp cell migration proliferation and differentiation. J Dent Res 1985;64:541–8.

CHAPTER

30

Management of Discolored Teeth

Chapter Outline

- Classification of Discoloration
- Etiology
- Bleaching
- Bleaching Agents
- Bleaching Techniques
- Home Bleaching Technique
- In-office Bleaching
- Bleaching of Nonvital Teeth
- Effects of Bleaching Agents on Tooth and its Supporting Structures

Introduction

Teeth are polychromatic so color varies among the gingival, incisal, and cervical areas according to the thickness, reflections of different colors, translucency, and thickness of enamel and color of dentin **(Fig. 30.1)**. Thickness of enamel is greater at the occlusal/incisal third of the tooth and thinner at the cervical third. That is why teeth are more darker on cervical one third than at middle or incisal one third. Normal color of primary teeth is bluish white, whereas color of permanent teeth is grayish yellow, grayish white, or yellowish white. With age, the color of teeth changes to more yellow or grayish yellow due to increase in dentin thickness and decrease in enamel thickness.

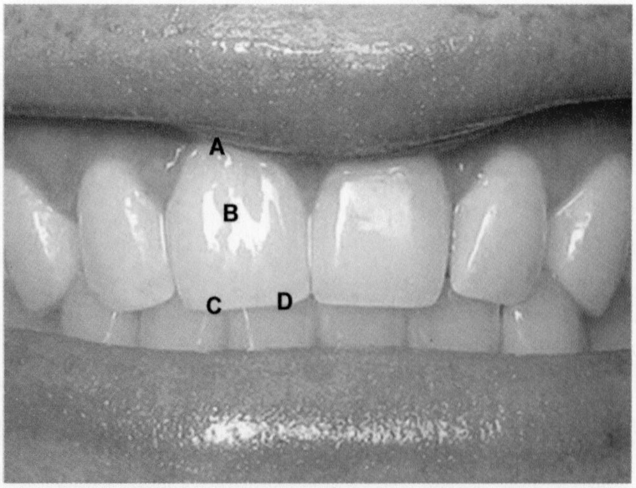

Figs. 30.1 Normal anatomical landmarks of tooth: A. Cervical margin, B. Body of tooth, C. Incisal edge, D. Translucency of enamel.

Classification of Discoloration

Color of the teeth is influenced by a combination of their intrinsic color and presence of any extrinsic stains on the tooth surface. Intrinsic tooth color is associated with light scattering and adsorption properties of enamel and dentine, where dentine plays a major role in determining the overall shade. Extrinsic stains form due to smoking, dietary intake of tannin-rich foods, use of some cationic agents like chlorhexidine, or metal salts like tin and iron. So, discoloration of teeth can be classified as:

- Intrinsic discoloration
- Extrinsic discoloration
- Combination of both

Intrinsic Stains

Preeruptive Causes

These are incorporated into the deeper layers of enamel and dentin during odontogenesis and alter the development and appearance of the enamel and dentin.

Alkaptonuria

Dark brown pigmentation of primary teeth is commonly seen in alkaptonuria. It is an autosomal recessive disorder resulting into complete oxidation of tyrosine and phenylalanine causing increased level of homogentisic acid.

Etiology

Intrinsic stains		Extrinsic stains	
Preeruptive	Posteruptive	Daily acquired stains	Chemicals

• Disease
  – Alkaptonuria
  – Hematological disorders
  – Diseases of enamel and dentin
  – Liver diseases
• Medications
  – Tetracycline and fluorosis stain
	• Pulpal changes
	• Trauma
	• Dentin hypercalcification
	• Dental caries
	• Restorative materials and operative procedures
	• Aging
		• Plaque
		• Food and beverages
		• Tobacco use
		• Poor oral hygiene
		• Swimmer's calculus
		• Gingival hemorrhage
			Chlorhexidine
			Metallic stains

Hematological Disorders

❑ *Erythroblastosis fetalis:* It is a blood disorder of neonates due to Rh incompatibility. In this, stain does not involve teeth or portions of teeth developing after cessation of hemolysis shortly after birth. Stain is usually green, brown, or bluish in color

❑ *Congenital porphyria:* It is an inborn error of porphyrin metabolism, characterized by overproduction of uroporphyrin. Deciduous and permanent teeth may show a red or brownish discoloration. Under ultraviolet light, teeth show red fluorescence

❑ *Sickle cell anemia:* It is inherited blood dyscrasia characterized by increased hemolysis of red blood cells. In sickle cell anemia infrequently the stains of the teeth are similar to those of erythroblastosis fetalis, but discoloration is more severe, involves both dentitions and does not resolve with time

Diseases of Enamel and Dentin

Amelogenesis imperfecta (AI): It comprises a group of conditions that demonstrate developmental alteration in the structure of the enamel in the absence of a systemic disorders. AI has been classified mainly into hypoplastic, hypocalcified, and hypomaturation type **(Figs. 30.2A to D)**.

Fluorosis: In fluorosis, staining is due to excessive fluoride uptake during development of enamel. Excess fluoride induces a metabolic change in ameloblast and the resultant enamel has a defective matrix and an irregular, hypomineralized structure **(Fig. 30.3)**.

Fluorosis staining manifests as:
❑ Gray or white opaque areas on teeth
❑ Yellow to brown discoloration on a smooth enamel surface **(Fig. 30.4)**
❑ Moderate and severe changes showing pitting and brownish discoloration of surface **(Fig. 30.5)**
❑ Severely corroded appearance with dark brown discoloration and loss of most of enamel

Enamel hypoplasia and hypocalcification due to other causes **(Figs. 30.6A to C)**:
❑ Vitamin D deficiency results in characteristic white patch hypoplasia in teeth

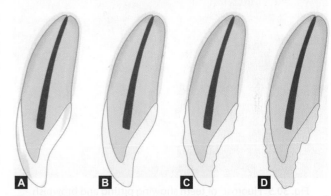

Figs. 30.2A to D Amelogenesis imperfecta: (A) Normal enamel; (B) Hypocalcified enamel; (C) Hypoplastic, pitted enamel; (D) Hypomaturation enamel.

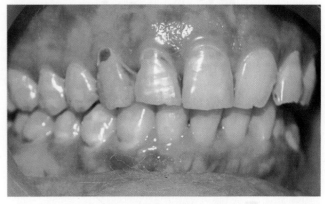

Fig. 30.3 Clinical picture showing fluorosis of teeth in form of hypomineralized brownish discoloration.

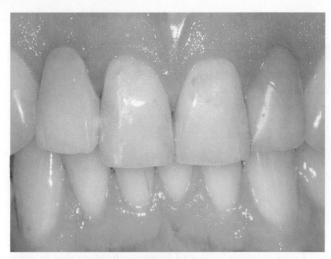

Fig. 30.4 Fluorosis of teeth showing yellow to brown discoloration of teeth.

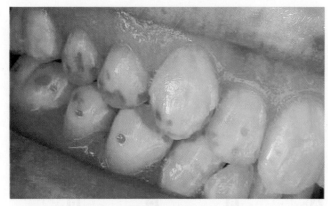

Fig. 30.5 Fluorosis of teeth showing pitting and brownish discoloration.

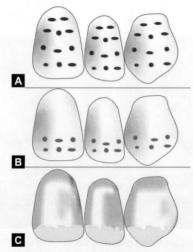

Figs. 30.6A to C (A) Amelogenesis imperfecta (hypoplastic, pitted); (B) Acquired enamel hypoplasia; (C) Amelogenesis imperfecta (snowcapped).

- Vitamin C deficiency together with vitamin A deficiency during formative periods of dentition resulting in pitting type appearance of teeth
- Childhood illnesses during odontogenesis, such as exanthematous fevers, malnutrition, and metabolic disorder also affect teeth

Dentinogenesis imperfecta (DI): It is an autosomal dominant development disturbance of the dentin which occurs along or in conjunction with AI **(Figs. 30.7A to C)**. Color of teeth in DI varies from gray to brownish violet to yellowish brown with a characteristic usual translucent or opalescent hue.

Tetracycline and minocycline: Unsightly discoloration of both dentitions results from excessive intake of tetracycline and minocycline during the development of teeth. Chelation of tetracycline molecule with calcium in hydroxyapatite crystals forms tetracycline orthophosphate which is responsible for discolored teeth **(Fig. 30.8)**.

Classification of tetracycline staining according to developmental stage, banding and color (Jordun and Boksman, 1984):
- First degree (mild)—yellow to gray, uniformly spread through the tooth. No banding
- Second degree (moderate)—yellow brown to dark gray, slight banding, if present
- Third degree (severe staining)—blue gray or black and is accompanied by significant banding across tooth
- Fourth degree—stains that are so dark that bleaching is ineffective, totally

Severity of pigmentation with tetracycline depends on three factors:
1. Time and duration of administrations
2. Type of tetracycline administered
3. Dosage

Posteruptive Causes

- **Pulpal changes:** Pulp necrosis usually results from bacterial, mechanical, or chemical irritation to pulp. In this, disintegration products enter dentinal tubules and cause discoloration **(Figs. 30.9 and 30.10)**

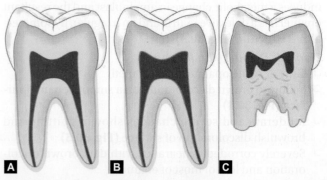

Figs. 30.7A to C (A) Normal tooth; (B) Dentinogenesis imperfecta; (C) Dentin dysplasia.

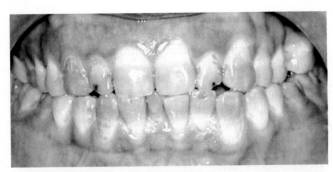

Fig. 30.8 Photograph showing tetracycline stains.

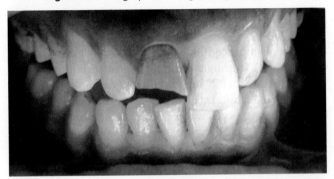

Fig. 30.9 Discoloration of right maxillary central incisor due to pulp necrosis.

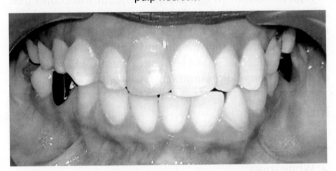

Fig. 30.10 Loss of translucency of right maxillary central incisor due to pulp necrosis.

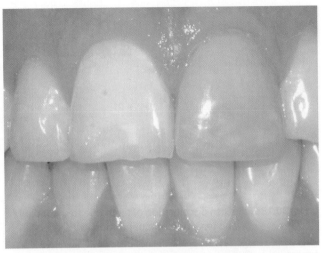

Fig. 30.11 Discolored left maxillary central incisor due to traumatic injury followed by pulp necrosis.

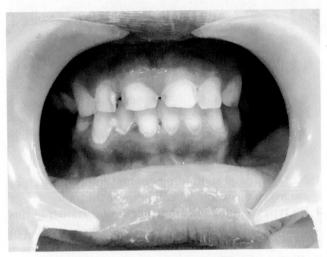

Fig. 30.12 Discolored appearance of teeth due to caries.

- **Trauma:** Accidental injury to tooth can cause pulpal and enamel degenerative changes that may alter color of teeth **(Fig. 30.11)**. Pulpal hemorrhage leads to grayish discoloration and nonvital appearance. Injury causes hemorrhage which results in lysis of RBCs and liberation of iron sulfide which enter dentinal tubules and discolor surrounding tooth
- **Dentin hypercalcification:** Dentin hypercalcification results when there are excessive irregular elements in the pulp chamber and canal walls. It causes decrease in translucency and yellowish or yellow brown discoloration of the teeth
- **Dental caries:** In general, teeth present a discolored appearance around areas of bacterial stagnation and leaking restorations **(Fig. 30.12)**
- **Restorative materials and dental procedures:** Discoloration can also result from the use of endodontic sealers and restorative materials

- **Aging:** Color changes in teeth with age result from surface and subsurface changes. Age-related discoloration is because of
  - *Enamel changes:* Both thinning and texture changes occur in enamel
  - *Dentin deposition:* Secondary and tertiary dentin deposits, pulp stones cause changes in the color of teeth **(Figs. 30.13 and 30.14)**
  - **Functional and parafunctional changes:** Tooth wear may give a darker appearance to the teeth because of loss of tooth surface and exposure of dentin which is yellower and is susceptible to color changes by absorption of oral fluids and deposition of reparative dentin **(Fig. 30.14)**

Extrinsic Stains

Classification of Extrinsic Stains (Nathoo in 1997)

- **N1 type dental stain (direct dental stain):** Here colored materials bind to the tooth surface to cause discoloration. Tooth has same color, as that of chromogen

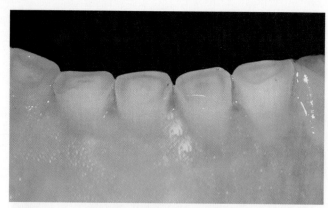

Fig. 30.13 Yellowish discoloration of teeth due to secondary and tertiary dentin deposition.

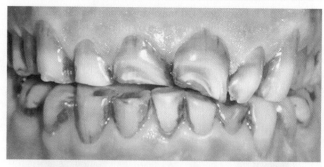

Fig. 30.14 Discoloration of teeth resulting from tooth wear and aging.

❑ **N2 type dental stain (direct dental stain):** Here chromogen changes color after binding to the tooth
❑ **N3 type dental stain (indirect dental stain):** In this type, prechromogen (colorless) binds to the tooth and undergoes a chemical reaction to cause a stain

Daily Acquired Stains

❑ **Plaque:** Pellicle and plaque on tooth surface gives rise to yellowish appearance of teeth
❑ **Food and beverages:** Tea, coffee, red wine, curry, and colas if taken in excess cause discoloration
❑ **Tobacco use:** It results in brown to black appearance of teeth
❑ **Poor oral hygiene manifests as:**
  • Green stain
  • Brown stain
  • Orange stain
❑ **Swimmer's calculus:**
  It is yellow to dark brown stain present on facial and lingual surfaces of anterior teeth. It occurs due to prolonged exposure to pool water
❑ Gingival hemorrhage

Chemicals

❑ **Chlorhexidine stain:** The stains produced by use of chlorhexidine are yellowish brown to brownish in nature

❑ **Metallic stains:** These are caused by metals and metallic salts introduced into oral cavity in metal containing dust inhaled by industry workers or through orally administered drugs

Stains caused by different metals
• Copper dust—green stain
• Iron dust—brown stain
• Mercury—greenish black stain
• Nickel—green stain
• Silver—black stain

Bleaching

Bleaching is a procedure which involves lightening of the color of a tooth through the application of a chemical agent to oxidize the organic pigmentation in the tooth.

Goal of bleaching is to restore the normal color of a tooth by lightening the stain with a powerful oxidizing agent, also known as a bleaching agent.

Mechanism

Mechanism of bleaching is mainly linked to degradation of high molecular weight complex organic molecules that reflect a specific wavelength of light, which is responsible for color of stain **(Fig. 30.15)**. Resulting degradation products are of lower molecular weight and composed of less complex molecules that reflect less light, resulting in a reduction or elimination of discoloration.

Indications

❑ Generalized staining
❑ Age-related discolorations
❑ White spots
❑ Mild tetracycline staining
❑ Mild fluorosis without pitting

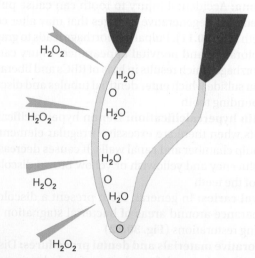

Fig. 30.15 Schematic representation of mechanism of bleaching.

□ Acquired superficial staining; dietary staining (tea/coffee)
□ Stains from smoking tobacco
□ Color changes related to pulpal trauma or necrosis.

Contraindications

Poor Case Selection

Patient having emotional or psychological problems is not right choice for bleaching.

Dentin Hypersensitivity

Hypersensitive teeth need to provide extra protection before going for bleaching.

Extensively Restored Teeth

These teeth are not good candidate for bleaching because of insufficient enamel to respond properly to bleaching. In teeth with large composite restorations, the restoration becomes more evident after bleaching.

Teeth with Hypoplastic Marks and Cracks

Application of bleaching agents increases the contrast between white opaque spots and normal tooth structure. In these cases, bleaching can be done in conjunction with microabrasion, ameloplasty, and composite resin bonding.

Defective and Leaky Restorations

Defective and leaky restorations are not good candidate for bleaching. If discoloration is from metallic salts particularly silver amalgam, dentinal tubules of the tooth become saturated with alloys and no amount of bleaching will significantly improve the shade.

Defective Obturation

If root canal is not well-obturated, then refilling must be done before attempting bleaching.

▌Bleaching Agents

Different types of bleaching agents are available commercially. These bleaching agents may contain the following components.

Hydrogen Peroxide

□ Used in concentration ranging from 5% to 35%
□ H_2O_2 has low molecular weight so can penetrate dentin and release oxygen
□ It is clear, colorless, odorless liquid stored in light proof bottles
□ If stored properly, its shelf life is 3–4 months but decomposes rapidly in presence of organic debris and an open air
□ Should be handled carefully to prevent direct contact with mucous membrane
□ Can be used alone or in combination with sodium perborate

Sodium Perborate

□ Available as white powder in granular form
□ Mainly three types: sodium perborate monohydrate, trihydrate, and tetrahydrate and these three types vary in oxygen content.
□ When mixed with superoxol, it decomposes into sodium metaborate, water, and oxygen

Carbamide Peroxide

□ Also known as urea hydrogen peroxide
□ Used in concentrations ranging from 3% to 45%
□ It decomposes into urea, ammonia, carbon dioxide, and hydrogen peroxide **(Flowchart 30.1)**
□ Carbopol (polyacrylic acid polymer) is used as a thickening agent. It prolongs the release of active peroxide
□ For gel preparations, glycerine, propylene glycol, sodium stannate, citric acid, and flavoring agents are added

Flowchart 30.1 Mechanism of action of carbamide peroxide

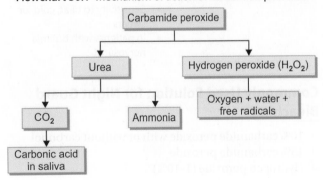

Bleaching Techniques (Flow chart 30.2)

Flowchart 30.2 Bleaching technique

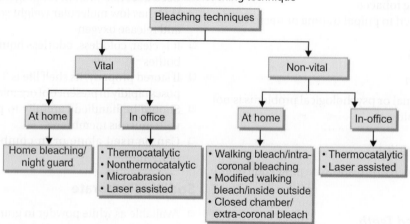

```
                    Bleaching techniques
                    /                    \
                Vital                   Non-vital
                /    \                   /        \
          At home   In office      At home      In-office
             |          |             |             |
    Home bleaching/  • Thermocatalytic  • Walking bleach/intra-   • Thermocatalytic
      night guard    • Nonthermocatalytic  coronal bleaching      • Laser assisted
                     • Microabrasion    • Modified walking
                     • Laser assisted     bleach/inside outside
                                        • Closed chamber/
                                          extra-coronal bleach
```

Home Bleaching Technique

Home bleaching technique is also called night guard bleaching.

Indications	Contraindications
• Age-related discolorations • Mild generalized staining • Mild tetracycline staining • Mild fluorosis • Acquired superficial staining stains from smoking tobacco • Color changes related to pulpal trauma or necrosis	Teeth with • Insufficient enamel for bleaching • Cracks and fracture lines • Inadequate or defective restorations • Large pulp chamber • Severe fluorosis and pitting hypoplasia • Noncompliant patients • Severe tetracycline staining • Sensitivity to heat, cold, or sweets • In patients with bulimia nervosa

Commonly Used Solution for Night Guard Bleaching

❏ 10% carbamide peroxide with or without carbopol
❏ 15% carbamide peroxide
❏ Hydrogen peroxide (1–10%)

Factors Affecting Prognosis

❏ History or presence of sensitive teeth
❏ Extremely dark gingival third of tooth visible during smiling
❏ Extensive white spots
❏ Translucent teeth
❏ Excessive gingival recession and exposed root surfaces

Steps of Tray Fabrication

❏ Take the impression and make a stone model
❏ Trim the model
❏ Place the stock out resin and cure it
❏ Apply separating media
❏ Choose the tray sheet material
❏ Nature of material used for fabrication of bleaching tray is flexible plastic. Most common tray material used is ethyl vinyl acetate
❏ Cast the plastic in vacuum tray forming machines
❏ Trim and polish the tray
❏ Checking the tray for correct fit, retention, and overextension
❏ Demonstrate the amount of bleaching material to be placed

Thickness of Tray

❏ Standard thickness of tray is 0.035 in **(Fig. 30.16).**

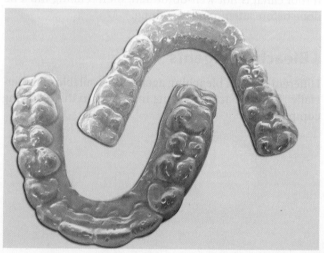

Fig. 30.16 Photograph showing bleaching trays.

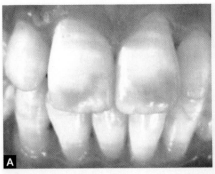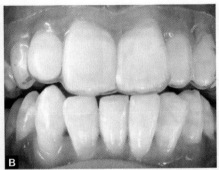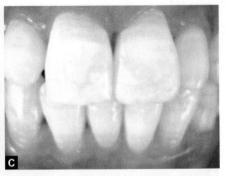

Figs. 30.17A to C Bleaching with night guard: (A) Preoperative photograph; (B) Bleaching with night guard; (C) Postoperative photograph.
Courtesy: Jaidev Dhillon.

- Thicker tray, that is, 0.05 in. is indicated in patients with breaking habit
- Thinner tray, that is, 0.02 in. thick is indicated in patients who gag

Treatment Regimen

- Patient is instructed to brush the teeth before tray application
- Patient is instructed to place enough bleaching material into the tray to cover the facial surfaces of the teeth. After seating tray in mouth, the extra material is carefully wiped away **(Figs. 30.17A to C)**
- Wearing the tray during day time allows replenishment of the gel after 1–2 h for maximum concentration. Overnight use causes decrease in loss of material due to decreased salivary flow at night
- While removing the tray, patient is asked to remove the tray from second molar region in peeling action. This is done to avoid injury to soft tissues
- Patient is instructed to rinse off the bleaching agent and clean the tray
- Duration of treatment depends upon original discoloration, duration of bleaching, patient compliance, and time of bleaching
- Patient is recalled for periodic checkups for assessing bleaching process.

Maintenance

Additional rebleaching can be done every 3–4 years if necessary with duration of 1 week.

Side Effects

- Gingival irritation—painful gums after a few days of wearing trays
- Soft tissue irritation—from excessive wearing of the trays or applying too much bleach to the trays
- Altered taste sensation—metallic taste immediately after removing trays
- Tooth sensitivity—most common side effect

Advantages	Disadvantages
• Simple method for patients to use • Simple for dentists to monitor • Less chair time and cost-effective • Patients can bleach their teeth at their convenience	• Patient compliance is mandatory • Color change is dependent on amount of time the trays are worn • Chances of abuse by using excessive amount of bleach for too many hours per day

In-Office Bleaching

Thermocatalytic Vital Tooth Bleaching

Indications	Contraindications
• Superficial stains **(Figs. 30.18A and B)** • Moderate-to-mild stains **(Figs. 30.18C and D)**	• Tetracycline stains • Extensive restorations • Severe discolorations • Extensive caries • Patient sensitive to bleaching agents

Equipment Needed

- Power bleach material
- Tissue protector
- Energizing/activating source
- Protective clothing and eyewear
- Mechanical timer

Light Sources

Conventional bleaching light

- Uses heat and light to activate bleaching material
- More heat is generated during bleaching
- Causes tooth dehydration
- Uncomfortable for patient
- Slower in action

Tungsten halogen curing light

- Uses light and heat to activate bleaching solution
- Application of light 40–60 s per application per tooth
- Time consuming

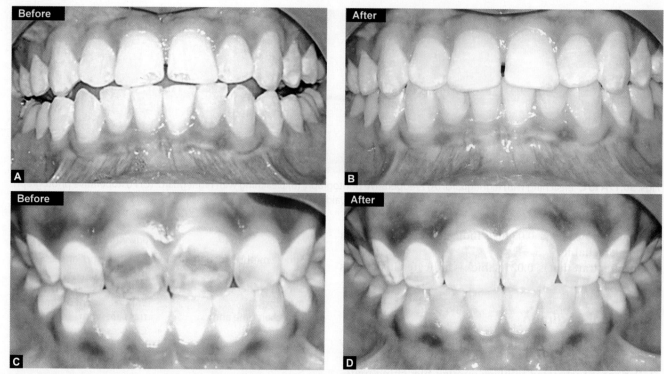

Figs. 30.18A to D (A) Photograph showing superficial stains on maxillary anteriors; (B) Postoperative photograph after thermocatalytic bleaching; (C) Maxillary central incisors showing discoloration; (D) Postoperative photograph after thermocatalytic bleaching.

Xenon plasma arc light
- High intensity light, so more heat is liberated during bleaching
- Application requires 3 s per tooth
- Faster bleaching
- Action is thermal and stimulates the catalyst in chemicals
- Greater potential for thermal trauma to pulp and surrounding soft tissues

Argon and CO₂ laser
- True laser light stimulates the catalyst in chemical so there is no thermal effect
- Requires 10 s per application per tooth

Diode laser light
- True laser light produced from a solid state source
- Ultrafast
- Requires 3–5 s to activate bleaching agent
- No heat is generated during bleaching

Procedure
- Pumice the teeth to clean off any debris present on the tooth surface
- Isolate the teeth with rubber dam and protect the gingival tissues with orabase or vaseline. Protect patient's eyes with sunglasses

- Saturate the cotton or gauze piece with bleaching solution (30–35% H_2O_2) and place it on the teeth
- Depending upon light, expose the teeth **(Fig. 30.19)**. The temperature of device should be maintained between 52 and 60°C (125–140°F)
- Change solution in between after every 4–5 min. The treatment time should not exceed 30 min
- Remove solution with the help of wet gauge
- Remove solution and irrigate teeth thoroughly with warm water
- Polish teeth and apply neutral sodium fluoride gel
- Instruct the patient to use fluoride rinse on daily basis
- Second and third appointment is given after 3–6 weeks. This will allow pulp to settle

  Figures 30.20A to D show bleaching of teeth by thermocatalytic vital bleaching technique.

Advantages	Disadvantages
• Patient preference • Less time than overall time needed for home bleaching • Patient motivation • Protection of soft tissues	• More chair time • More expensive • More frequent and longer appointment • Dehydration of teeth • Safety considerations

Nonthermocatalytic Bleaching

In this technique, heat source is not used.

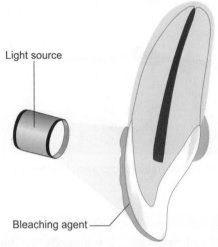

Fig. 30.19 Thermocatalytic technique of bleaching for vital teeth.

Commonly used solutions for bleaching	
Name	*Composition*
Superoxol	5 parts H$_2$O$_2$:1 part ether
McInnes solution	5 parts of HCl (36%) (etches the enamel)
	1 part of 0.2% ether (cleans the tooth surface)
	5 parts 30% H$_2$O$_2$ (bleaches the enamel)
Modified McInnes solution (in this sodium hydroxide is added in the solution)	H$_2$O$_2$ (30%)
	NaOH (20%) because of its highly alkaline nature, it dissolves calcium of tooth at slower rate. Mix 1 part of H$_2$O$_2$ and 1 part of NaOH along with ether (0.2%)

Steps

- Isolate the teeth using rubber dam
- Apply bleaching agent on the teeth for 5 min

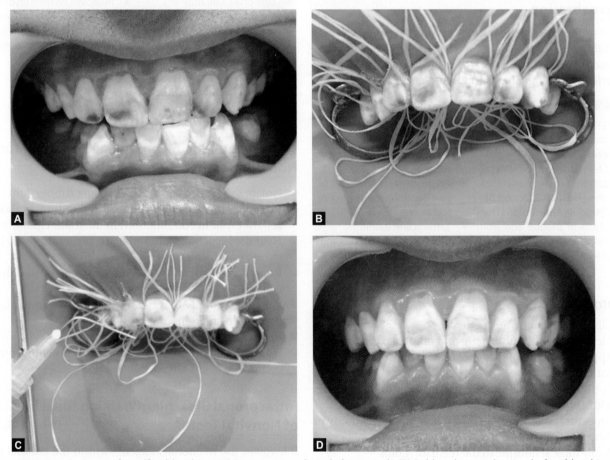

Figs. 30.20A to D Steps of in-office bleaching: (A) Preoperative clinical photograph; (B) Rubber dam application before bleaching; (C) Application of bleaching agent; (D) Postoperative photograph after bleaching.
Courtesy: Jaidev Dhillon.

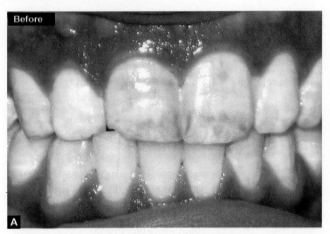
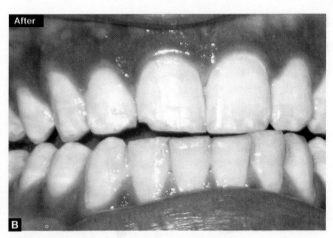

Figs. 30.21A and B (A) Preoperative photograph showing discolored 11, 21; (B) Postoperative photograph after microabrasion.

- Wash the teeth with warm water and reapply the bleaching agent until the desired color is achieved
- Wash the teeth and polish them

Microabrasion

It is a procedure in which a microscopic layer of enamel is simultaneously eroded and abraded with a special compound (usually contains 18% of hydrochloric acid) leaving a perfectly intact enamel surface behind.

Indications	Contraindications
• Stains and discoloration limited to superficial enamel only • Stains due to hypomineralization or hypermineralization **(Figs. 30.21A and B)** • Decalcification lesions from stasis of plaque and from orthodontic bands • Areas of enamel fluorosis	• Deep enamel and dentin stains • Deep enamel hypoplastic lesions • Amelogenesis imperfecta and dentinogenesis imperfecta cases • Tetracycline staining • Carious lesions underlying regions of decalcification • Age-related staining

Protocol

- Clinically evaluate the teeth
- Clean teeth with rubber cup and prophylaxis paste
- Apply petroleum jelly to the tissues and isolate the area with rubber dam
- Apply microabrasion compound to areas in 60 s intervals with appropriate rinsing
- Repeat the procedure if necessary. Check the teeth when wet
- Rinse teeth for 30 s and dry
- Apply topical fluoride to the teeth for 4 min
- Re-evaluate the color of the teeth. More than one visit may be necessary sometimes

Advantages	Disadvantages
• Minimum discomfort to patient • Less chair side time • Useful in removing superficial stains • Resultant tooth surface is shiny and smooth in nature	• Not effective for deeper stains • Removes enamel layer • Yellow discoloration of teeth has been reported in some cases after treatment

Bleaching of Nonvital Teeth

Thermocatalytic Technique of Bleaching for Nonvital Teeth

- Isolate the tooth to be bleached using rubber dam
- Place bleaching agent (superoxol and sodium perborate separately or in combination) in the tooth chamber
- Heat the bleaching solution using bleaching stick/light curing unit
- Repeat the procedure till the desired tooth color is achieved
- Wash the tooth with water and seal the chamber using dry cotton and temporary restorations
- Recall the patient after 1–3 weeks
- Do the permanent restoration of tooth using suitable composite resins afterwards

Intracoronal Bleaching/Walking Bleach of Nonvital Teeth

It involves use of chemical agents within the coronal portion of an endodontically treated tooth to remove tooth discoloration **(Fig. 30.22 A and B)**.

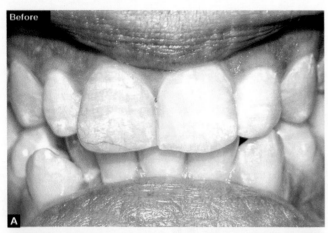

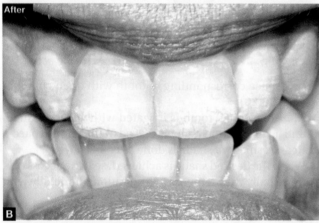

Figs. 30.22A and B (A) Preoperative photograph showing discolored 11; (B) postoperative photograph showing 11 after walking bleach.

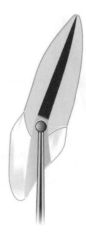

Fig. 30.23 Removal of coronal gutta-percha using rotary instrument.

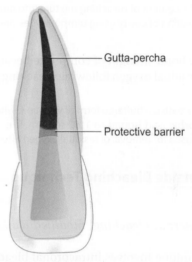

Gutta-percha

Protective barrier

Fig. 30.24 Placement of protective barrier over gutta-percha.

Indications	Contraindications
• Discolorations of pulp chamber origin	• Superficial enamel discoloration
• Moderate-to-severe tetracycline staining	• Defective enamel formation
• Dentin discoloration	• Presence of caries
• Discoloration not agreeable to extracoronal bleaching	• Unpredictable prognosis of tooth

Steps

❑ Take the radiographs to assess the quality of obturation. If found unsatisfactory, retreatment should be done
❑ Evaluate the quality and shade of restoration, if present. If restoration is defective, replace it
❑ Evaluate tooth color with shade guide
❑ Isolate the tooth with rubber dam
❑ Prepare the access cavity, remove the coronal gutta-percha, expose the dentin, and refine the cavity **(Fig. 30.23)**
❑ Place mechanical barriers of 2 mm thick, preferably of glass ionomer cement, zinc phosphate, IRM,

polycarboxylate cement, or MTA on root canal filling material **(Fig. 30.24)**. The coronal height of barrier should protect the dentinal tubules and conform to the external epithelial attachment
❑ Now mix sodium perborate with an inert liquid (local anesthetic, saline, or water) and place this paste into pulp chamber **(Fig. 30.25)**. In case severe stains add 3% hydrogen peroxide to make a paste
❑ After removing the excess bleaching paste, place a temporary restoration over it. Apply pressure with the gloved finger against the tooth until the filling has set because filling may get displaced due to release of oxygen
❑ Recall the patient after 1–2 weeks, repeat the treatment until desired shade is achieved
❑ Restore access cavity with composite after 2 weeks

Complications of Intracoronal Bleaching

❑ External root resorption
❑ Chemical burns if using 30–35% H_2O_2 so gingival should be protected using petroleum jelly or cocoa butter.

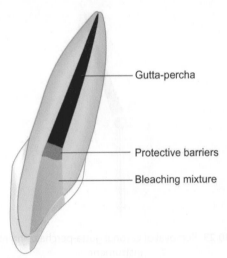

Fig. 30.25 Placement of bleaching mixture into pulp chamber and sealing of cavity using temporary restoration.

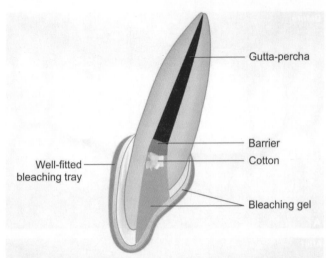

Fig. 30.26 Inside/outside techniques in this tray is sealed over an open internal access opening, with a cotton pellet placed in open access cavity.

❑ Decrease bond strength of composite because of presence of residual oxygen following bleaching procedure

> Sodium ascorbate is a buffered form of vitamin C which consists of 90% ascorbic acid bound to 10% sodium. It is a powerful antioxidant used for removal of residual oxygen after bleaching.

Inside/Outside Bleaching Technique

Synonyms

Internal/external bleaching, modified walking bleach technique.

This technique involves intracoronal bleaching technique along with home bleaching technique. This is done to make the bleaching program more effective. This combination of bleaching treatment is helpful in treating difficult stains, for specific problems like single dark vital or nonvital tooth and to treat stains of different origin present on the same tooth.

Procedure

❑ Assess the obturation by taking radiographs
❑ Isolate the tooth and prepare the access cavity by removing gutta-percha 2–3 mm below the cementoenamel junction
❑ Place the mechanical barrier, clean the access cavity and place a cotton pellet in the chamber to avoid food packing into it
❑ Evaluate the shade of tooth
❑ Check the fitting of bleaching tray and advise the patient to remove the cotton pellet before bleaching
❑ Instructions for home bleaching. Bleaching syringe can be directly placed into chamber before seating the tray or extrableaching material can be placed into the

tray space corresponding to tooth with open chamber **(Fig. 30.26)**
❑ After bleaching, tooth is irrigated with water, cleaned, and again a cotton pellet is placed in the empty space
❑ Reassessment of shade is done after 4–7 days
❑ When the desired shade is achieved, seal the access cavity initially with temporary restoration and finally with composite restoration after ≥2 weeks

Advantages
- More surface area for bleach to penetrate
- Treatment time in days rather than weeks
- Decreases the incidence of cervical resorption
- Uses lower concentration of carbamide peroxide

Disadvantages
- Noncompliant patients
- Overbleaching by overzealous application
- Chances for cervical resorption is reduced but still exist

Closed Chamber Bleaching/Extracoronal Bleaching

In this technique, instead of removing the existing restoration, the bleaching paste is applied to the tooth via bleaching tray.

Indications of Closed Chamber Technique

❑ In case of totally calcified canals in a traumatized tooth
❑ As a maintenance bleaching treatment several years after initial intracoronal bleaching
❑ Treatment for adolescents with incomplete gingival maturation
❑ A single dark nonvital tooth where the surrounding teeth are sufficiently light or where other vital teeth are also to be bleached

Laser-Assisted Bleaching Technique

This technique achieves power bleaching process with the help of efficient energy source with minimum side effects. Laser whitening gel contains thermally absorbed crystals, fumed silica, and 35% H_2O_2. In this, gel is applied and is activated by light source which in further activates the crystals present in gel, allowing dissociation of oxygen and therefore better penetration into enamel matrix. The following lasers have been approved by FDA for tooth bleaching:

❑ Argon laser
❑ CO_2 laser
❑ GaAlAs diode laser.

Argon Laser

❑ Emits wavelength of 480 nm in visible part of spectrum
❑ Activates the bleaching gel and makes the darker tooth surface lighter
❑ Less thermal effects on pulp as compared to other heat lamps.

CO_2 Laser

❑ Emits a wavelength of 10,600 nm
❑ Used to enhance the effect of whitening produced by argon laser
❑ Deeper penetration than argon laser thus more efficient tooth whitening
❑ More deleterious effects on pulp than argon laser

GaAlAs Diode Laser (Gallium-Aluminum-Arsenic)

Emits a wavelength of 980 nm.

Effects of Bleaching Agents on Tooth and its Supporting Structures

Tooth Hypersensitivity

Tooth sensitivity is common side effect of external tooth bleaching. Higher incidences of tooth sensitivity (67–78%) are seen after in-office bleaching with hydrogen peroxide in combination with heat. The mechanism responsible for external tooth bleaching though is not fully established, but it has been shown that peroxide penetrated enamel, dentin and pulp. This penetration was more in restored teeth than that of intact teeth.

Effects on Enamel

Studies have shown that 10% carbamide peroxide significantly decreased enamel hardness. But application of fluoride showed improved remineralization after bleaching.

Effects on Dentin

Bleaching has shown to cause uniform change in color through dentin.

Effects on Pulp

Penetration of bleaching agent into pulp through enamel and dentin occurs resulting in tooth sensitivity. Studies have shown that 3% solution of H_2O_2 can cause transient reduction in pulpal blood flow and occlusion of pulpal blood vessels.

Effects on Cementum

Recent studies have shown that cementum is not affected by materials used for home bleaching. But cervical resorption and external root resorption in teeth has been seen in teeth treated by intracoronal bleaching using 30–35% H_2O_2.

Cervical Resorption

More serious side effects such as external root resorption may occur when a higher than 30% concentration of hydrogen peroxide is used in combination with heat. Hydroxyl groups may be generated during thermocatalytic bleaching, especially where ethylenediamine tetraacetic acid has been used previously to clean the tooth. Hydroxyl ions may stimulate cells in the cervical periodontal ligament to differentiate into odontoclasts, which begin root resorption in the area of the tooth below the epithelial attachment.

Mucosal Irritation

A high concentration of hydrogen peroxide (30–35%) is caustic to mucous membrane and may cause burns and bleaching of the gingiva.

Genotoxicity and Carcinogenicity

Hydrogen peroxide shows genotoxic effect as free radicals released from hydrogen peroxide (hydroxyl radicals, perhydroxyl ions and superoxide anions) are capable of attacking DNA.

Toxicity

The acute effects of hydrogen peroxide ingestion are dependent on the amount and concentration of hydrogen peroxide solution ingested. Signs and symptoms usually seen are ulceration of the buccal mucosa, esophagus and stomach, nausea, vomiting, abdominal distention and sore throat.

Bleaching is safe, economical, conservative, and effective method of decoloring the stained teeth due to various reasons.

It should always be given a thought before going for more invasive procedure like veneering or full ceramic coverage, depending upon specific case.

Effects on Restorative Materials

Application of bleaching on composites has shown the following changes:
- Increased surface hardness
- Surface roughening and etching
- Decrease in tensile strength
- Increased microleakage
- No significant color change of composite material itself other than the removal of extrinsic stains around existing restoration

▌Conclusion

Bleaching is safe, economical, conservative, and effective method of decoloring the stained teeth due to various reasons. It should always be given a thought before going for more invasive procedure like veneering or full ceramic coverage, depending upon specific case. It can be performed in office or at home as per patient's requirements. However, as with any dental procedure, bleaching involves risks. Clinician should inform their patients about the possible changes that may occur on their dental tissues and restorations after bleaching procedure so as to compare risk versus benefit of the procedure.

▌Questions

1. What are different etiological factors responsible for discoloration of teeth?
2. Define bleaching. Explain the mechanism of bleaching and classify different bleaching procedures.
3. How will you bleach a nonvital central incisor tooth?
4. Discuss advantages and disadvantages of bleaching. How will you bleach a nonvital central incisor?
5. Enumerate the causes of discoloration of teeth? What methods are used to achieve normal color of teeth? Describe the methods used to bleach the vital teeth.
6. Write short notes on:
   a. Contraindication of bleaching.
   b. Night guard vital bleaching technique.
   c. Walking bleach.
   d. In-office bleach.
   e. Effects of bleaching on teeth.

▌Bibliography

1. Goldstein RE. Bleaching teeth: new materials, new role. J Am Dent Assoc 1988 Feb;116(2):156.
2. Haywood VB, Heymann HO. Nightguard vital bleaching: how safe is it?. Quintessence Int 1991;22:515–23.
3. Haywood VB. Historical development of whiteners: clinical safety and efficacy. Dent Update 1997;24(3):98-104
4. Laser assisted bleaching: an update. J Am Dent Assoc 1998;129:1484–7.
5. Nathanson D. Vital tooth bleaching: sensitivity and pulpal considerations. J Am Dent Assoc 1997;1281:41–4.
6. Settembrini L1, Gultz J, Kaim J, Scherer W. A technique for bleaching non-vital teeth: inside/outside bleaching. J Am Dent Assoc 1997;128(9):1283-4.
7. Watts A, Addy M. Tooth discolouration and staining: a literature review. Br Dent J 2001;190:309–16.

Root Resorption

Introduction

Resorption is a condition associated with either physiologic or a pathologic process resulting in a loss of dentin, cementum, and/or bone. It causes loss of the tooth structure either internal or external which may lead to extraction of the tooth if not treated well at the time. There are many classifications and terms coined for resorption defects depending upon their location and etiology. Etiology of any resorption defect is inflammation which starts from injury in form of dental trauma, surgical procedures, chemical injury from bleaching agents or excessive pressure from impacted tooth. Tooth can be saved if treatment is given at initial stage but if resorption continues without treatment, it may lead to extraction of the tooth. Identification of stimulating factors and removal of the etiology are the main requirements to render proper treatment to the tooth undergoing resorption.

Definition

According to American Association of Endodontics in 1944 (Glossary—Contemporary Terminology for Endodontics), *resorption is defined as* "A condition associated with either a physiologic or a pathologic process resulting in the loss of dentin, cementum or bone."

Root resorption is the resorption affecting the cementum or dentin of the root of tooth. Resorption is a perplexing problem for which etiologic factors are vague.

External resorption: When resorption is initiated in periodontium and initially affects the external surface of the tooth.

Internal resorption: When resorption is initiated within the pulp space affecting the internal dentin surface.

Etiology of Root Resorption

Local	Systemic	Idiopathic

• Trauma
• Periapical pathology
• Cysts and tumors
• Impacted tooth
• Intracoronal bleaching
	• Paget's disease
	• Hormonal imbalance:
	  – Hyperthyroidism
	  – Hypothyroidism
	  – Hypo and hyper pituitarism	

Classification of Resorption (Flowchart 31.1)

Cohen's classification of root resorption
- ❑ According to nature
  - • Physiologic [(in deciduous teeth during eruption of permanent teeth (**Figs. 31.1A to C**)]
  - • Pathologic (in teeth due to underlying pathology)
- ❑ According to anatomic region of occurrence
  - • Internal
  - • External
- ❑ Based on cause
  - • Local
    - – Inflammatory
      - a. External
      - b. Internal
    - – Pressure
      - a. Orthodontic tooth movement
      - b. Impacted tooth
    - – Dentoalveolar ankylosis
  - • Systemic
  - • Idiopathic

Flowchart 31.1 Lindskog classification of root resorption.

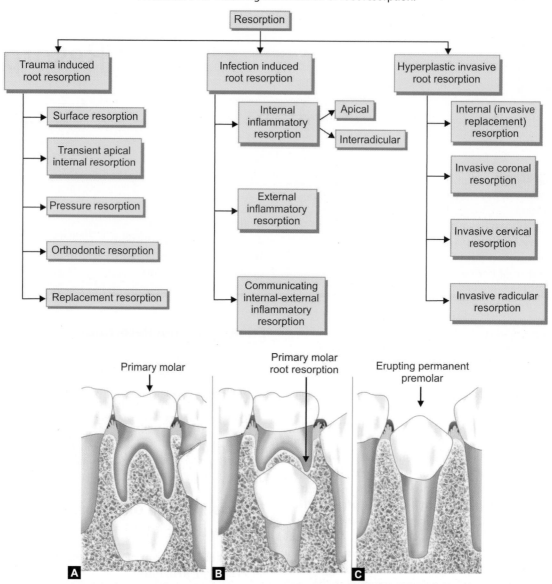

Figs. 31.1A to C Primary tooth is lost naturally due physiological root resorption caused by pressure of erupting permanent tooth. (A) Permanent tooth bud under primary tooth; (B) eruption of permanent tooth with simultaneous root resorption of primary tooth; (C) loss of primary tooth with eruption of permanent tooth.

Andreasen classification of root resorption

- ❑ *Internal resorption*
  - Root canal replacement resorption
  - Internal inflammatory resorption
- ❑ *External resorption*
  - Surface resorption
  - Inflammatory resorption
  - Replacement resorption
  - Dentoalveolar ankylosis

Protective Mechanism Against Resorption

There are few hypotheses which tell the protective mechanism against resorption. These are as follows.

Remnant of Epithelial Root Sheath

Remnants of epithelial root sheath surround the roots like a net and impart resistance to resorption and subsequent ankylosis

Intrinsic Factors

Intrinsic factors found in predentin and cementum act as inhibitor of resorption

Presence of Osteoprotegerin (OPG)

OPG a member of tumor necrosis factor (TNF) binds to receptor activator of NF-κB ligand and reduces its concentration and further inhibits its ability to stimulate osteoclast production (osteoclastogenesis) and subsequently inhibits resorption

Anti-Invasion Factors

Low-molecular-weight proteolytic activity inhibitor is present in cartilages, blood vessel walls and teeth. It causes loss of ruffled border, attachment ability of osteoclasts to bone and thus bone resorption

Intermediate Cementum

Presence of hyaline layer of Hopewell-Smith (*intermediate cementum*) is hypercalcified in relation to adjacent dentin and cementum. It prevents development of inflammatory resorption in replanted teeth with pulpal pathosis, possibly by forming a barrier against egress of noxious agents from the dentinal tubules to the PDL

Anti-Resorptive Factors

Like estrogen, calcitonin, platelet-derived growth factor, calcium, tumor growth factor, interlukin,-17 etc.

Cells Involved in Root Resorption

Clast Cells

Odontoclasts, Dentinoclasts, Osteoclasts, and Cementoclasts

All these cells belong to the group of clast cells and they have a common origin, that is, circulating monocytes which form macrophages. When the inflammation gets out of control, these monocytes/macrophages join to form *giant cells* (Fig. 31.2). These are highly vacuolated and contain numerous mitochondria. Majority of odontoclasts have 10 or fewer nuclei, that is, 96% are multinucleated and rest 4% are mononucleated.

Oligonuclear odontoclasts are cells with <5 nuclei. They resorb more dentin per nucleus when compared with cells with higher number of nuclei.

Monocytes and Macrophages

Monocytes and macrophages along with osteoclasts are found in tissue surfaces adjacent to bone, for example, in resorpting surfaces of rheumatoid arthritis, periodontal diseases, periradicular granulomas, cysts and in metastatic

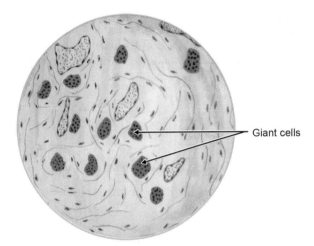

Fig. 31.2 Diagram showing giant cells.

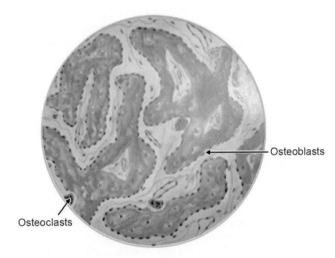

Fig. 31.3 Structure of bone showing osteoclasts and osteoblasts.

bone tumors. Though macrophages have structure (**Fig. 31.3**) similar to osteoclasts and like osteoclasts, can become multinucleated giant cells, macrophages lack a ruffled border, that is, attached to hard tissue substrates during resorption and do not create lacunae on the dentinal surface.

Mechanism of Root Resorption

Resorption of hard tissue takes place in two events:
1. Degradation of inorganic crystal structures—hydroxyapatite
2. Degradation of the organic matrix—principally Collagen Type 1

Degradation of the Inorganic Crystal Structures

The degradation of inorganic structures initiates when pH is 3–4.5 at the site of resorption. This is created by the polarized proton pump formed in ruffled border of the clast cells. Below the pH of 5, the dissolution of hydroxyapatite occurs.

Enzymes carbonic anhydrase II which catalyzes the conversion of CO_2 and H_2CO_3 intracellularly also maintains an acidic environment at the site of resorption which is a readily available source of H^+ ions. The enzyme acid phosphatase also favors the resorption process.

$$CO_2 + H_2O \rightarrow H_2CO_3$$
$$H_2CO_3 \rightarrow H^+ + HCO_3^-$$

Degradation of the Organic Matrix

Three main enzymes involved in this process are collagenase, matrix metalloproteinases (MMP) and cysteine proteinases.

Collagenase and MMP act at a neutral or just below neutral pH—7.4. They are found more toward the resorbing bone surface where the pH is near neutral, because of the presence of the buffering capacity of the resorbing bone salts. MMP is more involved in odontoblastic action. Cysteine proteinases are secreted directly into the osteoclasts into the clear zone via the ruffled border. Cysteine proteinases work more in an acidic pH and near the ruffled border, the pH is more acidic.

Factors regulating resorption	
Systemic	*Local*
• **PTH** favors resorption by stimulating osteoclasts and formation of multinucleated giant cells • **1,2,5-dihydroxy vitamin D$_3$** increases resorption activity of osteoblasts • **Calcitonin** inhibits resorption by suppressing osteoclastic cytoplasmic mobility of ruffled border	• Interleukin 6 • Interleukin 1 • Tumor necrosis factor-α • Prostaglandin • Bacterial toxins • Macrophage stimulating factor

PTH: parathyroid hormone.

Diagnosis of Resorption

Clinically: Pink spot in case of internal resorption

Imaging
- Conventional radiograph
- Digital radiographs
- CT scan
- Rapid prototyping tooth model
- Cone beam computed tomography (CBCT)

Vitality testing
If tooth is vital: Internal root resorption or subepithelial external root resorption.

If tooth is nonvital: External inflammatory root resorption with infected pulp or internal root resorption with necrotic coronal pulp.

Internal Resorption

According to **Shafer**, "internal resorption is an unusual form of tooth resorption that begins centrally within the tooth, apparently initiated in most cases by a peculiar inflammation of the pulp." It is characterized by oval-shaped enlargement of root canal space (**Fig. 31.4**).

Synonyms of internal resorption
- Chronic perforating hyperplasia of the pulp
- Internal granuloma
- Odontoblastoma
- Pink tooth of mummery

Etiology

Though etiology is unknown but it is most often seen in the following cases:
- Long-standing chronic inflammation of the pulp
- Caries-related pulpits
- Traumatic injuries
  - Luxation injuries
- Iatrogenic injuries
  - Preparation of tooth for crown
  - Deep restorative procedures
  - Application of heat over the pulp
  - Pulpotomy using $Ca(OH)_2$
- Idiopathic

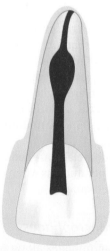

Fig. 31.4 Internal resorption showing oval-shaped enlargement of root canal space.

Clinical Features

❑ Internal root resorption is usually asymptomatic until root is perforated. It is detected coincidentally by routine radiographs

❑ Patient may complain of pain when the lesion perforates and tissue is exposed to oral fluids (**Fig. 31.5**)

❑ Most commonly affected teeth are maxillary central incisors

❑ Usually single tooth is involved but sometimes multiple teeth are also involved

❑ It occurs in permanent as well as in deciduous teeth. In primary teeth, it spreads more rapidly

❑ Granulation tissue can clinically manifest itself as a "pink spot" where crown dentin destruction is severe leading to pink tooth appearance (**Fig. 31.6**).

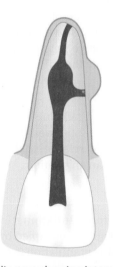

Fig. 31.5 Line diagram showing internal resorption with root perforation.

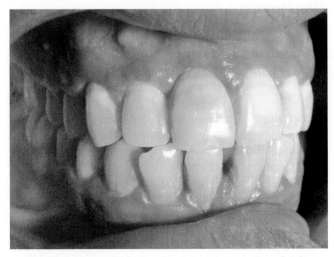

Fig. 31.6 Photograph showing internal resorption of right maxillary central incisor resulting in pink tooth appearance.

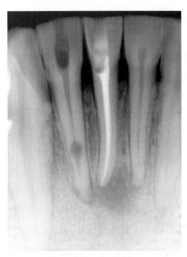

Fig. 31.7 Radiograph showing oval radiolucent enlargement of pulp space in mandibular lateral incisor with internal resorption.

Radiographic Features

Outline of lesion: Lesion appears as uniform, round-to-oval radiolucent enlargement of the pulp space (**Fig. 31.7**).

Outline of root canal: There is distortion of original root canal outline.

Radiographs are taken from different angles to show the resorptive lesion in the central location.

Types of Internal Resorption

❑ Internal replacement resorption
❑ Internal inflammatory resorption

Internal Replacement Resorption (Metaplastic Resorption)

Resorption of dentin and subsequent deposition of hard tissues are found that resembles bone or cementum or osteodentin, but not dentin. They represent areas of destruction and repair. This occurs mainly due to low grade irritation of pulpal tissue.

Etiology

❑ Trauma
❑ Extreme heat to the tooth
❑ Chemical burns
❑ Pulpotomy procedures

Radiographic Features

Radiographically, the tooth shows enlargement of the canal space. This space latter gets engorged with a material of radiopaque appearance giving the expression of hard tissue.

Histopathology

Histological studies of internal resorption demonstrate replacement of normal pulp tissue by a periodontal-like connective tissue with both osteogenic and resorptive potential.

Origin of metaplastic hard tissue

- Metaplastic hard tissue formed in replacement resorption is produced by postnatal dental pulp stem cells present in apical part of root canal as reparative response to restorative insult
- Both granulation tissue and metaplastic hard tissue are nonpulpal in origin and might be derived from cells that transmigrated from vascular compartment from periodontium.

Internal Inflammatory Resorption

This is that form of internal resorption in which progressive loss of dentin is present without deposition of any form of hard tissue in the resorption cavity.

Pathophysiology (Fig. 31.8)

- Long-standing injury leads to chronic pulp inflammation and circulatory changes within the pulp. Active hyperemia with high oxygen pressure supports and induces the osteoclastic activity
- *Electric activity:* Piezoelectricity arising due to increased blood flow adds to the resorptive process
- Sudden trauma leads to intrapulpal hemorrhage, which latter organizes to form clot and forms the granulation tissue. Proliferating granulation tissues compresses the dentinal walls and stimulate the formation of odontoblasts which differentiate from the connective tissue. Thereby, the resorption process starts.

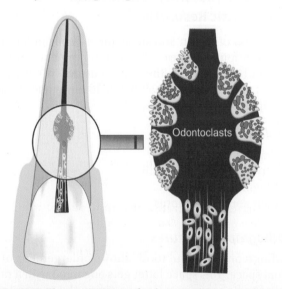

Fig. 31.8 Chronic irritation of pulp can induce osteoclastic activity in pulp, resulting in internal inflammatory resorption.

- According to **Heithersay**, the internal resorption may result from collateral blood supply via an interconnecting large accessory canal, which provides a vascular bed for the process

Clinical Features

Clinical characteristics of internal root resorption are dependent on the development and location of the resorption.

- It is asymptomatic in most of the cases, but when resorption is actively progressing, it may present symptoms of pulpitis
- If it occurs in or near the crown, a pinkish or reddish color is seen through the crown and appears gray/dark gray if the pulp becomes necrotic
- In advance cases of resorption, perforation of the root is usually followed by the development of a sinus tract
- Internal resorption is active only in teeth where a part of the pulp remains vital. Therefore, pulp tests may show different responses, a positive pulp test if the coronal pulp is vital, or a negative pulp test if the coronal pulp becomes necrotic while the apical pulp is vital

Radiographic Features

It presents round or ovoid radiolucent area in the central portion of the tooth with smooth well-defined margins. The defect does not change its relation to the tooth, when the rays are projected from an angulation.

Histology

Pulp tissue shows chronic inflammation reaction and resorption lacunae irregularly occupied by "dentinoclasts" similar to osteoclasts. The granulation tissue present in this type of resorption is highly proliferating in nature.

Classification

> **Internal inflammatory resorptions may be classified according to location as**
> - Apical
> - Intraradicular

Apical internal inflammatory resorption

- Seen in teeth with inflammatory periapical pathologies
- *Management:* There are two approaches to the endodontic management of apical internal resorption:
  - To extend instrumentation only to the position of the resorption with the expectation that removal of microorganisms followed by root canal filling, hard tissue repair will occur in the resorbed apical region of the tooth
  - To enlarge and prepare the apical region, either with hand or rotary filing techniques, to include the

resorbed region and then root fills to the root canal "terminus"

Intraradicular inflammatory resorption

- Internal resorption fully contained within an otherwise intact root will be referred to as intraradicular internal inflammatory resorption
- This can be recognized as round- or oval-shaped radiolucencies contained within the root
- A common finding is a large accessory canal communicating from the periodontal ligament to the resorbed area; this may have allowed the passage of a collateral blood supply which probably played an important role in the development and maintenance of the internal resorptive process
- Treatment is endodontic therapy. The obturation of the canal can be done by using vertically condensed guttapercha, obtura, or microseal technique

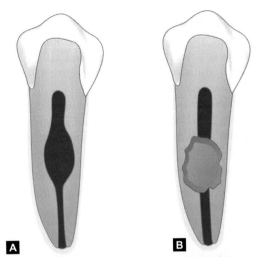

Figs. 31.9A and B (A) Internal resorption; (B) external resorption.

Differences between internal and external resorption (Figs. 31.9A and B)		
	Internal resorption	*External resorption*
Definition	• Internal resorption is the resorption that begins centrally within the tooth, apparently initiated by a peculiar inflammation of the pulp	• It is defined as loss of tooth substance from outer surface of the tooth, arising from a tissue reaction in periodontal or pericoronal tissue
Canal shape	• It is characterized by oval-shaped enlargement of root canal space • Causes expansion of the canal	• Canal shape is not altered • Defect is separate and is superficial on root lateral to the canal
Pink tooth of mummery	• Pathognomic feature • Hyperplastic vascular pulp tissue showing through the tooth	• Pink tooth not seen • Pulp is nonvital consisting of granulation tissue
Symmetry	• Symmetric defect though may be eccentric	• Usually asymmetrical
Margins	• Smooth and well defined	• Rough with moth eaten appearance
Radiographic appearance	• Ballooning of canal space • Lesion appears close to canal even if angulation of radiograph changes • Root canal and resorptive defect appears contiguous • Does not involve bone so radiolucency is confined to root. Bone resorption is seen if lesion perforates the root	• Scooped out areas on the root surface • Lesion moves away from canal as the angulation changes • Root canal can be seen running through the defect • It involves resorption of bone, so radiolucency appears both in root and bone
Pulp vitality test	• Pulp is vital unless it gets involved	• Pulp is nonvital as it commonly involves infected pulp space

Management of Internal Root Resorption

- Early diagnosis is important to prevent the weakening of the remaining root structure by the resorptive process
- Conventional root canal therapy should be instituted as soon as the diagnosis of internal resorption is made
- If the apical third is not involved, then the cases are treated as usual and the resorbed area is filled with warm gutta-percha technique

- Teeth with perforation often need both surgical and nonsurgical procedures

Treatment options in teeth with internal resorption
- Without perforation: *Endodontic therapy*
- With perforation
  - *Nonsurgical*: Ca(OH)$_2$ therapy—obturation
  - *Surgical*:
    - ◆ Surgical flap
    - ◆ Root resection
    - ◆ Intentional replantation

Management of Nonperforating Resorption

Pulp removal and canal preparation: Removal of all inflamed tissue from the resorptive defect is the basis of the treatment. But sometimes complete extirpation of the inflamed tissue may become difficult by hand instruments. Evidence shows that ultrasonic instruments can give better results as compared to hand instruments. Ultrasonic vibration is unparalleled in its ability to enhance cleaning with irrigant (**Fig. 31.10**).

Canal obturation: Because of the size, irregularity and in accessibility of the resorption defects, obturation of the canal may be technically difficult.

Canal apical to the defect is filled with solid gutta-percha while the resorptive area is usually filled with material that will flow in the irregularities. The warm gutta-percha technique, thermoplasticized gutta-percha technique and the use of chemically plasticized gutta-percha are methods of obturation to be used (**Figs. 31.11 to 31.15**).

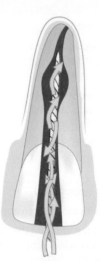

Fig. 31.10 Use of ultrasonics helps in better cleaning of canal.

Various materials used include:
- MTA
- Glass ionomer cement
- Super EBA
- Hydrophilic plastic polymer (2-hydroxyethyl methacrylate with barium salts)
- Zinc oxide eugenol and zinc acetate cement
- Amalgam alloy
- Thermoplasticized gutta-percha administered either by injection or condensation techniques

Management of Perforating Internal Resorption

When the internal root resorption has progressed through the tooth into the periodontium, there are additional problem of periodontal bleeding, pain and difficulty in obturation. Presence of a perforation cannot be determined radiographically unless a lateral radiolucent lesion is present adjacent to the lesion. Clinically in some cases, a sinus tract may be present and there will be continued hemorrhage in the canal after the pulp is removed.

Nonsurgical repair

Indications of nonsurgical repair:
- When the defect is not extensive
- When defect is apical to epithelial attachment
- When hemorrhage can be controlled

In this technique, after thorough cleaning and shaping of the canal, the intracanal calcium hydroxide dressing is placed and over it a temporary filling is placed to prevent interappointment leakage.

Patient is recalled after 3 months for replacement of calcium hydroxide dressing and for radiographic confirmation of the barrier formation at the perforation site. Afterwards, 2 months recall visits are scheduled until there is a radiographic barrier at resorption defect. After the barrier is formed, the canal is obturated with gutta-percha as in the nonperforating internal resorption.

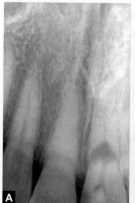 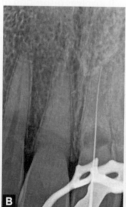 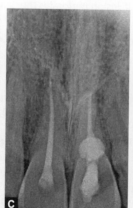 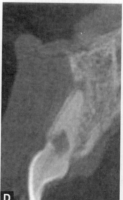 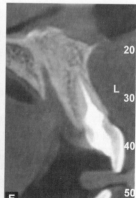

Figs. 31.11 A to D Management of internal resorption case of maxillary central incisor: (A) Preoperative radiograph of central incisor showing internal resorption defect; (B) Working length radiograph; (C) Obturation of canal by Obtura II; (D and E) Confirmation of internal resorption before and after on CBCT.

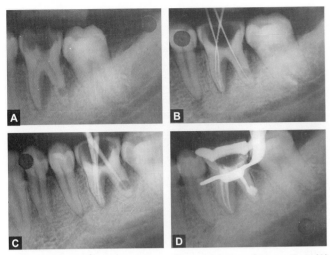

Figs. 31.12A to D Management of 36 with internal resorption. (A) Preoperative radiograph; (B) Working length radiograph; (C) Master cone radiograph; (D) Obturation by themoplasticized gutta-percha.
Courtesy: Jaidev Dhillon

Surgical repair

If it is not possible to get access to the lesion through the canal, surgical repair of the defect should be considered. Treatment options in surgical repair can be

- *Surgical flap:* Defect is exposed to allow good access. The resorptive defect is curetted, cleaned and restored using an alloy, composite, glass ionomer cement, super EBA, MTA, biodentine, etc. Final obturation is done using gutta-percha

- *Root resection:* If the resorbed area is located in the apical third, root may be resected coronal to the defect and apical segment is removed afterwards. Following root resection, retrofilling is done. If one root of a multirooted tooth is affected, root resection may be considered based on anatomical, periodontal and restorative parameters

- *Intentional replantation:* If the perforating resorption with minimal root damage occurs in an inaccessible area, intentional replantation may be considered.

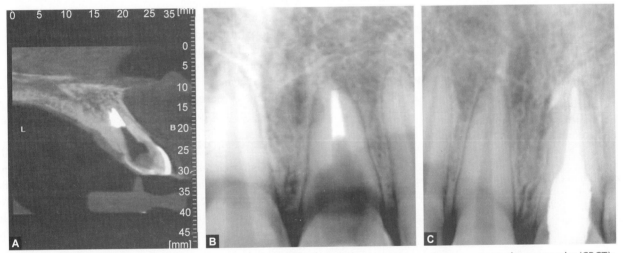

Figs. 31.13A to C Management of internal resorption with MTA and obtura using cone beam computed tomography (CBCT): (A) CBCT view of internal resorption; (B) MTA plug at apical part of root; (C) Postobturation radiograph.
Courtesy: Anil Dhingra

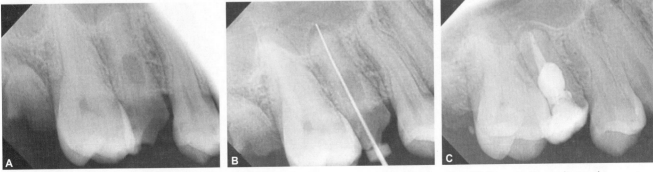

Figs. 31.14A to C Management of maxillary second premolar with internal resorption. (A) Preoperative radiograph; (B) Working length radiograph; (C) Obturation by themoplasticized gutta-percha.
Courtesy: Punit Jindal

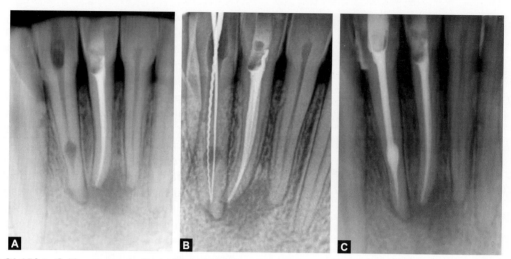

Figs. 31.15A to C Management of mandibular lateral incisor with internal resorption: (A) Preoperative radiograph; (B) Working length radiograph; (C) Obturation by themoplasticized gutta-percha.

External Root Resorption

External root resorption is defined as loss of tooth substance from outer surface of the tooth, arising from a tissue reaction in periodontal or pericoronal tissue **(Figs. 31.16A and B)**.

Classification
According to Rita F-Ne, Gutman et al. (Quintessence International, 1999), external resorption is of three types:
- **S**urface resorption
- **I**nflammatory root resorption
- **R**eplacement resorption

According to Cohen, on the basis of the location:
- Cervical
- Lateral
- Apical

External resorption may be found in the following conditions:
- Periodontal disease
- Luxation injuries
- Hypoparathyroidism
- Hyperparathyroidism
- Turner syndrome
- Paget disease
- Gaucher disease
- Radiation therapy

Surface Resorption (Fig. 31.17)

External surface resorption is a transient phenomenon in which the root surface undergoes spontaneous destruction and repair. It is the least destructive form of external root resorption and is a self-limiting process; hence, it requires no treatment.

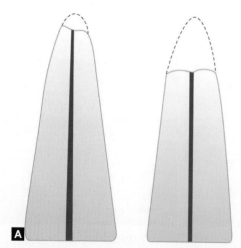

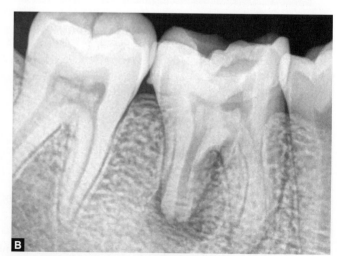

Figs. 31.16A and B External resorption: (A) Schematic representation of external root resorption; (B) Radiograph showing external root resorption of distal root of mandibular first molar.

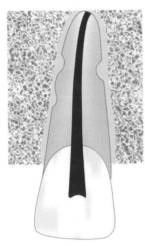

Fig. 31.17 Surface resorption.

Etiology

- As part of the repair process
- Indirect physical injury, caused by physiologic function, to localized areas of periodontal ligament or cementum on root surface
- In trauma, it occurs because of direct mechanical contact of the root surface and alveolar bone proper

Clinical Evaluation

No significant signs of external surface resorption are detectable on the supragingival portion of the tooth.

Radiographic Evaluation

External surface resorption is usually not visible on radiographs because of its small size. Later, it appears as small excavations on the lateral surface or at the root apex resulting in the appearance of shorter roots.

Histologic Evaluation

Small, superficial lacunae in the cementum and outermost layer of dentin are seen which are simultaneously being repaired with new cementum.

Classification

Surface resorption can be
- Transient
- Progressive

Transient surface resorption: In this type, the tooth has a vital, healthy pulp that has recovered from traumatic event. In such cases, the resorbed area will be restored completely to normal surface contour by deposition of new cementum.

Progressive surface resorption: In this type, the surface resorption is the beginning of more destructive resorption, either inflammatory resorption or replacement resorption.

Treatment

No treatment is indicated.

External Inflammatory Root Resorption (Fig. 31.18)

It is the most common and most destructive type of resorption and is thought to be caused by presence of infected or necrotic pulp tissue in the root canal. It is best described as a bowl-shaped resorptive defect that penetrates dentin (**Fig. 31.19**).

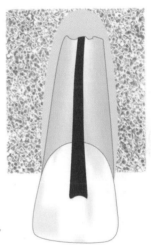

Fig. 31.18 External inflammatory resorption.

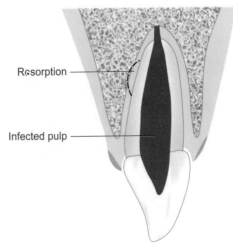

Resorption

Infected pulp

Fig. 31.19 Progression of inflammatory root resorption. It forms a bowl-shaped resorptive defect which penetrates dentin.

Etiopathology

❑ Injury or irritation to the periodontal tissues where the inflammation is beyond repair

❑ Trauma leads to pulpal necrosis which may further cause periodontal inflammation due to the passage of the toxins and microorganisms from the infected pulp, lateral canals, apical foramen, accessory canals, dentinal tubules where there is a discontinuity of cementum

❑ Orthodontic tooth movement using excessive forces (**Fig. 31.20**)

❑ Trauma from occlusion—leading to periodontal inflammation

❑ Avulsion and luxation injuries

❑ Pressure resorption occurring from pressure exerted by tumors, cysts and impacted teeth (**Fig. 31.21**)

❑ In the initial stages, bowl-shaped lacunae are seen in cementum and dentin, if not controlled, it may resorb the entire root in latter stages

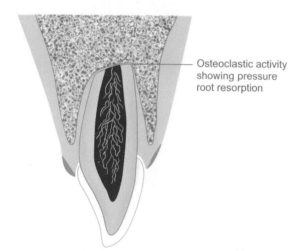

Osteoclastic activity showing pressure root resorption

Fig. 31.20 Orthodontic tooth movement resulting in inflammatory resorption.

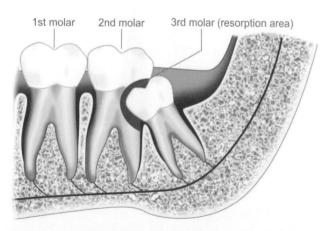

1st molar   2nd molar   3rd molar (resorption area)

Fig. 31.21 External inflammatory root resorption resulting due to pressure exerted by impacted 3rd molar.

Clinical Features

❑ Patient gives history of trauma

❑ Signs of necrotic pulp/irreversible pulpitis

❑ Tooth is usually mobile

❑ Inflammation of periodontal tissue

❑ Percussion sensitivity is present

Radiographic Features (Figs. 31.22A to C)

Bowl-like radiolucency with ragged irregular areas on the root surface is commonly seen in conjunction with loss of tooth structure and alveolar bone. Small lesion of external root resorption usually go undetected.

Histologic Evaluation

Histologically, EIRR is represented by a bowl-shaped resorption area into cementum and dentin with inflammation of adjacent periodontal tissue and infected or necrotic pulp in the root canal.

Types of external inflammatory root resorption			
	Apical	*Lateral*	*Cervical*
Etiology	Mainly trauma, inflammation is confined to apical area (**Fig. 31.23**)	Seen in luxation and avulsion cases	Injury to attachment apparatus below epithelial attachment, for example, in orthdontic tooth movement, bleaching of nonvital tooth
Features	Root resorption at apical area	Cemental loss is there, bacterial toxins pass through dentinal tubules and stimulate inflammatory response in periodontal ligament	It is usually destructive, and there is invasion of root by fibrovascular tissue from PDL
Clinical features	Symptoms same as apical periodontitis	Usually asymptomatic, in later stages tender on percussion	Asymptomatic, probing may show profuse bleeding, in long-standing cases pink tooth appearance which can be confused with internal resorption

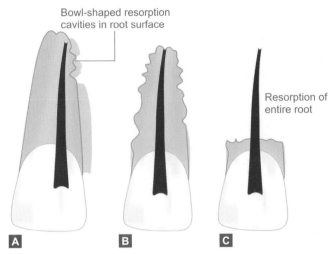

Bowl-shaped resorption cavities in root surface

Resorption of entire root

Figs. 31.22A to C External inflammatory root resorption: (A) In initial stages, bowl-shaped resorption cavities are seen in root surface; (B) More of resorption; (C) Complete resorption of root in later stages.

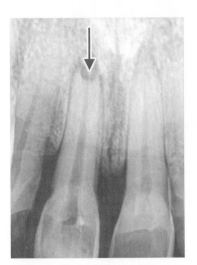

Fig. 31.23 Radiograph showing apical root resorption in maxillary central incisor.

Treatment (Figs. 31.24 and 31.25)

Treatment of external inflammatory root resorption is dependent on the etiology:

☐ If it is because of orthodontic treatment, remove the pressure of orthodontic movement to arrest resorption

☐ In cervical resorption
  • If pulp is vital and treatment of cervical resorption is unlikely to cause pulpal injury, restore the defect and carry on baseline thermal and electrical pulp tests for records
  • If treatment of the cervical resorption is likely to cause pulpal injury, restore the defect and perform endodontic treatment

☐ If pulp is nonvital, restore the defect and perform endodontic treatment. If required, calcium hydroxide dressing is also given

☐ In case of infected gingival tissues, remove plaque and calculus and maintain periodontium

☐ Calcitonin can also be used as an interim root canal medicament to assist in the inhibition of osteoclastic bone and dentin resorption

Replacement Resorption/Dentoalveolar Ankylosis (Fig. 31.26)

This is similar to ankylosis, but there is presence of an intervening inflamed connective tissue, always progressive and highly destructive. In this, tooth becomes a part of the alveolar bone remodeling process and thus, progressively resorbed. Ankylosis may be transient or progressive.

In the transient type, <20% of the root surface becomes ankylosed. In such cases, reversal may occur, resulting in re-establishment of a periodontal ligament connection between tooth and bone.

In the progressive type, tooth structure is gradually resorbed and replaced with the bone.

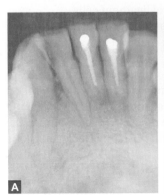
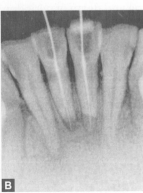
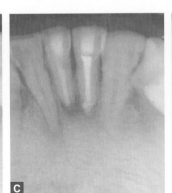
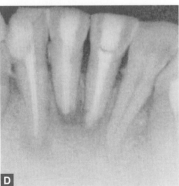

Figs. 31.24A to D Management of external inflammatory root resorption of mandibular central incisors. (A) Preoperative radiograph showing external root resorption involving roots of mandibular central incisors; (B) Working length radiograph; (C) Postobturation radiograph; (D) Follow-up radiograph after 3 months.
Courtesy: Jaidev Dhillon

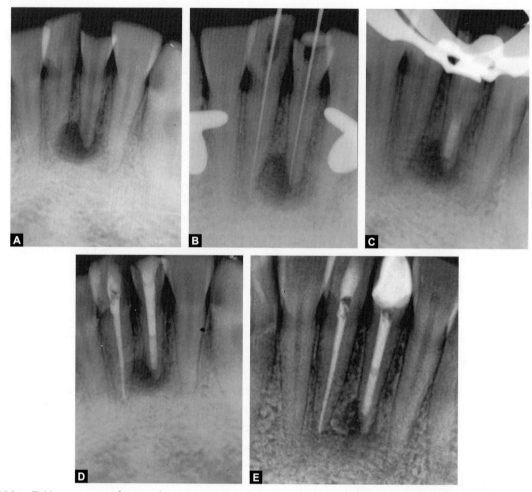

Figs. 31.25A to E Management of external root resorption of mandibular incisors: (A) Preoperative radiograph; (B) Working length radiograph; (C) MTA plug at the apical third; (D) Postobturation radiograph; (E) Follow-up after 3 months.
Courtesy: Jaidev Dhillon

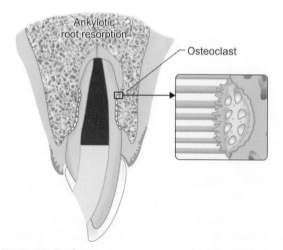

Fig. 31.26 Replacement resorption resulting in ankylosis.

Etiopathogenesis

❑ Replacement resorption occurs after a severe dental injury like intrusive luxation or avulsion resulting in drying and death of periodontal ligament cells

❑ An inflammatory process removes the necrotic debris from the root surface which results in root surface devoid of cementum

❑ To compensate this, cell in vicinity of root surface try to repopulate it. Cells which form bone move across the socket wall and colonize the damaged root wall. By this, bone comes in direct contact with root without an intermediate attachment apparatus resulting in dentoalveolar ankylosis

Histological Examination

❑ Direct fusion between dentin and bone without separating cemental or periodontal ligament layer

❑ Active resorption lacunae with osteoclasts are seen in conjunction with apposition of normal bone laid by osteoblasts

Clinical Features

- Replacement resorption is usually asymptomatic
- Infraocclusion, incomplete alveolar process development (if the patient is young) and absence of normal mesial drift
- Pathognomonic feature is immobility of affected tooth and a distinctive metallic sound on percussion.

Radiographic Features

Moth eaten appearance with irregular border, absence of periodontal ligament and lamina dura are seen in radiographs of an ankylosed tooth.

Diagnosis

- Lack of mobility and high-pitched metallic sound on percussion
- Radiographically, loss of periodontal ligament space with replacement by bone and uneven contour of root is indicative of ankylosis

Treatment

Currently, there is no treatment for replacement resorption. To slowdown the resorptive process, root surface is treated with fluoride solution prior to replantation if extraoral time for tooth was >2 h and it was not kept moist to protect the periodontal ligament.

Prevention

The following points should be considered in cases of avulsion:

- Immediate replantation without much of extraoral dry time
- Proper extraoral storage to prevent dehydration
- In case of extended period of extraoral time, soak the tooth in fluoride gel

Cervical Root Resorption (Extracanal Invasive Resorption)

According to Cohen, it is the type of inflammatory root resorption occurring immediately below the epithelial attachment of tooth. Epithelial attachment need not be always exactly at the cervical margin but can also be apical to the cervical margin (**Fig. 31.27**). So the term "cervical" is a misnomer.

Etiology

According to *Heithersay*, etiology can be

- Orthodontic treatment
- Trauma

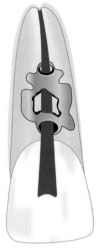

Fig. 31.27 Extracanal invasive resorption.

- Bleaching of nonvital teeth
- Periodontal treatment
- Bruxism
- Idiopathic

Etiopathogenesis

Though it is a relatively common occurrence, it is not well recognized and often classified as idiopathic resorption because of difficulty in establishing a cause and effect relation. It appears to originate in the cervical area of the tooth below the epithelial attachment and often proceeds from a small surface opening to involve a large part of dentin between the cementum and the pulp.

The resorption can proceed in several directions due to its invasive nature, hence the term ***invasive resorption.*** It can extend coronally under the enamel, giving the tooth a pink spot appearance. Because cervical resorption is not always associated with infected or necrotic pulp, the treatment options vary accordingly.

Theories of Cervical Root Resorption

- Some procedures like bleaching, trauma, or orthodontic treatment cause alteration in the organic and inorganic cementum, finally making it more inorganic. This makes the cementum less resistant to resorption
- Immunological system senses the altered root surface, as a different tissue, attacks as a foreign body

Clinical Features

- Initially, the cervical root resorption is asymptomatic in nature. Pulp is vital in most of the cases
- It initially starts as a small lesion, progress and reaches the predentin. Predentin is more resistant to resorption,

spreads laterally in apical and coronal direction "enveloping" the root canal

- In long-standing cases, extensive loss of tooth structure is replaced by granulation tissues which undermines the enamel in due course giving rise to pink spot appearance. It is misdiagnosed as internal resorption, but confirmed with a radiograph. Rarely, it perforates into the tooth causing secondary involvement of pulp

Heithersay's Classification (Fig. 31.28)

Class I: A small invasive resorptive lesion near cervical area with shallow penetration into dentin.

Class II: Well-defined resorptive defect close to coronal pulp chamber, but little or no involvement of radicular dentin.

Class III: Deep resorptive lesion involving coronal pulp and also coronal-third of the root.

Class IV: Resorptive defective extending beyond coronal-third of root canal.

Frank's Classification of Cervical Root Resorption (Figs. 31.29A to C)

- *Supraosseous:* Coronal to the level of alveolar bone
- *Intraosseous:* Not accompanied by periodontal breakdown
- *Crestal:* At the level of alveolar bone

Radiographic Features

Radiographically, one can see the moth eaten appearance with the intact outline of the canal. Because bone is often involved, resorption may give the appearance of an infrabony pocket.

Treatment

Main aim of the treatment is to restore the lost tooth structure and to disrupt the resorptive process. Since pulp is mostly vital, repair of resorbed area without removing the pulp is done. Heithersay recommended topical application of *90% solution of trichloroacetic acid* (to cause coagulation

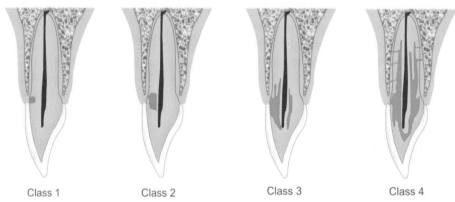

Class 1   Class 2   Class 3   Class 4

Fig. 31.28 Heithersay's classification of cervical root resorption.

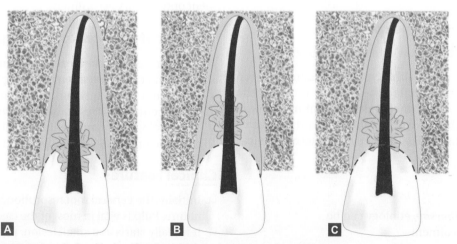

Figs. 31.29A to C Frank's classification of cervical root resorption: (A) Supraosseous; (B) Intraosseous; (C) Crestal extracanal invasive resorption.

and necrosis of necrotic tissue), curettage and then restoration with glass ionomer cement. If symptoms of pulpitis develop later, endodontic treatment is done.

Conclusion

Tooth resorption is a perplexing problem where the etiologic factors are vague and less clearly defined. For the best treatment outcome, the clinician should have a very good knowledge of the etiopathology of resorptive lesions. Early diagnosis and prompt treatment in such cases are the key factors which determine the success of the treatment. More clinical studies and research with animal models are required to explain more about this phenomenon scientifically.

Questions

1. Define and classify root resorption. Write in detail about internal resorption.
2. Classify external root resorption. Write in detail about replacement resorption.
3. Write short notes on
   - Differential diagnosis of internal and external resorption.
   - Cervical root resorption.

Bibliography

1. AAE Glossary of Endodontic Terms. American Association of Endodontists website. 2014. Accessed July 29, 2016.
2. Gartner AH, Mack T, Somerlott RG, Walsh LC. Differential diagnosis of internal and external root resorption. J Endod. 1976;2(11):329–334.
3. Kuo T-C, Cheng Y-A, Lin C-P. Clinical management of severe external root resorption. Chin Dent J. 2005;24(1):59–64.
4. Maria R, Mantri V, Koolwal S. Internal resorption: A review and case report. Endodontology. 2010;22(1):100–108.

CHAPTER

32

Crack Tooth Syndrome and Vertical Root Fracture

Chapter Outline

- ❑ Definition
- ❑ Classification

- ❑ Vertical Root Fracture (VRF)

Cracked teeth or incompletely fractured teeth are commonly seen by clinicians in routine practice. The severity and treatment of the fracture can range from infraction line, needing minimum treatment, to severe, requiring endodontic treatment or even extraction. Patients usually present extended history of pain of varying intensity; the origin of which may be difficult to locate. Most common chief complaint in these cases is intermittent pain on biting. Symptoms normally depend on the extent and direction of the crack and the tissues involved. Cracks in teeth may occur in both horizontal and vertical directions involving the crown and/or root. Etiology of these fractures is usually occlusal forces and iatrogenic procedures.

▍Definition

Many authors gave different definitions for cracks in teeth, for example, Gibbs first described incomplete fracture of posterior teeth as "cuspal fracture odontalgia," Cameron as "cracked tooth syndrome," and Ellis as incomplete tooth fracture.

Crack tooth syndrome is defined as "incomplete tooth fracture extending through body of the tooth causing pain of idiopathic origin." The fracture commonly involves enamel and dentin but sometimes pulp and periodontal structure may also get involved.

Synonyms of Crack Tooth Syndrome

- ❑ Incomplete tooth fracture
- ❑ Tooth infraction
- ❑ Split tooth syndrome
- ❑ Green stick fracture
- ❑ Hairline fracture
- ❑ Cuspal fracture odontalgia

Etiology

Etiology of cracked tooth syndrome is not specific but is commonly seen to be associated in teeth with large and complex restorations, leaving the teeth more susceptible to cracks. Moreover, stressful lifestyle, parafunctional habits, and high masticatory forces are important contributing factors. Etiological factors for cracked teeth can be classified as following:

Etiology of the cracked tooth syndrome			
S. no.	Etiology	Factors	Examples
1.	Restorative procedures	• Inadequate tooth preparation • Stress concentration	• Overpreparation of cavities • Insufficient cuspal protection • Physical forces during placement of restoration, e.g., amalgam • Nonincremental placement of composite restorations
2.	Occlusal	• Masticatory trauma • Parafunction	• Excessive biting force • Eccentric contacts and interferences • Bruxism
	Miscellaneous	• Thermal cycling • Dental instruments	• Enamel cracks • Cracking associated with high speed handpieces

Table 32.1: American Association of Endodontists classifications of cracked teeth

	Craze line	Cuspal fracture	Cracked tooth	Split tooth	Vertical root fracture
Origin	Crown	Crown and cervical margin of root	Crown only or crown to root extension	Crown and root	Only root
Direction	Variable	Mesiodistal and faciolingual	Mesiodistal	Mesiodistal	Faciolingual
Origin	Occlusal surface	Occlusal surface	Occlusal surface	Occlusal surface	Root (any level)
Etiology	Occlusal forces	Undermined cusp, damaging habits	Damaging habits, weakened tooth structure	Damaging habits, weakened tooth structure	Wedging posts, obturation forces, excessive root-dentin removal
Symptoms	Asymptomatic	Pain on biting and sensitivity to cold	Acute pain on biting and sharp pain to cold	Pain on chewing	None to slight. Mimics periodontal disease
Identification	Direct visualization, transillumination	Visualize, remove restoration	Remove restoration, pain on biting	Remove restoration	• Radiograph • Reflect flap and transilluminate
Pulp status	Vital	Usually vital	Variable	Mostly root canal treated	Root canal treated
Prognosis	Excellent	Good	Questionable	Poor, unless crack terminates subgingivally	Poor

Classification

American Association of Endodontists (AAE) divided cracks into five types which are described in **Table 32.1.**

Clinical Symptoms

❑ Sharp pain on biting, which may get worse if the biting force is increased. "Rebound pain" i.e. sharp, fleeting pain occurs when the biting force is released from the tooth.

❑ Pain on biting occurs because fractured segments of the tooth move independently of each other, causing sudden movement of fluid within the dentinal tubules. This stimulates the A delta fibers in the dentin-pulp complex causing pain. Pain when releasing biting pressure on an object occurs because when biting down, the segments are usually moving apart and thereby reducing the pressure on the nerves in the dentin. When the bite is released, the "segments" come back together sharply increasing the pressure in the nerves causing pain.

❑ Sharp pain on eating or drinking cold and/or sugary substances because of stimulation of A delta fibers due to dentinal fluid movement.

❑ If the fracture propagates into the pulp, it may result in pulpitis or necrosis. If the crack propagates further into the root, a periodontal defect may develop or even a vertical root fracture **(Figs. 32.1A to E).**

❑ Patient may have difficulty in identifying the affected tooth as there are no proprioceptive fibers in the pulp

❑ Pulp is usually vital.

❑ Tooth is not tender to percussion in an axial direction

❑ Tooth often has an extensive intracoronal restoration or history of extensive dental treatment involving repeated occlusal adjustments or replacement of restorations, which fail to eliminate the symptoms **(Figs. 32.1A to E).**

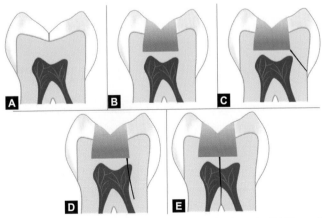

Figs. 32.1A to E Progression chart of cracked teeth. (A) Natural tooth; (B) Tooth with large restoration; (C) Oblique fracture; (D) Fracture reaching pulp; (E) Fracture splitting tooth.

Diagnosis

The patient with cracked tooth syndrome gives history of variable signs and symptoms which are difficult to diagnose. Even the radiographs are inconclusive. The careful history of the patient, examination, diagnostic tests, radiographs, and sometimes surgical exposure are needed for accurate diagnosis of cracked tooth syndrome.

Clinical Examinations

For definite diagnosis, one should obtain adequate information from patient history and clinical examination.

Chief Complaint

Patient usually complains of pain on chewing and sensitivity to cold and sweets. If these symptoms are associated with non-carious teeth, one should consider the possibility of infraction.

History of Patient

Patient should be asked about
- Previous trauma if any
- Details regarding dietary habits
- Presence of abnormal habits like bruxism, etc.

Visual Examination

One should look for presence of
- Large restoration
- Wear facets and steep cusps
- Cracked restoration
- Gap between tooth structure and restoration
- Sometimes removal of restoration is required for examination of fracture line in a cavity

Tactile Examination

While carrying out tactile examination, one should gently pass the tip of sharp explorer along the tooth surface, it may catch the crack.

Periodontal Probing

Thorough periodontal probing along the involved tooth may reveal a narrow periodontal pocket.

Bite Test

Orange wood stick, rubber wheel, or the tooth slooth are commonly used for detecting cracked tooth. Tooth slooth is small pyramid shaped, plastic bite block with small concavity at the apex which is placed over the cusp and patient is asked to bite upon it with moderate pressure and release. *Pain during biting or chewing especially upon the release of pressure is classic sign of cracked tooth syndrome.*

Transillumination

Use of fiber-optic light to transilluminate a fracture line is also a method of diagnosing cracked tooth syndrome.

Use of Dyes

Staining of fractured teeth with a dye such as methylene blue dye can aid in diagnosis. Dye can be directly applied to the tooth to identify fracture (**Fig. 32.2A**), or it can be incorporated into a temporary restoration like zinc oxide eugenol and placed in the prepared cavity (**Fig. 32.2B**) or patient can be asked to chew a disclosing tablet (**Fig. 32.2C**). The dark stain present on the fracture line helps in detecting the fracture.

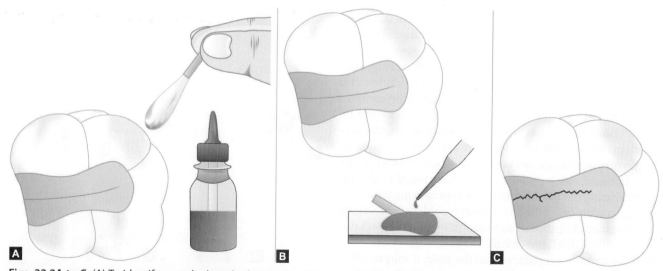

Figs. 32.2A to C (A) To identify a cracked tooth, dye can be directly applied to the tooth; (B) Dye can be incorporated in a temporary restoration and placed in prepared cavity; (C) Patient can be asked to chew a disclosing tablet, dark line on fracture area indicates crack.

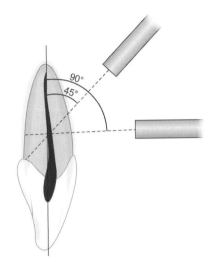

Fig. 32.3 Taking radiographs at more than one angle can help in locating the crack.

Radiographs

□ Radiographs are not of much help, especially if the crack is mesiodistal in direction. Even the buccolingual cracks will only appear if there is actual separation of the segments or the crack happens to coincide with the X-ray beam

□ Taking radiographs from more than one angle can help in locating the crack **(Fig. 32.3)**

□ A tooth with crack may show widened periodontal ligament space and diffused radiolucency especially with elliptical shape in apical area.

Surgical Exposure

If a fracture is suspected, a full thickness mucoperiosteal flap should be reflected for visual examination of root surface.

Differential Diagnosis of Cracked Tooth Syndrome

Crack tooth should be differentiated from a fractured cusp. The tooth crack occurs more toward the center of the occlusal surface as compared to the cusp fracture which is more peripheral in position. To differentiate a cracked tooth from a fractured cusp, if a crack has been detected, use wedging to test the movement of the segments. If there is no movement with wedging forces, it indicates a cracked tooth. A fractured cusp may break off under slight pressure with no further mobility. If fracture splits the tooth then tooth will show mobility with wedging force.

It should be differentiated from dentinal hypersensitivity, reversible pulpitis, acute periodontal disease, fractured restoration, postoperative sensitivity associated with microleakage from recently placed composite resin restorations, and areas of hyperocclusion from restorations, pain from bruxism, orofacial pain, or atypical facial pain. Possibility of cracked tooth syndrome should be considered when there is pain on biting. If crack involves pulp, patient may have spontaneous pain or thermal sensitivity which lingers even after removal of the stimulus.

Treatment of Cracked Teeth

See **Flowchart 32.1**.

Flowchart 32.1 Treatment plan for a fractured tooth.

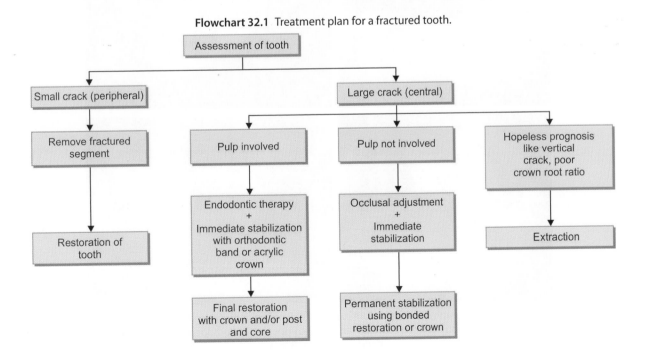

- Urgent care of the cracked tooth involves immediate reduction of its occlusal contacts by selective grinding of tooth at the site of the crack or its antagonist
- Definitive treatment of the cracked tooth aims to preserve the pulpal vitality by providing full occlusal coverage for cusp protection
- When crack involves the pulpal floor, endodontic access is needed but one should not make attempts to chase down the extent of crack with a bur, because the crack may become invisible long before it terminates. Endodontic treatment can alleviate irreversible pulpal symptoms
- If the crack is partially visible across the floor of the chamber, the tooth may be bonded with a temporary crown or orthodontic band. This will aid in determining the prognosis of the tooth and protect it from further deterioration till the endodontic therapy is completed (**Figs. 32.4 and 32.5**)

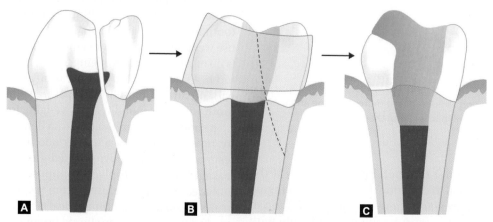

Figs. 32.4A to C (A) If crack is visible across the floor of pulp chamber; (B) Tooth is bonded with orthodontic band; (C) Keeping orthodontic band in place, endodontic therapy is completed.

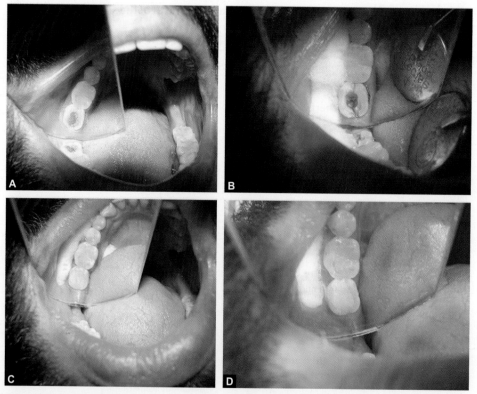

Figs. 32.5A to E (A) Preoperative photograph showing fracture in molar; (B) Banding done, amalgam restoration removed and fracture line seen (C) Restoration done with flowable and Z350 composite; (D) Post operative photograph
Courtesy: Poonam Bogra.

□ Apical extension and future migration of the crack apically onto the root determines the prognosis. If the fracture is not detected, pulpal degeneration and periradicular pathosis may be the initial indication that complete vertical fracture is present. Depending upon the extensions of the crack and symptoms, the treatment may involve extractions, root resection, or hemisection

Prevention

□ Awareness of existence and etiology of cracked tooth syndrome is important for its prevention
□ Perform conservative tooth preparation if possible
□ Line angles should be rounded instead of sharp to avoid stress concentration
□ Incorporate adequate cuspal coverage if required
□ Cast restorations should fit passively to avoid building of hydraulic pressure during placement
□ Pins should be placed at appropriate distance from the enamel to avoid stress concentration
□ Remove eccentric contacts and adjust occlusion for patients with a history of cracked tooth syndrome to reduce the risk of crack formation

Vertical Root Fracture (VRF)

According to the AAE, a "true" vertical root fracture is defined as a complete or incomplete fracture initiated from the root at any level, usually directed buccolingually".

These have incidence of 2.3% in total fractured teeth with the highest incidence in endodontically treated teeth in patients older than 40 years of age.

VRF can occur at any phase of root canal treatment, that is, during biochemical preparation, obturation, or during post-placement. This fracture results from wedging forces within the canal. These excessive forces exceed the binding strength of existing dentin causing fatigue and fracture (**Fig. 32.6**).

Etiology

The most common reasons for VRF are
□ Excessive dentin removal during biomechanical preparation
□ Weakening of tooth during post-space preparation

Factors which predispose the VRF:
□ *Anatomy of root:* Roots with narrow mesiodistal diameter than buccolingual dimensions, are more prone to fracture, for example, roots of premolars and mesial roots of mandibular molar. Presence of root curvatures and depressions make roots more prone to fracture
□ *Amount of remaining tooth structure:* Lesser is the amount of remaining tooth structure, more are the chances of VRF

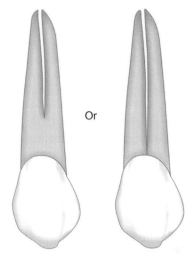

Fig. 32.6 Diagrammatic representation of vertical root fracture.

□ *Presence of pre-existing cracks:* Cracks present in dentin before treatment may later propagate to result in VRF
□ *Loss of moisture in dentin:* Though loss of moisture is not a main etiological factor, it can be a predisposing factor for VRF
□ *During obturation:* Use of a spreader results in generation of stresses during lateral compaction of gutta-percha due to wedging effect of spreader on canal walls or through gutta-percha results in root fracture
□ *Pathogenesis:* As vertical root fracture progresses to the periodontal ligament, soft tissue grows into the fracture space causing separation of the root segments. When it communicates with the oral cavity through the gingival sulcus, bacteria enter the fracture area and initiate inflammatory process in periodontal tissue causing disintegration of adjacent periodontal ligament, alveolar bone loss, and formation of granulation tissue.

Classification of Vertical Root Fracture (Flowchart 32.2)

Flowchart 32.2 Classification.

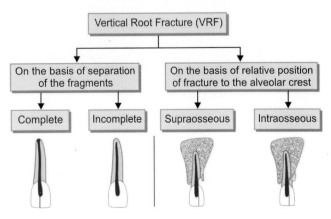

Signs and Symptoms

Following signs and symptoms are seen in cases of VRF:

- Pain and swelling due to local chronic inflammation in response to infection. Pain is usually mild to moderate in nature, mostly accompanied by a bad taste. Palpation shows swelling and tenderness over the root itself, especially near the gingival area **(Fig. 32.7)**
- Sudden crunching sound accompanied by pain
- Sinus tract commonly seen close to the gingival margin. Presence of two sinus tracts, i.e. at both buccal and lingual surface or multiple sinus tracts is the pathognomonic feature of vertical root fracture. In case of nonvital teeth, sinus tracts are located more apically (differential diagnosis)
- Presence of deep, narrow, isolated periodontal pockets in an otherwise normal periodontal condition.
- Sharp cracking sound during obturation or post cementation
- Bleeding or lack of resistance within the canal during obturation

Diagnosis

It is difficult to diagnose a case with VRF because of the following reasons:

- Signs and symptoms of VRF like pain on mastication, mobility, presence of sinus tract, bony radiolucency, and spontaneous dull pain can also be seen in failed root canal treatment or in periodontal disease
- VRF is not detected during or immediately after root canal treatment. It may take years to diagnose VRF.

Following steps should be carried out to diagnose a case of vertical root fracture:

History

- History of pain, swelling, presence of sinus tract, endodontic treatment, facial trauma, and dislodged restoration may suggest VRF
- Thorough clinical examination including age, involved tooth, history of previous dental treatment help reaching the diagnosis. Rapid deterioration of endodontic status of a tooth after a long time without symptoms, or re-appearance of radiolucencies after healing has previously taken place, is indicative of fracture.

Clinical Tests

- Direct visualization with good illumination and magnification is important to see the crack
- Transillumination test is done by exposing fiberoptic light on tooth. Light is deflected at the crack, reducing its transmission through the tooth, making the fractured segment appear darker
- Staining the fracture line using dyes help the clinician to visualize a crack
- Bite test using tooth slooth, rubber wheels, and cottonwood sticks can be used to reproduce the pain on chewing.
- Periodontal probing shows presence of narrow, isolated, periodontal defect in the gingival attachment **(Fig. 32.8)**
- Pulp testing usually shows nonvital tooth because fracture line may extend to the pulp causing inflammation and necrosis. This is especially helpful in diagnosing fracture in otherwise sound tooth.

Radiographic Examination

i. Tracing the sinus tract using gutta-percha and taking radiograph helps to detect its origin.

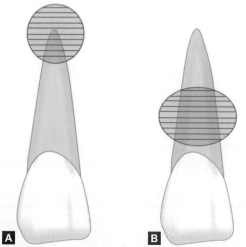

Figs. 32.7A and B Schematic representation of swelling. (A) In case of periapical lesion; (B) In case of vertical root fracture.

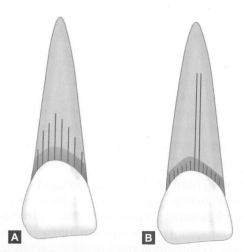

Figs. 32.8A and B Schematic representation of probing pattern. (A) In case of periodontal lesion, generalized pocket depth; (B) In case of vertical root fracture, deep, narrow isolated pocket.

ii. "Halo-like" radiolucency running around whole of the root surface is a classic sign of VRF. Radiolucent area may travel almost completely up the side of the root, resulting in a "J-type" lesion **(Fig. 32.9)**.

iii. Isolated V-shaped bone loss which is wider coronally, narrowing towards the apex is important sign of VRF.

iv. Fracture line can be seen on the tooth as vertical line along the root, root canal filling, or post present in the tooth.

v. If separation of fragments occurs in a direction other than parallel to the X-ray beam, overlapping of fragments may result in double images of the external root surface.

vi. Extrusion of obturating material may occur into the fracture site which can be seen on radiograph.

vii. Widening of periodontal ligament space along with bone loss is seen in cases of VRF. In case of periapical lesion, bone loss occurs apically without destruction of the lamina dura along the root surface

viii. Furcation bone loss in otherwise sound molars without periapical or periodontal disease may indicate VRF.

Cone Beam Computerized tomography (CBCT)

CT gives three-dimensional view of the tooth. It shows separation of the adjacent root segments seen on at least two adjacent sections without continuation of the hypo-attenuated line into the contiguous tissue.

Surgical Exposure

Surgical exposure helps in definitive diagnosis if VRF is suspected from clinical and radiographic signs. After soft tissue retraction, visualization of the fracture line, probing over the fracture line can confirm the VRF.

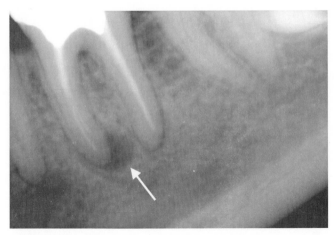

Fig. 32.9 Halo appearance of mesial root of mandibular 1st molar with VRF.

Treatment of Vertical Root Fracture

It involves extraction in most of the cases. In multirooted teeth root, resection or hemisection can be tried. Other treatment options include retention of the fractured fragment and placement of calcium hydroxide or cementation of the fractured fragments.

Recently, repair of root fracture have been tried by binding them with the help of adhesive resins, glass ionomers and lasers. But to date, no successful technique has been reported to correct this problem.

Prevention of VRF

Prevention of root fracture basically involves avoidance of the causes of root fracture.

Principles to prevent root fracture are to
❑ Avoid weakening of the canal wall
❑ Minimize the internal wedging forces

The following points should be kept in mind before during and after endodontic therapy:
❑ Evaluate the tooth anatomy before taking treatment
❑ Preserve as much tooth structure as possible during biomechanical preparation
❑ Use only optimal force during obturation for compaction of gutta-percha
❑ Use posts and pins if indicated
❑ Use posts with passive fits and round edges so as to reduce stress generation

❚ Conclusion

Early recognition of cracked tooth syndrome helps to prevent further propagation of crack into the pulp or sub-gingivally. The clinician should be aware of the existence of crack tooth syndrome and able to differentiate it from other mimicking conditions. A good history, careful clinical examination, inspection, along with some tests help to reach the diagnosis. The treatment of crack tooth depends on the position and extent of the crack. Treatment options vary from a simple restoration to placement of an extracoronal restoration with adequate cuspal protection.

❚ Questions

1. What is cracked tooth syndrome? How can you diagnose a case with cracked tooth?
2. What is vertical root fracture? What are signs and symptoms, radiographic features of VRF?
3. Describe cracked tooth syndrome and their management.
4. Discuss endodontic perforations and their prognosis and their treatment.

▌Bibliography

1. Ailor JE. Managing incomplete tooth fractures. J Am Dent Assoc. 2000;131:1168–74.
2. Alex JM, Bill K. Diagnosis and management of teeth with vertical root fractures. Aust Dent. 1999;44(2):75–87.
3. Banerji S, Mehta SB, Millar BJ. Cracked tooth syndrome. Part 1: aetiology and diagnosis. Br Dent J. 2010;208:459–63.
4. Cameron CE. Cracked-tooth syndrome. J Am Dent Assoc. 1964;68:405–11.
5. Lynch CD, McConnell RJ. The cracked tooth syndrome. J Can Dent Assoc. 2002; 68(8):470–5.
6. Dhawan A, Gupta S, Mittal R. Vertical root fractures: an update review. J Res Dent 2014; 2(3): 107-13.
7. Grossman LI. Endodontic practice. Philadelphia, PA: Lea and Febiger; 1978.
8. Swepston JH, Miller AW. The incompletely fractured tooth. J Prosthet Dent. 1985;55:413–16.
9. Wiene FS. Endodontic therapy. 6th ed. St Louis, MO: Mosby; 2004.

Geriatric Endodontics

Geriatric is a Greek word where **geras** means old and **iatro** means doctor. Geriatric dentistry is providing dental care to older adults involving diagnosis, prevention, management and treatment of problems associated with older age. In general, geriatric dental treatment starts at the age of 65 years. With improvement in health care facilities and awareness, not only older age group is going to increase but also their dental needs will continue to increase. By this age, teeth have experienced decades of dental disease, restorative and periodontal procedures. These all have an adverse effect on the pulp, periradicular and surrounding tissues. The combination of an increase in pathosis and dental needs along with greater expectations has resulted in more endodontic procedures for older adults. Before considering endodontic treatment in older teeth, we will discuss age change in teeth and surrounding tissues.

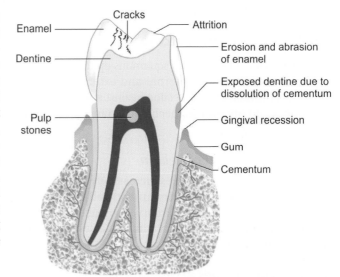

Fig. 33.1 Age changes in enamel, pulp, dentin and cementum.

Age Changes in the Teeth (Fig. 33.1)

Macroscopic Changes

❑ Changes in form and color
❑ Wear and attrition of teeth
❑ Causes for change in color of teeth:
- Decrease in thickness of dentin
- General loss of translucency
- Pigmentation of anatomical defects
- Corrosion products
- Inadequate oral hygiene

Age Changes in Enamel

❑ Changes in enamel are based on ionic exchange mechanism
❑ Decrease in permeability of enamel

❑ Enamel becomes more brittle with age
❑ Enamel exhibits attrition, abrasion and erosion

Age Changes in Cementum

❑ Thickness of cementum increases with age
❑ It becomes more susceptible to resorption
❑ There is increased fluoride and magnesium content of cementum with age

Age Changes in Dentin

❑ Physiologic secondary dentin formation
❑ Gradual obliteration of dentinal tubules

- Dentin sclerosis
- Occlusion of dentinal tubules by a gradual deposition of the peritubular dentin

Clinical Implications of Age Changes in Dentin

- Obliteration of the tubules leads to reduction in sensitivity of the tissue
- Reduction in dentin permeability prevents the ingress of toxic agents
- Addition of more bulk to the dentin reduces pulpal reactions and chances of pulp exposures

Age Changes in Pulp

- Size of pulp cavity decrease due to secondary dentin formation
- Difference between dental pulp of old individuals and young teeth is due to more fibers and less cells
- Blood supply to teeth decreases with age
- Prevalence of pulp stones increases with age

Age Changes in Oral Mucosa

Oral cavity is lined by stratified squamous epithelium which forms a barrier between internal and external environment, thus providing the protection against entry of noxious substances and organisms, mechanical damage and fluid exchange.

Clinical Changes in Epithelium

With age, oral mucosa becomes increasingly thin, smooth and dry with loss of elasticity and stippling and thus becomes more susceptible to injury. Tongue exhibits loss of filiform papillae and deteriorating taste sensation and occasional burning sensation.

Histological Changes in Oral Mucosa

These are seen in epithelium and connective tissue.

Epithelial Changes

- Decreased thickness of epithelial cell layer
- Reduced keratinization
- Alteration in the morphology of epithelial–connective tissue interface
- Decrease in the length of rete pegs of oral epithelium have been reported with age
- Rate of cell renewal in human oral epithelia decreases with aging

Connective Tissue Change

- There is increase in number and density of elastin fibers
- Cells shrink in size and number and tend to become inactive

Age Changes in Periodontal Connective Tissue

- Gingival connective tissue becomes denser and coarsely textured upon aging
- Decrease in the number of fibroblasts
- Decrease in the fiber content
- Increase in the size of interstitial compartments containing blood vessels
- Evidence of calcification on and between the collagen fibers

Age Changes in Salivary Glands

There is diminished function of salivary glands with aging resulting in reduced salivation or xerostomia. This causes xerostomia, mouth soreness, burning or painful tongue, taste changes, chewing difficulty, problems with swallowing and talking.

Age Changes in Bone Tissue

- Cortical thinning
- Loss of trabeculae
- Cellular atrophy
- Sclerosis of bone

Endodontic Challenges in Geriatric Patients (Fig. 33.2)

Primary function of teeth is mastication, thus the loss of teeth leads to detrimental food changes and reduction in health. The needs, expectations, desire, demands of older

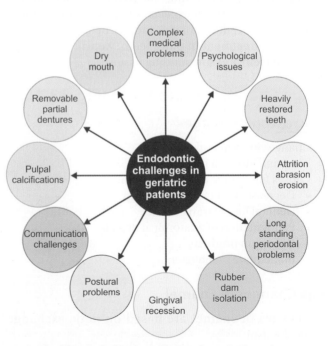

Fig. 33.2 Endodontic challenges in geriatric patients.

patients thus exceeds for those of any age group. Quality of life for older patients can be improved by preventing the loss of teeth through endodontic treatment and can add a large and impressive value to their overall dental, physical and mental health. Root canal treatment can be offered as a favorable alternative to the terms of extraction and cost of replacement.

Diagnosis and Treatment Plan

Chief Complaint of Geriatric Patients

The most common reason for pain in old age patients is pulpal or periapical problem that requires either root canal treatment or extraction. Older patients are more likely to have or already had root canal treatment and have a more realistic perception about treatment comfort. By and large, the pain associated with vital pulps seems to be reduced with aging and severity seems to diminish over the time suggesting a reduced pulp volume. Patient explains regarding complaint, stimulus, or irritant that causes pain, nature of pain, etc. This information is useful in determining whether the source is pulpal or periapical and if these problems are reversible or not.

Past Dental History

Dentist should ask the patients past dental history so as to access the patient's dental status and plan future treatment accordingly. From dental history, the clinician can assess the patient's knowledge about dental treatment and his psychological attitude, expectations from dental treatment.

Medical History

Dentists should recognize that the biologic or functional age of an individual is far more important than chronological age. As most of the old-aged people suffer from one or the other medical problems, a medical history should be taken prior to starting any treatment for geriatric patients.

A standardized form should be used to identify any disease or therapy that would alter treatment plan or its outcome. Aging usually causes changes in cardiovascular, respiratory, central nervous system that result in most drug therapy needs. The renal and liver function of the patients should be considered while prescribing drugs as they have some action on these organs.

Examination of the Patient

Extraoral and intraoral clinical examination provides dentist useful information regarding the disease and previous treatment done. Common observations in geriatric patients:

- **Missing teeth:** In older patients, usually some of teeth get extracted. Missing teeth indicate the decrease in functional ability, resulting in loss of chewing ability. This reduced chewing ability leads to a higher intake of more refined soft carbohydrate diet and sugar intake to compensate for loss of taste and xerostomia. All these lead to increased susceptibility to dental decay
- **Gingival recession:** It results in exposure of cementum and dentin and thus making them more prone to decay and sensitivity (**Figs. 33.3A and B**)
- **Root caries (Fig. 33.4):** It is very common in older patients and is difficult to treat; the caries excavation is irritating to the pulp and often results in pulp exposures or reparative dentin formation makes the canal negotiation difficult
- **Attrition, abrasion and erosion** expose the dentin and allow the pulp to respond with dentinal sclerosis and reparative dentin which may completely obliterate the pulp (**Figs. 33.5 and 33.6**)

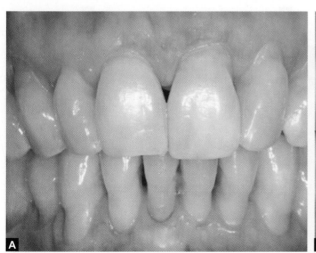 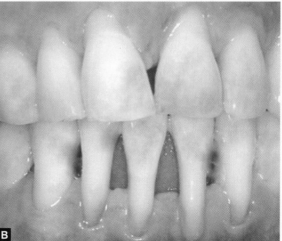

Figs. 33.3A and B Gingival recession is commonly seen in geriatric patients.

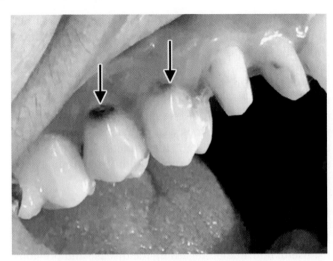

Fig. 33.4 Photograph showing root caries.

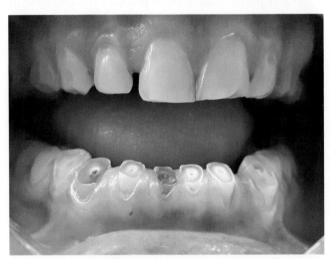

Fig. 33.5 Photograph showing attrition of mandibular anterior teeth resulting in pulp exposure.

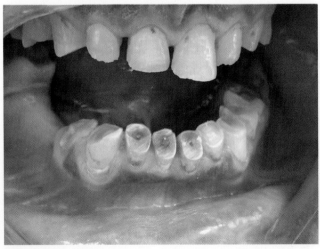

Fig. 33.6 Attrition of teeth resulting in multiple pulp exposure.

- With increasing age, the size of *pulp cavity decreases* due to reparative dentin formation **(Figs. 33.7A and B)**
- *Continued cementum deposition* is seen with increasing age thus moving cementodentinal junction (CDJ) farther from the radiographic apex **(Figs. 33.8A and B)**
- *Calcifications* are observed in the pulp cavity which can be due to caries, pulpotomy, or trauma and is more of linear type. The lateral and accessory canals can be calcified, thus decreasing their clinical significance
- *Reduced tubular permeability* is seen because dentinal tubules become occluded with advancing age
- *Missing and titled teeth* in older patients result in change in the molar relationship, biting pattern which can cause temporomandibular joint (TMJ) disorders
- *Reduced mouth opening* increases the working time and decreases the accessibility for treatment
- **Presence of *multiple restorations*** indicates a history of repeated dental treatment. Pulpal injury in older age patients is the mainly because of *marginal leakage* and microbial contamination of cavity walls

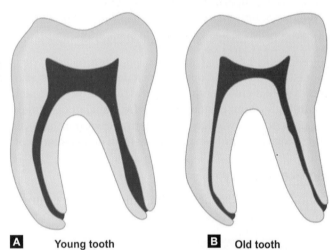

A Young tooth   **B** Old tooth

Figs. 33.7A and B Size of pulp cavity is smaller in older tooth as compared to young tooth.

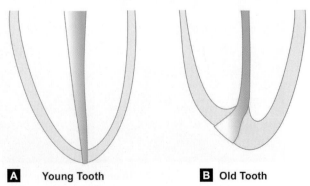

A Young Tooth   **B** Old Tooth

Figs. 33.8A and B With increasing age, CDJ moves away from apex due to continued cementum deposition.

Pulp Vitality Tests

Pulp vitality tests like cold test, heat test, electric pulp test and test cavity tell status of the pulp, but these tests are not very accurate because of extensive calcification and reduced size of pulp cavity.

Radiographs

Radiographs help the clinician to identify the status of tooth and then plan the treatment. But while taking radiographs of geriatric patients, the following problems are encountered:

❑ Presence of tori, exostoses, denser bone requires increased exposure times for proper diagnostic contrast
❑ Older patients may be less capable of assisting in film placement so film holders should be used to secure the position of film.

Common Radiographic Observations in Geriatric Patients

❑ Receded pulp cavity which is accelerated by reparative dentin **(Figs. 33.9A to C)**
❑ Presence of pulp stones and dystrophic calcification
❑ Receding pulp horns can be noted in the radiograph
❑ Deep proximal or root decay may cause calcification of pulp cavity
❑ A midroot disappearance of a detectable canal may indicate bifurcation rather than calcification
❑ In cases where the vitality tests do not correlate with the radiographic findings, one should consider the presence of odontogenic and nonodontogenic cysts and tumors
❑ In teeth with root resorption along with apical periodontitis, shape of apex and anatomy of foramen may change due to inflammatory osteoclastic activity
❑ In teeth with hypercementosis, the apical anatomy may become unclear

Treatment Plan

Considerations for endodontic treatment in geriatric patients:

❑ Irrespective of age, main aim of treatment is removal of pain and infection so as to restore teeth to normal health and function
❑ For medically compromised or cognitively impaired cardiac patients and neuropsychiatric patients, it is safe and better to start treatment only after a valid consent is obtained from the particular doctors
❑ Depending on the length of the appointment, morning appointments are preferable though some patients prefer late morning or early afternoon visits to allow "morning stiffness" to dissipate
❑ Single appointment procedures are better, as these patients may have physical problems and require transportation or physical assistance to get into the office
❑ Because of reduced blood supply, pulp capping is not as successful in older teeth as in younger ones, therefore, not recommended
❑ Endodontic surgery in geriatric patients is not as viable an alternative as for a younger patient

Anesthesia

❑ Older patients are less anxious about dental treatment because of low conduction velocity of nerves, limited extension of nerves into dentin and dentinal tubules are more calcified
❑ In older patients, the width of periodontal ligament is reduced which makes the needle placement for intraligamentary injection more difficult. Only smaller amounts of anesthetic should be deposited and the depth of anesthesia should be checked before repeating the procedure
❑ Intrapulpal anesthesia is difficult in older patients as the volume of pulp chamber is reduced

Isolation

❑ Rubber dam is the best method of isolation. If the tooth is badly mutilated making the rubber dam placement difficult, then consider multiple tooth isolation with saliva ejector

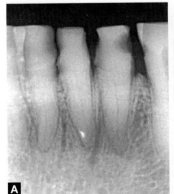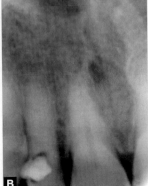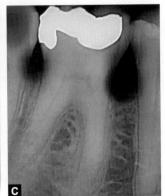

Figs. 33.9A to C Radiographs of (A) Mandibular incisors; (B) Maxillary lateral incisor (C) Mandibular first molar showing narrow and calcified canals.

Access to Canal Orifice

❏ One of the most difficult parts in the treatment of older patients is the identification of the canal orifices
❏ Obtaining access to the root canal and making the patients to keep their mouth open for a longer period of time is a real problem in older patients
❏ Radiograph should be taken to determine canal position, root curvature, axial inclinations of root and crown and extent of the lesion
❏ In case of compromised access for preparation, coronal tooth structure or restorations need to be sacrificed. Endodontic microscopes can be of greater help in identifying and treating narrow geriatric canals

Cleaning and Shaping

❏ Calcified canals in geriatric patients are more difficult to locate and penetrate. Canals seem to be longer due to cementum deposition
❏ DG 16 explorer is used for initial assessment of the orifice
❏ Use of broaches for pulp tissue extirpation is avoided in older patients, because very few canals of older teeth have adequate diameter to allow safe and effective uses of broaches
❏ NiTi instruments are used for cleaning and shaping in crown down technique rather than stainless steel hand files. This saves time, provides flexibility of NiTi and avoids tiredness of hand while working in sclerosed canals
❏ One should prefer rotary NiTi files with no rake angle in crown down technique
❏ It is difficult to locate apical constriction in these patients because of reduced periapical sensitivity in older patients, reduced tactile sense of the clinician and limited use of apex locator in heavily restored teeth

Obturation

For obturation, those obturation techniques are employed which do not require large midroot taper. Lateral compaction technique is preferred in these patients.

Prognosis of Endodontic Treatment

In case of vital pulp, the prognosis depends on many local and systemic factors.
In case of nonvital pulp, the repair is slow because of
❏ Arteriosclerotic changes in blood vessels
❏ Decreased rate of bone formation and resorption
❏ Increased mineralization of bone
❏ Altered viscosity of connective tissue

Endodontic Surgery

Indications

❏ Irrespective of age, indications are same as discussed in Chapter 25
❏ Medical history is important in older patients
❏ Following local anatomic considerations should be considered in elderly patients:
  • Increased incidence of dehiscence of roots and exostoses
  • Apically positioned muscle attachment
  • Less resilient tissue
  • Decreased resistance to reflection
  • Ecchymosis and delayed healing are common postoperative findings

▌Conclusion

Geriatric dentistry is a specialized multidisciplinary branch of general dentistry designed to provide dental services to elderly patients. With the increase in life expectancy, the demand for geriatric dentistry is increasing. It means, the dental practioners are expected to take care of more geriatric patients in future. Due to presence of age-related physiological and psychological changes, medical conditions, the management of the elderly population differs from that of the general population. Since oral health is directly associated with general well being of patient, dental care should be included into overall health management of all geriatric patients. Dentist should make an attempt to meet the needs of elderly patients, provide necessary infrastructure, and offer them empathetic care to ensure satisfaction.

▌Questions

1. What are age changes of dental tissue?
2. What all factors to be taken care of while dealing with a geriatric patient?
3. How will you diagnose and plan endodontic treatment in geriatric patient? What challenges are faced by clinician while managing the patient?

▌Bibliography

1. Charles H Rankin. Geriatrics in Endodontics. Tuft University 2007.
2. Geriatric Endodontics : Meeting the Challenge. Australian Dental Association. 2009.
3. Holm-Pedersen P, Loe H. Textbook of geriatric dentistry. 2nd edition London: Wiley; 1997.
4. Mulligan R. Geriatrics: contemporary and future concerns. Dent Clin N Am 2005;49:11–3.
5. Papas AS, Niessen LC, Chauncey HH. Geriatric dentistry—aging and oral health. St. Louis, MO: Mosby Yearbook; 1991.
6. Walton RE. Endodontic considerations in the geriatric patients. Dent Clin N Am 1997;41:795–816.

Lasers in Endodontics

Lasers in dentistry are considered to be a new technology which is being used in clinical dentistry to overcome some of the drawbacks posed by conventional dental procedures. This technology was first used for dental application in 1960 but its use has rapidly increased in the last few decades.

Laser is an acronym for "*Light Amplification by Stimulated Emission of Radiation.*" The application of lasers is almost in every field of human endeavor from medicine, science and technology to business and entertainment over the past few years.

▮ History

1960	Albert Einstein	Theory of spontaneous emission of radiation
1960	Theodore Maiman	First demonstrated laser function and developed working laser device known as ruby laser
1961	Snitzer	Developed neodymium laser
1964	Stern, Sognnaes and Goldman	Laser in dentistry
1965	Leon Goldman	Exposure of vital tooth to laser
1965	Taylor et al.	Studied histological effects on pulp
1966	Lobene et al.	Use of CO_2 lasers in dentistry
1971	Weichman and Johnson	First use of lasers in endodontics and used high-power infrared CO_2 laser to seal the apical foramen in vitro

1974	Yamamoto et al.	Nd:YAG in prevention of caries
1977	Lenz et al.	First application in oral and maxillofacial surgery
1979	Adrian and Gross	Sterilization of dental instruments by argon laser
1985	Shoji et al.	Laser aided pulpotomy
1985	Pick et al.	First in periodontal surgery
1986	Zakariasen et al.	Sterilization of root canals by CO_2 laser
1988	Miserendino	Laser apicoectomy, i.e., endodontic application of CO_2 laser for periapical surgery
1993	Paghdiwala	Root resection of endodontically treated teeth by erbium:YAG
1994	Morita	Nd:YAG laser in endodontics
1998	Mazeki et al.	Root canal shaping with Er:YAG laser

The first *laser or maser* as it was initially called, developed by *Theodore H Maiman* in 1960. Maser like laser is an acronym for "Microwave amplification by stimulated emission of radiation." This laser constructed by Maiman was a pulsed ruby laser.

The second laser to be developed was the neodymium laser by *Snitzer* in 1961. The first report of laser exposure to a vital human tooth was given in 1965 by *Leon Goldman*. In 1965, *Taylor and associates* reported the histologic effect of ruby laser on the dental pulp. From the 1960s to the early 1980s, dental researchers continued to search for other type

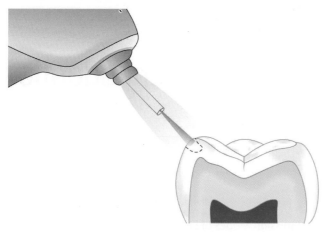

Fig. 34.1 Laser beam produces precised and clean cavity cutting with minimal tooth loss.

of lasers. *Lobene et al.* in 1966 researched about the CO_2 laser which has wavelength of 10.6 µm which can be well absorbed by enamel, so considered suitable for sealing of pits and fissures, welding of ceramics to enamel, or prevention of dental caries.

The advantages of CO_2 laser was first applied to periodontal surgery by Pick et al. in 1985. Sufficient research exists to predict that current laser systems such as erbium:YAG, holmium:YAG, Nd:YAG and excimer have the potential to replace the dental drill for a number of cases **(Fig. 34.1)**.

Classification of Laser

- ❑ *According to ANSI and OHSA standards, lasers are classified as:*
  - **Class I:** These are low-powered lasers that are safe to use, for example, laser beam pointer
  - **Class IIa:** Low-powered visible lasers that are hazardous only when viewed directly for longer than 1,000 s, for example, He–Ne lasers
  - **Class IIb:** Low-powered visible lasers that are hazardous when viewed for >0.25 s
  - **Class IIIa:** Medium-powered lasers that are normally hazardous if viewed for <0.25 s without magnifying optics
  - **Class IIIb:** Medium-powered lasers that can be hazardous if viewed directly
  - **Class IV:** High-powered lasers (0.5 W), can cause ocular, skin and fire hazards.
- ❑ *Based on the wavelength of the beam:*
  - **Ultraviolet rays:** 140–400 nm
  - **Visible light:** 400–700 nm
  - **Infrared:** 700 to microwave spectrum.
- ❑ *Based on penetration power of beam:*
  - **Hard:** Increased penetration power
    - For example, Nd:YAG, argon
  - **Soft lasers:** Decreased penetration power
    - For example, diode, GA–Sa, He–Ne lasers.
- ❑ *Based on pulsing:*
  - **Pulsed:** The beam is not continuous, i.e., it is of short duration
  - **Nonpulsed:** The beam is continuous and is of fixed duration.
- ❑ *According to type of laser material used:*
  - **Gas lasers:** CO_2 lasers, argon lasers, He–Ne lasers
  - **Liquid lasers:** Ions of rare earth or organic fluorescent dyes are dissolved in a liquid, for example, dye lasers
  - **Solid state lasers:** Ruby lasers, Nd:YAG lasers
  - **Semiconductor lasers:** Gallium, Arsenide.

Principles of Laser Beam

The common principle on which all lasers work is the generation of monochromatic, coherent and collimated radiation by a suitable laser medium in an optical resonator **(Fig. 34.2)**.

Monochromatic: Light produced by a particular laser is of a characteristic wavelength. If the light produced is in the visible spectrum (400–750 nm), it will be seen as a beam of intense color. It is important to have this property to attain high spectral power density of the laser.

Coherence: A laser produces light waves that are physically identical. They are all in phase with one another, that is, they have identical amplitude and identical frequency.

In an ordinary light source, much of the energy is lost as out of phase waves cancel each other. Coherency is a property unique to lasers. The light waves produced by a laser are a specific form of electromagnetic energy.

Collimation: Collimation refers to the beam having specific spatial boundaries. These boundaries ensure that there is a constant beam size and shape that is emitted from the laser unit **(Fig. 34.3)**.

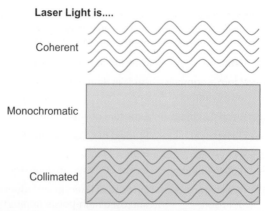

Fig. 34.2 Common principles on which all lasers work is generation of monochromatic, coherent and collimated beam.

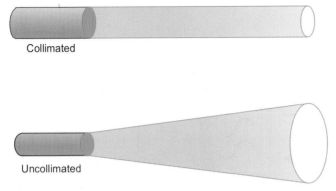

Collimated

Uncollimated

Fig. 34.3 Collimated and uncollimated beam.

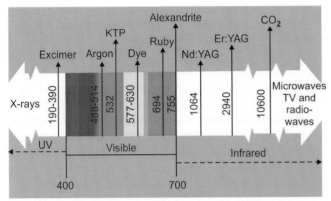

Fig. 34.4 Schematic representation of electromagnetic spectrum showing lasers of different wavelengths.

The main differentiating characteristic of lasers is wavelength which depends on the laser medium and excitation diode, i.e., continuous wave or pulsed mode. Laser is classified in three groups according to wavelength spectrum under which it falls **(Fig. 34.4):**

❑ Ultraviolet (UV range) approx 140–400 nm
❑ Visible light (VIS range) approx 400–700 nm
❑ Infrared (IR range) approx 700–microwave spectrum
  The shorter the wavelength, more energetic is the light.

Comparison between ordinary visible light and LASER light	
Visible light	*LASER light*
Polychromatic	Monochromatic
Non-directional and non-focused	Unidirectional-collimated and highly focused
Unorganized	Organized and efficient
Incoherent	Coherent
Low intensity—0.1 W/cm^2	High intensity—108–1016 W/cm^2

■ Laser Physics

The basic units or quanta of light are called photons. Photons behave like tiny wavelets similar to sound wave

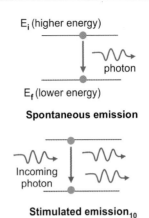

Spontaneous emission

Stimulated emission$_{10}$

Fig. 34.5 Spontaneous emission occurs when electron makes unstimulated transition to lower energy levels. Stimulated emission occurs when an incoming photon induces the electron to change energy levels.

pulses. If a photon is absorbed, its energy is not destroyed but rather used to increase the energy level of the absorbing atom. The photon then ceases to exist and an electron within the atom jumps to a higher energy level. This atom is thus pumped up to an excited state from the resting ground state. In the excited state, the atom is unstable and will soon spontaneously decay back to the ground state, releasing stored energy in the form of an emitted photon. This process is called *spontaneous emission*. The spontaneously emitted photon has a longer wavelength and less energy than the absorbed photon. The difference in the energy is usually turned into heat **(Fig. 34.5)**.

The process of lasing occurs when an excited atom can be stimulated to emit a photon before the process occurs spontaneously. When an atom in the excited state becomes irradiated with a photon of light energy of the same wavelength and frequency that was previously absorbed, as it returns to its resting state, it will emit two photons of light energy of the same direction in spatial and temporal phase. This is the stimulated emission of radiation.

If a collection of atoms is more that are pumped up into the excited state than remain in the resting state, the spontaneous emission of a photon of one atom will stimulate the release of a second photon in a second atom and these two photons will trigger the release of two more photons. These four then yield eight, eight yields sixteen and the cascading reaction follows to produce a brief intense flash of a monochromatic and coherent light.

Basic Components of Laser (Fig. 34.6)

1. *Laser medium or active medium*—This consists of chemicals that used to fill the optical cavity. The active medium contains atoms which can emit light by stimulated emission. The active medium can be solid,

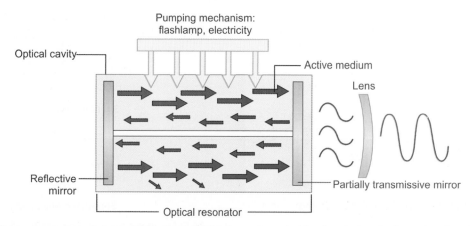

Fig. 34.6 Schematic representation of gas or solid, active-medium laser. At each side of optical cavity (contains chemicals which can emit light stimulated emission) two mirrors are there parallel to each other which act as optical resonator reflecting the waves back and forth and help to collimate and amplify the laser beam. Another components are cooling system and focusing lenses.

liquid, gas and plasma. Lasers are generally named for material of active medium which can be container of gas, a crystal, or a solid-state semiconductor.

2. ***Excitation mechanism***—Pump energy into active medium by one or more of three basic methods: optical, electrical, or chemical.

3. ***Optical resonator***—Lasers reflects the laser beam through active medium for amplification. It also helps to prevent the scattering of radiation in the optical cavity.

4. ***Optical cavity***—In this, all the other components of laser are housed. An optical cavity is at the center of the device. The core of cavity is comprised of chemical elements, molecules, or compounds and is called the active medium.

5. ***Optical mirror***—These are totally reflective and partially transmissive mirrors placed parallel to each other. These act as optical resonator reflecting the waves back and forth and help to collimate and amplify the laser beam.

6. ***Lens***—It helps in convergence of light to a focal point. The size and shape of the lens determine the focal length and spot size. Spot size measures the surface area on which laser is concentrated. It is directly related to efficiency. Smaller spot size is ideal for incision and bigger one for ablation and hemostatic procedures. Laser beam can be focused through a lens to achieve a converging beam which has high intensity to form a focal spot. When the laser is moved away from the tissue and away from the focal point, the beam is defocused, becomes more divergent, and therefore delivers less energy to the surgical site (**Fig. 34.7**).

Power Density

Power density is simply the concentration of photons in a unit area. Photons concentration is measured in watts and area in square cm.

Therefore, $PD = W/cm^2$
$$= W/pr^2 \ (r = \text{beam diameter}/2)$$

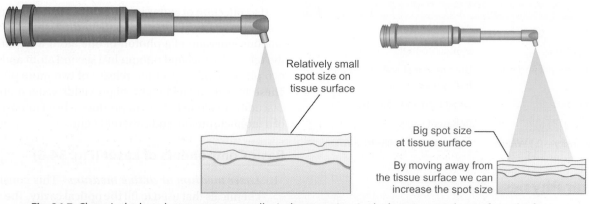

Relatively small spot size on tissue surface

Big spot size at tissue surface

By moving away from the tissue surface we can increase the spot size

Fig. 34.7 Closer is the laser beam to target, smaller is the spot size. As the laser is moved away from the focus, the beam gets divergent and spot size increases.

From the beam profile, we know that the power density in the center of the spot is higher and that at the edge of the spot approaches zero.

Power density can be increased significantly by placing a lens in the beam path because the light is monochromatic and collimated.

Power density can be increased by the wattage but increasing the power by 10 changes the power density by 10. But decreasing area by 10 increases the power density by 100.

Type of Lasers (Figs. 34.8A and B)

Carbon Dioxide Lasers

- Developed by Patel et al. in 1964
- Wavelength—10.6 μm
- Highly absorbed by soft and hard tissues with shallow depth of penetration
- Ideal laser for soft tissues
- Limited penetration depth (0.2–0.3 mm)
- Focused beam—fine dissection
- Defocused beam—ablates the tissue.

Uses

It has been used successfully in soft tissue surgery such as:
1. Gingivectomy
2. Soft tissue surgery (**Figs. 34.9 to 34.11**)
3. Frenectomy
4. Removal of benign and malignant lesion
5. Excisional biopsy
6. Incisional biopsy.

Neodymium:Yttrium Aluminum-Garnet Lasers

- Developed by Geusic in 1964
- Wavelength—1.06 μm
- Penetration depth—0.5–4 mm
- First laser exclusively for dentistry
- Affinity for pigmented tissues
- Penetrates wet tissues more rapidly
- Ideal for root canal sterilization and soft tissue procedures.

Uses

Nd:YAG laser is used for
- Vaporizing carious tissue
- Sterilizing tooth surfaces
- Cutting and coagulation of dental soft tissue
- Sulcular debridement
- Treat dentinal hypersensitivity
- Remove extrinsic stains
- Prepare pits and fissures for sealants.

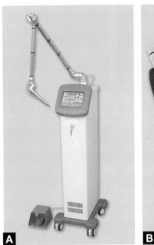
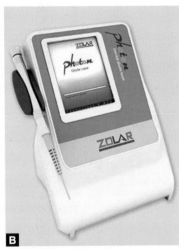

Figs. 34.8A and B (A) CO_2 laser; (B) Diode laser.

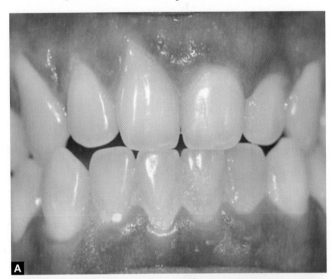

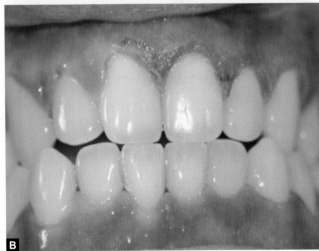

Figs. 34.9A and B Gingivoplasty by Laser: (A) Preoperative photograph; (B) Postoperative photograph.
Courtesy: Sanjay Jain.

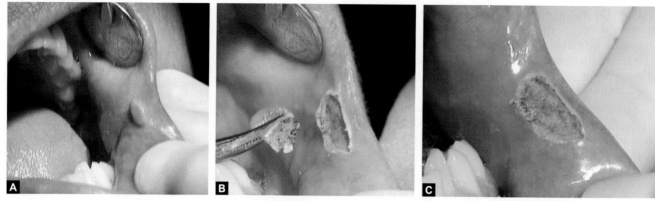

Figs. 34.10A to C Management of fibroma by laser treatment: (A) Preoperative photograph;
(B) Excision of fibroma by laser; (C) Postperative photograph.
Courtesy: Sanjay Jain.

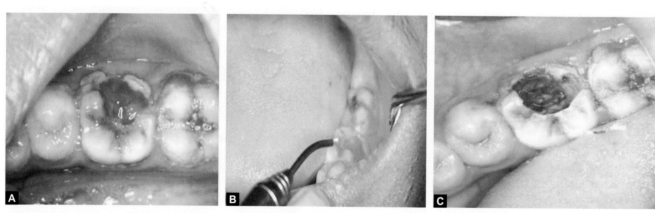

Figs. 34.11A to C Management of Pulp polyp by Laser; (A) Preoperative photograph;
(B) Laser treatment of pulp polyp; (C) Postperative photograph.
Courtesy: Sanjay Jain.

Argon Lasers

❑ Two emission wavelength used in dentistry
❑ Delivered through fibro-optic system
❑ Blue wavelength—488 nm—mainly used for composite curing
❑ Green wavelength—510 nm—used for soft tissue procedure and coagulation
❑ Absorbed by hemoglobin tissue and melanin cells.

Uses

❑ Composite curing
❑ Acute inflammatory periodontal lesion
❑ Hemangioma
❑ Caries detection.

Emission Modes of Laser

❑ **Continuous:** The beam transmitted at one power continuously as long device is active, for example, CO_2 and diode lasers

❑ **Gated pulse mode:** The periodic alteration of laser being on or off like blinking of an eye. It is activated by opening or closing of shutter in front of the beam path
❑ **Free running pulse mode:** Here a large peak energy of laser light is emitted for a short time followed by long time when laser is off, for example, Nd:YAG, Er:YAG lasers.

Laser Interaction with Biological Tissues

When laser interacts the tissues, it can be absorbed, reflected, scattered or transmitted **(Fig. 34.12)**. The type of interaction between a laser beam and any tissue is determined by the wavelength of the laser beam, the operation mode of the laser, the amount of energy applied, and tissue characteristics.

Absorption

Here specific molecules in the tissue known as chromophores absorb photons and produce photochemical,

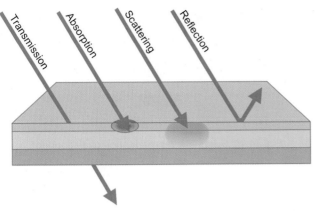

Fig. 34.12 When light encounters matter, it can be reflected, scattered, absorbed, or transmitted.

photothermal, photomechanical and photoelectrical effects.

Photochemical Effects

The basis of the photochemical effect is the absorption of the laser light without any thermal effect leading to change in the chemical and physical properties of atoms and molecules.

Photochemical effects include biostimulation, that is, stimulatory effect of lasers on biochemical and molecular processes that normally occur in the tissues such as healing and repair.

Photothermal Interaction

In this interaction, laser light energy absorbed by tissue substances and molecules become transformed into heat energy which produces the tissue effect. The amount of laser light absorbed into the tissue depends on:
- The wavelength of radiant energy from the laser
- Power density
- Pulse duration
- Spot size
- Composition of target tissue: High water content of most oral tissue is responsible for absorption of radiant energy in the target region.

Thermal effects of laser irradiation at different temperature range			
Temperature <60°C	*Temperature >60°C*	*Temperature <100°C*	*Temperature >100°C*
• Tissue hyperthermia • Enzymatic changes • Edema	Protein denaturation	• Tissue dehydration • Blanching of tissue	• Super heating causes vaporization • Tissue ablation and shrinkage

Photomechanical Interaction

Laser energy can be converted into acoustical energy which upon impact, creates a shock wave that disrupts the target tissue. This mechanical disruption occurs whenever the photon energy of beam exceeds target tissues. It has three interrelated phases, i.e. ionization, plasma formation and shockwave generation.

Photoelectrical Interaction

This includes photoplasmolysis which explains how tissue is removed by formation of electrically charged ions which exist in a semigaseous high-energy state.

Reflection

The laser beam gets reflected back with no absorption and interaction with tissues. This reflected beam results in undesirable effects of laser.

Transmission

In this laser energy can pass through superficial tissues to interact with deeper tissues. Nd: YAG and diode lasers show deeper penetration due to tissue transmission.

Scattering

Once the laser energy enters the target tissue, it scatters in different directions. This property is not helpful but can help with biostimulative properties sometimes.

▌Laser Safety in Dental Practice

The surgical lasers currently used in dentistry generally fall in class IV category which is considered the most hazardous group of lasers. Following hazards are seen with lasers in dentistry:
- **Ocular hazards:** Retinal and corneal injury occurs either by direct emission or from the laser.
- **Tissue hazards:** Temperature rise of 21°C above normal body temperature can cause denaturation of cellular enzymes which interrupt basic metabolic processes.
- **Environmental hazards:** These non-beam hazards can be production of smoke, toxic gases and chemicals
- **Electrical hazards:** These can occur in form of electric shock, fire, or explosion.

▌Laser Safety

To avoid an electrical hazard, the operatory must be kept dry.
- Use eyewear for protecting eyes **(Fig. 34.13)**
- Ventilation and evacuation to prevent airborne contamination
- Avoid highly reflective instruments and mirror surfaces.

Advantages of Lasers
• Less bleeding • Less pain • No need for anesthesia • No noise • Faster healing • Less chances of infection

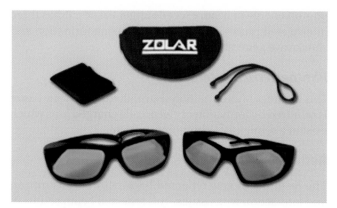

Fig. 34.13 Protective eyewear for use of laser.

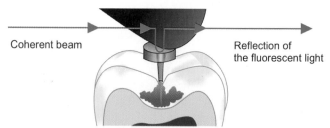

Coherent beam   Reflection of
                                 the fluorescent light

Fig. 34.14 Schematic representation of diagnodent.

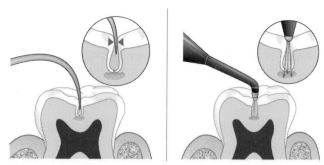

Figs. 34.15 (A) Tip of explorer does not detect the cavity until cavity is large enough; (B) Diagnodent can detect caries even at early stage.

Applications of Lasers

Laser Doppler Flowmetry

Laser doppler flowmetry (LDF) detects blood circulation in pulp to check the vitality. It is a reliable and comfortable method for the patient.

Diagnodent

It is based on the principle, that is, bacterial metabolites within caries produce fluorescence which is enhanced by laser light **(Fig. 34.14)**.

Advantages of diagnodent
- Easy detection of ICEBERG syndrome—90% of the caries is within proximal area—they will be detected with diagnodent
- Helps in early detection of fissure caries and calculus **(Figs. 34.15A and B)**

Thermal Testing

In this pulsed Nd:YAG laser is applied on the tooth. Pain produced by laser is mild and tolerable when compared to conventional pulp tester.

Pulp Capping and Pulpotomy

The first laser pulpotomy was performed by Shoji using CO_2 lasers in 1985. Following this, studies have been done using Nd:YAG, Ga–As semiconductor and Ar lasers. Lasers have advantages of less chair side time, noninvasive and enhanced patient cooperation

1. *Indirect pulp capping*: Commonly used lasers are Nd:YAG, Ga–As, argon laser and CO_2 lasers
2. *Direct pulp capping*: Commonly used lasers for direct pulp capping are CO_2, Nd:YAG, argon and Er:YAG laser.

Advantages of laser-assisted root canal treatment over conventional root canal treatment
- Laser-assisted treatment is precise and more accurate
- Causes reduction of ≥99.7% bacterial count from root canals
- It causes better disinfection of the canals
- Laser has ability to reach and clean the accessory canal, so the sealer can penetrate and can cause better seal of root canal
- It is less aggressive than conventional method, resulting in less bleeding, reduced inflammation, less postoperative discomfort and infection

3. *Root canal treatment*:
   - **Modification of root canal walls:** Laser is used for the removal of the smear layer and its replacement with the uncontaminated chemical sealant or sealing by melting the dentinal surface. The removal of smear layer and debris by lasers is possible; however, it is hard to clean all root canal walls because the laser is emitted straight ahead, making it impossible to irradiate lateral wall
   - **Sterilization of root canals:** Traditionally, endodontic techniques use hand and rotary instruments along with irrigants to clean, shape and disinfect the root canal system. Nowadays, laser energy is used to increase cleaning ability, remove smear layer and for disinfection of the root canal system **(Fig. 34.16)**. Studies have shown that efficiency of lasers increased in combination with 5.25% sodium hypochlorite and

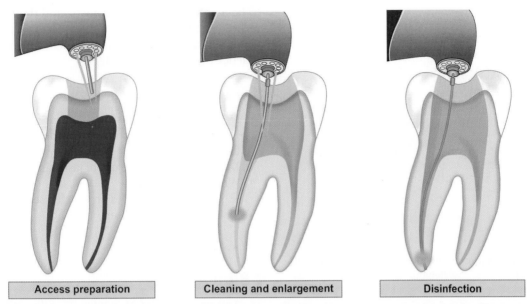

| Access preparation | Cleaning and enlargement | Disinfection |

Fig. 34.16 Laser beam causes removal of smear layer and better disinfection of root canals due to greater penetration power in the dentinal tubules.

17% EDTA and 10% citric acid. The use of chelating agents facilitates the laser light to penetrate deep into dentinal walls up to 1 mm depth. This is known as laser activated irrigation which is considered to be more effective than traditional techniques and ultrasonic methods. Commonly used laser for sterilization are Nd:YAG, argon CO_2, Er:YAG and semiconductor diode

- **Photoactivated disinfection (PAD):** It uses photodynamic therapy or light-activated therapy. It is a combination of photosensitizing dye and a laser beam which kills bacteria, destroys collagen and carious dentin
- **Root canal shaping and obturation:** Ar, CO_2 and Nd:YAG lasers are used to soften gutta-percha for vertical compaction. Obturation with AH plus and composite resin is activated with argon lasers. Lasers initiate photopolymerization by activation of composite resin.

4. *Treatment of incomplete fracture:* Lasers are using in repairing incomplete vertical fractures by causing fusion of the fracture.

5. *Apicoectomy:*
   - If laser is used for surgery, a bloodless surgical field is easier to achieve. If the cut surface is irradiated, it gets sterilized and sealed
   - Clinically, the use of Er:YAG laser resulted in improved healing and diminished postoperative discomfort.

6. *In periodontology:* It causes bacterial reduction in gingival pockets before root planning and decontamination of the root canals after root planning, crown lengthening and depigmentation procedures **(Fig. 34.17).**

7. *Treatment of dental hypersensitivity:* The lasers used for the treatment of dental hypersensitivity are divided into two groups:
   - Low output power lasers (He–Ne and Ga, Al, As lasers)
   - Middle output power lasers (Nd:YAG and CO_2 lasers)
   - In case of low output power lasers, a small fraction of the laser energy is transmitted through enamel or dentin to reach the pulp tissue. He:Ne laser affects the peripheral Aδ or C-fiber nociceptor

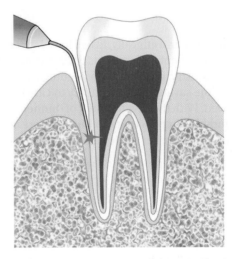

Fig. 34.17 Schematic representation of decontamination of root surface by laser.

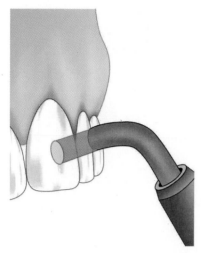

Fig. 34.18 Schematic representation of use of laser for teeth whitening.

- Laser energy of Nd:YAG is indicating thermally mediated effects and pulpal analgesia. Using CO_2 lasers mainly seal the dentinal tubules as well as reduce the permeability.

8. ***Sterilization of instruments:*** Argon, CO_2 and Nd:YAG lasers have been used successfully to sterilize dental instruments.

9. ***Teeth whitening:*** The whitening effect of the laser is achieved by a chemical oxidation process **(Figs. 34.18)**. Once the laser energy is applied, H_2O_2 breaks down to H_2O and free O_2 radical which combines with and thus remove stain molecules. The energy of CO_2 laser is emitted in the form of heat. This energy can enhance the effect of the whitening after initial argon laser process.

Conclusion

If used cautiously and ethically, lasers have been an essential tool in many dental treatments. With the introduction of lasers in dentistry, the complex procedures have become easier and time saving. Thus the ability to care for patients has improved. With the development of thinner, more flexible and durable laser fibers, its applications are increasing in endodontics. A further area of future growth is expected to be a combination of diagnostic and therapeutic laser techniques. Looking to the future, it is expected that laser technologies will become an indispensable part of dental practice over the next decade.

Questions

1. Define and classify lasers.
2. Define and classify lasers. Write briefly on laser physics and types of lasers.
3. Describe in detail the use of lasers in endodontics.
4. Write short notes on:
   - Common principles on which laser work
   - Tissue effects of laser
   - Principles of laser
   - Laser safety.

Bibliography

1. Arakawa S, Cobb CM, Repley JW, Killoy WJ, Spencer P. Treatment of root fracture by CO_2 and Nd:YAG lasers: an *in vitro* study. J Endod 1996;22:662–7.
2. Bader G, Lajeune S. Prospective study of two retrograde endodontic apical preparations with and without the use of CO_2 laser. Endod Dent Traumatol 1998;14:75–8.
3. Hardee MW, Miserendino LJ, Kos W, Walia H. Evaluation of the antibacterial effects of intracanal Nd:YAG laser Irradiation. J Endod 1994;20:377–80.
4. Kaba K, Kimura Y, Matsumoto K, et al. A histopathological study of the morphological changes at the apical seat and in the periapical region after irradiation with a pulsed Nd:YAG laser. Int Endod J 1998;31:415–20.
5. Kouchi Y, Ninomiya J, Yasuda H, et al. Location of *Streptococcus mutans* in the dentinal tubules of open infected root canals. J Dent Res 1980;59:2038–46.
6. Levy G. Cleaning and shaping the root canal with a Nd:YAG laser beam: a comparative study. J Endod 1992;18:123–7.
7. Midda M, Renton-Harper P. Lasers in dentistry. Br Dent J 1991;168:343–6.
8. Moritz A, Schoop U, Goharkhay K, Sperr W. The CO_2 laser as an aid in direct pulp capping. J Endod 1998;24:248–51.
9. Takeda FH, Harashima T, Kimura Y, Matsumoto K. Efficacy of Er:YAG laser irradiation in removing debris and smear laser on root canal walls. J Endod 1998;24:548–51.
10. Wigdor H, Abt E, Ashrafi S, Walsh JT. The effect of lasers on dental hard tissues. J Am Dent Assoc 1993;124:65–70.

Bioceramics in Endodontics

The term "bioceramic" refers to biocompatible material which is composed of ceramic as one of its constituents. These materials mainly consist of alumina and zirconia, bioactive glass, glass ceramics, coatings and composites, hydroxyapatite, and resorbable calcium phosphates. In dentistry, they are used as compositions of implants and periodontal surgeries, such as alveolar ridge augmentation. In endodontics, first use of bioceramics was mineral trioxide aggregate (MTA) which was used for perforation repair and root end filling. The promising clinical results achieved during the last two decades by MTA encouraged the evolution of new endodontic materials with improved biologic, physical, and chemical properties. At present, there are more than 20 types of bioceramic materials which with properties comparable to MTA.

Classification

Bioceramics can be classified as:

Bioinert

These are noninteractive with biological systems, i.e., they do not demonstrate osteoconductive or osteoinductive properties but allow growth of fibrous tissues around the material, for example, alumina, and zirconia.

Bioactive

These show interfacial interactions with surrounding tissue, i.e., they have osteoinductive and osteoconductive properties, for example, hydroxyapatites, bioactive glasses, and glass ceramics.

Biodegradable, Soluble, or Resorbable

These are broken down by the body and degraded; the resorbed material is eventually replaced by endogenous tissue, for example, tricalcium silicates and calcium phosphate.

Rationale of Using Bioceramics

Currently, bioceramics are used in most of the treatments like pulp capping, apexification, root-end fillings, perforation repair, and pulp regeneration. The main rationale of using bioceramics in endodontics is their positive involvement in dental pulp pathology. When pulp experiences trauma or injury or pulp capping is done, growth factors released both by injury and protective pulp dressing play an essential role in organizing the cell differentiation and whole dentin-pulp complex regeneration.

Within 24 hours after injury, there occurs an increased release of growth factors like FGF-2, VEGF, and PDGF in pulp tissue. These cause neoangiogenesis that is important for recovering the locally destroyed blood vessels and for stem cells recruitment. In this, mainly fibroblasts are involved though endothelial cells also interact.

MTA and MTA-based materials have capability to join to fibroblasts, endothelial cells, and growth factors by discharging transforming growth factor (TGF)-β1 from injured pulp cells. Since pulp damage causes loss of primary odontoblasts, other cells are required for dentinogenesis, which is done by differentiation of DPSC into odontoblast-like cells. MTA and MTA-like materials are conducive in promoting the proliferation and differentiation of DPSC and subsequently reparative dentinogenesis. During setting of MTA, calcium ions are released that stimulate signaling molecules like interleukins (IL-1α and IL-1β), TGF-β, etc. which control the cell growth and differentiation.

Moreover, MTA acts as bioactive material due to release of calcium hydroxide and calcium silicate hydrate during hydration reaction of calcium silicates.

Advantages of Bioceramics

❑ Act as regenerative scaffold of resorbable lattices which provide a framework which eventually dissolves as the body rebuilds tissue
❑ Intrinsic osteoinductive ability because of their tendency to absorb osteoinductive chemicals if bone healing is taking place adjacent to it
❑ Biocompatible due to their similarity with hydroxyapatite
❑ Antibacterial properties due to release of calcium ions
❑ Ability to achieve an optimal hermetic seal and form a chemical bond with the tooth structure
❑ Radiopaque in nature.

▌ Bioceramics Available in Endodontics

Calcium silicate-based cements: Portland cement (PC), MTA, biodentine.

Sealers: Endo CPM Sealer, MTA Fillapex, BioRoot RCS, TechBiosealer.

Calcium phosphates/tricalcium phosphate/hydroxyapatite-based: Mixture of calcium silicates and calcium phosphates—iRoot BP, iRoot BP Plus, iRoot FS EndoSequence BC Sealer, BioAggregate

▌ Portland Cement

Portland cement (PC) is obtained from the calcination of the mixture of limestones and silicon-argillaceous materials. The calcined product is then finely grounded and mixed with water for use.

Heating at 1500° + blending + grinding
Clay + limestone ⟶ ===Portland cement

Composition

Portland cement consists of:
❑ Tricalcium silicate   50%
❑ Dicalcium silicate   25%
❑ Tetracalcium aluminoferrite 10%
❑ Tricalcium aluminate   10%
❑ Gypsum   5%

Advantages

❑ Sealing ability is almost the same as that of MTA if used as root end filling material
❑ Antibacterial properties—It shows antibacterial and antifungal properties similar to MTA against *Enterococcus faecalis, Staphylococcus aureus, Pseudomonas aeruginosa,* and *Candida albicans*
❑ Particle size—It is larger than MTA.

Disadvantages

❑ Safety concerns due to higher amount of lead and arsenic released from PC
❑ Higher solubility endangers long-term seal of the restoration
❑ Excessive setting expansion may cause crack formation in the tooth
❑ Biomineralization is not as effective as with MTA
❑ Very low radiopacity, cannot be appreciated on radiograph.

▌ Mineral Trioxide Aggregate (MTA) (Fig. 35.1)

It was introduced by Dr. Torabinejad in 1993 as the first bioceramic material used in endodontics. It is osseoconductive, inductive, and biocompatible. Till 2002, only gray MTA was available, later white MTA was introduced as ProRoot MTA (Dentsply) so as to overcome discoloration of tooth due to gray MTA.

Types of MTA

It is available as gray and white MTA.
❑ **Gray MTA:** It contains tetracalcium aluminoferrite which is responsible for gray discoloration in gray MTA
❑ **White MTA:** It is tooth colored with smaller particle size

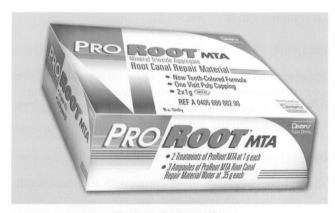

Fig. 35.1 ProRoot MTA.
Courtesy: Dentsply.

Composition of MTA

Portland cement	75%

(responsible for setting and biologic properties)

Bismuth oxide	20%

(provides radiopacity)

Gypsum	5%

(determines setting time)

Portland cement consists of:

- Tricalcium silicate: It is the main component in formation of calcium silicate hydrate which gives early strength to the cement
- Dicalcium silicate: It hydrates slower than tricalcium silicate and is responsible for late strength
- Tetracalcium aluminoferrite: It is present in gray MTA. It balances the heat which occurs during setting
- Tetracalcium aluminate: It forms 20% of the cement. During hydration, it reacts with calcium sulfate.

Setting of MTA

MTA is called hydraulic silicate cement because it sets and is stable under water. It primarily relies on hydration reaction for setting. When mixed with water, MTA sets by process of hydration. Chemical reaction leading to setting of the cement is called **"hydration."** Hydration reaction is divided into different steps including mixing process, sleep process, setting process, cooling process and condensation process **(Fig. 35.2)**.

During mixing, aluminate and gypsum dissolve in water and react. Then aluminates dissociated from cement forms a gel-like layer around the powder particles to prevent fast reaction of aluminates and, thus, rapid setting of cement.

During sleep process, cement can be transported, placed, or processed. In this, cement components dissolve and saturate with water calcium in the cement and hydroxyl ions.

Setting process starts when the water of cement is oversaturated with soluble calcium ions, new hydration products begin to form. Amount of new products formed in the setting period increases constantly resulting in solidification of the cement.

Cooling process occurs when cement has become saturated in terms of components. Cement gains strength in this period.

In concentration process, reaction slows down and the heat output is reduced. Hydration products continue to generate and develop slowly and cement reaches the most rigid state.

Manipulation of MTA

To prepare MTA, a small amount of liquid and powder are mixed to putty consistency. Since MTA mixture is a loose granular aggregate (like concrete cement), it does not stick very well to any instrument. It cannot be carried out in cavity with normal cement carrier, and thus has to be tried with messing gun, amalgam carrier, or especially designed carrier **(Figs. 35.3A and B)**. Once MTA is placed, it is compacted with burnishers and micropluggers. Unless compacted very lightly, the loosely bound aggregate will be pushed out of the cavity. Next, a small damp cotton pellet is used to gently clean the resected surface and to remove any excess MTA from cavity.

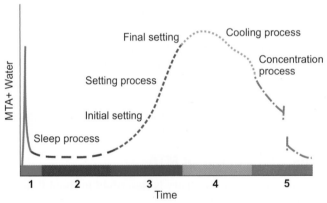

Fig. 35.2 Setting reaction of MTA showing different stages.

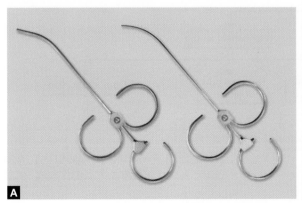

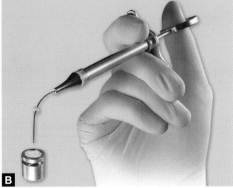

Figs. 35.3A and B MTA carrier gun.

Properties

❑ Compressive strength: It takes 3–4 hours to set MTA. Compressive strength is 40 MPa immediately after setting and 70 MPa after 21 days. It is equal to IRM and super EBA but less than that of amalgam
❑ pH of MTA is 12.5 (when set), so it has properties similar to calcium hydroxide
❑ Setting time is 2 hours and 45 minutes
❑ Contrast to $Ca(OH)_2$, it produces hard setting nonresorbable surface
❑ It sets in a moist environment (hydrophilic in nature)
❑ It has low solubility
❑ It shows resistance to marginal leakage
❑ It also reduces bacterial migration due to release of calcium ions and high pH
❑ It exhibits excellent biocompatibility in relation with vital tissues.

Difference between Gray and White MTA

Gray MTA	White MTA
• Contains tetracalcium aluminoferrite (ferrous oxide) which is responsible for gray discoloration • Large particle size • Greater compressive strength • Longer setting time	• Ferrous oxide is replaced with magnesium oxide, so no tooth discoloration • Smaller particle size • Less compressive strength • Shorter setting time

Advantages of MTA

❑ Water-based chemistry, requiring moisture for setting
❑ Excellent biocompatibility
❑ Normal healing response without inflammation
❑ Least toxic of all the filling materials

❑ More radiopaque than calcium hydroxide
❑ Bacteriostatic in nature due to high pH
❑ Resistance to marginal leakage
❑ Excellent sealing ability
❑ Produces artificial barrier against which obturating material can be condensed
❑ Vasoconstrictive, so beneficial for hemostasis, especially in cases of pulp capping.

Disadvantages of MTA

❑ Difficult handling characteristics due to its sandy nature
❑ Long setting time (2 hours 45 minutes)
❑ Expensive
❑ Discoloration potential of gray MTA
❑ Known solvent is present so difficult to remove after curing.

Precautions to Be Taken for MTA

❑ MTA material should be kept in closed container to avoid moisture contamination
❑ MTA must be stored in dry area
❑ MTA material should be immediately placed after mixing with liquid to prevent dehydration during setting
❑ Do not irrigate after placing MTA, and remove excess water with moist cotton pellet
❑ Adding too much or too little liquid will reduce the ultimate strength of the material
❑ MTA material usually takes 3–4 hours but the working time is about 5 minutes. If more working time is needed, the mixed material should be covered with a moist gauge pad to prevent evaporation.

Indications of Use of MTA

The use of MTA in dentistry is described in the following flowchart:

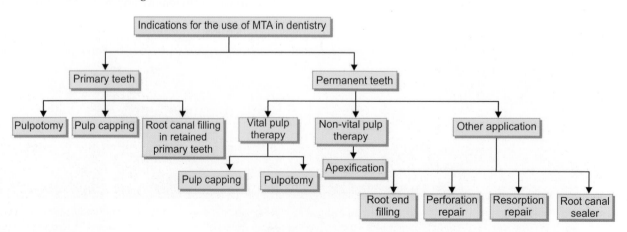

Contraindications of Use of MTA

It is not indicated for obturation of primary teeth which are expected to exfoliate because it resorbs very slowly.

Clinical Applications of MTA (Fig. 35.4)

Pulp Capping

By placing MTA over the exposed area allows healing and preservation of vital pulp without further treatment. Rinse the cavity with sodium hypochlorite to disinfect the area. Mix the MTA with enough sterile water to give it a putty consistency. Apply it over the exposed pulp and remove the excess. Blot the area dry with a cotton pellet and restore the cavity with an amalgam or composite filling material.

Apexogenesis

Vital pulp—isolate the tooth with a rubber dam and perform a pulpotomy procedure. Place the MTA over the pulp stump and close the tooth with temporary cement until the apex of the tooth close.

Apexification

Nonvital pulp—isolate the tooth with a rubber dam and perform root canal treatment. Mix the MTA and compact it to the apex of the tooth, creating a 2 mm thickness of plug. Wait for it to set; then fill in the canal with cement and gutta-percha (**Figs. 35.5 and 35.6**).

Internal and External Root Resorption

In internal resorption cases, after cleaning and shaping, prepare a putty mixture of MTA and fill the canal with it, using a plugger or gutta-percha cone and obturate the canal. In the case of external resorption, complete the root canal therapy for that tooth. Raise a flap and remove the defect on the root

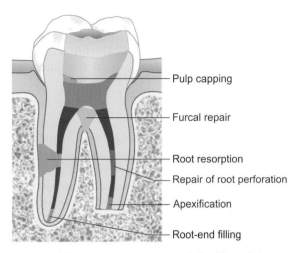

Fig. 35.4 Schematic representation of clinical applications of MTA.

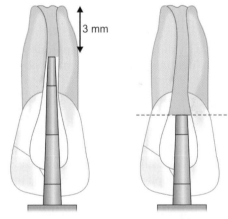

Fig. 35.5 Schematic representation of apexification of tooth by creating 2–3 mm thick plug at the apex and then backfilling with gutta-percha.

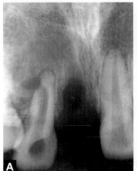 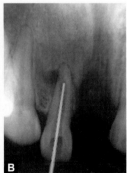 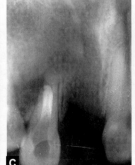 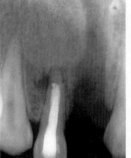 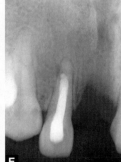

Figs. 35.6A to E Management of case with MTA: (A) radiograph showing maxillary incisor with open apex and periradicular radiolucency associated with it; (B) Working length radiograph; (C) MTA plug placed apically; (D) Backfilling with gutta-percha; (E) Radiograph after 9 months showing decrease in size of radiolucency.
Courtesy: Manoj Hans.

surface with a round bur. Mix the MTA in the same manner as above and apply it to the root surface. Remove the excess cement and condition the surface with tetracycline. Graft the defect with decalcified freeze dried bone allograft and a calcium sulfate barrier.

Perforation

Complete the cleaning and shaping of the perforated canal. If perforation is at mid-to-apical third, then follow the directions for treating an internal resorption. If perforation is closer to coronal third, then obturate the canal with gutta-percha, remove the gutta-percha below the perforation and fill MTA in the canal with a plugger.

Root-End Filling

Prepare a class I cavity at the root end, mix MTA and condense it into the cavity using a small plugger. Remove the excess cement with the help of moist gauge.

Biodentine (Fig. 35.7)

Biodentine is a calcium silicate-based product, specifically designed as a "dentine replacement" material.

Composition

Powder: Tricalcium silicate, dicalcium silicate, calcium carbonate, and oxide filler and zirconium oxide. Tricalcium silicate and dicalcium silicate are core materials, zirconium oxide provides radiopacity, and iron oxide is responsible for shade.

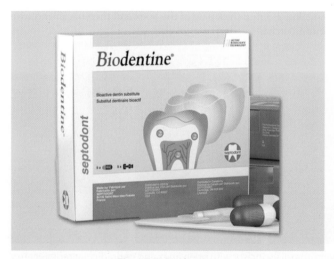

Fig. 35.7 Biodentine.

Liquid: Liquid consists of Calcium chloride as an accelerator, hydrosoluble polymer as a water reducing agent and water. Setting period is 9–12 minutes. On mixing, it forms calcium silicate hydrate and leaches calcium and hydroxide in solution.

Manipulation

Take capsule powder and liquid and manipulate it in amalgamator for 30 seconds.

On mixing, the following reaction products are formed:

- CSH gel is the matrix of the cement and crystals of $CaCO_3$ are filling spaces between gel of the cement
- Calcite has two phases as an active agent and as filler
- Final set cement structure consists of unreacted particles of the cement, CSH gel, and calcium hydroxide.

Setting Time

Initial setting time is 8–9 minutes and final setting time is up to 20 minutes. It can be accelerated by using calcium chloride.

Properties

Compressive Strength

Compressive strength of biodentine is >100 MPa and reaches >200 in 24 hours. It becomes 300 MPa almost the same as dentin after 30 days.

Density and Porosity

Use of hydrosoluble polymer in biodentine reduces the amount of water which has positive influence on density. Lower porosity causes better mechanical strength.

Microhardness

Microhardness of biodentine is more than BioAggregate, IRM, and glass ionomer cement.

Adhesion

It's because of two mechanisms:
1. Ion exchange between cement and dental tissues
2. Physical processes of crystal growth within the dentinal tubules leading to micromechanical tag formation.

Ion Release

It releases calcium and hydroxyl ions. High calcium release is due to presence of calcium silicate, calcium chloride, and calcium carbonate.

Antibacterial Properties

It shows antibacterial property due to release of calcium hydroxide and pH of 12 which inhibits microorganisms and disinfects dentin.

Radiopacity

It is radiopaque but it's not sufficient to well distinguish limits of the material in tooth structure. In biodentine, zirconium oxide is used as a radiopacifier rather than bismuth oxide which is used in other materials because zirconium oxide is biocompatible and bioinert material with favorable mechanical properties and resistance to corrosion.

Remineralization

Biodentine causes remineralization because of
❑ Ability to release calcium, this calcium helps in differentiation, proliferation, and mineralization of pulp cells
❑ Calcium and hydroxide ions increase the activity of alkaline phosphatase, pyrophosphatase, TGF-β, and osteopontin. TGF-β is responsible for remineralization of reparative dentin.

Advantages of Biodentine

❑ Helps in dentine remineralization
❑ Preserves pulp vitality and promotes pulp healing
❑ Replaces dentin with same mechanical properties
❑ Indicated for root and crown repair
❑ Good handling and manipulation
❑ Short setting time
❑ Adhesion to dentin
❑ Biocompatible
❑ Antibacterial.

▍Bioceramic-Based Root Canal Sealers

The main functions of root canal sealers are to seal off the voids, form a bond between the core of the filling material and the root canal wall, and act as a lubricant. Sealers have been classified according to chemical composition as zinc oxide eugenol, calcium hydroxide, glass ionomer, silicone, resin, and bioceramic-based sealers.

MTA-based sealers (Figs. 35.8A to F)
❑ MTA as sealer
❑ ProRoot Endo Sealer
❑ Fillapex
❑ CPM sealer
❑ MTA Obtura
❑ MTAS experimental sealer
❑ F-doped MTA cements.

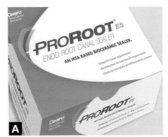
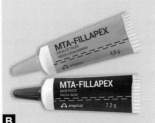
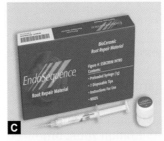
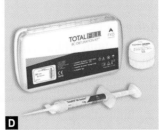
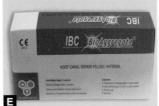
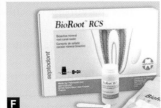

Figs. 35.8A to F Commercially available bioceramic sealers.

Properties

Biocompatibility

Bioceramic-based root canal sealers are biocompatible which is mainly due to the presence of calcium phosphate in the sealer.

Flow

Flow of a sealer allows it to fill canals, isthmus, accessory canals, and voids between the master and accessory cones. According to ISO 6786/2001, a root canal sealer should have a flow rate of not <20 mm. Bioceramic-based sealers meet the ISO requirements of flow.

Retreatability

Bioceramic sealers are difficult to remove from the root canals during retreatment and post-space preparation.

Solubility

iRoot SP and MTA-Fillapex are highly soluble and do not meet ANSI/ADA requirements. MTA-Angelus has low solubility which is consistent with ANSI/ADA requirements.

Radiopacity

Bioceramic sealers are radiopaque due to presence of bismuth trioxide and barium sulfate.

Antimicrobial Properties

Bioceramic sealers are antimicrobial in nature due to their alkalinity and release of calcium ions which stimulates repair by the deposition of mineralized tissue.

Adhesion

Sealing ability of bioceramic-based sealers is because of following three mechanisms:

1. Diffusion of the sealer particles into the dentinal tubules and form mechanical interlocking bonds
2. Infiltration of sealer's mineral content into intertubular dentin forming mineral infiltration zone, produced after denaturing the collagen fibers with a strong alkaline sealer
3. Reaction of phosphate with calcium silicate hydrogel and calcium hydroxide, produced by reaction of calcium silicates in the presence of dentin's moisture, resulting in the formation of hydroxyapatite along the mineral infiltration zone.

Conclusion

When compared to conventional materials used in endodontic treatments, bioceramic cements are not only biocompatible but also bioactive as they proved to be involved in controlling the tissue healing and pulp regeneration. Seeing the advantages of bioceramics, recent studies favor bioceramic materials even if not many products are available for use. Being biocompatible and bioactive materials, these are used in root perforations, large apical foramens, and root resorptions. MTA or MTA-like cements have been used as materials of choice in regenerative endodontics, vital pulp therapy, and periradicular surgery due to their clinical success rate. Based on in-progress technology of fabrication, it is expected that the newer bioceramic cements will overcome drawbacks of previous ones, mainly the discoloration problem. With further research, bioceramics has the potential to become the preferred materials for the various endodontic procedures.

Questions

Write short notes on:
- MTA
- Advantages of bioceramics in endodontics
- Biodentine
- Bioceramic sealers
- Clinical applications of MTA.

Bibliography

1. Altan H, Tosun G. The setting mechanism of mineral trioxide aggregate. J Istanb Univ Fac Dent 2016;50:65–72. http://dx.doi.org/10.17096/jiufd.50128.
2. Berzins DW. Chemical properties of MTA. In: Torabinejad M, editor. Mineral trioxide aggregate. Properties and clinical applications. Oxford: Wiley Blackwell; 2014. pp. 17–35.
3. Camilleri J, Sorrentino F, Damidot D. Investigation of the hydration and bioactivity of radiopacified tricalcium silicate cement, biodentine and MTA angelus. Dent Mater 2013;29:580–93.
4. Ford TR. Physical and chemical properties of a new root-end filling material. J Endod 1995;21:349–53.
5. Grech L, Mallia B, Camilleri J. Characterization of set intermediate restorative material, biodentine, BioAggregate and a prototype calcium silicate cement for use as root-end filling materials. Int Endod J 2013;46:632–41.
6. Parirokh M, Torabinejad M. Calcium silicate-based cements. In: Torabinejad M, editor. Mineral trioxide aggregate. Properties and clinical applications. Oxford: Wiley Blackwell; 2014. pp. 281–332.
7. Ribeiro CS, Kuteken FA, Hirata Jr R, Scelza MF. Comparative evaluation of antimicrobial action of MTA, calcium hydroxide and Portland cement. J Appl Oral Sci 2006;14:330–3.
8. Sarkar NK, Caicedo R, Ritwik P. Physicochemical basis of the biologic properties of mineral trioxide aggregate. J Endod 2005;31:97–100.
9. Tziafas D, Pantelidou O, Alvanou A. The dentinogenic effect of mineral trioxide aggregate (MTA) in short-term capping experiments. Int Endod J 2002;35:245–54.
10. Zhu L, Yang J, Zhang J, Peng B. A comparative study of BioAggregate and ProRoot MTA on adhesion, migration and attachment of human dental pulp cells. J Endod 2014;40:1118–23.

Vital Pulp Therapy

Once the pulp gets exposed, the aim of the treatment is to promote pulp tissue healing and preserve pulp vitality. Young permanent teeth are teeth which have recently erupted and where apical physiological root closure has not occurred. Normal physiological closure may take 2–3 years after eruption. In such teeth, if there is an injury to the pulp, the aim of the treatment is to preserve the pulp vitality and promote healing. Vital pulp therapy procedures involve removal of irritants of the pulp and placement of a protective material directly or indirectly over the pulp followed by tight-sealed restoration. Vital pulp therapy is performed to treat reversible pulpal injury to promote root formation and apical closure. Nonvital pulp therapy, that is, apexification and pulpectomy are indicated if irreversible damage to pulp has occurred.

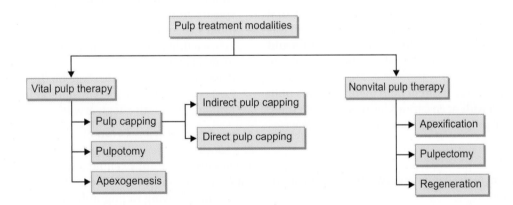

Vital Pulp Therapy

Definition: Vital pulp therapy is defined as a treatment that aims to preserve and maintain pulp tissue that has been compromised but not destroyed by caries, trauma, or restorative procedures.

It is specially indicated for young permanent teeth because of the high healing capacity of pulp tissue compared to older patients. Dental pulp forms secondary dentin, peritubular dentin, and reparative dentin in response to biologic and pathologic stimuli; it also keeps the dentin moist which in turn ensures resilience and toughness of the dentin. Also, the vital pulp provides the protective resistance to mastication forces compared to endodontically treated tooth. So, it is always preferred to maintain the vitality of the pulp unless it is unavoidable.

One should take care that management of deep carious lesion approaching the pulp necessitates the removal of

Table 36.1: Difference between infected and affected dentin.

Infected dentin	Affected dentin
• Soft, demineralized dentin invaded with bacteria	• Demineralized dentin but not invaded by bacteria
• Soft leathery tissue which can be flaked easily	• Does not flake easily though soft in nature
• Irreversible denaturation of collagen	• Uninterrupted collagen cross-linking
• Cannot be remineralized	• Can be remineralized
• Caries detecting dyes can stain	• Does not stain

infected dentin while keeping the affected dentin to avoid inadvertent pulp exposure. Table 36.1 summarizes the differences between affected and infected dentin.

Commonly used techniques for vital pulp therapy are pulp capping and pulpotomy.

Pulp Capping

Pulp capping is the procedure used in dental restorations to prevent pulp from degeneration after being exposed or accidental exposure during tooth preparation. It can be of two types: indirect and direct pulp capping.

Indirect Pulp Capping (IPC)

Indirect pulp capping is a procedure performed in a tooth with deep carious lesion adjacent to the pulp. In this procedure, caries near the pulp is left in place to avoid pulp exposure and is covered with a biocompatible material.

According to Cohen, indirect pulp therapy avoids pulp exposure in teeth with deep carious lesions in which there is no evidence of pulp degeneration or periapical disease.

Rationale

❑ Decalcification of the dentin precedes bacterial invasion within the dentin
❑ Removal of outer carious dentin removes majority of bacteria reducing further decalcification of deeper dentin
❑ Sealing the lesion to allow the pulp to generate reparative dentin

Objective

❑ Arrest carious process
❑ Promote dentinal sclerosis
❑ Stimulate promotion of reactionary dentin
❑ Remineralization of carious dentin while preserving pulp vitality

Indications

❑ Deep carious lesion near the pulp tissue but not involving it
❑ No history of spontaneous toothache or history of mild discomfort from chemical and thermal stimuli
❑ No tenderness to percussion

Contraindications

❑ Presence of pulp exposure
❑ Radiographic evidence of pulp pathology
❑ History of spontaneous toothache
❑ Tooth sensitive to percussion
❑ Mobility present
❑ Root resorption or radicular disease is present radiographically

Clinical Technique

In 1938, Bodecker introduced the stepwise excavation (SWE) technique for the treatment of teeth with deep caries for preservation of pulp vitality where exposure of pulp is probable.

Two-appointment Technique (Figs. 36.1A to C)

First sitting

❑ Anesthetize the tooth and apply rubber dam to isolate it
❑ Remove soft, necrotic, and infected caries either with spoon excavator **(Fig. 36.2)** or round bur using a slow speed handpiece. Use fissure bur and extend it to sound tooth structure
❑ Leave a thin layer of dentin and some amount of caries to avoid exposure
❑ Place calcium hydroxide paste on the exposed dentin
❑ Cover calcium hydroxide with durable interim restoration
❑ Evaluate the tooth after 6–8 weeks

Second visit (6–8 weeks later)

If a tooth has been asymptomatic, the surrounding soft tissues are free from swelling and the temporary filling is intact, the second step can be performed.

❑ Obtain bitewing radiograph to assess the presence of reparative dentin
❑ Give local anesthesia and apply rubber dam
❑ Take care while removing restoration and calcium hydroxide dressing
❑ Remove the remaining affected carious dentin which appears hydrated and flaky. The area around the potential exposure should appear whitish and may be soft (predentin) and should not be disturbed
❑ Gently clean and dry the cavity
❑ Cover the entire floor with a hard-setting calcium hydroxide dressing

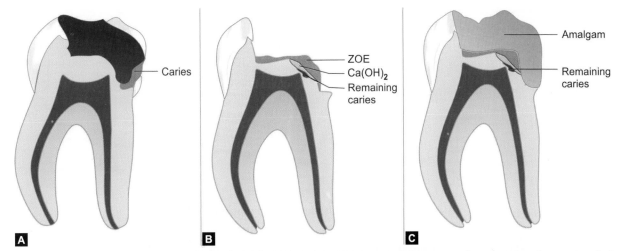

Figs. 36.1A to C Schematic representation of indirect pulp capping: (A) Indirect pulp capping is done in cases when carious lesion is quite close to the pulp; (B) Placement of calcium hydroxide and zinc oxide eugenol dressing after excavation of soft caries; (C) Permanent restoration of tooth.

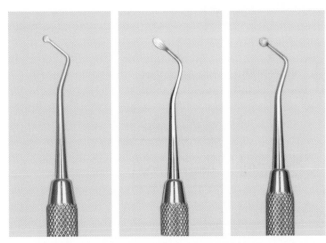

Fig. 36.2 Spoon excavators for removing deep caries.

❑ Place reinforced zinc oxide eugenol or glass ionomer cement over calcium hydroxide and give final restoration with composite or amalgam over it

One-appointment Technique

❑ Anesthetize the tooth and apply rubber dam to isolate it
❑ Remove soft, necrotic, and infected caries either with spoon excavator or large round bur using a slow-speed hand piece. Remove all soft moist and leathery texture of dentin
❑ Leave a thin layer of dentin and some amount of caries to avoid exposure
❑ Place calcium hydroxide paste on the exposed dentin
❑ Cover the calcium hydroxide with durable interim restoration. Ensure proper seal of the restoration

The removal of bacteria and substrate together with an effective seal of restoration provides the suitable environment for pulp to recover by laying down secondary dentin.

It is difficult to state which treatment approach is better because no high-quality randomized clinical trials are available. The need to uncover the residual dentin to remove dehydrated dentin and view the sclerotic changes has been questioned. The second entry subjects the pulp to potential risk of exposure owing to overzealous re-excavation.

Factors Affecting Success of IPC

❑ If remaining dentin thickness is approximately 0.5–2 mm, prognosis is better
❑ Choice of indirect pulp capping agent; though many new materials have been introduced, calcium hydroxide has been used successfully due to its high pH and hard tissue formation

Ideal Requirements of a Pulp Capping Agent

Cohen and Combe gave the following requirements of an ideal pulp capping agent:
❑ Should maintain pulp vitality
❑ Should be bactericidal or bacteriostatic in nature
❑ Should be able to provide bacterial seal
❑ Should stimulate reparative dentin formation
❑ Should be radiopaque in nature
❑ Should be able to resist the forces under restoration

Materials used for Pulp Capping (Fig. 36.3)

❑ Calcium hydroxide
❑ Mineral trioxide aggregate (MTA)
❑ Biodentine
❑ BioAggregate

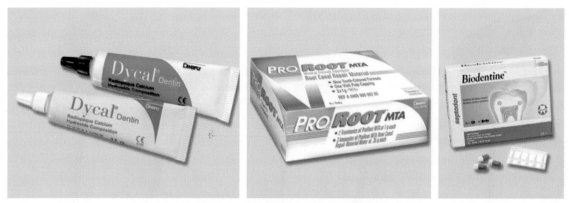

Fig. 36.3 Materials used for pulp capping.

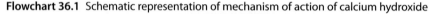

Flowchart 36.1 Schematic representation of mechanism of action of calcium hydroxide

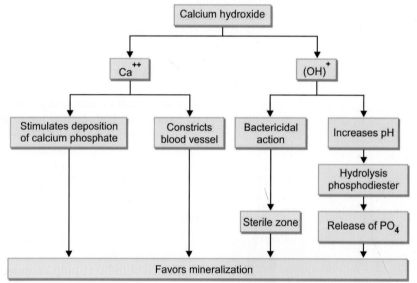

- Bonding systems
- Tricalcium phosphate

Calcium hydroxide

It was introduced by Hermann in 1920. It is most commonly used for pulp capping because, along with blocking the dentinal tubules, it helps in neutralizing the attack of inorganic acids from restorative materials.

Mechanism of action of calcium hydroxide

Calcium hydroxide has a high alkaline pH of 12.5 which is responsible for its antibacterial activity and its ability to form hard tissue. Though calcium ions from calcium hydroxide do not directly contribute to formation of hard tissue, they stimulate the repair process (**Flowchart 36.1**).

Mechanism of hard tissue formation is not known but can be considered due to combination of its direct effects and indirect effects due to high pH (**Flowchart 36.2**).

Histology of healing with calcium hydroxide (Fig. 36.4)
Zone of obliteration

- Pulp tissue immediately in contact with calcium hydroxide is completely distorted because of its caustic effect of drug
- This zone consists of debris, dentinal chips, blood clot, and particles of calcium hydroxide

Zone of coagulation necrosis

- A weaker chemical effect reaches subjacent, more apical tissue and results in zone of coagulation necrosis and thrombosis
- This is also called as *Stanley's mummified zone and Schroder's layer of firm necrosis*

Line of demarcation

- This line forms between the deepest level of zone of coagulation necrosis and adjacent vital pulp tissue
- This is formed by the reaction of calcium hydroxide with tissue proteins to form proteinate globules

Flowchart 36.2 Showing mechanism of action of hard tissue formation due to high pH and its direct effects.

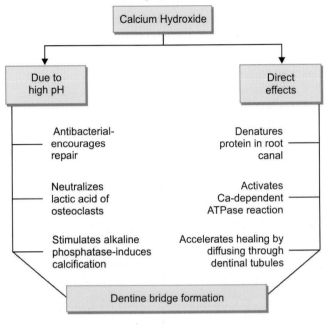

MTA

It was developed by Torabinajad in 1990s. It contains
- Tricalcium silicate
- Dicalcium silicate
- Tricalcium aluminate
- Bismuth oxide
- Calcium sulfate
- Tetracalcium aluminoferrite

Properties
- pH of MTA is 12.5 and sets in a moist environment (hydrophilic in nature)
- Contrast to calcium hydroxide, it produces hard-setting nonresorbable surface and low solubility
- It is antibacterial
- Induces pulpal cell proliferation and stimulate hard tissue formation

Mechanism of action is not yet known. It is thought that when tricalcium oxide comes in contact with tissue fluids it releases calcium hydroxide which causes hard tissue formation.

Advantages	Disadvantages
• Promotes healing and repair • High pH stimulates fibroblasts and neutralizes acids • Bactericidal and bacteriostatic • Stops resorption process	• Does not exclusively stimulate dentinogenesis • Degrade upon tooth flexure • May degrade acid etching • Does not adhere to tooth structure • Can cause primary tooth resorption

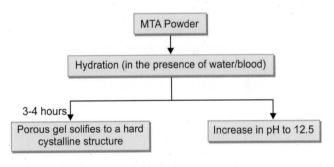

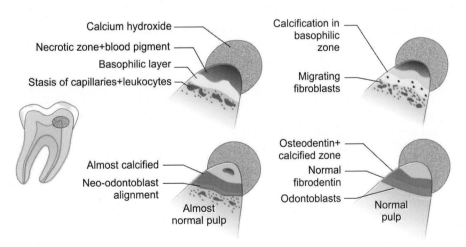

Fig. 36.4 Schematic representation of healing with calcium hydroxide.

Advantages	Disadvantages
• Excellent biocompatibility • Normal healing response without inflammation • More radiopaque than calcium hydroxide • Bacteriostatic in nature due to high pH • Excellent sealing ability • Vasoconstrictive and beneficial for hemostasis, especially in cases of pulp capping	• Difficult handling characteristics • Long setting time (2 h 45 min) • Expensive

Tricalcium phosphate

It is used in bone regeneration procedures. It shows formation of dentinal bridge by direct apposition on the pulpal wall.

Biodentine

Its powder consists of tricalcium silicate, dicalcium silicate, calcium carbonate, and zirconium oxide. Liquid consists of hydrosoluble polymer and calcium chloride. Hydration of tricalcium silicate causes formation of hydrated calcium silicate gel and calcium hydroxide. It stimulates release of TGF-β from pulp cells which cause dentine bridge formation. Biodentine is both a dentin substitute base and a cement for maintaining pulp vitality and stimulating hard tissue formation.

Bioaggregate

It consists of bioceramic nanoparticles. Its powder and liquid are mixed to form a thick paste like consistency for use.

Direct Pulp Capping

Direct pulp capping (DPC) involves the placement of biocompatible material over the site of pulp exposure to maintain vitality and promote healing.

When a small mechanical exposure of pulp occurs during cavity preparation or following a trauma, an appropriate protective base should be placed in contact with the exposed pulp tissue to maintain the vitality of the remaining pulp tissue.

Rationale

To encourage young and healthy pulp to initiate a dentin bridge and form a wall over the exposure site.

Objective

The objective of DPC is to seal the pulp against bacterial leakage, protect the pulp from thermal stimulus, encourage the pulp to wall off the exposure site by initiating a dentin bridge, and maintain the vitality of the underlying pulp.

Indications

☐ Small pinpoint (<1 mm) mechanical exposure of pulp surrounded by sound dentin during tooth preparation
☐ Traumatic injury (<24 h) with pinpoint exposure
☐ No or minimal bleeding at the exposure site

Contraindications

☐ Carious or wide pulp exposure
☐ Spontaneous and nocturnal toothache
☐ Uncontrolled bleeding at the exposure site
☐ Radiographic evidence of pulp pathology
☐ Excessive tooth mobility
☐ Purulent or serous exudates from exposure site

Clinical Procedure (Flowchart 36.3 and Fig. 36.5)

Flowchart 36.3 Direct pulp capping.

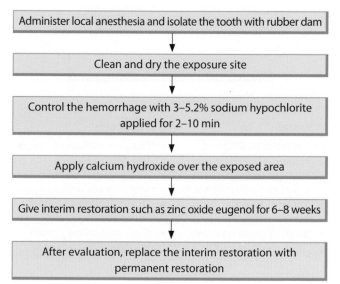

Factors affecting success of pulp capping

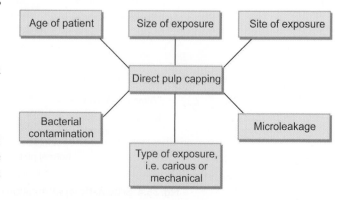

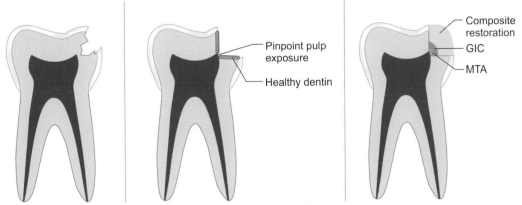

Fig. 36.5 Schematic representation of direct pulp capping.

☐ **Type of exposure:** Prognosis is good if exposure is mechanical. In case of carious exposure, opt for endodontic treatment

☐ **Type of restoration:** Restoration which provides hermetic seal shows better results when compared to temporary restoration

☐ **Area of exposure:** Prognosis of pulp capping is inversely proportional to the area of mechanical exposure. If exposure is <1 mm, go for DPC, if it is 1–2 mm, choice is pulpotomy

☐ **Class of restoration:** Better prevention of microleakage in class I restoration shows better prognosis than class II, III, IV, and MOD restorations

☐ **Choice of pulp capping agent:** Calcium hydroxide is tried and tested material for successful capping procedures due to its high pH and the ability to form dentinal bridge

☐ **Time lapse between exposure and treatment:** If time gap is up to 48 hours, perform partial pulpotomy; if it is >48 hours, opt for complete pulpotomy or pulpectomy

☐ **Bacterial contamination:** Prognosis is poor in case of bacterial contamination of exposure

Why DPC is not Recommended in Primary Teeth?

Many researchers have given different reasons for not indicating DPC in primary teeth. Following are some of the reasons:

1. *McDonalds (1956):* Localization of infection and inflammation in primary teeth is poorer than in permanent teeth
2. *Rayner and Southam (1979):* Effects of dentinal caries are seen very rapidly in primary teeth than the permanent teeth
3. *Kennedy and Kopel (1985):* Due to presence of thin enamel and dentinal layers, primary pulp gets rapidly affected by caries. Once the pulp gets exposed by caries, prognosis for DPC is poor

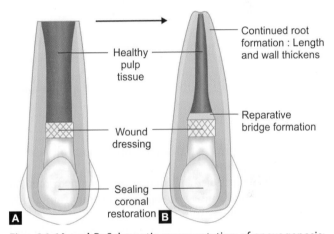

Figs. 36.6A and B Schematic representation of apexogenesis: (A) Young permanent tooth with immature root and open apex; (B) Shows root formation of reparative dentin and thickening of root canal wall after apexogenesis procedure.

4. *Kennedy (1985):* Undifferentiated mesenchymal cells may differentiate into osteoclasts in response to pulp capping material resulting in internal resorption
5. *Stanley (1985):* Primary teeth show incidences of increased resorption because of already happening root resorption process

▌Apexogenesis

Apexogenesis is defined as the treatment of vital pulp by capping or pulpotomy to permit continued growth of root and closure of root apex **(Figs. 36.6A and B)**.

▌Pulpotomy

According to Finn (1995), pulpotomy refers to complete removal of the coronal portion of the dental pulp followed by placement of a suitable medicament that will promote healing and preserve tooth vitality.

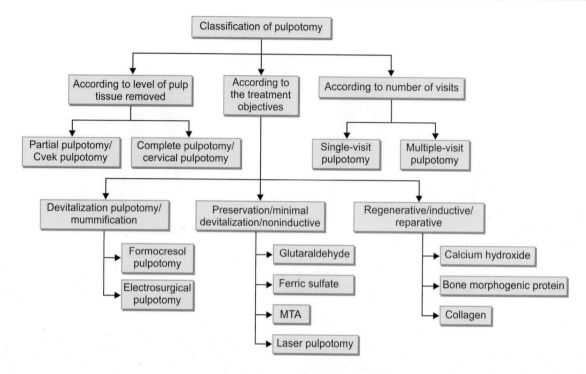

Rationale

- Maintain integrity of radicular pulp tissue to allow continued root growth
- Pulp of immature teeth has significant reparative potential
- Pulp revascularization and repair occurs more efficiently in tooth with open apex
- Root-end closure occurs in a tooth with vital pulp and minimum inflammation.

Objectives

- To maintain vitality of the pulp to help root maturation
- Promote root-end closure and natural apical constriction
- Sustain a viable Hertwig's epithelial root sheath to allow root development
- Form a dentinal bridge at the site of pulpotomy.

Indications

- Traumatized or pulpally involved vital permanent tooth with open apex
- Clinical and radiographic signs of radicular pulp vitality
- Pain, if present, is neither spontaneous nor persists after removal of the stimulus
- No or easy-to-control hemorrhage from amputation site.

Contraindications

- Symptoms of irreversible pulpitis
- Nonrestorable crown structure
- Pulp necrosis with radiolucency in furcal or periradicular areas

- Presence of purulent discharge
- Spontaneous pain
- Tenderness to percussion
- Mobility.

Criteria for Successful Pulpotomy

- No radiographic evidence of internal root resorption
- No radiographic sign of periradicular periodontitis
- Tooth should respond to pulp testing
- Tooth should be asymptomatic.

Cvek Pulpotomy/Partial Pulpotomy/Calcium Hydroxide Pulpotomy/Young Permanent Partial Pulpotomy

It was given by Cvek in 1993. Cvek showed that, with pulp exposures resulting from traumatic injuries, pulpal changes are characterized by a proliferative response with inflammation extending only a few millimeters into the pulp, whereas in teeth with carious exposure of the pulp, it may be necessary to remove pulpal tissue to a greater depth to reach noninflamed tissue.

Procedure (Figs. 36.7 A to C)

- Anesthetize and isolate the tooth
- Remove carious lesion with a slow speed round bur
- Remove the coronal pulp and control hemorrhage using sodium hypochlorite and moistened cotton pellets with slight pressure.

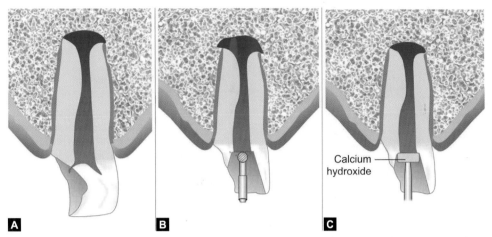

Figs. 36.7A to C (A) Partial pulpotomy is indicated in patients with incomplete root formation; (B) preparation of cavity 1–2 mm deep into pulp; (C) placement of calcium hydroxide over pulp.

- Place calcium hydroxide or MTA over the amputation site
- If calcium hydroxide is placed, recall the patient, check dentin bridge formation, and place permanent restoration

Cervical Pulpotomy/Complete Pulpotomy

- In young permanent teeth, cervical pulpotomy is performed to allow root maturation. The procedure is performed in teeth in which it is assumed that healthy pulp tissue, with a potential to produce a dentin bridge and complete the formation of the root, still remains in the canal
- The technique is same as that of partial pulpotomy except that it is up to root orifice (**Figs. 36.8A to C**).

Formocresol Pulpotomy

It was introduced in 1904 by Buckley. He found that equal parts of formalin and tricresol would react chemically with the products of pulp inflammation to form a non-infective compound of a harmless nature. Sweet popularized this technique in 1930. It is preferred in primary teeth due to high (98%) clinical and radiographic success rate.
- Buckley's formocresol consists of
- Formaldehyde 19%
- Tricresol 35%
- Glycernin 15%
- Water 31%

Technique of formocresol pulpotomy is shown in **Flowchart 36.4** and **Figures 36.9A to D**.

Mechanism of Action

Formocresol is an efficient bactericide. It has the ability to prevent tissue autolysis by the complex chemical binding

Flowchart 36.4 Clinical procedure of formocresol pulpotomy

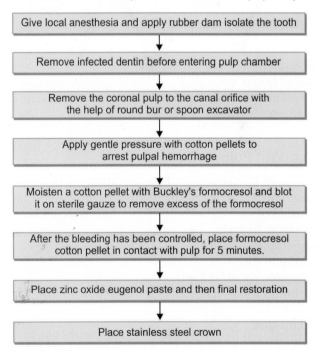

Give local anesthesia and apply rubber dam isolate the tooth
↓
Remove infected dentin before entering pulp chamber
↓
Remove the coronal pulp to the canal orifice with the help of round bur or spoon excavator
↓
Apply gentle pressure with cotton pellets to arrest pulpal hemorrhage
↓
Moisten a cotton pellet with Buckley's formocresol and blot it on sterile gauze to remove excess of the formocresol
↓
After the bleeding has been controlled, place formocresol cotton pellet in contact with pulp for 5 minutes.
↓
Place zinc oxide eugenol paste and then final restoration
↓
Place stainless steel crown

of formaldehyde with peptide groups of side chain amino acids without changing the basic structure of protein molecule.

After 7 days of application, pulp shows three distinct zones:
1. Broad eosinophilic zone of fixation
2. Broad pale-staining zone with poor cellular definition
3. Zone of inflammation diffusing apically into normal pulp tissue. After 60 days, in a limited number of samples, the remaining tissue was believed to be completely fixed, appearing as a strand of eosinophilic fibrous tissue

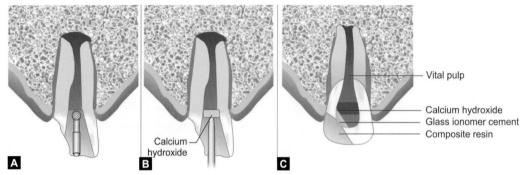

Figs. 36.8A to C Showing Complete pulpotomy. (A) Removal of coronal pulp up to the level of roof orifices; (B) Placement of Ca(OH)$_2$ over exposed pulp; (C) Tooth restored with final restoration.

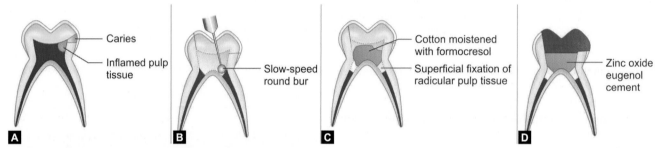

Figs. 36.9A to D Schematic representation of formocresol pulpotomy: (A) Tooth showing deep caries with inflamed pulp tissue; (B) remove coronal pulp till orifice of the canals using round bur; (C) Place a cotton pellet moistened with formocresol on pulp tissue; (D) Place zinc oxide eugenol dressing.

Two-Visit Pulpotomy

It is used in cases of profuse and difficult-to-control bleeding. In this, paraformaldehyde paste is used which consists of:

Paraformaldehyde—1 g
Lignocaine—0.06 g
Carmine—10 g
Propylene glycol—0.5 mL
Carbowax 1500—1.3 g

Technique

The procedure is same as for one-visit formocresol pulpotomy till hemorrhage control except for the following changes:

- ❑ Place cotton pellet moistened with paraformaldehyde over the pulpal exposure
- ❑ Place paraformaldehyde mixed with zinc oxide eugenol for 1–2 weeks. Formaldehyde vapors fix the tissues
- ❑ At the <u>second</u> visit, remove the cotton pellet and clean the pulp chamber with hydrogen peroxide. Alternatively, use an antiseptic dressing (equal parts of eugenol and formocresol with zinc oxide)

- ❑ Place IRM or glass ionomer cement over it
- ❑ Restore the tooth with stainless steel crown

Other Materials Used for Pulpotomy

- ❑ Glutaraldehyde
- ❑ Ferric sulfate
- ❑ MTA
- ❑ Bone morphogenic proteins
- ❑ Laser
- ❑ Electrosurgical pulpotomy

Glutaraldehyde

It was suggested by Gravemade. Glutaraldehyde (2–4%) produces rapid superficial fixation of underlying pulpal tissue. Unlike formocresol, a large percentage of the underlying pulpal tissue remains vital and free from inflammation. A narrow zone of eosinophilic, stained and compressed, fixed tissue is found directly beneath the area of application that bends into vital, normal appearing tissue apically. With time, glutaraldehyde fixed zone is replaced through macrophagic action with dense collagen tissues; thus, the entire root canal tissue is vital.

Glutaraldehyde versus formocresol

Formocresol	Glutaraldehyde
Absorbs and distributes throughout the body within minutes of placement	It does not perfuse the pulp tissue to the apex and shows less systemic distribution immediately after application
Cause changes in vascular activity as it diffuses toward the apex	It is more active chemically and forms cross linkages but its penetration is more limited
Formaldehyde is tissue bond with only small fraction being metabolized	It gets eliminated primarily in urine and exhaled gases; 90% of the drug is gone within 3 days
It is 15–20 times more toxic than glutaraldehyde	No or very little toxic effects

Ferric sulfate pulpotomy

Ferric sulfate has been used due to its hemostatic effect. Due to its effect of controlling hemorrhage, it might minimize the chances of inflammation and internal resorption. In this, remove coronal pulp, achieve hemostasis with wet cotton pellet, and place 15.5% solution of ferric sulfate over the pulp stump for 10–15 seconds. Then rinse the pulp stump, dry with cotton pellet, and cover with zinc oxide eugenol and followed by permanent restoration.

Calcium hydroxide pulpotomy

Harmann (1930) demonstrated the formation of reparative dentin over amputated vital pulps capped with calcium hydroxide. Calcium hydroxide is not a preferred dressing for pulpotomies in primary teeth because of limited clinical success rate. Heilig et al. (1984) suggested that internal resorption results from the "embolization" process by which particles of calcium hydroxide work their way deep into the pulp tissue, forming focal points of inflammation.

Technique: Place calcium hydroxide paste in chamber and press it with sterile cotton pledget. Over it place resin modified glass ionomer restoration.

MTA pulpotomy

MTA is more recent material used for pulpotomies with a high rate of success.

It has excellent biocompatibility, an alkaline pH, radiopacity, high sealing ability, and promotes regeneration of the original tissues when placed in contact with the dental pulp or periradicular tissues.

Technique: Isolate the tooth with a rubber dam and remove coronal pulp. Place the MTA over the pulp stump and close the tooth with temporary cement until the apex of the tooth close.

Bone morphogenic proteins (BMPs)

BMPs stimulate the induction and differentiation of mesenchymal cells with varying degrees of dentinal bridge formation.

Laser pulpotomy

Laser (erbium family, diode, Nd:YAG, CO_2) can be used for coagulation of pulp tissue over the pulp stump before the placement of zinc oxide eugenol or IRM. Clinical studies show either no significant difference between laser pulpotomy or conventional pulpotomy or in favor of laser pulpotomy.

After removal of coronal pulp, hemorrhage is controlled with the laser and capping material like MTA, zinc oxide, eugenol, or IRM is applied.

Electrosurgical pulpotomy

After removal of the coronal pulp, remaining tissues are cauterized with electrocautery unit. Pulp chamber is filled with zinc oxide eugenol or IRM. It is a non-pharmacological method; cautery carbonizes and heat denatures the pulp and bacterial contamination.

Apexification (Root-End Closure)

Apexification is the process of inducing the development of the root and the apical closure in an immature pulpless tooth with an open apex **(Figs. 36.10A and B)**. It is different from apexogenesis in that in latter root development occurs by physiological process.

Apexification is defined as the method to induce a calcific barrier across an open apex of an immature pulpless tooth. Apexification is most commonly performed in traumatized incisors which have lost vitality, carious exposure, and in teeth with variations such as dens invagination with an immature root. Apex in young permanent teeth may present two morphological variations; divergent with flaring apical foramen (blunderbuss apex) and parallel to convergent apex. In both cases, conventional root canal cannot be performed.

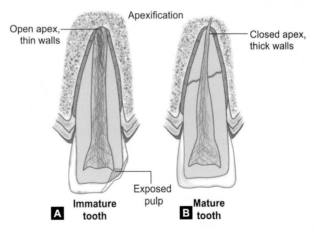

Figs. 36.10A and B (A) An immature tooth has an open apex and thin walls; (B) A mature tooth has a closed apex and thick walls.

Objectives of Apexification

The main objective of apexification is to achieve an apical stop for obturating material. This apical step can be obtained by
❑ Inducing natural calcific barrier at apex or short of apex
❑ Forming an artificial barrier by placing a material at or near the apex
❑ Inducing the natural root lengthening by stimulating Hertwig's epithelial root sheath

Rationale of Apexification

The main aim of apexification is to preserve the Hertwig's root sheath and apical pulp tissue. It is based on the fact that after completion of root formation. Hertwig's epithelial root sheath (HERS) disintegrates and its remnants remain at apical end of root. HERS is considered to be highly resistant to infection, so even if tooth is nonvital, viable HERS may be present at the apex which can help in further root development.

In apexification, it is always suggested to complete biomechanical preparation 2 mm short of the radiographic apex to avoid any trauma to apical pulp or HERS tissue present in that area.

In cases when damage has already occurred to HERS, root formation cannot take place of its own. In such cases, an artificial barrier is created by placing a material in the apical portion.

Hard barrier or calcific barrier which is formed in apexification has shown to possess "*Swiss cheese configuration.*" It may mimic dentin or cementum or bone.

Indications

In young permanent tooth with blunderbuss canal having:
❑ Symptoms of irreversible pulpits
❑ Necrotic pulp
❑ Pulpoperiapical pathology with swelling, tenderness, or sinus

Contraindications

❑ Teeth with vital pulp
❑ Teeth with very short roots and compromised periodontium

Materials Used for Apexification

❑ Calcium hydroxide
❑ Calcium hydroxide in combination with other drugs like
- Camphorated paramonochlorophenol
- Cresanol
- Anesthetic solution
- Normal saline
- Ringer's solution
❑ Zinc oxide paste
❑ Antibiotic paste
❑ Tricalcium phosphate
❑ Collagen calcium phosphate gel
❑ MTA
❑ Osteogenic protein I and II

Technique

Purpose of apexification is to induce root-end closure. It can be achieved in two ways viz; long-term procedure using calcium hydroxide dressing to allow the formation of a hard tissue barrier or as a short-term procedure creating an apical plug of MTA.

Long-Term Apexification Using Calcium Hydroxide

Apexification is traditionally performed using a calcium hydroxide dressing that disinfects the root canal and induces apical closure. High pH and low solubility retains its antimicrobial effect for long time.

Calcium hydroxide assists in debridement of the root canal because it increases the dissolution of necrotic tissue when used alone or in combination with sodium hypochlorite. This procedure requires multiple visits and could take a year or more to achieve complete apical barrier that will allow root canal filling using gutta-percha and sealer. The time needed for apexification depends on the stage of root development and the status of the periapical tissue.

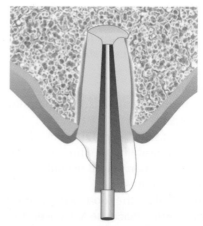

Fig. 36.11 Adjust the final working length 2 mm short of radiographic apex.

Clinical technique of apexification using Calcium Hydroxide is shown in **Flowchart 36.5, Figures 36.12 and 36.13.**

Types of Closure Which Can Occur during Apexification (Figs. 36.14A to D)

❑ Root-end development in normal pattern
❑ Apex closes but is wider at the apical end

❑ Development of calcific bridge just coronal to the apex
❑ Formation of thin barrier at or close to the apex

The time taken for this process for completion may range from 6 weeks to 18 months. The final obturation of the canal should be carried out when there is

❑ Absence of any symptoms
❑ Absence of any fistula or sinus
❑ Absence or decrease in mobility
❑ Evidence of firm stop both clinically as well as radiographically

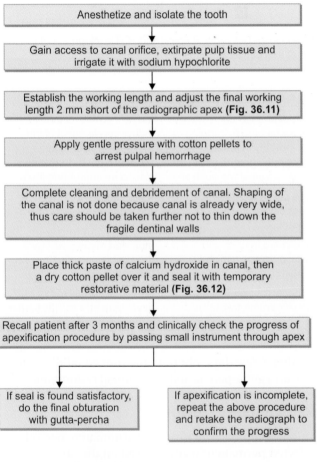

Flowchart 36.5 Showing apexification procedure using calcium hydroxide

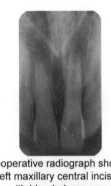

Preoperative radiograph showing left maxillary central incisor with blunderbuss canal

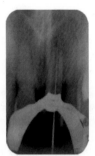

Working length radiograph with distal angulation of file

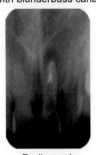

Radiograph showing MTA placement

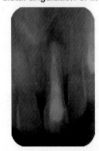

Radiograph showing obturation and composite reinforcement of coronal third of tooth

Figs. 36.13 Management of left maxillary central incisor by calcium hydroxide apexification.

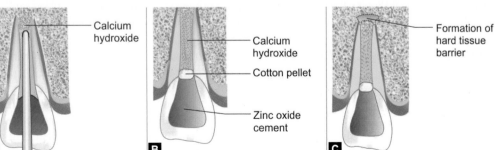

Figs. 36.12A to C (A) Placement of calcium hydroxide in the canal; (B) restoration of the tooth with zinc oxide cement; (C) formation of hard tissue barrier at apex.

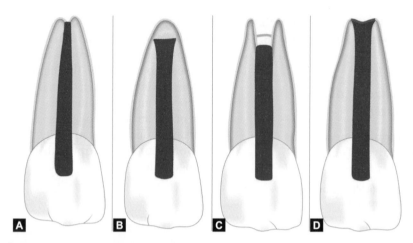

Figs. 36.14A to D (A) Root-end development in normal pattern; (B) Apex closes but wider at apical end; (C) Development of calcific bridge coronal to apex; (D) Formation of thin barrier close to apex.

POINTS TO REMEMBER

- Obturation in such teeth using lateral condensation is not advocated because the lateral pressure during compaction of gutta-percha may fracture the teeth. In such teeth, vertical compaction method of obturation is preferred
- Since the dentinal walls are weak in such cases, restoration should be designed to strengthen the tooth. To strengthen the root, gutta-percha should be removed below the alveolar crest, the dentin is acid etched and then composite resin is placed. Placement of posts in such cases should be avoided as far as possible

Short-Term Apexification with MTA (One-Visit Apexification)

MTA reduces the time needed for completion of the root canal treatment and restoration of the tooth. Apical barrier is achieved in one visit and the entire treatment is completed in a few visits. Care should be taken to perform complete debridement and disinfection of root canal and dentin walls because it is very difficult to remove MTA after it sets; if at all retreatment is required, it is done by apical surgery. Advantages of this technique are that patient compliance is less crucial, dentin does not lose its physical properties, and it allows earlier restoration and thus minimizing the likelihood of root fracture.

MTA Apexification Technique (Figs. 36.15 A to C)

- ❑ Carry the MTA using special carrier and compact 2-mm thick plug of MTA into the apical 4–5 mm using hand condensers or ultrasonic activation
- ❑ Cover MTA with wet cotton pellet and seal the tooth with a temporary restoration

Differences between apexogenesis and apexification

It is defined as the treatment of a vital pulp by capping or pulpotomy in order to permit continued growth of the root and closure of the open apex	It is defined as a method to induce development of the root apex of an immature pulpless tooth by formation of osteocementum/bone-like tissue
It is physiological process of root development in vital tooth	It is the method of inducing the regenerative potential in a nonvital tooth
Indicated in teeth with vital pulp and minimal inflammation	Indicated in cases where irreversible pulpal damage is present
Normal root-end development takes place	Instead of normal root development, a calcific barrier is formed at the apex

- ❑ After a few days, obturate the root canal filling using warm gutta-percha and give coronal restoration.

▌ Revascularization

This new approach for treatment of immature necrotic and infected permanent teeth is based on the observation of spontaneous revascularization that occasionally occurs in the immature teeth after traumatic injury. With revascularization, root lengthening and apical closure with thickening of the canal walls is expected, thus improving the long term of the young tooth. The nature of the hard tissue formed is not clear and can be cementum-like instead of dentin. The first step of the treatment is disinfection of the root canal space with sodium hypochlorite and using intracanal medicament like triple antibiotic paste. This combination

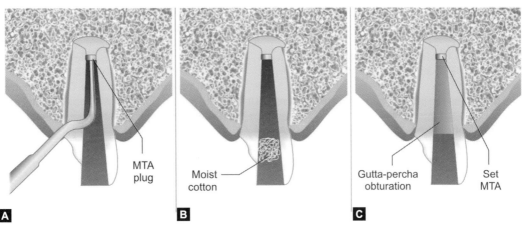

Fig. 36.15 (A) Placing MTA at apex of tooth, creating a 2 mm thickness of the plug; (B) Seal the cavity with moist cotton because MTA needs moisture for setting; (C) After confirming final set of MTA, obturate the canal using gutta-percha.

contains metronidazole, ciprofloxacin, and minocyclin which is effective in disinfection of immature infected root canals and well tolerated by vital pulp tissue. After disinfection, bleeding is induced into the canal space through the apical foramen to create a scaffold on which a new tissue will grow and repopulate the canal space. Over it, MTA is placed and final restoration is given.

Revascularization has been covered in detail in this in chapter 37.

Coronal Restoration

- ❑ Restoration of the immature tooth following obturation with gutta-percha should be designed to strengthen the tooth as much as possible
- ❑ Placement of posts within the canal should be avoided unless no other means of restoration is possible
- ❑ Preparation of a post space has been shown to significantly weaken the remaining tooth structure, whereas acid etching and placement of a composite resin strengthen the tooth, making it more resistant to fracture
- ❑ In the apexified tooth, the gutta-percha should be removed below the alveolar crest, the dentin acid etched, and bonded composite resin placed to strengthen the root

Conclusion

It has been accepted that maintaining and regenerating pulp vitality is important for long-term tooth viability. Complete pulp regeneration and revascularization can be achieved after successful vital pulp therapy if vital pulp is in the canal.

At the present time, stem cell-based tissue engineering approaches provide the most promising solution. Prognosis of vital pulp procedures has shown different results due to methodological variations between the different studies. Status of the pulp tissue and type of coronal restoration has a significant influence on the results. Among the different materials used, MTA appears to be more effective than calcium hydroxide for maintaining long-term pulp vitality in pulp capping and pulpotomy procedures. Further research and clinical trials are also needed to develop case selection guideline, treatment approaches, and materials needed to maximize clinical success.

Questions

1. What are the indications and contraindications of pulpotomy?
2. What is apexification? Explain in detail about the technique of apexification.
3. Describe apexogenesis and apexification for immature maxillary central incisors.
4. Write short notes on
   - Indirect pulp capping
   - Direct pulp capping
   - MTA.

Bibliography

1. Accorinte ML, Holland R, Reis A, et al. Evaluation of mineral trioxide aggregate and calcium hydroxide cement as pulp-capping agents in human teeth. J Endod. 2008;34:1–6.
2. Aguilar P, Linsuwanont P. Vital pulp therapy in vital permanent teeth with cariously exposed pulp: a systematic review. J Endod. 2011;37:581–7.

3. Bakland LF. Endodontic considerations in dental trauma. In: Ingle JF, Bakland IF, editors. Endodontics. 5th ed. London: BC Decker; 2002. pp. 829–31.

4. Casamassimo P, Fields H, McTigue D, Nowak A. Pediatric dentistry infancy through adolescence. 5th ed. Elsevier; 2013.

5. Fuks AB. Pulp therapy for the primary and young permanent dentitions. Dent Clin North Am. 2000;44:571–96.

6. Grossman LI. Endodontic practice. 11th ed. Philadelphia, PA: Lea and Febiger; 1998.

7. Hargreaves KM, Cohen S, Berman LH. Cohen's pathways of the pulp. 10th ed. St. Louis, MO: Mosby Year Book; 2011.

8. Pitt Ford TR. Apexification and apexogenesis. In: Walton RE, Torabinejad M, editors. Principles and practical of endodontics. 3rd ed. Philadelphia, PA: WB Sanders; 2002. pp. 373–84.

9. Rafter M. Apexification: a review. Dent Tramatol. 2005;21:1–8.

10. Torabinejad M, Hong CU, McDonald F, Pitt Ford TR. Physical and chemical properties of a new root-end filling material. J Endod. 1995;21:349–53.

Regenerative endodontics is one of the most thrilling developments in endodontics which uses the concept of tissue engineering to restore the root canals to a healthy state, allowing for continued development of the root and surrounding tissue. This development in the regeneration of a functional pulp–dentin complex gave a hope to retain the natural dentition.

Regenerative endodontics employs the role of tissue engineering which employs the use of stem cells. Stem cell is a special kind of cell that has a unique capacity to renew itself and give rise to specialized cell types. Although most cells of the body, such as heart cells or skin cells, are committed to perform a specific function, a stem cell is uncommitted and remains uncommitted, until it receives a signal to develop into a specialized cell.

▌ Definition of Tissue Engineering

The first definition of tissue engineering given by Langer and Vacanti is that "as an *interdisciplinary field that applies the principles of engineering and life sciences toward the development of biological substitutes that restore, maintain, or improve tissue function or a whole organ.*"

MacArthur and Oreffo defined tissue engineering as "*understanding the principles of tissue growth and applying this to produce functional replacement tissue for clinical use.*"

▌ Strategies of Stem Cell Technology

Three strategies to stem cell technology (**Figs. 37.1A to C**)
1. Conductive
2. Inductive
3. Cell-base transplantation

Conductive

Conductive approach utilizes biomaterials in a passive manner to facilitate the growth or regenerative capacity of existing tissue. An example of this is guided tissue regeneration in which the appropriate use of barrier membranes promotes predictable bone repair and new attachment with new formation of cementum and periodontal ligament fibers.

Inductive

Induction approach involves activating the cells in close proximity to the defect site with specific biological signals like bone morphogenic proteins (BMPs). Urist first

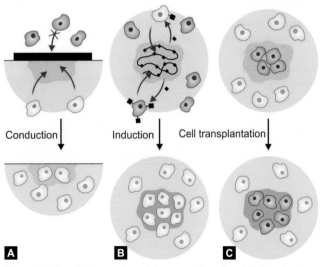

Figs. 37.1A to C Strategies of tissue engineering: (A) Conduction; (B) Induction; (C) Cell transplantation.

showed that new bone could be formed at nonmineralizing or ectopic sites after implantation of powdered bone containing BMPs, which turned out to be the key elements for inducing bone formation. Limitation of this technique is that the inductive factor for a particular tissue may not be known.

Cell-Base Transplantation

This approach involves direct transplantation of cells grown in the laboratory.

▌ Triad of Tissue Engineering (Fig. 37.2)

Tissue engineering employs the use of three materials: (1) Stem cells/Progenitor cells, (2) Morphogens/Signaling molecules/Growth factors and (3) Scaffold/Matrix

Stem Cells/Progenitor Cells

Stem cells are undifferentiated cells that divide and respond to specialized cell on response to morphogens. Progenitor cells retain the differentiation potential and high proliferation capability but have lost the self-replication property unlike stem cells.

Unique Characteristics of Stem Cells

- ❑ They exist as undifferentiated cells and maintain this phenotype by the environment and/or the adjacent cell populations until they are exposed to and respond to the appropriate signals
- ❑ Ability to self-replicate for prolonged periods
- ❑ Maintain their multiple differentiation potential throughout the life of the organism

Categories of Stem Cells According to their Source

- ❑ *Autologous cells:* These are obtained from the same individual to whom they will be reimplanted. Advantage

of autologous stem cells is that they have minimum problems with rejection and pathogen transmission; however, the disadvantage is limited availability

- ❑ *Allogeneic cells:* These are obtained from the body of a donor of the same species
- ❑ *Xenogeneic cells:* These are those isolated from individuals of another species. In particular, animal cells have been used quite extensively in experiments aimed at the construction of cardiovascular implants
- ❑ *Syngeneic or isogenic cells:* These are isolated from genetically identical organisms, such as twins, clones, or highly inbred research animal models
  - Primary cells are from an organism
  - Secondary cells are from a cell bank

Categories of stem cells according to their potency:

Stem cell type	Differentiation	Source
Totipotent	Can differentiate into a new organism	Cells from early embryos (1–3 days)
Pluripotent	Can differentiate into nearly all cells but not entire organism	Blastocyst (5–14 days)
Multipotent	In limited range of cells	Fetal tissue, cord blood dental pulp stem cells

Stem Cell Markers

Every cell in body is coated with specialized proteins on their surface called receptors that have capability of selectively binding to other "signaling" molecules. The stem cell markers are similar to these cell surface receptors. Each cell type, for example, a liver cell, has a certain combination of receptors on their surface that makes them distinguishable from other kinds of cells. Researchers use the signaling molecules that selectively adhere to the receptors on the surface of the cell as a tool that allows them to identify stem cells. The signaling molecules have the ability to fluoresce or emit light energy when activated by an energy source such as an ultraviolet light or laser beam **(Fig. 37.3)**. Thus, stem cell markers help in identification and isolation of stem cells.

Isolation of Stem Cells

Stem cells can be identified and isolated from mixed cell population by the following four techniques:

1. By staining the cells with specific antibody markers and using a flow cytometer. This process is called fluorescent antibody cell sorting (FACS)
2. Physiological and histological criteria. This includes phenotype, chemotaxis, proliferation, differentiation and mineralizing activity
3. Immunomagnetic bead selection
4. Immunohistochemical staining

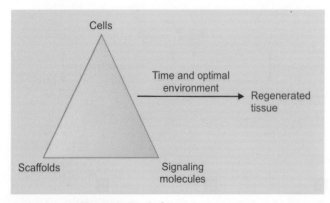

Fig. 37.2 Triad of tissue engineering.

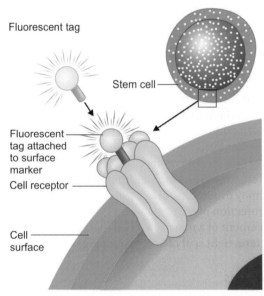

Fig. 37.3 Identification of cell surface markers using fluorescent tags.

Tooth bud tissues containing stem cells are dissociated enzymatically and mechanically and filtered to remove even small clumps of cells, generating single cell suspensions. The tissue is then plated in vitro and cultured to eliminate differentiated cell types. The resultant culture contains enriched dental stem cell population.

Morphogens/Signaling Molecules/ Growth Factors

These trigger the differentiation of selected mesenchymal stem cells into odontoblast-like cells.

Functions
- ❏ To stimulate division of neighboring cells and those infiltrating the defect [example: growth factors—platelet-derived growth factor (*PDGF*)]
- ❏ To stimulate the differentiation of certain cells along a specified pathway (example: differentiation factors—*BMP*)
- ❏ To stimulate angiogenesis
- ❏ To serve as chemoattractants for specific cell types

Different types of morphogens are
- BMPs
- Fibroblast growth factors (FGFs)
- Hedgehog proteins (Hhs)
- Tumor necrotic factor (TNF)
- Transforming growth factor (TGF)
- Insulin-like growth factor (IGF)
- Colony stimulating factor (CSF)
- Epidermal growth factor (EGF)
- Interleukins (IL)
- PDGF
- Nerve growth factor (NGF)

} Embryonic tooth development

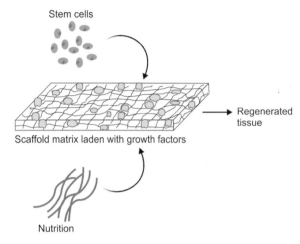

Fig. 37.4 Schematic representation of scaffold matrix.

Scaffold/Matrix

Scaffold provides a physicochemical and biological three-dimensional microenvironment for cell growth and differentiation, promoting cell adhesion and migration (**Fig. 37.4**). Scaffold is used to guide, organize, provide physical and chemical signals and help in growth and differentiation of cells.

Tissues are composed of cells, insoluble extracellular matrix (ECM) and soluble molecules serving as regulators of cell functions. ECM consists of collagen, glycoprotein and proteoglycan and it is important for growth and function of different cells involved. Plasma-rich protein (PRP) is autologous, easy-to-prepare scaffold rich in growth factors, degrades and form three-dimensional fibrin network.

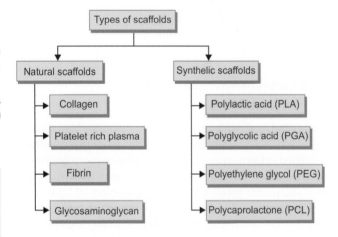

Types of scaffolds

Natural scaffolds
- Collagen
- Platelet rich plasma
- Fibrin
- Glycosaminoglycan

Synthelic scaffolds
- Polylactic acid (PLA)
- Polyglycolic acid (PGA)
- Polyethylene glycol (PEG)
- Polycaprolactone (PCL)

▮ Regenerative Endodontics Procedures

Definition

Regenerative endodontics is defined as biologically based procedures designed to physiologically replace damaged tooth structures, including dentin and root structures, as

Flowchart 37.1 Schematic representation showing goals of regenerative endodontics.

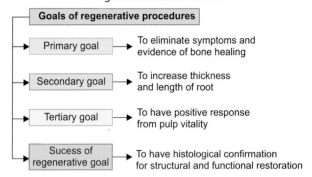

well as the pulp–dentin complex. According to the American Association of Endodontists' Clinical Considerations for a Regenerative Procedure, the primary goal of the regenerative procedure is elimination of clinical symptoms and resolution of apical periodontitis and secondary goal is thickening of canal walls and continued root maturation **(Flowchart 37.1)**. Thus, primary goal is same as that of endodontic treatment but difference between the two is that after disinfecting the canals in endodontic treatment, roots are filled with biocompatible materials and in regenerative procedure, roots are filled with the host's own vital tissue.

Different techniques of tissue engineering applied for regenerative endodontics are
- ❑ Root canal revascularization via blood clotting
- ❑ Postnatal stem cell therapy
- ❑ Pulp implantation
- ❑ Scaffold implantation
- ❑ Injectable scaffold delivery
- ❑ Three-dimensional cell printing
- ❑ Gene delivery

Root Canal Revascularization via Blood Clotting

In non-vital teeth with immature root, materials like calcium hydroxide, MTA, biodentine and other bioactive materials were used to form an apical barrier against which obturation could be done. But each material comes with its own advantages and disadvantages. Problems with calcium hydroxide are like long treatment time occupying canal space physically it so no room for vital tissue to proliferate; high pH may cause necrosis of tissue and barrier formation is often porous and non-continuous. MTA is placed in the apical-third of the immature root to create a stop for the filling material but it does not allow new tissue to grow into the root canal thus the root remains thin and weak. Hence, apexification does not lead to continued root formation or thickening of the root canal wall, leading to the risk of an undesirable side effect

of a short and weakened root that is susceptible to fracture. An alternative treatment regime is preferred to overcome these problems, that is, pulp revascularization.

Definition

Revascularization is the procedure to re-establish vitality in a non-vital tooth to allow repair and regeneration of tissue. It allows further development of root and dentin structure with a better long-term prognosis.

In teeth with open apices and necrotic pulp, some vital pulp tissue and Hertwig's epithelial root sheath remains which may proliferate once the canal is disinfected.
- ❑ Disinfection of root canal
- ❑ Placement of a matrix in canal for tissue growth
- ❑ Bacteria tight seal of access opening

Indications

- ❑ The teeth that present with symptoms of acute or chronic apical periodontitis (i.e., pain, diffuse facial and/or mucosal swelling, tenderness to percussion, or intraoral sinuses)
- ❑ Radiographically, the tooth had an immature apex, either blunderbuss or in the form of a wide canal with parallel walls and an open apex. On electric pulp test, the affected tooth is non-vital
- ❑ Teeth with apical opening more than 1 mm show greater success with revascularization procedures by encouraging ingrowth of tissue into root canal space

Technique (Fig. 37.5)

First appointment
- ❑ After anesthetizing, isolate the tooth with rubber dam
- ❑ Prepare access cavity and gently flush the canal 5.25% with sodium hypochlorite solution
- ❑ Dry the canal using sterile paper points
- ❑ Place a mixture of ciprofloxacin 200 mg, metronidazole 400 mg and minocycline 100 mg in root canal 2 mm from the working length and leave for 7 days
- ❑ Seal the tooth with sterile sponge and temporary filling
- ❑ Recall after 3–4 weeks

Second appointment
- ❑ Evaluate the patient for resolution of signs and symptoms of infection like pain, swelling, sinus, etc.
- ❑ Repeat antimicrobial treatment if required
- ❑ Isolate the tooth and copiously irrigate it with 5.25% NaOCl and gently place the small hand file to remove the antimicrobial dressing
- ❑ Dry the canal using sterile paper points
- ❑ Introduce a size no. 40 K-file into the root canal 2 mm beyond the working length to induce some bleeding into the root canal

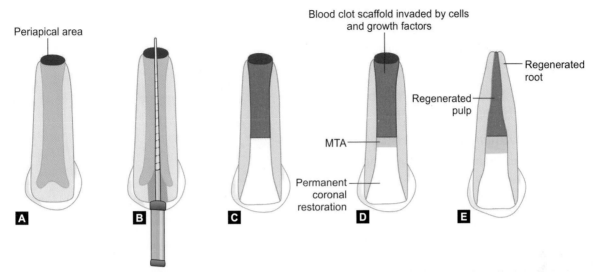

Figs. 37.5A to E Line diagram showing pulp revascularization procedure: (A) Tooth showing immature apex with wide canal and open apex; (B) Endodontic file in the canal, 2 mm beyond the established working length to induce bleeding; (C) Allow the blood clot to form 3 mm below CEJ; (D) Place MTA over clot; (E) Regenerated root showing thickening of canal walls and closure of apex.

❑ Allow the bleeding to reach a level 3 mm below the cementoenamel junction (CEJ) and leave the tooth for 15 min so that a blood clot is formed. Blood clot acts as a scaffold and source of growth factors to facilitate regeneration and repair of the tissue into the canal

❑ Place mineral trioxide aggregate over the clot carefully up to the level of CEJ followed by a wet cotton pellet and restore it with a temporary dressing material

❑ After 1 week, restore the tooth with a composite restoration and recall the patient for clinical and radiographical evaluation

❑ Patients are recalled after a minimum of 1 year. The criteria of success are
  • Lack of symptoms
  • Radiographic evidence of increased root length
  • Radiographic evidence of increased root canal thickness

Mechanism of Revascularization

❑ Few cells remain at the apical end of the root canal. These cells might proliferate into the newly formed matrix and differentiate into odontoblasts under the organizing influence of cells of Hertwig's epithelial root sheath, which are quite resistant to destruction, even in the presence of inflammation. The newly formed odontoblasts can lay down atubular dentin at the apical end, causing apexogenesis as well as on lateral aspects of dentinal walls of the root canal, reinforcing and strengthening the root

❑ Continued root development due to multipotent dental pulp stem cells (DPSCs), which are present in permanent

teeth and might be present in abundance in immature teeth. These cells from the apical end might be seeded onto the existing dentinal walls and might differentiate into odontoblasts and deposit tertiary or atubular dentin

❑ Stem cells in the periodontal ligament can proliferate, grow into the apical end and within the root canal and deposit hard tissue both at the apical end and on the lateral root walls

❑ Root development could be attributed to stem cells from the apical papilla or the bone marrow. Instrumentation beyond the confines of the root canal to induce bleeding can also transplant mesenchymal cells from the bone into the canal lumen. These cells have an excellent proliferative capacity. Transplantation studies have shown that human stem cells from bone marrow can form bone or dentin in vivo

❑ Blood clot itself being a rich source of growth factors could play important role in regeneration. These include PDGF, vascular factor and tissue growth factor and could stimulate differentiation, growth and maturation of fibroblasts, odontoblasts, cementoblasts, etc. from the immature undifferentiated mesenchymal cells in the newly formed tissue matrix.

Advantages of Revascularization Procedure

❑ Short treatment time, after control of infection, it can be completed in single visit

❑ Approach is simple and can be completed without using expensive biotechnology

❑ Continued root development and strengthening of root as a result of reinforcement of lateral dentinal walls by deposition of hard tissue

□ Regeneration of tissue in root canal systems by a patient's own blood cells avoids the possibility of immune rejection and pathogen transmission from replacing the pulp with a tissue engineered construct

□ Cost-effective

□ Obturation of canal not required so avoids root fracture by forces of lateral compaction technique

Limitations of Revascularization Procedure

□ Composition of cells found in fibrin clot is unpredictable resulting in variations in treatment outcome

□ Crown discoloration, development of resistant bacterial strains and allergic reactions to intracanal medications

□ Entire canal may get calcified compromising esthetics and not allowing future endodontic treatment if required

□ Long-term clinical results not available

□ Post and core not possible because vital tissues in apical two third of canal can't be compromised for post placement

Postnatal Stem Cell Therapy

There are two stem cells categories according to their origin:

□ Embryonic stem cells (pluripotent): These can be isolated from normal blastocyst and can give rise to all derivatives of three layers. These are highly plastic and can give rise to any kind of specialized cell type and yet maintain their undifferentiated state pluripotent cells.

□ Postnatal cells: These can be collected directly from the bone marrow or umbilical cord blood. These are less plastic and have limited life cycle and thus have limited potential of differentiation than embryonic stem cells.

Stem cells of dental origin (Fig. 37.6)
• Postnatal dental pulp stem cells (DPSCs)
• Stem cells obtained from deciduous teeth (SHED)
• Periodontal ligament stem cells (PDLSCs)
• Dental follicle progenitor stem cells (DFPCs)
• Stem cells from the apical papilla (SCAP)

Dental Pulp Stem Cells (DPSCs)

Dental pulp contains the dentinogenic progenitors, i.e., DPSCs that are responsible for dentin repair. These can regenerate a dentin–pulp-like complex which is composed of mineralized matrix with tubules lined with odontoblasts and fibrous tissue containing blood vessels in an arrangement similar to the dentin–pulp complex is found in normal human teeth. Stem Cells from Human Exfoliated Deciduous Teeth (SHED) These are the cells present in living pulp remnants of exfoliated deciduous tooth consisting of connective tissue, blood vessels and odontoblasts. These can differentiate into odontoblast-like cells that form dentin-like structures.

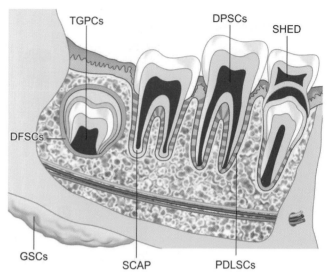

Fig. 37.6 Line diagram showing different types of stem cells of dental origin.

Periodontal Ligament Stem Cells (PDLSC)

These are present in enzymatically digested PDL (Periodontal ligament) and can form cementum/PDL-like structure as thin layer of cementum that interfaced with dense collagen fibers, similar to Sharpey's fibers. Their differentiation is believed to be due to Hertwig's epithelial root sheath cells.

Dental Follicle Precursor Cells (DFPCs)

These are derived from developing tissue and have shown greater plasticity than other dental stem cells. They can differentiate into odontoblasts in vitro.

Stem Cells from Apical Papilla (SCAP)

These are found in apical papilla found at apices of developing teeth at the junction of apical papilla and dental pulp. Apical papilla is important for development of root. It is the soft tissue present at the apices of developing permanent teeth, lying apical to epithelial diaphragm. An apical cell rich zone is present between apical papilla and pulp. These cells can undergo odontoblastic, osteogenic, or neurogenic differentiation.

In postnatal stem cell therapy, cells are injected in disinfected root canal (**Fig. 37.7**). This approach is quick, easy to deliver and relatively painless.

Pulp Implantation

Here replacement pulp tissue is transplanted in disinfected root canal. This pulp tissue is got from stem cells which are grown in a laboratory. This pulp tissue is grown in sheets in vitro on biodegradable polymer nanofibers. These sheets are rolled together to form a 3-D pulp tissue which can be implanted into root canal system (**Fig. 37.8**). But this

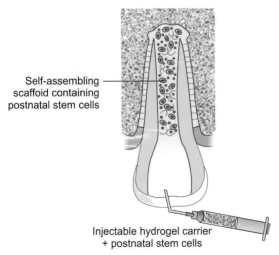

Self-assembling
scaffoid containing
postnatal stem cells

Injectable hydrogel carrier
+ postnatal stem cells

Fig. 37.7 Postnatal stem cell therapy.

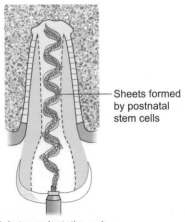

Sheets formed
by postnatal
stem cells

Pulp transplantation using
stem cell grown in sheets

Fig. 37.8 Pulp implantation using stem cells grown in sheets.

procedure does not ensure that cells properly adhere to the root canal walls. Moreover, sheets of cells lack vascularity so only apical part of root canal receives these cellular constructs.

Scaffold Implantation

During dental pulp regeneration, an ideal scaffold should also ensure good neurovascular supply to new pulp tissue, for example, DPSCs are seeded on three-dimensional polyglycolic acid matrix and grown in vitro and then surgically implanted.

Three-Dimensional Cell Printing

This technique is used to precisely position the cells and thus constructed tissue mimics the natural dental pulp tissue structure. Here an inkjet device is used to disperse the layers of cells suspended in a hydrogel to recreate dental pulp tissue. But for this, precise 3-D models for individual pulp cavity and an effective delivery system are required.

Injectable Scaffold

Here polymerizable hydrogels alone or containing cell suspensions are delivered by injections. This may promote regeneration by providing substitute for Extracellular matrix (ECM) but has low cell survival and has limited control over tissue formation.

Gene Therapy

It is the means of delivering genes for growth factors, morphogens and ECM molecules to somatic cells of individual resulting in the therapeutic effect. Gene can induce a natural biological process by expressing a molecule involved in regenerative response for the target tissue.

▌ Conclusion

Due to emergence of regenerative endodontic procedures, clinician should re-evaluate the current clinical protocols while treatment planning of some clinical cases is done. This is especially important when dealing with immature teeth which carry potent stem cells which can enable the tissue to regenerate and repair better than mature tissues.

▌ Questions

1. Define tissue engineering. What are strategies of stem cell technology?
2. What are bioactive molecules in restorative dentistry?
3. Write short notes on:
   - Regenerative endodontics
   - Pulp revascularization.

▌ Bibliography

1. Baum BJ, Mooney DJ. The impact of tissue engineering on dentistry. J Am Dent Assoc 2000;131:309–18.
2. Freitas Jr RA. Nanodentistry. J Am Dent Assoc 2000; 131:1559–65.
3. Hochman R. Neurotransmitter modulator (TENS) for control of dental operative pain. J Am Dent Assoc 1988;116:208–12.
4. West JL, Halas NJ. Applications of nanotechnology to biotechnology. Curr Opinbiotechnol 2000;11:215–17.

CHAPTER
38

Magnification

Chapter Outline

- Definitions
- Loupes
- Surgical Operating Microscope
- Endoscope
- Orascope

The concept of magnifications was introduced in medicine during the late 19th century. Carl Nylen is father of microsurgery, he first used a binocular microscope for ear surgery in 1921. Apotheker and Jako first introduced the microscope in dentistry in 1978. Nowadays, many advancements have been done to improve the visualization and magnification. Introduction of loupes, microscopes, endoscopes, etc. enables the clinician to magnify an object beyond that perceived by a human eye.

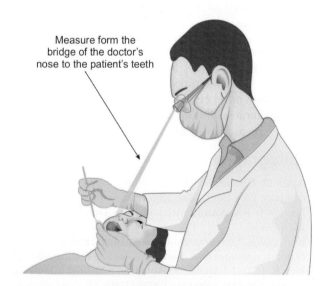

Measure form the bridge of the doctor's nose to the patient's teeth

Fig. 38.1 Working distance is measured from bridge of operator's nose to teeth of patient.

Definitions

Magnification: It is defined as making an object bigger in size.

Differentiation: It is defined as making something distinct.

Field of view: The area which is visible through optical magnification.

Working distance: The distance measured from the clinician's eye to the treatment field **(Fig. 38.1)**.

Depth of field: It refers to the ability of the lens system to focus on the objects which are both near and far without changing the loupe position.

Loupes

These are most commonly used for magnification. Basically, loupes consist of two monocular microscopes, with side-by-side convergent lenses which are angled to focus on an object to form magnified images. These can provide magnifications ranging from ×1.5 to ×10. Though loupes are most commonly used but main disadvantage is that eyes converge to view an image resulting in eye strain, fatigue and even vision changes. Three types of loupes are commonly used in dental practice.

Simple Loupes (Fig. 38.2)

Simple loupes consist of a pair of single, positive, side-by-side meniscus lenses. Each lens has two refracting surfaces, with

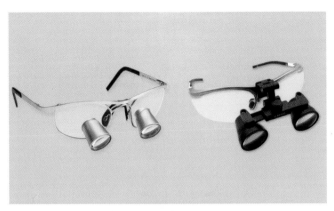

Fig. 38.2 Simple loupes.

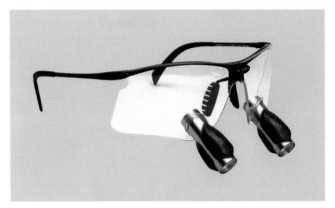

Fig. 38.4 Prism loupes.

Surgical Operating Microscope

Microscope consists of lenses which allow stereoscopic vision with magnification of ×4–40 with an excellent illumination of the working area. Since light beam falls parallel into the retina of the clinician, so convergence is not required causing minimum tiring of the muscles.

Classification of Dental Operating Microscope

Based on use:
- Surgical microscope
- Examination microscope

Based on installation (Figs. 38.6 A to C)
- Floor mounted
- Ceiling mounted
- Wall mounted

Based on magnification
- Lower magnification (2.5–8×)
- Midrange magnification (8–14×)
- Higher range magnification (14–30×).

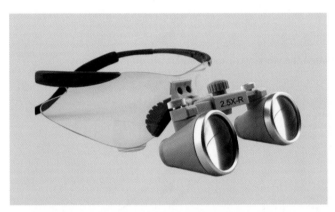

Fig. 38.3 Compound loupes.

one occurring as light enters the lens and the other when it leaves. These are cost-effective but have poor resolution and are subjected to spherical and chromatic aberrations causing image distortion.

Compound Loupes or Telescopic Loupes (Fig. 38.3)

These are also called through the lens (TTL) which consist of multiple lenses with intervening air spaces which allow adjustment of magnification, working distance and depth of field without increase in size or weight.

Prism Loupes (Fig. 38.4)

These are most advanced loupes available which lengthen the light path through a series of mirror reflections within by virtually folding the light so that the barrel of the loupe can be shortened. They produce better magnification, larger fields of view, wider depths of field and longer working distance. If compared, longer working distance produces less strain on eye muscles than close-up viewing **(Fig. 38.5)**.

Parts of an Operating Microscope

Microscope consists of:
- Supporting structure
- Body of the microscope
- Source of light.

Supporting Structure

Supporting structure is to keep the microscope stable and easy to handle. It can be mounted on the floor, ceiling, or wall. Stability of setup can be increased by decreasing the distance between the fixation point and body of microscope.

Body of the Microscope (Fig. 38.7)

It consists of lenses and prisms which produce magnification and stereopsis. The body is made of eyepieces, binoculars, magnification changer factor and the objective lens.

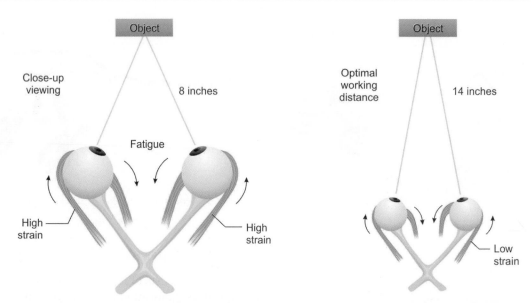

Fig. 38.5 Schematic representation showing relation between the working distance and strain on eye muscles.

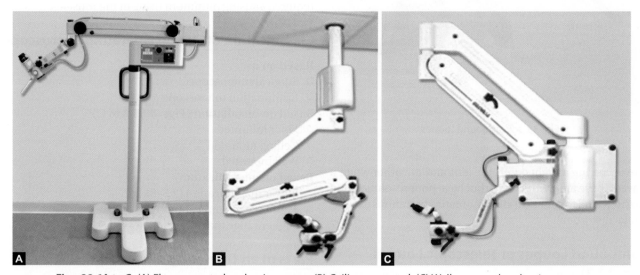

Figs. 38.6A to C (A) Floor-mounted endomicroscope; (B) Ceiling mounted; (C) Wall-mounted endomicroscope.

Eyepieces are usually available in powers of 10, 12.5, 16 and 20×. *Binoculars* hold the eyepieces and are available in different focal lengths. Longer is the focal length of binocular, better is the magnification with smaller field of vision.

Magnification changers are available as three or five step manual changers providing the option of four different magnification levels.

Objective lens determines the working distance between the microscope and the surgical field. The range of focal length is from 100 to 400 mm. Most of the endodontists use a 200-mm lens which focuses at about 8 inches.

All lenses of microscope, like objective lens, eyepiece lenses, magnification lenses, etc., have many layers of an antireflective coating on both surfaces, which absorb only a minimum amount of light so don't decrease the illumination of the operative field.

How Does SOM Work?

It is discussed under four headings:
1. Magnification
2. Illumination
3. Documentation
4. Accessories.

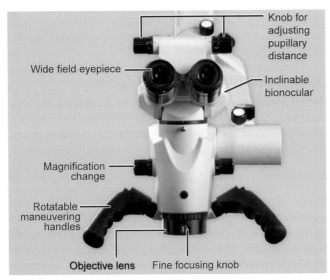

Fig. 38.7 Body of the microscope.

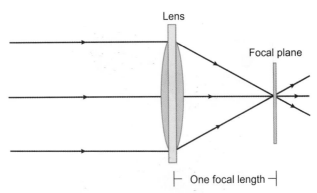

Fig. 38.8 Focal length is the between principal focus and the optical center of lens.

Magnification

Magnification is determined by:
- Power of eyepiece
- Focal length of binoculars
- Focal length of objective lens
- Magnification change factor.

Power of eyepiece: Eyepiece has diopter settings ranging from −5 to +5. These are used to adjust for accommodation, which is ability to focus the lens of eyes.

Increase in power of eyepiece increases the magnification but decreases the field of view.

Focal length of binoculars: Binoculars hold the eyepieces. The interpupillary distance is set by adjusting the distance between binocular tubes.

Increase in focal length increases the magnification but decreases the field of view.

Focal length of objective lens (Fig. 38.8): Focal length of objective lens determines the operating distance between the lens and surgical field. If objective lens is removed, the microscope focuses at infinity and performs as pair of field binoculars.

For SOM, a variety of objective lenses is available with focal length ranging from 100 to 400 mm.

Magnification changers: These are available as three- or fivestep manual changers or power zoom-changers, located within the head of microscope.

Illumination

Commonly used light source is 100 W Xenon–halogen bulb. The intensity of light can be controlled by rheostat. This light is reflected through condensing lens to a series of prisms and then through objective lens to surgical field area. On reaching surgical field, it is again reflected back through objective lens through magnification changer lenses, through binoculars and then exits to eyes as two separate beams of light. This results in stereoscope effect which allows the clinician to see depth of the field.

Illumination with operating microscope is coaxial with line of sight. This means that light is focused between the eyepieces such that a dentist can look at surgical site without seeing the shadow.

Documentation

The ability to produce quality video slides is directly related to magnification and illumination system. The adapter attaches video camera to beam splitter. It also provides the necessary focal length so that camera records an image with same magnification and field of view as seen by operator.

Accessories

- Bicycle style handles attached at bottom of head to facilitate movement during surgery
- Eyepiece with reticle field for alignment during videotaping and photography
- Observation ports for helping in teaching situations
- LCD screen so as to provide view to patient as well as to assistant.

Positioning of Operating Microscope

It consists of
- **Operator positioning:** Most preferable position is 11 or 12'o clock position with hips perpendicular to the floor and knees perpendicular to the hips (**Fig. 38.9**)
- **Tentative patient positioning:** Patient is positioned in Trendelenburg position and chair is raised until patient is in focus
- **Focusing of operating microscope:** Move the microscope up and down till working area comes into the focus

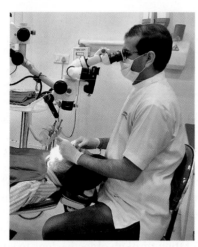

Fig. 38.9 Photograph showing position of operator while using endomicroscope.

- **Adjustment of interpupillary distance (IPD):** Interpupillary distance is the key adjustment for using any magnification system. To understand your IPD, focus both the binocular eyepieces to initially see two images or circles and adjust it to the point, where they merge and become one circle. This point is identified as the IPD and used as a permanent reference for the use of magnifications
- **Final positioning of the patient:** Adjust the patient for optimal focusing. For maxillary teeth, position should be horizontal and for mandibular teeth, it should be Trendelenburg
- **Fine focus adjustment:** Adjust the focus for sharp magnification. Working area in focus to operator should be in same focus to the assistant for video camera.

Fundamental Prerequisites for Optimal Use of Microscope

Vision

With microscope, it is almost impossible to do endodontic treatment using direct vision. So, front surface good quality mirror which is silvered on the surface of glass should be used for having best quality undistorted reflected image.

Lightening

Adequate lightening is also mandatory for using a microscope. Inbuilt lightening system is usually present in microscope, but if necessary an auxiliary light can also be used. This can be placed perpendicular to long axis of the tooth at the level of pulp chamber.

Patient Compliance

Patient compliance is must for use of microscope. Even a slight movement of patient's head can affect field of vision

adversely. For optimal view through microscope, patient needs to have extended neck. This can be achieved by providing a U-shaped inflatable pillow.

Cooperation from Dental Assistance

Dental assistant can also be helpful in increasing the efficiency of clinician. Use of secondary eyepiece from microscope provides better view of root canals. A dental assistant should be given adequate training for use of microscope.

Rubber Dam Placement

Rubber dam placement is necessary because direct viewing with microscope is difficult. So if mirror is used without using rubber dam, due to exhalation of patient, mirror would fog immediately. This would affect visualization. For absorbing bright reflected light and to accentuate tooth structure, use of blue or green rubber dam sheet is recommended.

Mouth Mirror Placement

Mouth mirror should be placed slightly away from the tooth. If it is placed close to tooth, it will make use of endodontic instruments difficult.

Indirect View and Patient Head Position

Mirror should be placed at 45° to the microscope. For indirect viewing, patient's head should be positioned such that it form 90° angle between binocular and the maxillary arch.

Instruments

Clinician should possess microinstruments for locating canals, use of files called micro-openers, micromirrors and other microinstruments is recommended (**Fig. 38.10**).

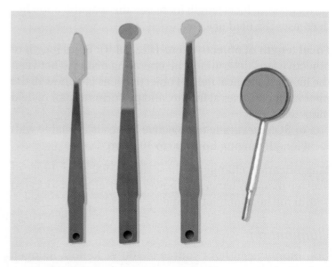

Fig. 38.10 Microinstruments used with endomicroscope.

Uses of SOM

SOM is useful in all aspects of endodontic therapy from diagnosis to evaluation of final obturation.

☐ **Diagnosis (Figs. 38.11A to C)**
- It allows calcified, irregularity positioned, or accessory canals to be found with ease and thereby increasing the success rate and decreasing stress
- SOM helps to detect microfractures which are not visible with naked eye
- Missing canals (most common MB2 of maxillary molar) can be successfully located by use of endomicroscope.

☐ **Removal of foreign materials** like cast post and filling material can be made easy due to better vision

☐ **Endodontic retreatment** involving the removal of screw posts, separated instruments, silver points can be guided by use of endomicroscope

☐ **Perforation repair** can be precisely done by use of SOM by accurate placement of the repair material and by précised manipulation of the tissue

☐ **Evaluation of the canal preparation** can be accurately done by use of endomicroscope

☐ SOM is also useful in **evaluation of the final obturation of root canals.** With the help of SOM, one can assess the irregularly shaped and poorly obturated canals and quality of apical seal

☐ **Intracanal isthmus communication** and canal anatomy can be well assessed by use of endomicroscope **(Figs. 38.12A and B).**

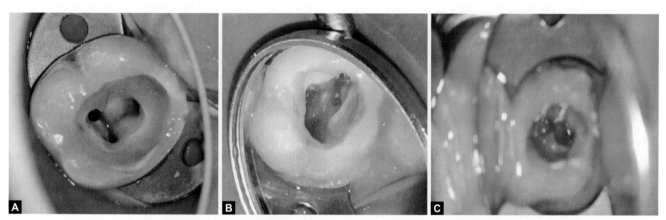

Figs. 38.11A to C Endomicroscope showing: (A) Dentinal map in mandibular first molar; (B) MB2 canal in maxillary first molar; (C) Fractured instrument in MB2.

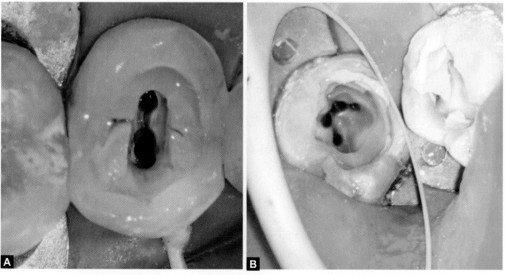

Figs. 38.12A and B Canal anatomy can be better appreciated under magnification.

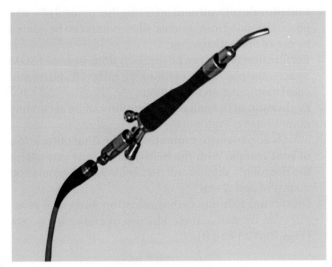

Fig. 38.13 Endoscope.

Endoscope (Fig. 38.13)

It was introduced in endodontics in 1979. Endoscope consists of glass rods, camera, light source and a monitor. Endoscope offers a better magnification than loupes or a microscope. It is mainly used during surgical endodontic treatment.

Advantage

Provides better view to surgical site in nonfixed field of vision.

Disadvantage of endoscope

Requires hemostasis of operating field.

Orascope

Orascope is a fiber optic endoscope. Since fiber optics are made up of plastics, so they are small, flexible and light weight. It is mainly used for intracanal visualization. An orascope consists of 10,000 parallel visual fibers. Quality of image produced by orascope is directly related to number of fibers.

Advantage

Better imaging of apical third of canal.

Disadvantages

❏ Canal must be enlarged to number 90 file in coronal 15 mm of canal
❏ Presence of sodium hypochlorite blurs the image.

Conclusion

In endodontics, along with other advancements, micro-surgical procedures coupled with microscopic magnification offer an absolute clinical accuracy. The use of surgical microscopes has brought revolutionary transformation in predictable success of the endodontic procedures. In spite of their significant cost, learning new techniques with their use, and their peculiar appearance to patients, magnifying loupes and endomicroscope assist the endodontists in producing higher-quality dentistry. Working under magnification is useful, and clinicians should give strong consideration to adopting the concept.

Question

1. Write short notes on:
   - Endomicroscope
   - Loupes.

Bibliography

1. Barrows MJ, BeGole EA, Wenckus CS. Effect of magnification on locating the MB2 canal in maxillary molars. J Endod 2002;28:324–7.
2. Carr GB. Microscopes in endodontics. J Calif Dent Assoc 1992;20:55–61.
3. Coeth de CArvalho MC, Zuolo ML. Orifice locating with a microscope. J Endod 2000;26:532–4.
4. Cohen ES. Microsurgery. Cohen ES, ed. Atlas of cosmetic and reconstructive periodontal surgery. 3 rd edition. Italy: B C Decker Inc; 2007. pp. 433-8.
5. Kanca J, Jordan PG. Magnification systems in clinical dentistry. J Can Dent Assoc 1995;61:851–6.
6. Kim S, Kratchman S. Modern endodontic surgery concepts and practice: a review. J Endod 2006;32:601–23.
7. Kim S. Microscope in endodontics. Dent Clin North Am 1997;41:481–97.
8. Kim S. The microscope and endodontics. Dent Clin North Am 2004;48:11–8.
9. Pecora G, Baek SH, Rethnam S, Kim S. Barrier membrane technique in endodontic microsurgery. Dent Clin North Am 1997;41:585–602.
10. Pecora G andreana S. Use of dental operating microscope in endodontic surgery. Oral Surg Oral Med Oral Pathol 1993;75:751–8.
11. Rubinstein R. The anatomy of the surgical operating microscope and operating positions. Dent Clin North Am 1997;41:391–4.

Ethics in Endodontics

Ethics is a moral concept that has been considered worthy of major contemplation since the beginning of human life on earth.

The word "ethics" is derived from the Greek word "ethos" meaning custom or character.

Nature of Ethics

- ❑ It is related with evaluation of human conduct and standard for judging whether actions performed are right or wrong
- ❑ It is the philosophy of human conduct, away from stating and evaluating principles by which problems of behavior can be solved
- ❑ It is an attempt to determine the goals of living.

Principles of Ethics

The principles of ethics for dental profession should be considered as guidelines for the dentist in treating patients. The dentist has to work on some principles for providing service to the patient, community, and his/her profession.

Related to Patient

The primary duty of dentist is to provide care to patients irrespective of nationality, socioeconomic status, race, etc.

- ❑ Dentist should not hesitate in referring specialist for treatment of patient
- ❑ Dentist should inform the patient of all the possible treatment options

- ❑ Proposed comprehensive treatment plan and options should be explained to the patient before starting and after the procedure
- ❑ Any complication which may occur during or after the dental procedure should be explained to the patient.

Related to Community

- ❑ Dentist should provide knowledge about the prevention, prophylaxis, and treatment of dental diseases
- ❑ Dentist should know the attitude and needs of the people
- ❑ Dentists may advance their reputation through professional services to patients and to society and assume a responsible role in the community.

Related to Profession

- ❑ Dentist should update his knowledge and skill by continuing dental education programs
- ❑ Dentist should maintain honor, morality, and integrity of the profession and should avoid any misconduct
- ❑ Dentist should support advancement of their profession through membership at scientific and professional organization
- ❑ Dentist should respect other opinions given by other dental professionals.

Root Canal Ethics

In present situation, patients are more keen to understand what the problem is and the possible treatment options to save the teeth. Before commencing a treatment, the dentist should take treatment records as well as informed consent of the patient which are the most important tools in the prevention of dental malpractice claim.

Treatment Records

Each dentist should have standardized protocol for diagnosis and management of pulpal and periapical diseases. In addition to established standardized protocol, the endodontist should record written documentation of the treatment provided. It includes the following procedure:

- A detailed written medical history should be taken if medical consultation is required, and consultant's remarks should be recorded in the file
- The chief complaint of patient should be recorded in his or her own words and treatment should be planned accordingly
- The dental history of the patient should also be recorded. If any treatment previously given affects the present outcome of the treatment, it should be explained to the patient and recorded in the performa
- The extraoral and intraoral examination should be conducted and recorded in the performa
- An important part of performa, that is, examination of affected tooth/teeth should be done thoroughly. Both subjective and objective tests related to diagnosis and treatment should be done and recorded in the performa. If required, a dental specialist can be referred. Radiographs of good diagnostic quality should be taken and interpreted. The dentist should record the findings of radiographs in the performa
- A detailed pulpal and periodontal examination should be done and recorded in the performa
- Provisional diagnosis and proposed treatment plan should be presented to the patient. It should be recorded in the performa also
- The medication, if prescribed, should also be recorded in the dental performa
- The informed/written consent regarding the treatment outcomes should be recorded and included in the performa
- Final prognosis/outcomes should be clearly mentioned
- The dentist should always sign the performa.

Common Elements of Negligence and Malpractice

- Failure to meet the standard of care
- Failure to diagnose properly
- Use of poor standard dental materials
- Failure to refer
- Use of infected/unsterilized instruments
- Overinstrumentation and formation of abscess/sinus.

Common Malpractice Errors Against Endodontics

- Failure to meet the standard of care
- Instrument separation
- Treating a wrong tooth
- Performing procedure not up to mark
- Failure to get informed consent
- Paresthesia.

Informed Consent

As a general rule, the information presented to a patient must be presented in a terminology that is easily understood by the patient. The dentist should tell advantages, risks and cost related to patient's problems. Informed consent should also be duly signed by the patient and date should also be recorded. Failure to provide the adequate information to the patient is also a breach of code. The written, informed consent should include the following:

- The diagnosis for each affected tooth should be recorded
- The treatment plan should be recorded in brief
- The date on which consent was taken should be recorded in the consent form
- The potential complication which may occur during or after the treatment should be written in consent form
- The success rate of treatment should also be mentioned in the consent form
- Alternative treatment options, such as tooth extraction, or no treatment should be told to the patient and should also be mentioned in the consent form
- The patient or his/her guardians should sign the consent form along with date.

No specific form should be used in every case. In endodontics, the incidence of complications is relatively low if done by specialist. The endodontist should tell the patient about the following facts:

- Despite best efforts by endodontist, few cases of root canal failure are reported
- Sometimes overextensions occur in root canal therapy. If it is minor, then no treatment is required because these cases heal well and remain asymptomatic
- Slight-to-moderate pain may occur after root canal therapy
- A file may break in canal during root canal therapy, then, patient should be informed about this occurrence
- Perforation may also occur during root canal therapy. Tell the patient about the perforation and explain him/her that it can be repaired with newer materials.

Dental Negligence

Dental negligence is defined as a violation of the standards of care. In a layman term, malpractice means negligence. Dental negligence occur mainly due to two reasons—either a clinician does not possess a required qualification or despite of qualification, he or she acts carelessly.

Related to Local Anesthesia

There are certain problems that can occur while injecting local anesthesia in patients. Some cases that can lead to allegations of negligence are:
- Syncope (fainting)
- Fracture of the needle in situ
- Hematoma
- Trismus
- Drug allergy
- Injection of incorrect solution
- Infection
- Injection of expired solution.

Syncope (Fainting)

Although syncope usually occurs in the dental clinic, it can be reduced if proper counseling of the patient is done before initiating treatment.

Doctor should explain each and every step of the dental procedure to the patient.

If at all it happens even after taking proper care, the clinician and his assistant should be ready to manage the situation effectively.

Fracture of the Needle in Situ

Incidence of fracture of the needle has been reduced in modern era because of wider availability of disposable needles and syringes. In the past, reuse of the needles and syringes was the main reason for this problem.

Several other conditions, such as hematoma, trismus and, drug allergy, may also make the conditions worse for dentist in the dental clinic. So, good communication and rapport between the practitioner and the patient is the key factor in these circumstances to prevent the allegation of negligence.

The injection of an incorrect or expired solution causing harm is considered as an indefensible action. Such occurrences should be avoided in the dental office or extra care should be taken during injection of local anesthetic.

Thermal or Chemical Burns (Iatrogenic Problems)

Both thermal and chemical burns are also a part of dental negligence.

Thermal Burns

Thermal burns can occur due to overheated instruments such as handpieces or when instruments are insufficiently cooled after sterilization. These can cause burns on the lips, oral mucosa, and cheeks. To prevent or minimize such occurrences
- All rotary instruments such as air rotor/handpiece should be properly maintained and oiling should be done regularly
- Burs used in these handpieces should be new and sharp
- Excessive pressure should not be applied during cutting
- Irrigation with normal saline should be done during surgical extractions.

Any instrument which appears warm to the operator's hands is likely to retain some heat which can cause problem when applied to oral structure immediately. It is usually found that claims based on these findings are difficult to defend. So, these circumstances should be avoided.

Chemical Burns

Chemical burns are also common in the dentist's clinic. These can be avoided by the following steps:
- Provide proper training of dental assistants
- Avoid use of strong chemicals in the oral cavity
- Avoid overuse of chemicals
- Avoid carrying the chemicals over patient's face
- Accidental ingestion or inhalation.

Sometimes incidents such as accidental ingestion or inhalation of certain objects may occur, for example,
- A portion of tooth
- Burs
- Endodontic instruments such as file or reamer
- Crown/bridge.

It is the dentist's responsibility to make all provisions so that no instrument or object is ingested or inhaled. To prevent this, dentist should take the following precautions:
- Use of rubber dam
- Use of floss to tie endodontic instruments and rubber dam clamps.

If claims are made for this negligence, heavy compensation has to be paid because these cases are truly a case of negligence on the part of dentist.

Poor Quality of Radiographs

An improper radiographic film or poorly developed film can also lead to allegation of negligence which is difficult to refute. So, treatment provided on the basis of poor quality of radiographs should be repeated.

Since radiographs are only two-dimensional views of three-dimensional objects, in some cases it becomes necessary to take different radiographs in different angulations. Unable to take the radiographs is also liable to cause allegation of negligence.

Failure to Provide Adequate Care

Failure to provide adequate care and treatment to a patient is also a part of dental negligence. Commonly seen cases of dental negligence performed by most of dentist in practice are
❏ Failure to use rubber dam while performing endodontics
❏ Failure to take good quality radiographs
❏ Failure to periodically check the water unit connected to the dental unit
❏ Failure to record and probe the periodontal pockets
❏ Failure to follow barrier technique such as use of sterilized gloves, face masks, instruments, use of protective eye shields and disposal of waste.

Negligence Related to Patient

Patient also has to follow some rules of behavior while undergoing treatment. In accepting treatment, the patient should
❏ Cooperate during and after treatment
❏ Follow home-care instructions given by dentist
❏ Immediately inform any change in health status
❏ Pay his/her bills timely.

Depending upon treatment, additional warranties may exist. If patient does not follow any of these instructions or instruction given by dentist, these should be recorded in patient's record.

Malpractice and the Standard of Care

Good endodontic practice is defined as standard of reasonable care legally to be performed by a reasonably careful clinician.

A good clinician always maintains records. Records are considered as a single most evidence which a dentist can present in the court.

The law recognized that there are differences in the abilities of doctors with same qualification as there are also differences in the abilities of people engaged in different activities. To practice the profession, the clinician does not require extraordinary skills. In providing dental services to the community, the doctor is entitled to use his/her brain for judgment of cases and providing optimal care. For preventing malpractice, certain guidelines should be followed:
❏ Do not provide treatment beyond your ability even if patient insists
❏ For patients requiring specialty care, refer them to a specialist
❏ In patients where certain diagnostic tests are required for his/her care, if he/she refuses for that, clinician should not undertake treatment otherwise the clinician will be at risk.

Standard of Care Set by Endodontists

Endodontists set a high standard of care as compared to general dentist. Endodontists should not forget their general dentist norms as these are required during care of endodontic treatment also.

After referral from the dentist, take new radiographs if required.

Endodontists should not provide rubber stamp treatment for what the clinician has asked. He/she should record complete medical and dental history before doing a thorough clinical examination. Endodontist should examine specific tooth/teeth along with general oral condition of the patient.

An endodontist should expose a new radiograph to know the status of tooth/teeth before starting a treatment.

Abandonment

By initiating endodontic treatment, the dentist has taken the legal responsibility to complete the case or the case can further be referred to a specialist. He should also be responsible for postoperative emergency care. If the dentist fails to comply with his or her obligation to complete the treatment, he/she can be exposed to liability on the basis of abandonment. A dentist/endodontist if wants to end his or her treatment obligation may have several reasons like patient:
❏ Failed to keep appointments
❏ Failed to cooperate
❏ Failed to follow home-care instructions
❏ Failed to give payment at time.

To avoid abandonment claim, several precautionary measures need to be taken. These are:
❏ No law can force the dentist to treat all patients despite severe pain, infection, or any other emergency condition. A dentist can do the emergency treatment, if patient and dentist both are interested but dentist should write clearly in the patient's record that he has given emergency treatment only
❏ Reasonable notice should be given to patient, if patient is willing to seek endodontic treatment from somewhere else. The dentist should provide copies of treatment record and radiographs.

Regardless of the justification given for treatment cessation, a dentist/endodontist who fails to follow the proper procedures may incur liability on the ground of abandonment. For prevention of abandonment claim, reasonable notice should be given to the patient. The following points should be taken care of while preparing a notice:
❏ Notify the patient if the dentist plans to terminate the treatment
❏ Appropriate valid reasons for not continuing the treatment should be given in detail, for example, if patient

is not following instruction properly, the notice should include instruction in writing

❑ Provide all details about the treatment, that is, treatment records and diagnostic radiographs
❑ Dentist should provide emergency care during the intermediate time
❑ A patient can contact any time regarding previous treatment given by dentist.

The card should be signed properly mentioning the contact number also.

Malpractice Cases

Injury from Slips of the Drill

A slip of the drill is usually the result of operator's error. It can cause injury to tongue, oral mucosa, and lips. To avoid malpractice claim, the dentist should follow these steps:
❑ Inform the patient about incident and explain its remedy
❑ Refer the patient to a specialist like an oral and maxillofacial surgeon or plastic surgeon
❑ Dentist should bear the expenditure
❑ Call the patient for periodic checkup.

Inhalation or Ingestion of Endodontic Instruments

Rubber dam should be used in every conditions and its use is mandatory for endodontic work. It not only reduces the chances of aspirating or swallowing endodontic instruments but also reduces the microbial contamination. If patient swallows or aspirates dental instrument, it is operator's fault. He should follow the following steps:
❑ Inform the patient about the incident and should regret what has happened
❑ Refer the patient immediately for medical care
❑ Pay all the bills of patient.

Broken File

These incidents usually occur in routine endodontic practice. But to avoid malpractice claims, you have to follow some guidelines. Before going into discussion about these guidelines, consider some facts about broken or separated instruments:
❑ Multiple use can result in fatigue of the instruments which further lead to failure of these instruments
❑ Failure to follow the manufacturer's instructions regarding use of the instruments can lead to failure
❑ Manufacturing defect may also lead to failure
❑ Teeth with separated files may remain asymptomatic and functional for years.

When an instrument gets separated in a tooth, dentist should follow some guidelines which are as follows:
❑ Explain the patient about the incident
❑ Show the remaining part of endodontic instruments to the patient and assure that tooth will remain asymptomatic
❑ Dental assistant should place the part of endodontic instrument and radiographs in the treatment record for future reference
❑ Dentist should reassure the patient that he/she would follow this case closely.

Perforations

Any dentist who is performing endodontic treatment can cause perforation. It usually occurs in or around furcal floor. Despite getting panic at the time of incident, dentist should follow some basic steps:
❑ Explain the patient about the incident that despite of best effort, perforation has occurred
❑ Record the findings in treatment records of the patient
❑ Assure that it can be quickly repaired with newer materials
❑ Follow-up the case regularly.

Overextensions

Overextensions usually happen to every dentist. The irony about overextensions is that no one agrees on exactly where overextensions begin. Does it begin at the apex? 1 mm beyond the apex or 2 mm? Rather than going into controversial discussion, we should follow some basic steps which are as follows:
❑ Explain the incident to the patient and mention patient that some of the biocompatible material has gone beyond the end of the root
❑ There can be little more numbness for few days
❑ Mostly these cases heal asymptomatically
❑ Follow-up the case closely.

Conclusion

The dentist as a health professional holds a special position of trust within society. Therefore, society affords the profession certain privileges that are not available to members of the public at large. In return, the profession makes a commitment to society that its members will stick to high ethical standards of conduct. Having sociability, availability, and ability helps make you a better practitioner. To practice within the standard of care and communicate appropriately will help you avoid litigation. One must maintain character with integrity at all times along with adhering to ethical guidelines and have moral behavior.

Questions

1. What are principles of endodontic ethics?
2. Mention different malpractice cases.

Bibliography

1. Bailey B. Informed consent in dentistry. J Am Dent Assoc 1985;110:709.
2. Cohen S, et al. Endodontic complications and the law. J Endod 1987;13:191.
3. Ingle JI, Bakland LK, Decker BC. Endodontics. 6th edition. Elsevier; 2008.
4. Row AHR. Damage to the inferior alveolar nerve during or following endodontic treatment. Br Dent J 1983;153:306.
5. Weichman JA. Malpractice prevention and defense. Calif Dent Assoc J 1975;3:58.

Page numbers followed by *f* refer to figure, *fc* refer to flowchart, and *t* refer to table.